Recent Progress in Particle Toxicology

Recent Progress in Particle Toxicology

Edited by Lucy Malone

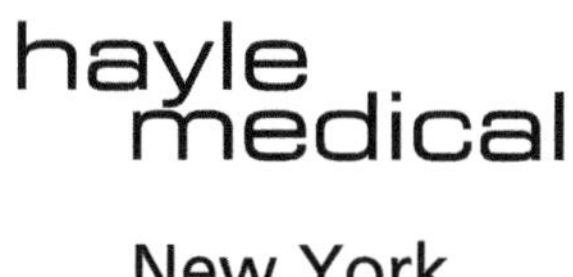

New York

Hayle Medical,
750 Third Avenue, 9th Floor,
New York, NY 10017, USA

Visit us on the World Wide Web at:
www.haylemedical.com

ISBN: 978-1-63241-860-9

Cataloging-in-Publication Data

Recent progress in particle toxicology / edited by Lucy Malone.
p. cm.
Includes bibliographical references and index.
ISBN 978-1-63241-860-9
1. Particles--Toxicology. 2. Pulmonary toxicology. I. Malone, Lucy.
RC720 .R43 2020
616.200 471--dc23

Table of Contents

Preface

Over the recent decade, advancements and applications have progressed exponentially. This has led to the increased interest in this field and projects are being conducted to enhance knowledge. The main objective of this book is to present some of the critical challenges and provide insights into possible solutions. This book will answer the varied questions that arise in the field and also provide an increased scope for furthering studies.

The inhalation of harmful airborne particles may result in adverse health conditions and pathological changes in the respiratory tract. It is often seen that noxious inhaled particles activate an inflammatory pulmonary response, which can initiate a sub-chronic or chronic pulmonary disease. These conditions may include silicosis, pneumonitis, chronic obstructive pulmonary disease, asbestosis, emphysema, fibrosis, asthma or cancer. The severity of a particle-induced pathology is dependent on the exposure time and concentration as well as particle size, structure and composition. Airborne particles may include combustion-derived particles from welding, cigarette smoke, traffic and industry, etc. as well as biological particles such as pollen and fungi. Research on particle toxicology attempts to investigate the effects of individual particles and sources. This enables better predictability of newly generated particles. In vivo toxicological studies screen for long-term effects in the respiratory tract. Such studies include the histopathological analysis of the lungs for investigating adverse effects of particles. This book provides comprehensive insights into the field of particle toxicology. The topics included herein are of utmost significance and bound to provide incredible insights to readers. It will prove to be immensely beneficial to students and researchers in toxicology.

I hope that this book, with its visionary approach, will be a valuable addition and will promote interest among readers. Each of the authors has provided their extraordinary competence in their specific fields by providing different perspectives as they come from diverse nations and regions. I thank them for their contributions.

Editor

Preface

1

Diesel engine exhaust accelerates plaque formation in a mouse model of Alzheimer's disease

Maja Hullmann[1], Catrin Albrecht[1], Damiën van Berlo[1,7], Miriam E. Gerlofs-Nijland[2], Tina Wahle[1], Agnes W. Boots[1,3], Jean Krutmann[1,4], Flemming R. Cassee[2,5], Thomas A. Bayer[6] and Roel P. F. Schins[1*]

Abstract

Background: Increasing evidence from toxicological and epidemiological studies indicates that the central nervous system is an important target for ambient air pollutants. We have investigated whether long-term inhalation exposure to diesel engine exhaust (DEE), a dominant contributor to particulate air pollution in urban environments, can aggravate Alzheimer's Disease (AD)-like effects in female 5X Familial AD (5XFAD) mice and their wild-type female littermates. Following 3 and 13 weeks exposures to diluted DEE (0.95 mg/m^3, 6 h/day, 5 days/week) or clean air (controls) behaviour tests were performed and amyloid-β (Aβ) plaque formation, pulmonary histopathology and systemic inflammation were evaluated.

Results: In a string suspension task, assessing for grip strength and motor coordination, 13 weeks exposed 5XFAD mice performed significantly less than the 5XFAD controls. Spatial working memory deficits, assessed by Y-maze and X-maze tasks, were not observed in association with the DEE exposures. Brains of the 3 weeks DEE-exposed 5XFAD mice showed significantly higher cortical Aβ plaque load and higher whole brain homogenate Aβ42 levels than the clean air-exposed 5XFAD littermate controls. After the 13 weeks exposures, with increasing age and progression of the AD-phenotype of the 5XFAD mice, DEE-related differences in amyloid pathology were no longer present. Immunohistochemical evaluation of lungs of the mice revealed no obvious genetic background-related differences in tissue structure, and the DEE exposure did not cause histopathological changes in the mice of both backgrounds. Luminex analysis of plasma cytokines demonstrated absence of sustained systemic inflammation upon DEE exposure.

Conclusions: Inhalation exposure to DEE causes accelerated plaque formation and motor function impairment in 5XFAD transgenic mice. Our study provides further support that the brain is a relevant target for the effects of inhaled DEE and suggests that long-term exposure to this ubiquitous air pollution mixture may promote the development of Alzheimer's disease.

Keywords: Diesel engine exhaust, Inhalation, Particulate matter, 5XFAD mice, Alzheimer's disease, Amyloid-β, Behaviour

* Correspondence: Roel.Schins@uni-duesseldorf.de
[1]IUF - Leibniz Research Institute for Environmental Medicine, Auf'm Hennekamp 50, 40225 Düsseldorf, Germany
Full list of author information is available at the end of the article

Background

An increasing number of studies indicates that chronic exposure to ambient particulate matter (PM) may have toxic effects on the nervous system. In urban environments, diesel engine exhaust (DEE) emissions represent a dominant source of the particulate fraction of air pollution [1]. Inhalation toxicology studies in rodents have shown that markers of neuroinflammation and neurotoxicity are induced upon exposures to PM [2–4] and DEE [5–9]. These experimental findings are in line with a growing number of epidemiological studies that demonstrated associations between exposure to PM or traffic-related air pollution and cognitive function or cognitive decline [10–16].

Meanwhile, the specific concern has risen that long-term exposure to particulate air pollution could contribute to the pathogenesis of Alzheimer's disease (AD) [17–19]. AD is the most common cause of dementia worldwide affecting millions of people. AD is clinically characterised by progressive loss of memory associated with cognitive deficits extending to language skills, decision-making ability, movement and recognition [20]. Neuropathologically, this disease is characterised by the presence of neurofibrillary tangles, intracellular aggregates consisting of hyperphosphorylated Tau proteins and extracellular amyloid plaques, associated with widespread loss of neurons in brain [21]. A major component of the amyloid plaques is the hydrophobic 4kD Amyloid-β peptide (Aβ), which is generated by sequential proteolysis of the amyloid precursor protein (APP) by β- and γ-secretase (reviewed in [22]). The β-secretase cuts APP at the N terminus of the Aβ domain and subsequent cleavage by the γ-secretase at the C terminus of Aβ domain generates a series of Aβ peptides of 38–43 amino acids in length [23]. A strong genetic association between early onset familial forms of AD (FAD) and the 42 amino acid Aβ species (Aβ42) has been demonstrated (reviewed in [24]). FAD-related autosomal dominant mutations in the genes for Presenilin (PS) 1 and 2, subunits of the γ-secretase complex, or in the gene for APP are known to elevate the production of Aβ42 [22]. As Aβ42 is more fibrillogenic than shorter Aβ peptides, increased levels of Aβ42 are thought to drive the formation of the insoluble fibrils that compose amyloid plaques [25].

The earliest clues for a link between (particulate) air pollution exposure and AD came from studies from Calderón-Garcidueñas et al. [26] who compared brain autopsies from lifelong residents from cities with severe air pollution versus cities with low levels of air pollution [26, 27]. Besides markers of inflammation and DNA damage, they found augmented Aβ42 protein levels in frontal cortex, hippocampus and olfactory bulb among the individuals from the highly polluted cities. More recently, they also showed increased presence of markers of oxidative stress, inflammation and neurodegeneration as well as Aβ diffuse plaques in brain autopsies of children and young adults from highly polluted regions. This led the authors to suggest that air pollution plays a role in central nervous system (CNS) damage at a young age with potential development of AD [28]. Experimental clues have become available from Levesque et al. [8] who detected enhanced Aβ42 levels in brains of rats exposed to DEE and Bhatt et al. [29] who showed increased levels of Aβ40 and β-secretase in mice exposed to concentrated PM. The effect of air pollution and dementia is further supported by a recent critical systemic review [30] and outcomes from a major population-based neurological diseases cohort study, showing an association of residential proximity to major roadways with dementia among 243,611 incident cases [16]. Regarding observed epidemiological associations between PM and AD, it has been stated that: "If these data reflect causality, PM exposure would be one of few AD risk factors that are not only widespread, but that also can be modified at the population level using regulatory intervention" [18].

Whether and how long-term exposure to air pollution particles could contribute to pathogenesis of AD is not clear yet. Therefore, we performed a sub-chronic whole-body DEE inhalation study in female transgenic 5X Familial Alzheimer's Disease (5XFAD) mice and their female wildtype (WT) littermate controls. We hypothesized that DEE could accelerate AD-like effects in this transgenic mouse model. Following exposures for 3 or 13 weeks to DEE or clean air (controls), the mice were subjected to behaviour tests, and then analysed for Aβ plaque formation in hippocampus and cortex. To evaluate the potential involvement of peripheral inflammation, which has been discussed to be involved in AD-pathogenesis [31–33], the mice were also evaluated for the presence of pulmonary histopathology and markers of systemic inflammation.

Methods

Animals

Female 5XFAD transgenic mice were used as a model for AD. These mice overexpress the 695 amino acid isoform of the human amyloid precursor protein (APP695) carrying Swedish (K670 N), London (V717I) and Florida (I716V) mutations as well as the human PS1 (M146 L; L286 V) mutations [34, 35]. The mice develop a specific phenotype showing high APP expression levels, amyloid deposition beginning with two month of age and memory impairments and motor deficits [34, 36]. Breeding was performed by mating heterozygote transgenic founders with C57Bl/6 J wild-type (WT) mice to obtain littermate controls for the experiments. Only female mice were used for the study in view of the reported sex-specific differences in age- and treatment related Aβ development [37]. The mice were handled according to guidelines of the Society for Laboratory Animals Science (GV-SOLAS). The study was approved by the Animal Ethics Committee (IUCAC) of the Dutch National Vaccine Institute (NVI, Bilthoven, Netherlands) (project number 201000169). All animals included in this study were born within a time range of 4 days, and age was 10 weeks when inhalation exposures started. Temperature and the relative humidity in the inhalation units [38] were controlled at 22 ± 2 °C and at 40–70%, respectively. Lighting was artificial with a sequence of 12 h light (06:00–18:00) and 12 h dark. Commercially available rodent food pellets and water were provided ad libitum.

Diesel engine exhaust (DEE) exposure and characterisation of the test atmosphere

All animals were exposed in whole body inhalation chambers in separate inhalation units (2 mice per cage, and a maximum of 10 per unit) for 5 days/week, for 6 h a day during either 3 or 13 weeks. The design of the study is depicted in Fig. 1. Animals were exposed to control (conditioned, purified and HEPA-filtered) air or to DEE diluted by mixing the freshly generated exhaust from a stationary diesel engine (Common-rail motor, 100 kVA, 35 KW load) with conditioned purified air. Particle number and mass concentrations were determined continuously using a condensation particle counter (CPC model 3022A, TSI St. Paul, MN, USA), and a Tapered Element Oscillating Microbalance (TEOM 1400a, Rupprecht & Patashnick, Albany, NY, USA), respectively. The particle size distribution was measured 3–4 times during exposure by a Scanning Mobility particle Sizer (SMPS 3080 with CPC 3788, TSI Inc. Shoreview, MN, USA) Time-integrated particle concentrations were analyzed by gravimetric analyses using particles collected on 47 mm Teflon filters. Carbon monoxide and nitrogen oxides were measured continuously by a Gas Filter Correlation CO analyzer (Thermo Electron instr Model 48, Madison, WI, USA) and a Chemiluminescense NO/NOx analyzer (Advancend Pollution Instruments Model 200E, San Diego, Ca, USA). Exposure characteristics are shown in Table 1.

Behaviour tests

The behaviour tests were performed during the week after the last exposure, starting on the third day after the last exposure day (see Fig. 1). Motor coordination and grip strength of the mice were tested using a string suspension task. Therefore, a 2 mm broad and 35 cm long cotton string was stretched between two vertical poles above a cushioned bottom. The animals were carried by their tails and permitted to grasp the string by their forepaws before their release. A rating system from 0 to 5 was assigned to each animal during a single 60 s session [39], as follows: 0, unable to hang on the string; 1, hangs only by forepaws; 2, attempting to climb the string; 3, climbing the string with four paws successfully; 4, moving laterally along the string; 5, escaping to one of the platforms at the end of the string. The Y-maze and Cross (X)-maze tasks were applied to reflect spatial working memory of mice by spontaneous alternation, based on the natural affinity of mice to explore a novel environment [40]. For both mazes, alternation percentages were calculated as % of the actual alternations to the possible arm entries. To avoid influence on the behaviour of the mice due to odour of mice tested before, the mazes were thoroughly cleaned after every trial with 70% ethanol.

Necropsy

Eleven days after the last exposure to the DEE or HEPA-filtered air, the mice were sacrificed by cervical

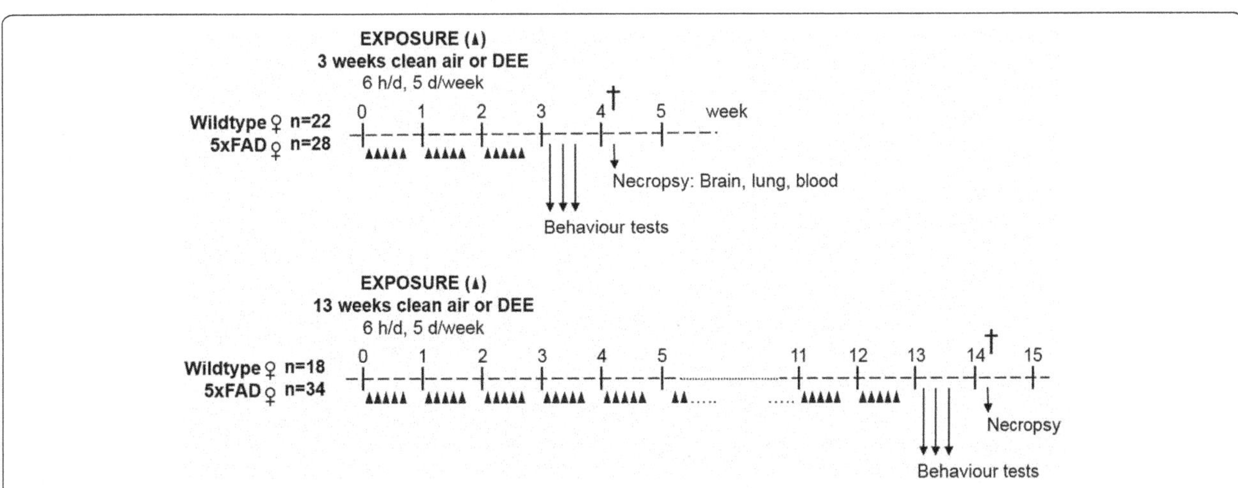

Fig. 1 Study design. Female 5X Familial AD (5XFAD) mice and wild-type (WT) female littermates were exposed for 3 or 13 weeks to clean air or diluted diesel engine exhaust (DEE). Animals were born within a time range of 4 days, and age was 10 weeks at exposure start

Table 1 Exposure characteristics based on measurements in three inhalation units

Parameter	Value
Mass concentration (mg/m^3)[a] [SD]	0.95 [5–12%[b]]
Number concentration[c] (#/cm^3) [SD]	$2.1 \cdot 10^6$ [$0.35 \cdot 10^6$]
Geometric mean size (nm), [geometric SD (nm)]	82 [1.75]
CO (ppm) [SD]	6.37 [1.37]
NO (ppm) [SD]	23.11 [5.50]
NO_2 (ppm) [SD]	1.56 [0.40]
NO_x (ppm) [SD]	24.59 [5.81]

[a]Time integrated Filter; [b]depending on the exposure unit; [c]CPC; *SD* standard deviation

dislocation and heparin-blood was immediately collected. After centrifugation at 2000 g, the plasma was stored at −80 °C until further analysis. Brains were carefully removed after opening of the scull and dissected. The left hemispheres were stored for immunohistochemical analyses after fixation with 4% paraformaldehyde at 4 °C and subsequent embedding in paraffin. The right hemispheres were snapfrozen for later analyses. Lungs were used for immunohistochemical analyses after perfusion and fixation in 10% formalin or dissected, followed by snapfreezing.

Immunohistochemical analyses of paraffin embedded slices

After sacrificing the animals and careful dissection of their brains, the right half of the brain was fixated in 4% buffered formalin at 4 °C for a minimum of 24 h. Dehydration was performed in a series of ethanol and followed by a transfer into xylene. Afterwards brains were embedded in paraffin. Four μm thick paraffin sections were cut using a sliding microtome, transferred on Superfrost Ultra Plus object slides and dried over night at 40 °C. Subsequently, sections were deparaffinised in xylene, followed by a rehydration in a series of ethanol (100%, 96%, 70%) and blocking of endogenous peroxidase by a treatment with 0.3% H_2O_2 in PBS. Antigen retrieval was performed by boiling slices in 10 mM citrate buffer, pH 6.0 followed by an incubation for 3 min in 88% formic acid. Unspecific antibody binding was blocked, via incubation in 10% fetal calf serum (FCS) and 4% skim milk in 0.01 M PBS before application of the primary anti human Aβ antibody (Merck Millipore, Darmstadt, Germany) diluted 1:1000 in 0.01 M PBS and 10% FCS, overnight in a humid chamber at room temperature. After washing slices were incubated with a biotinylated anti-mouse secondary antibody diluted 1:200 in 0.01 M PBS and 10% FCS, and the signal was detected via avidin-biotin-complex-method (ABC) by a Vectastain kit (Vectorlabs, Burlingame, USA) using diaminobenzidine (DAB, Sigma-Aldrich, Deisenhofen, Germany)) as chromogen and Hematoxylin for nuclear counterstaining. Light microscopical pictures from cortex and hippocampus were taken with 100 x or 50 x magnification, respectively, using a Zeiss Axiophot microscope equipped with AxioCam MRc (Carl Zeiss, Jena, Germany). Quantitative Aβ42 plaque analyses were performed via calculation of the % of total plaque load in the analysed area of the section. Plaque load was determined using ZEN 2011 image processing software (Zeiss) after a fixed adjustment of contrast threshold for stained Aβ42 plaques. In detail, the brain section was placed under the microscope at a magnification of 50×. For the analysis of the hippocampal area, this specific part was positioned in the middle of the focus and the region of interest was marked interactively for each animal. After analysis of the hippocampal region, the slide was shifted to a frontal cortex region, which was comparable for each animal. The objective was changed to a magnification of 100× and the complete image section was analysed. From each animal three brain slides with an interspace of approximately 30 μm were analysed and calculated as the % of total plaque load in the analysed area of the section.

Amyloid-β42 ELISA

Aβ40 and Aβ42 are the two major isoforms of amyloid-β. It has been shown that the transgenic 5XFAD mice produce Aβ42 in a highly predominant manner [34]. Thus, we determined only the levels of this isoform in the brains. The human Aβ42 ELISA was performed according to the manufacturer's manual (Thermo Fisher Scientific, Darmstadt, Germany). Therefore, frozen brain tissues were homogenised in a potter tissue grinder in 1500 μl Aβ42-ELISA homogenisation buffer (5 M guanidine HCl, 50 mM Tris HCl, pH 8.0), centrifuged for 15 min at 14,000 x g and supernatant was aliquoted and stored at −20 °C until further analysis. For the ELISA measurements, a 96-microtiter plate was pre-coated with a monoclonal antibody specific for the NH2-terminus region of human Aβ42. Protein concentrations were determined using the bicinchoninic acid method (Sigma Aldrich, Deisenhofen, Germany). Samples were diluted with Aβ42 ELISA reaction buffer (i.e. 0.2 g/L KCl: 0.2 g/L KH_2PO_4, 8.0 g/L NaCl, 1.150 g/L Na_2PO_4, 5% BSA, 0.03% Tween-20, 1 x protease inhibitor) at pH 7.4, in order to investigate to samples at the same total protein concentration. Fifty μl of Aβ peptide standards or samples were then incubated with 50 μl rabbit anti human Aβ42 detection antibody, specific for the COOH-terminus of the 1–42 Aβ sequence, by shaking for 3 h at room temperature. After washing, detection was performed using 100 μl anti rabbit IgG HRP solution followed by 100 μl stabilized Chromogen. After adding 100 μl stop solution optical density was measured at 450 nm and Aβ 42 concentrations was calculated using a serial dilution of the Aβ peptide standard.

Lung tissue analysis

Following sacrificing of the animals lungs were carefully removed and intratracheally fixed in 10% PBS-buffered Formalin (pH 7.4) at 4 °C for a minimum of 24 h. The dehydration occurred in a series of ethanol followed by a transfer into xylene. Lungs were then embedded in paraffin, sections were cut using a sliding microtome and shifted on Superfrost Ultra Plus object slides and dried over night at 40 °C. Afterwards slices were deparaffinised in xylene, followed by a rehydration in a series of ethanol (100%, 96%, 70%) and stained using haematoxylin-eosin (HE) for light microscopical evaluation.

Bio-Plex cytokine assay

Systemic inflammation was assessed by measurement of the concentrations of interleukin (IL)-1α, IL-1β, IL-6, IL-17, keratinocyte chemoattractant/interleukin-8 (KC/IL-8), macrophage inflammatory protein (MIP)-1α, MIP-1β, regulated on activation, normal T cell expressed and secreted (RANTES), monocyte chemoattractant protein-1 (MCP-1), granulocyte colony-stimulating factor (G-CSF) and granulocyte-macrophage colony-stimulating factor (GM-CSF), in mouse plasma using a Bio-Plex murine cytokine platform. The assay was performed according to manufacturer's instructions, as described previously [41]. Data were analysed with a Luminex 100 IS 2.3 system coupled to Bio-Plex Manager 4.1.1 software.

Statistical analyses

In the study design, the foreseen number of mice per treatment group (i.e. 10 per group for WT mice, 16 per group for 5XFAD mice) was based on power calculations, with the assumption that the DEE exposure would accelerate the progressive phenotype (i.e. plaques, behaviour effects) of the 5XFAD mice [36] by 3 months. During the actual inhalation experiments, due to technical problems two mice were excluded from the analyses. Combined with the genotyping verification, this resulted in the following animal numbers per group: WT 3 weeks clean air exposed (n = 12); WT 3 weeks DEE (n = 10); WT 13 weeks air (n = 10); WT 13 weeks DEE (n = 8); 5XFAD 3 weeks air (n = 14); 5XFAD 3 weeks DEE (n = 14); 5XFAD 13 weeks air (n = 16); 5XFAD 13 weeks DEE (n = 18). Data were analysed using IBM-SPSS (version 22) and are expressed as mean ± SEM unless stated otherwise. Data that were obtained for both 5XFAD and WT mice were evaluated by one-way analysis of variance (ANOVA) with post-hoc analysis according to Tukey's method. Possible interactions between genetic background and the DEE exposure were explored using additional 2-way ANOVA analysis. The 5XFAD-specific effect evaluations (i.e. effects of DEE exposure on amyloid plaque formation, whole brain Aβ42 protein levels and whole blood cytokine levels) were evaluated by Student's t-test. Differences were considered statistically significant at $p < 0.05$.

Results

Effects of DEE inhalation exposure on body and organ weights of 5XFAD and WT mice

The weights of the mice were determined prior to the exposures as well as after the 3 and 13 weeks exposures. Results are shown in Table 2. There were no statistically significant differences in body weights after the 3 weeks exposure for the 5XFAD mice compared to the WT mice of the respective exposure groups. However, at this time point the DEE-exposed 5XFAD mice weighed significantly less than the clean-air exposed WT mice (ANOVA-Tukey, $p < 0.001$). This was also confirmed by evaluation of the body weight gain during exposure. The mean weight gain of the WT controls was 3.9 g whereas the DEE-exposed 5XFAD mice only gained 1.9 g on average (see Table 2; ANOVA-Tukey, p = 0.012). Body weights did not significantly differ before the start of the inhalations. These findings suggests that the combination of the 3 weeks exposure to DEE and the genetic background has an adverse impact on weight gain for the mice at this developmental stage. A two-way ANOVA analyses revealed that there was no interaction between both factors (F = 0.003, $p > 0.1$). For the 13 weeks exposure groups, there was no influence of exposure, genotype or a combination of both factors on body weight. This suggests that the effect observed after the 3 weeks exposure is transient.

The weights of liver, lung, heart, kidneys and spleen of the mice were determined at sacrifice (see Table 2). No statistically significant differences in weights of these organs were found after the 3 and 13 weeks exposures. Thus, neither the exposure to the DEE, nor the genetic background had an influence on the weights of these organs.

Effects of DEE inhalation exposure on behaviour in 5XFAD and WT mice

The Y-maze and X-maze tasks were applied in this study to evaluate spatial working memory effects of the mice in association with the DEE exposure and genetic background. The string suspension task was performed to assess for grip strength and motor coordination. Results of these mouse behaviour tests are shown in Fig. 2. The total number of arm entries recorded during the 10 min interval for the Y-maze and X-maze tasks are shown in Table 3. After the 3 weeks exposure there were no statistically significant differences in spatial working memory between the four groups, as revealed from outcomes of

Table 2 Body and organ weights of the 5XFAD mice and their WT littermates after 3 or 13 weeks exposure to DEE of clean air

	3 weeks study				13 weeks study			
	Air		DEE		Air		DEE	
	WT	5XFAD	WT	5XFAD	WT	5XFAD	WT	5XFAD
Age (days)	101.6 ± 0.5	101.6 ± 0.5	101.5 ± 0.2	101.4 ± 0.1	171.0 ± 0.1	170.9 ± 0.2	170.6 ± 0.2	170.3 ± 0.1
Body weight, sacrifice (g)	23.5 ± 0.5	22.2 ± 0.4	21.9 ± 0.5	20.6 ± 0.3[a]	23.4 ± 0.7	23.6 ± 0.9	24.3 ± 0.7	23.6 ± 0.5
Body weight gain (g)[c]	3.9 ± 1.3	3.4 ± 1.0	2.6 ± 2.7	1.9 ± 0.8[b]	5.4 ± 0.6	4.7 ± 0.7	4.4 ± 0.3	4.9 ± 0.5
Liver/body weight (mg/g)	40.1 ± 3.37	45.69 ± 2.55	38.68 ± 1.66	43.24 ± 1.20	47.72 ± 4.40	43.13 ± 0.90	47.26 ± 1.99	44.20 ± 0.83
Lung/body weight (mg/g)	5.63 ± 0.14	5.64 ± 0.13	6.06 ± 0.52	5.86 ± 0.15	4.69 ± 1.04	6.48 ± 0.11	6.10 ± 023	6.09 ± 0.19
Heart/body weight (mg/g)	5.40 ± 0.24	5.28 ± 0.13	4.91 ± 0.21	5.35 ± 0.14	6.68 ± 0.36	5.81 ± 0.33	6.09 ± 0.24	6.11 ± 0.29
Kidney/body weight (mg/g)	11.31 ± 0.17	12.34 ± 0.29	12.39 ± 0.46	12.31 ± 0.19	10.98 ± 0.10	12.14 ± 0.33	12.33 ± 0.14	12.01 ± 0.30
Spleen/body weight (mg/g)	2.91 ± 0.13	2.85 ± 0.07	2.77 ± 0.09	3.01 ± 0.09	3.17 ± 0.22	3.74 ± 0.47	3.11 ± 0.09	3.26 ± 0.10

Data represent mean ± standard error. Statistical analysis was performed using ANOVA with Tukey post hoc evaluation
[a]versus clean air exposed WT mice (3 weeks), $p < 0.01$; [b]versus clean air exposed WT mice (3 weeks), $p < 0.05$
[c]Body weight gain at time interval between exposure start and sacrifice

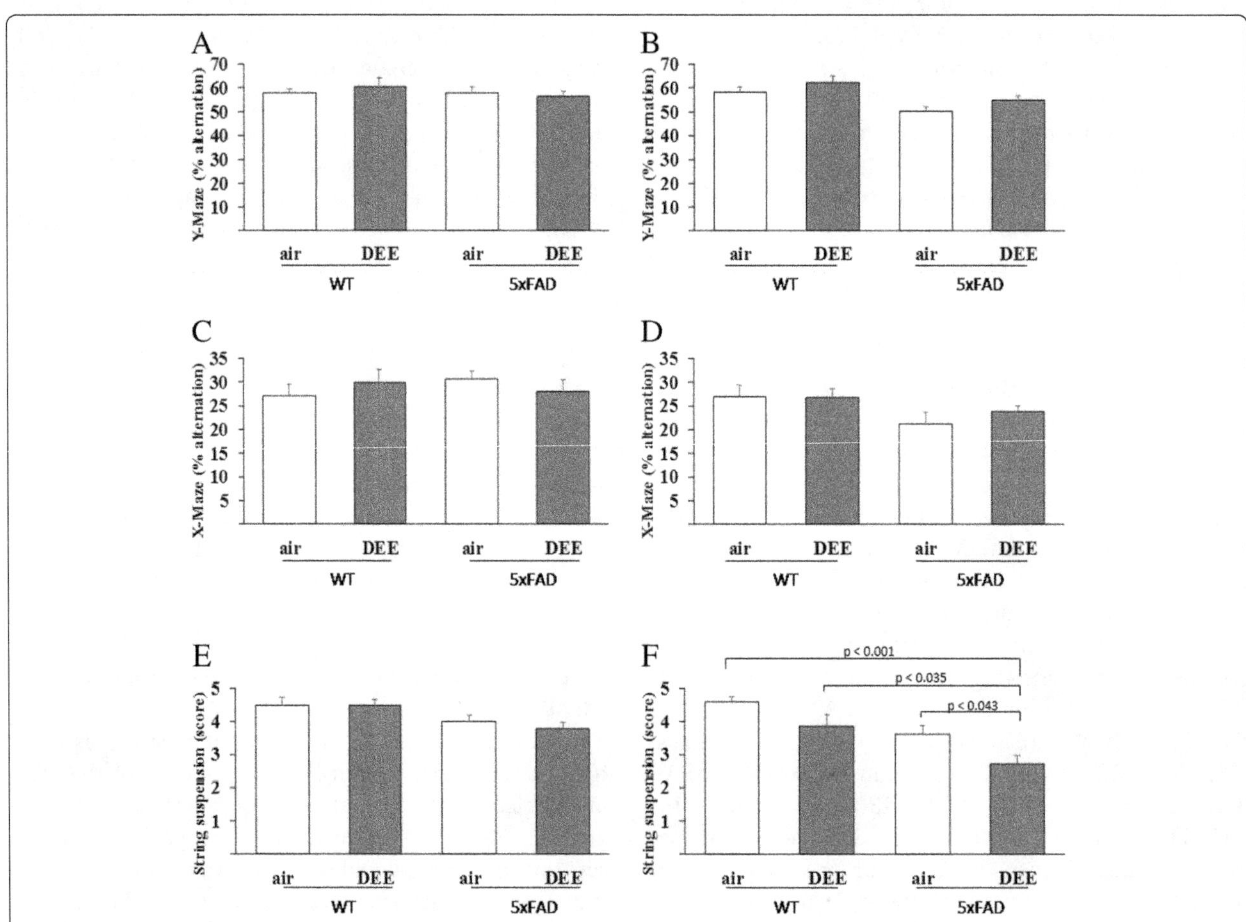

Fig. 2 Behaviour tasks performances of WT and 5XFAD mice following inhalation exposure to DEE or clean air. Data represent mean ± standard error of the % alternation in the Y-maze task (panels **a** and **b**), % alternation in the X-maze task (**c** and **d**) and the string suspension task score (**e** and **f**) following 3 weeks exposure (**a**, **c** and **e**) or 13 weeks exposure (**b**, **d** and **f**) to clean air or DEE as indicated in the figures

Table 3 Total number of arm entries in Y-maze and X-maze tasks

	3 weeks study				13 weeks study			
	Air		DEE		Air		DEE	
	WT $n = 12$	5XFAD $n = 14$	WT $n = 10$	5XFAD $n = 14$	WT $n = 10$	5XFAD $n = 16$	WT $n = 8$	5XFAD $n = 18$
Y-maze number of entries	41.5 ± 2.8	37.6 ± 3.2	39.0 ± 4.0	33.8 ± 2.8	46.2 ± 4.9	56.5 ± 3.5	51.3 ± 4.8	44.6 ± 3.9
X-maze number of entries	52.9 ± 3.9	47.6 ± 4.3	53.1 ± 5.8	44.4 ± 3.6	61.1 ± 4.4	77.2 ± 10.0	63.6 ± 5.6	56.1 ± 3.9

Data represent mean ± standard error. Statistical analysis was performed using ANOVA with Tukey post hoc evaluation

the Y-maze (see Fig. 2a) and X-maze tasks (panel c). The total number of arm entries also did not differ significantly between the treatment groups indicating overall similar explorative behaviour for both maze tasks (Table 3). There were also no statistically significant differences in the string suspension task (Fig. 2e). Irrespective of the genetic background of the mice, the 3 weeks inhalation exposure to DEE did not affect the performance in any of the three behaviour tasks.

Also in the 13-week study, there were no statistically significant differences in performance in spatial working memory tasks (see Fig. 2b and d for the Y-maze and X-maze task, respectively). For this time point, also the total number of arm entries did not differ in the Y-maze and X-maze task (Table 3), thus revealing similar explorative behaviour. Taken together, the sub-chronic (i.e. 13 week) inhalation study did not reveal any major adverse effect of the DEE on spatial working memory.

In contrast, with the string suspension task clear differences were found following the 13 weeks inhalation (see Fig. 2f). Both the genetic background and the DEE exposure affected the performance of the mice in this motor function assessment test. The 5XFAD mice that were exposed for 13 weeks to DEE performed significantly less than all three other groups (ANOVA-Tukey, $p < 0.001$ vs the clean-air exposed WT mice, $p = 0.035$ versus the DEE exposed WT mice and $p = 0.043$ vs the air exposed 5xFAD mice). A two-way ANOVA analysis revealed no significant background-by-exposure interaction (F = 0.099). Most importantly, the observed difference between the DEE-exposed 5XFAD mice and the clean air exposed 5XFAD littermates demonstrates that sub-chronic inhalation exposure to DEE aggravates the motor function phenotype of this transgenic mouse model of AD. Interestingly, the WT mice exposed to DEE also tended to perform less well in the string suspension task than the clean air-WT littermates, but this effect did not reach statistical difference ($p = 0.071$).

Effects of DEE inhalation exposure on Aβ plaque formation in the brains of 5XFAD mice

To evaluate the impact of the DEE exposure on plaque formation in 5XFAD mouse model parasagittal brain slices were stained with an antibody against Aβ42 and quantitative plaque analysis was performed with imaging software. Representative light microscopical pictures from cortex and hippocampus of 5XFAD brain slices stained for Aβ42 are shown in Fig. 3. The brains of selected WT animals were also stained, but no plaques could be detected (data not shown). Results of the plaque analyses are shown in Fig. 4. After the 3 weeks exposure, the level of plaque formation was found to

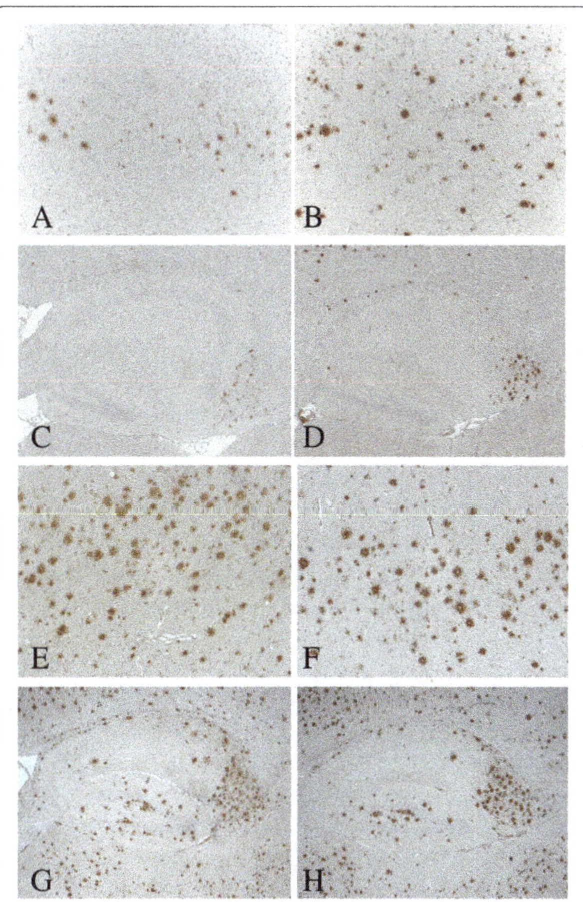

Fig. 3 Representative images showing amyloid-β plaque staining in cortex (**a**, **b**, **e** and **f**) and hippocampus (**c**, **d**, **g** and **h**) of brains sections from 5XFAD mice. The accumulation of Aβ42 (*reddish-brown* colour) was localised by immunohistochemistry in sections of paraffin-embedded brain hemispheres. Hippocampus (50 x magnification) and cortex (100 x magnification) from the same animal are shown for each time point and exposure. i.e. 3 weeks to clean air (**a** and **c**), 3 weeks to DEE (**b** and **d**), 13 weeks to clean air (**e** and **g**) and 13 weeks to DEE (**f** and **h**), respectively

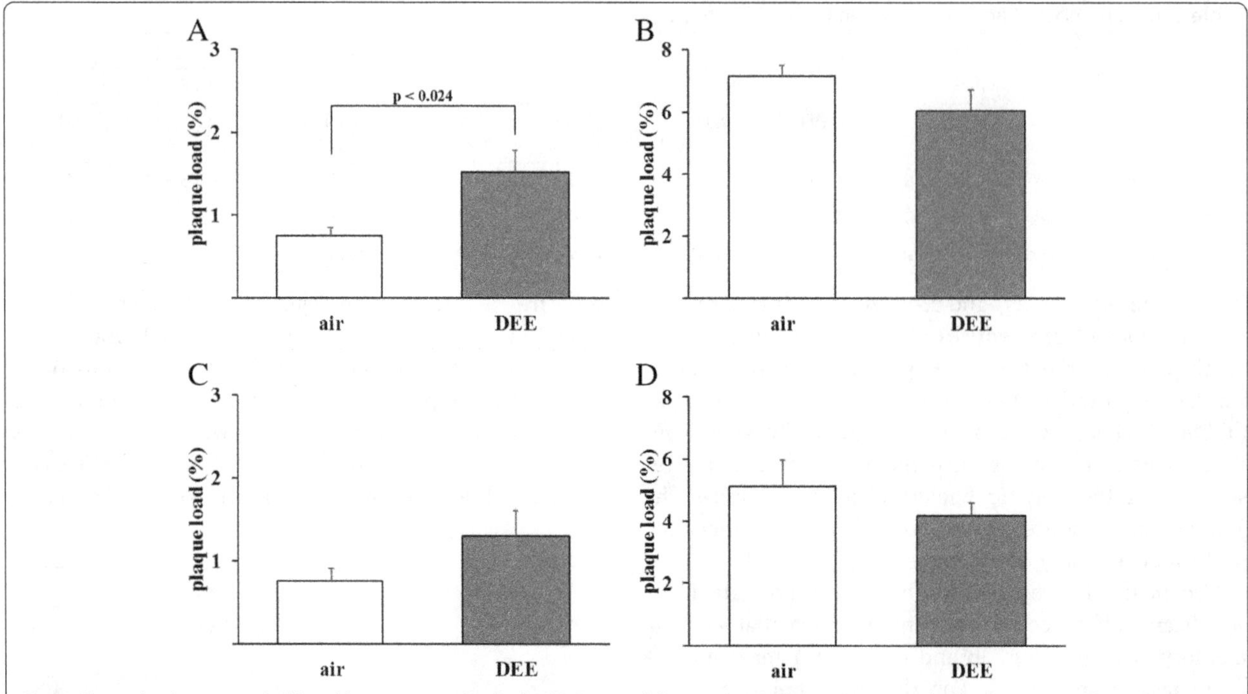

Fig. 4 Plaque load in cortex (**a**, **b**) and hippocampus (**c**, **d**) of 5XFAD mice following 3 weeks (**a**, **c**) or 13 weeks (**b**, **d**) exposure to DEE or clean air. Quantitative Aβ42 plaque analyses were performed via calculation of the % of total plaque load in the analysed area of the section (*n* = 11–16 mice per group)

differ between the DEE and the control group (See Fig. 4a and c). For the cortex region, there was a statistically significant difference in plaque formation between the DEE and clean-air exposed mice, Student's t-test, $p = 0.024$). For the hippocampus, the difference did not reach statistical significance. These data indicate that the inhalation exposure to DEE causes accelerated plaque formation in the 5XFAD mouse model. After the sub-chronic exposure (Fig. 4b and d) no statistically significant differences were observed. After the 13 weeks exposures, plaque density in cortex as well as hippocampus was by far more pronounced than after the 3 weeks exposure.

Since the 3 weeks DEE-exposed 5XFAD mice gained significantly less weight than the clean-air exposed WT littermates (see Table 2), the relation between body weight and plaque load was further explored in the 5XFAD animals. A Pearson correlation analysis revealed a significant inverse association between body weight and plaque load in cortex ($r = -0.467$, $p < 0.05$), but not in hippocampus ($r = -0.123$).

Effects of DEE inhalation exposure on human Aβ42 protein levels in 5XFAD mice

Human Aβ42 protein levels were determined in brain homogenates of the 5XFAD mice by ELISA. The applied ELISA method allowed for the detection of both soluble and insoluble Aβ42 fragments. Results are shown in Fig. 5. In line with the findings on plaque formation, mice that were exposed to DEE for 3 weeks showed markedly higher Aβ42 protein levels than the control mice (Student's t-test, $p < 0.001$). For this time point, the whole brain Aβ42 protein levels were significantly correlated with plaque load in cortex (Pearson $r = 0.710$, $p = 0.014$) as well as hippocampus ($r = 0.608$, $p = 0.047$). The 13 weeks inhalation study revealed no significant differences in Aβ42 levels between the DEE and clean air control littermates.

Pulmonary histology and systemic inflammation

To evaluate the pulmonary effects of the DEE exposure in the 5XFAD mice and WT littermates, lung sections were analysed. Representative pictures of HE-stained tissues are shown in Fig. 6. Histological evaluation of the mice lungs revealed no obvious differences in tissue structure related to DEE exposure or genetic background. The lungs of 5XFAD mice were also found to be comparable to those of their WT littermates. Deposition of clustered diesel exhaust particles could be clearly detected in the lungs of the DEE-exposed mice (see Fig. 6). However, these depositions were not associated with any obvious development of structural irreversible changes within the pulmonary tissues of the WT and 5XFAD mice.

A Bio-Plex murine cytokine platform was used to evaluate the levels of cytokines in the blood of DEE and clean air-exposed 5XFAD mice as an indicator of

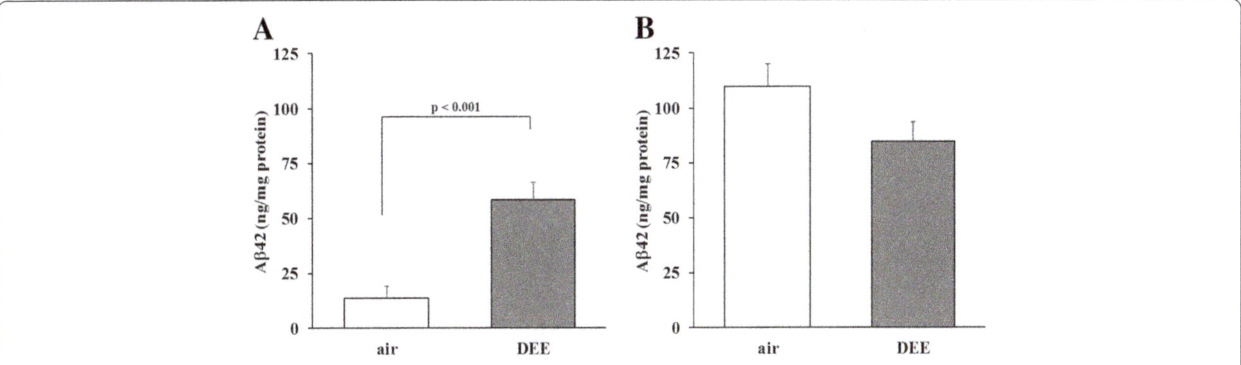

Fig. 5 Amyloid-β protein levels in mouse brain homogenates. Human Aβ42 protein levels were determined by ELISA following 3 (**a**) or 13 weeks (**b**) exposure to DEE or clean air (n = 5–8 mice per group)

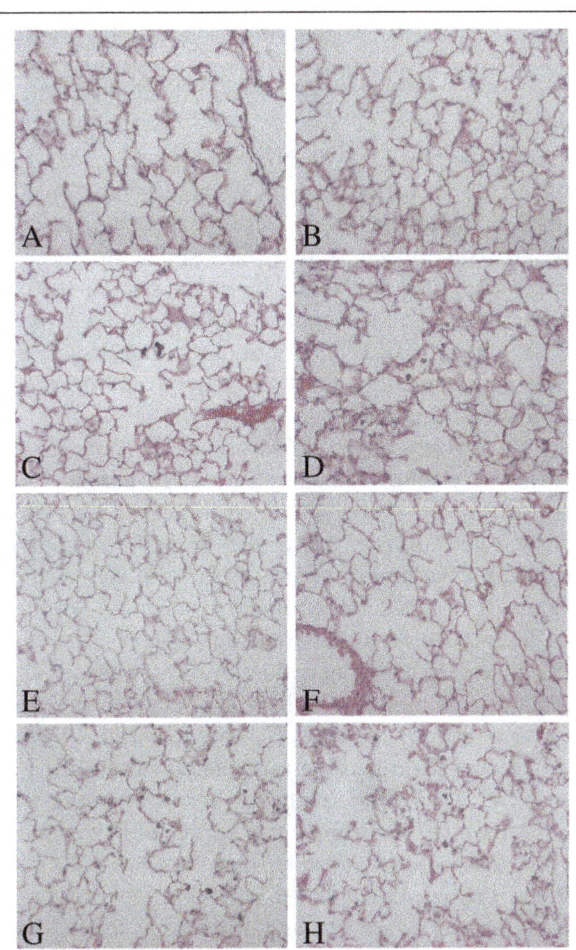

Fig. 6 Representative images of haematoxylin-eosin stained mouse lungs. Tissue sections shown are from: **a** 3 weeks clean air-exposed 5XFAD mouse; **b** 3 weeks clean air-exposed WT mouse; **c** 3 weeks DEE-exposed FAD mouse; **d** 3 weeks DEE-exposed WT mouse; **e** 13 weeks clean air-exposed 5XFAD mouse; **f** 13 weeks clean air-exposed WT mouse; **g** 13 weeks DEE-exposed 5XFAD mouse; **h** 13 weeks DEE-exposed WT mouse. Original magnification 640×

systemic inflammation. Results are shown in Fig. 7. The levels of the four cytokines that could be readily detected in the blood of the mice (i.e. IL-1β, RANTES, G-CSF and MCP-1) did not significantly differ between the DEE and sham exposure conditions. The levels of IL-1α, IL-6, IL-17, KC, GM-CSF, MIP-1α and MIP-1β were not consistently above detection limit. These findings indicated that the DEE inhalation exposure regime did not induce a sustained systemic inflammatory response.

Discussion

In the present study, we demonstrated that inhalation exposure to DEE leads to accelerated formation of Aβ-plaques as well as motor function impairment in 5XFAD mice. Studies in transgenic mouse models of AD, including the 5XFAD model, have contributed to the understanding of mechanisms involved in β-amyloid pathology [42–44]. The 5XFAD model has also been used to assess potential beneficial aspects of candidate-drugs or animal housing enrichment [45–48]. Factors that could accelerate AD-like pathology, like environmental toxicants or stress have been much less topic of investigation. Devi et al. [37] showed increased Aβ42 levels and accelerated Aβ plaque formation in the hippocampus of 3 months old female 5XFAD mice due to restraint stress, induced by placing them in plastic tubes for 5 days (6 h/day). In our study, accelerated plaque load and increased whole brain Aβ42 protein levels were detected in 15 weeks old female 5XFAD mice following 3 weeks DEE inhalation exposure. The results from Devi et al. [37] indicate that stress may also contribute to CNS pathologies in rodent inhalation studies, specifically in nose-only inhalation protocols, as this requires restraint of the animals. In the present study, a whole body inhalation approach was used with simultaneous exposure of littermates to DEE and clean air at otherwise identical conditions. Indeed, the specific caging, handling and treatment conditions of the 5XFAD mice may have led to differences in Aβ42 protein levels and extent of plaque load, when

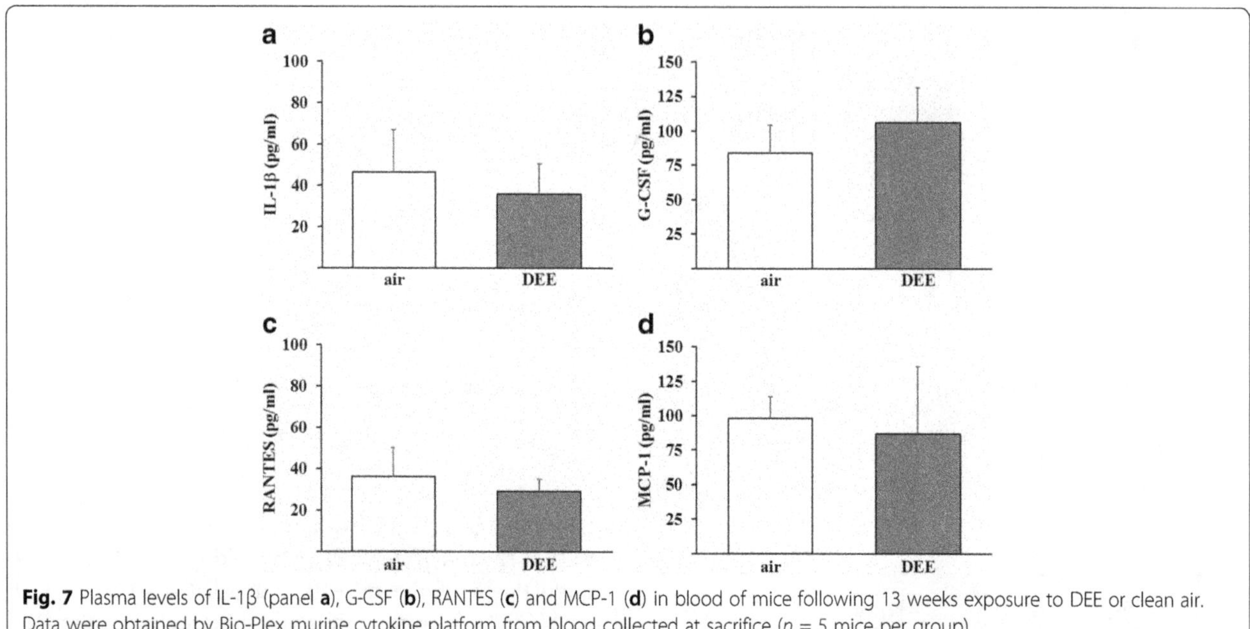

Fig. 7 Plasma levels of IL-1β (panel **a**), G-CSF (**b**), RANTES (**c**) and MCP-1 (**d**) in blood of mice following 13 weeks exposure to DEE or clean air. Data were obtained by Bio-Plex murine cytokine platform from blood collected at sacrifice (*n* = 5 mice per group)

compared to other studies with similar-aged 5XFAD mice. However, with our study design it can be assured that the observed effects in this AD mouse model were driven by the DEE inhalation per se.

Several other investigators have reported findings that support a role of DEE inhalation in AD pathogenesis. Levesque et al. [8] showed increased Aβ42 levels in frontal lobe of male Fischer 344 rats after 6 months exposure to DEE. Increased Aβ42 levels were also reported in a 90-day rat inhalation study with resuspended diesel exhaust particles, albeit at very high concentrations (>500 mg/m^3) [49]. Bhatt et al. [29] showed increased levels of Aβ40 and β-secretase in C57BL/6 mice following 9 months exposure to concentrated $PM_{2.5}$. To the best of our knowledge, the results of our study are the first to show an effect of DEE inhalation on actual Aβ plaque formation in mouse brain, and thus support the initial studies that suggested the link between ambient air pollution and Aβ plaque pathology in humans [26, 27].

Notably, in our study cortical plaque load and whole brain Aβ42 protein levels were inversely correlated with body weight following the 3 weeks exposures. This would suggest that the accelerated plaque formation could be the cause of, or the result of, impaired body weight gain in these young DEE-exposed 5XFAD mice. The absence of such associations in the 13 weeks exposed animals indicates the transient nature of this phenomenon. Significant lower body weights for the 5XFAD mice compared to their WT littermates were previously found starting at an age of 9 months [36]. We consider it unlikely that the amyloidogenic effect of the DEE is a mere indirect effect resulting from a direct adverse impact of DEE on body weight. Absence of effects of DEE inhalation on body weight has been demonstrated for inhalation studies in rats as well as mice at exposure concentrations that were similar to those in present study [50, 51]. Our data rather suggest that the weight changes are a secondary effect, resulting from a primary effect of DEE on plaque formation. However, a combined contribution of DEE and the 5XFAD background cannot be ruled out.

In the 13 weeks exposed 5XFAD mice, significant differences in plaque formation and Aβ42 protein levels were no longer observed. Levels of Aβ42 have been demonstrated to rise drastically in brain of 5XFAD mice within the first 6 months of age [34]. The marked differences in Aβ42 levels in the air-exposed (i.e. control) 5XFAD mice of different age (Fig. 5a versus b) confirm the rapid plaque development phenotype in this transgenic model. We therefore believe that the aggressive pathology of the 5XFAD model in the 13 weeks exposed mice saturated the early plaque-accelerating effect of the DEE. In line with this, recently, a long-term (i.e. 11 months) environmental enrichment was found to improve motor performance in 5XFAD mice, whereas this treatment failed to benefit working memory performance, anxiety and Aβ plaque load [47]. It was concluded that the relative fast and aggressive pathology of the 5XFAD model obscures interventions that are beneficial to disease progression [47]. Our study results indicate that this is also true for interventions that worsen disease hallmarks.

To assess effects of DEE inhalation exposure on cognition, Y-maze and X-maze tasks were performed, whereas motor function was evaluated by the string suspension. Importantly in this regard, all animals (i.e. including the clean air exposed "control" mice) were placed in the inhalation units with 2 animals per cage. Moreover, in concordance with conventional inhalation toxicology protocols, the mice were housed without inverted light conditions and exposed during daytime, i.e. during their sleep phase. Hence, also the post-exposure behaviour tasks were performed during daytime, while such testing is considered more suitable during the active phase for these night-active species [52]. These and further factors may very well have influenced the age of onset and extent of behaviour phenotype as reported for the 5XFAD mice in other studies. We did not observe significant behaviour impairments following the 3 weeks DEE exposure. Furthermore, no differences between the 5XFAD and WT littermates of the respective exposure groups were seen at this young-age (i.e. < 3 months) time point. The latter agrees with the pattern of age-dependent phenotype development of this transgenic model [34, 36, 44]. The 13 weeks DEE-exposure also did not cause statistically significant differences in the Y-maze and X-maze tasks. However, irrespective of the exposure condition the 5XFAD animals tended to show a slightly lower spatial working memory performance than the WT animals (see Fig. 2b and d for the Y-maze and X-maze task, respectively). Effects of age-differences among the different treatment groups could be excluded because of the littermate-study design.

However, significant effects of DEE on the performance in the string suspension task were found following the 13 weeks exposures. Thus, at this time point, an adverse impact on motor function was identified while differences in Aβ42 levels and plaque load were no longer present. As already mentioned, environmental enrichment of 5XFAD mice revealed a similar contrast [47]. In our hands, the DEE-exposed 5XFAD animals also performed less than their DEE-exposed WT littermates as well as the clean air-exposed WT littermates. Thus, apart from a specific effect of the DEE there also appeared to be a contribution of the transgenic background on motor function loss. Age-dependent performance impairment in the string suspension task by female 5XFAD mice has been described previously [36].

In our study, DEE inhalation exposure also tended to affect motor performance in the WT mice. Although the effect was not statistically significant, it suggests that DEE could cause motor impairments in other mouse strains. Indeed, others have shown locomotive activity effects in rats following exposure to DEE (6 mg/m^3, 8 h/day for 16 weeks) [53] or mice exposed to resuspended diesel exhaust particles (72 mg/m^3, 90 min/day for 4 days) [54]. Interestingly, decreased locomotor activity has also been shown in mice following prenatal exposure [55]. Sensory-motor impairments may occur due to axonal defects and these have been observed in studies with AD patients [56]. Axonopathy and deficits like swelling of accumulated motor proteins, organelles and vesicles have been detected in an APP transgenic mouse model carrying the Swedish mutation [57]. It has been demonstrated that 5XFAD mice develop, in addition to working memory deficits, an age-dependent motor phenotype. The motor phenotype correlates with spinal cord pathology, as demonstrated by abundant intraneuronal Aβ accumulation and extracellular plaque deposition [36].

The underlying molecular mechanisms of DEE-induced accelerated Aβ plaque deposition and motor impairment remain to be clarified. Two major principle pathways have been discussed whereby ultrafine air pollution particles may induce adverse effect in the CNS, namely a direct pathway whereby the particles physically enter the brain parenchyma, and an indirect pathway whereby peripheral effects contribute to neurotoxicity [19, 58]. Inhalation studies with PM and DEE have linked oxidative stress and associated induction of inflammation to pulmonary as well as cardiovascular effects [1, 59]. Systemic inflammation has been discussed to be involved in AD pathogenesis [31–33] and could thus provide a mechanism whereby inhaled DEE could affect the CNS indirectly. In our hands, the diluted DEE inhalations at a particle dose of 0.95 mg/m^3 did not cause notable irreversible pathological changes in the lungs of the mice of both backgrounds. The profile of blood inflammatory markers also did not differ between DEE and clean air-exposed mice. Taken together, our findings suggest that observed amyloidogenesis and motor function impairment effects were not mediated by strong pulmonary toxicity and/or systemic inflammatory responses. However, it should be emphasized that these analyses were performed 11 days after the last exposure (see also Fig. 1), and thus we cannot rule out the possible occurrence of mild and transient inflammatory effects during the DEE inhalations.

Induction of local oxidative stress and inflammation following direct translocation of the component of ultrafine carbonaceous particles of DEE into the brain represents the major alternative or complementary mechanism of action [19]. Inflammation and oxidative stress has been shown to trigger β-amyloid pathology (for review see [60, 61]), but brain tissue expression analyses of markers of these processes was not pursued in our study, in view of the considerable time interval between the last days of DEE exposure and tissue collection. However, brain-region specific inflammatory and oxidative stress responses have been demonstrated previously in a considerable number of rodent inhalation studies with PM ([2–4, 62] and DEE [5, 6, 8, 9, 63]. Translocation into the brain was firstly shown in a rat inhalation study for ultrafine ^{13}C particles [64], and recently regained major attention in a study were magnetite particles of proposed external origin were shown in human brains [65].

However, the potential contribution of non-particulate components within the DEE pollutant mixture should also be considered in our study. Apart from the carbonaceous particles and components (metals, organics) absorbed on their core, the exhaust of diesel also contains various non-particulate compounds including CO, NO_x, SO_2, and volatile organic compounds. The levels of the prevailing gases CO and NOx in the diluted DEE in the exposure units were of an order of magnitude at which adverse effects have been found to be absent (and even neuroprotective) in mice [66]. Findings from intratracheal instillation studies with diesel exhaust particles [7] or inhalation studies with resuspended particulates [49, 54] are in strong support for a role of the particle component of the DEE, although dosimetry aspects should be taken into account here. However, the effects observed in our present study could also have resulted from interactions among the various phases. This aspect has been elegantly addressed in a recent study by Tyler et al. [67] through the parallel testing of fine or ultrafine particles generated from gasoline or diesel emissions in either presence or absence of gaseous compounds. Interestingly, neuroinflammatory effects (i.e. cytokine expression in hippocampus) tended to be the strongest in the animals that were exposed to combination of ultrafine PM fraction and the gaseous components. The authors concluded their findings supported the observed epidemiological associations between roadway proximity and neurological outcomes, indicative of a dominant role for freshly generated ultrafine particles in the presence of combustion-derived gas phase pollutants [67].

Conclusions

We showed that DEE inhalation causes accelerated formation of Aβ-plaques and motor function impairment in 5XFAD transgenic mice. Our study provides further support that the brain is a relevant target for the effects of inhaled DEE and suggest that long-term exposure to this ubiquitous air pollution mixture may promote the development of AD. Our results should be viewed in the context of the recently published population-based findings on road proximity and incident dementia [16]. Further research is needed to determine the relevance of the applied dosimetry and animal model for humans in relation to relevant exposure situations. Toxicological investigations on the contributions of specific particulate versus non-particulate components of motor vehicle exhaust and other traffic-related stress factors (e.g. noise) to AD pathogenesis represent a major challenge.

Acknowledgements

The authors thank Prof. Sascha Weggen from the Department of Neuropathology, Heinrich-Heine-University Düsseldorf for fruitful discussions during the initiation of this study and Dr. Antje Hillmann for experimental and training support. We also thank John A. Boere, Paul H. Fokkens, and Daan L.A.C. Leseman (RIVM) as well as Christel Weishaupt, Gabriele Wick and Petra Gross (IUF) for technical support.

Funding

This work was supported by a grant from the Research Commission of the Faculty of Medicine of the Heinrich-Heine University Düsseldorf (Forschungskommission der medizinische Fakultät, FoKo 9772 365) and by the IUF-RIVM joint research project AIRBAG (AIR pollutants and Brain Aging research Group). MH received further financial support via the Research Training Group of the German Research Organisation (DFG Graduiertenkolleg 1033) and through a Josef Abel Research Stipend (IUF).

Authors' contributions

MH participated in the design and coordination of the study, the interpretation of results, carried out the behaviour studies and the ELISA and is co-writer of the manuscript. CA participated in the design, planning and coordination of the study, supervised tissue sectioning and processing, carried out the lung histopathology analysis and plaque load quantification, participated in the interpretation of the results and is co-writer of the manuscript. DvB participated in the tissue dissection, and provided advice regarding lung and brain tissue analyses. MEGN participated in the design of the study and coordinated the inhalation studies. TW made substantial contributions to the interpretation of the data and has been involved in critically revising the manuscript. AWB performed the luminex assay and interpretation of these data. JK, FRC and TAB participated in conceiving the study, its design and the interpretation of the results. PFRS devised the project, coordinated and supervised the study, performed the statistical analyses, and drafted the manuscript. All authors have read, reviewed, commented and approved the final version of the manuscript.

Competing interests

The authors declare that they have no competing interests.

Author details

[1]IUF - Leibniz Research Institute for Environmental Medicine, Auf'm Hennekamp 50, 40225 Düsseldorf, Germany. [2]National Institute for Public Health and the Environment, Bilthoven, The Netherlands. [3]Department of Pharmacology and Toxicology, NUTRIM School of Nutrition and Translational Research in Metabolism, Maastricht University, Maastricht, The Netherlands. [4]Medical Faculty, Heinrich-Heine-University, Düsseldorf, Germany. [5]Institute of Risk Assessment Sciences, Utrecht University, Utrecht, The Netherlands. [6]Department of Psychiatry and Psychotherapy, Division of Molecular Psychiatry, Georg-August-University Göttingen, University Medicine Göttingen, Göttingen, Germany. [7]Present address: Triskelion BV Utrechtseweg 48, 3704 HE Zeist, The Netherlands.

References

1. Donaldson K, Mills N, MacNee W, Robinson S, Newby D. Role of inflammation in cardiopulmonary health effects of PM. Toxicol Appl Pharmacol. 2005;207(Suppl 2):26–32.

2. Campbell A, Oldham M, Becaria A, Bondy SC, Meacher D, Sioutas C, et al. Particulate matter in polluted air may increase biomarkers of inflammation in mouse brain. Neurotoxicology. 2005;26:133–40.
3. Veronesi B, Makwana O, Pooler M, Chen LC. Effects of subchronic exposures to concentrated ambient particles. VII. Degeneration of dopaminergic neurons in Apo E–/– mice. Inhal Toxicol. 2005;17:235–41.
4. Guerra R, Vera-Aguilar E, Uribe-Ramirez M, Gookin G, Camacho J, Osornio-Vargas AR, et al. Exposure to inhaled particulate matter activates early markers of oxidative stress, inflammation and unfolded protein response in rat striatum. Toxicol Lett. 2013;222:146–54.
5. Van Berlo D, Albrecht C, Knaapen AM, Cassee FR, Gerlofs-Nijland ME, Kooter IM, et al. Comparative evaluation of the effects of short-term inhalation exposure to diesel engine exhaust on rat lung and brain. Arch Toxicol. 2010;84:553–62.
6. Gerlofs-Nijland ME, van Berlo D, Cassee FR, Schins RPF, Wang K, Campbell A. Effect of prolonged exposure to diesel engine exhaust on proinflammatory markers in different regions of the rat brain. Part Fibre Toxicol. 2010;7:12.
7. Levesque S, Taetzsch T, Lull ME, Kodavanti U, Stadler K, Wagner A, et al. Diesel exhaust activates and primes microglia: air pollution, neuroinflammation, and regulation of dopaminergic neurotoxicity. Environ Health Perspect. 2011;119:1149–55.
8. Levesque S, Surace MJ, McDonald J, Block ML. Air pollution & the brain: subchronic diesel exhaust exposure causes neuroinflammation and elevates early markers of neurodegenerative disease. J Neuroinflammation. 2011;8:105.
9. Cole TB, Coburn J, Dao K, Roqué P, Chang YC, Kalia V, et al. Sex and genetic differences in the effects of acute diesel exhaust exposure on inflammation and oxidative stress in mouse brain. Toxicology. 2016; doi:10.1016/j.tox.2016.11.010.
10. Chen JC, Schwartz J. Neurobehavioral effects of ambient air pollution on cognitive performance in US adults. Neurotoxicology. 2009; doi:10.1016/j.neuro.2008.12.011.
11. Ranft U, Schikowski T, Sugiri D, Krutmann J, Krämer U. Long-term exposure to traffic-related particulate matter impairs cognitive function in the elderly. Environ Res. 2009; doi:10.1016/j.envres.2009.08.003.
12. Power M, Weisskopf MG, Alexeeff SE, Coull BA, Spiro A 3rd, Schwartz J. Traffic-related air pollution and cognitive function in a cohort of older men. Environ Health Perspect. 2011; doi:10.1289/ehp.1002767.
13. Weuve J, Puett RC, Schwartz J, Yanosky JD, Laden F, Grodstein F. Exposure to particulate air pollution and cognitive decline in older women. Arch Intern Med. 2012; doi:10.1001/archinternmed.2011.683.
14. Ailshire JA, Crimmins EM. Fine particulate matter air pollution and cognitive function among older US adults. Am J Epidemiol. 2014; doi:10.1093/aje/kwu155.
15. Tzivian L, Dlugaj M, Winkler A, Weinmayr G, Hennig F, Fuks KB, et al. Long-term air pollution and traffic noise exposures and mild cognitive impairment in older adults: a cross-sectional analysis of the Heinz Nixdorf recall study. Environ Health Perspect. 2016; doi:10.1289/ehp.1509824.
16. Chen H, Kwong JC, Copes R, Tu K, Villeneuve PJ, van Donkelaar A, et al. Living near major roads and the incidence of dementia, Parkinson's disease, and multiple sclerosis: a population-based cohort study. Lancet. 2017; doi: 10.1016/S0140-6736(16)32399-6.
17. Block ML, Calderón-Garcidueñas L. Air pollution: mechanisms of neuroinflammation and CNS disease. Trends Neurosci. 2009; doi:10.1016/j.tins.2009.05.009.
18. Weuve J. Invited commentary: how exposure to air pollution may shape dementia risk, and what epidemiology can say about it. Am J Epidemiol. 2014; doi:10.1093/aje/kwu153.
19. Heusinkveld HJ, Wahle T, Campbell A, Westerink RH, Tran L, Johnston H, et al. Neurodegenerative and neurological disorders by small inhaled particles. Neurotoxicology. 2016; doi:10.1016/j.neuro.2016.07.007.
20. Förstl H, Kurz A. Clinical features of Alzheimer's disease. Eur Arch Psychiatry Clin Neurosci. 1999;249:288–90.
21. West MJ, Coleman PD, Flood DG, Troncoso JC. Differences in the pattern of hippocampal neuronal loss in normal ageing and Alzheimer's disease. Lancet. 1994;344:769–72.
22. Selkoe DJ. Alzheimer's disease: genes, proteins, and therapy. Physiol Rev. 2001;81:741–66.
23. Takami M, Nagashima Y, Sano Y, Ishihara S, Morishima-Kawashima M, Funamoto S, et al. Gamma-Secretase: successive tripeptide and tetrapeptide release from the transmembrane domain of beta-carboxyl terminal fragment. J Neurosci. 2009; doi:10.1523/JNEUROSCI.2362-09.2009.
24. Hutton M, Pérez-Tur J, Hardy J. Genetics of Alzheimer's disease. Essays Biochem. 1998;33:117–31.
25. Harper JD, Wong SS, Lieber CM, Lansbury PT. Observation of metastable Abeta amyloid protofibrils by atomic force microscopy. Chem Biol. 1997;4: 119–25.
26. Calderón-Garcidueñas L, Reed W, Maronpot RR, Henríquez-Roldán C, Delgado-Chavez R, Calderón-Garcidueñas A, et al. Brain inflammation and Alzheimer's-like pathology in individuals exposed to severe air pollution. Toxicol Pathol. 2004;32:650–8.
27. Peters A, Veronesi B, Calderón-Garcidueñas L, Gehr P, Chen LC, Geiser M, et al. Translocation and potential neurological effects of fine and ultrafine particles a critical update. Part Fibre Toxicol. 2006;3:13.
28. Calderón-Garcidueñas L, Kavanaugh M, Block M, D'Angiulli A, Delgado-Chávez R, Torres-Jardón R, et al. Neuroinflammation, hyperphosphorylated tau, diffuse amyloid plaques, and down-regulation of the cellular prion protein in air pollution exposed children and young adults. J Alzheimers Dis. 2012;28:93–107.
29. Bhatt DP, Puig KL, Gorr MW, Wold LE, Combs CK. A pilot study to assess effects of long-term inhalation of airborne particulate matter on early Alzheimer-like changes in the mouse brain. PLoS One. 2015; doi:10.1371/journal.pone.0127102.
30. Power MC, Adar SD, Yanosky JD, Weuve J. Exposure to air pollution as a potential contributor to cognitive function, cognitive decline, brain imaging, and dementia: a systematic review of epidemiologic research. Neurotoxicology. 2016; doi:10.1016/j.neuro.2016.06.004.
31. Perry VH. The influence of systemic inflammation on inflammation in the brain: implications for chronic neurodegenerative disease. Brain Behav Immun. 2004;18:407–13.
32. Johnston H, Boutin H, Allan SM. Assessing the contribution of inflammation in models of Alzheimer's disease. Biochem Soc Trans. 2011;39:886–90.
33. O'Banion MK. Does peripheral inflammation contribute to Alzheimer disease? Evidence from animal models. Neurology. 2014;83:480–1.
34. Oakley H, Cole SL, Logan S, Maus E, Shao P, Craft J, et al. Intraneuronal beta-amyloid aggregates, neurodegeneration, and neuron loss in transgenic mice with five familial Alzheimer's disease mutations: potential factors in amyloid plaque formation. J Neurosci. 2006;26:10129–40.
35. Ohno M, Chang L, Tseng W, Oakley H, Citron M, Klein WL, et al. Temporal memory deficits in Alzheimer's mouse models: rescue by genetic deletion of BACE1. Eur J Neurosci. 2006;23:251–60.
36. Jawhar S, Trawicka A, Jenneckens C, Bayer TA, Wirths O. Motor deficits, neuron loss, and reduced anxiety coinciding with axonal degeneration and intraneuronal Aβ aggregation in the 5XFAD mouse model of Alzheimer's disease. Neurobiol Aging. 2012; doi:10.1016/j.neurobiolaging.
37. Devi L, Alldred MJ, Ginsberg SD, Ohno M. Sex- and brain region-specific acceleration of β-amyloidogenesis following behavioral stress in a mouse model of Alzheimer's disease. Mol Brain. 2010; doi:10.1186/1756-6606-3-34.
38. Marra M, Rombout JA. Design and performance of an inhalation chamber for exposing laboratory animals to oxidant air pollutants. Inhal Toxicol. 1990;2:187–204.
39. Moran PM, Higgins LS, Cordell B, Moser PC. Age-related learning deficits in transgenic mice expressing the 751-amino acid isoform of human beta-amyloid precursor protein. Proc Natl Acad Sci U S A. 1995;92:5341–5.
40. Holcomb LA, Gordon MN, Jantzen P, Hsiao K, Duff K, Morgan D. Behavioral changes in transgenic mice expressing both amyloid precursor protein and presenilin-1 mutations: lack of association with amyloid deposits. Behav Genet. 1999;29:177–85.
41. Sabo-Attwood T, Ramos-Nino M, Bond J, Butnor KJ, Heintz N, Gruber AD, et al. Gene expression profiles reveal increased mClca3 (Gob5) expression and mucin production in a murine model of asbestos-induced fibrogenesis. Am J Pathol. 2005;167:1243–56.
42. Bayer TA, Wirths O. Intraneuronal Aβ as a trigger for neuron loss: can this be translated into human pathology? Biochem Soc Trans. 2011; doi:10.1042/BST0390857.
43. Bouter Y, Kacprowski T, Weissmann R, Dietrich K, Borgers H, Brauß A, et al. Deciphering the molecular profile of plaques, memory decline and neuron loss in two mouse models for Alzheimer's disease by deep sequencing. Front Aging Neurosci. 2014;6:75.
44. Richard BC, Kurdakova A, Baches S, Bayer TA, Weggen S, Wirths O. Gene dosage dependent aggravation of the neurological phenotype in the 5XFAD mouse model of Alzheimer's disease. J Alzheimers Dis. 2015; doi:10.3233/JAD-143120.
45. Hillmann A, Hahn S, Schilling S, Hoffmann T, Demuth HU, Bulic B, et al. No improvement after chronic ibuprofen treatment in the 5XFAD mouse model of Alzheimer's disease. Neurobiol Aging. 2012;33:833.e39–50.
46. Antonios G, Saiepour N, Bouter Y, Richard BC, Paetau A, Verkkoniemi-Ahola A, et al. N-truncated Abeta starting with position four: early intraneuronal

accumulation and rescue of toxicity using NT4X-167, a novel monoclonal antibody. Acta Neuropathol Commun. 2013; doi:10.1186/2051-5960-1-56.

47. Hüttenrauch M, Walter S, Kaufmann M, Weggen S, Wirths O. Limited effects of prolonged environmental enrichment on the pathology of 5XFAD mice. Mol Neurobiol. 2016;12 [Epub ahead of print].
48. McClure R, Ong H, Janve V, Barton S, Zhu M, Li B, et al. Aerosol delivery of Curcumin reduced Amyloid-β deposition and improved cognitive performance in a transgenic model of Alzheimer's disease. J Alzheimers Dis. 2017;55:797–811.
49. Durga M, Devasena T, Rajasekar A. Determination of LC50 and sub-chronic neurotoxicity of diesel exhaust nanoparticles. Environ Toxicol Pharmacol. 2015;40:615–25.
50. Mauderly JL, Bice DE, Carpenter RL, Gillett NA, Henderson RF, Pickrell JA, et al. Effects of inhaled nitrogen dioxide and diesel exhaust on developing lung. Res Rep Health Eff Inst. 1987;8:3–37.
51. Reed MD, Gigliotti AP, McDonald JD, Seagrave JC, Seilkop SK, Mauderly JL. Health effects of subchronic exposure to environmental levels of diesel exhaust. Inhal Toxicol. 2004;16:177–93.
52. Beeler JA, Prendergast B, Zhuang X. Low amplitude entrainment of mice and the impact of circadian phase on behavior tests. Physiol Behav. 2006;87: 870–80.
53. Laurie RD, Boyes WK, Wessendarp T. Behavioral alterations due to diesel exhaust exposure. Environ Int. 1981;5:357–61.
54. Hougaard KS, Saber AT, Jensen KA, Vogel U, Wallin H. Diesel exhaust particles: effects on neurofunction in female mice. Basic Clin Pharmacol Toxicol. 2009;105:139–43.
55. Suzuki T, Oshio S, Iwata M, Saburi H, Odagiri T, Udagawa T, et al. In utero exposure to a low concentration of diesel exhaust affects spontaneous locomotor activity and monoaminergic system in male mice. Part Fibre Toxicol. 2010; doi:10.1186/1743-8977-7-7.
56. Wirths O, Bayer TA. Motor impairment in Alzheimer's disease and transgenic Alzheimer's disease mouse models. Genes Brain Behav. 2008; doi:10.1111/j.1601-183X.2007.00373.x.
57. Stokin GB, Lillo C, Falzone TL, Brusch RG, Rockenstein E, Mount SL, et al. Axonopathy and transport deficits early in the pathogenesis of Alzheimer's disease. Science. 2005;307:1282–8.
58. Oberdörster G, Elder A, Rinderknecht A. Nanoparticles and the brain: cause for concern? J Nanosci Nanotechnol. 2009;9:4996–5007.
59. Quan C, Sun Q, Lippmann M, Chen LC. Comparative effects of inhaled diesel exhaust and ambient fine particles on inflammation, atherosclerosis, and vascular dysfunction. Inhal Toxicol. 2010;22:738–53.
60. Zhao Y, Zhao B. Oxidative stress and the pathogenesis of Alzheimer's disease. Oxidative Med Cell Longev. 2013; doi:10.1155/2013/316523.
61. Heneka MT, Carson MJ, El Khoury J, Landreth GE, Brosseron F, Feinstein DL, et al. Neuroinflammation in Alzheimer's disease. Lancet Neurol. 2015; doi:10. 1016/S1474-4422 (15)70016-5.
62. Fonken LK, Xu X, Weil ZM, Chen G, Sun Q, Rajagopalan S, et al. Air pollution impairs cognition, provokes depressive-like behaviors and alters hippocampal cytokine expression and morphology. Mol Psychiatry. 2011; doi:10.1038/mp.2011.76.
63. Oppenheim HA, Lucero J, Guyot AC, Herbert LM, McDonald JD, Mabondzo A, et al. Exposure to vehicle emissions results in altered blood brain barrier permeability and expression of matrix metalloproteinases and tight junction proteins in mice. Part Fibre Toxicol. 2013; doi:10.1186/1743-8977-10-62.
64. Oberdörster G, Sharp Z, Atudorei V, Elder A, Gelein R, Kreyling W, Cox C. Translocation of inhaled ultrafine particles to the brain. Inhal Toxicol. 2004; 16:437–45.
65. Maher BA, Ahmed IA, Karloukovski V, MacLaren DA, Foulds PG, Allsop D, et al. Magnetite pollution nanoparticles in the human brain. Proc Natl Acad Sci U S A. 2016; doi:10.1073/pnas.1605941113.
66. Li YS, Shemmer B, Stone E, Nardi MA, Jonas S, Quartermain D. Neuroprotection by inhaled nitric oxide in a murine stroke model is concentration and duration dependent. Brain Res. 2013; doi:10.1016/j. brainres.2013.02.031.
67. Tyler CR, Zychowski KE, Sanchez BN, Rivero V, Lucas S, Herbert G, et al. Surface area-dependence of gas-particle interactions influences pulmonary and neuroinflammatory outcomes. Part Fibre Toxicol. 2016;13:64.

2

An updated review of the genotoxicity of respirable crystalline silica

Paul J. A. Borm[1*], Paul Fowler[2] and David Kirkland[3]

Abstract

Human exposure to (certain forms of) crystalline silica (CS) potentially results in adverse effects on human health. Since 1997 IARC has classified CS as a Group 1 carcinogen [1], which was confirmed in a later review in 2012 [2]. The genotoxic potential and mode of genotoxic action of CS was not conclusive in either of the IARC reviews, although a proposal for mode of actions was made in an extensive review of the genotoxicity of CS by Borm, Tran and Donaldson in 2011 [3]. The present study identified 141 new papers from search strings related to genotoxicity of respirable CS (RCS) since 2011 and, of these, 17 relevant publications with genotoxicity data were included in this detailed review.

Studies on in vitro genotoxic endpoints primarily included micronucleus (MN) frequency and % fragmented DNA as measured in the comet assay, and were mostly negative, apart from two studies using primary or cultured macrophages. In vivo studies confirmed the role of persistent inflammation due to quartz surface toxicity leading to anti-oxidant responses in mice and rats, but DNA damage was only seen in rats. The role of surface characteristics was strengthened by in vitro and in vivo studies using aluminium or hydrophobic treatment to quench the silanol groups on the CS surface.

In conclusion, the different modes of action of RCS-induced genotoxicity have been evaluated in a series of independent, adequate studies since 2011. Earlier conclusions on the role of inflammation driven by quartz surface in genotoxic and carcinogenic effects after inhalation are confirmed and findings support a practical threshold. Whereas classic in vitro genotoxicity studies confirm an earlier no-observed effect level (NOEL) in cell cultures of 60-70 μg/cm^2, transformation frequency in SHE cells suggests a lower threshold around 5 μg/cm^2. Both levels are only achieved in vivo at doses (2–4 mg) beyond in vivo doses (> 200 μg) that cause persistent inflammation and tissue remodelling in the rat lung.

Keywords: Crystalline silica, Quartz, Nanoparticles, Genotoxicity, Risk assessment

Background

Prolonged chronic inhalation exposure to respirable crystalline silica (RCS) in the forms of quartz or cristobalite) can induce silicosis and, under certain circumstances, may also cause lung tumours. In 1997, the International Agency for Research on Cancer (IARC) classified crystalline silica (silica) as a Group I human carcinogen [1]. This classification was confirmed in a more recent review [2] but the pathogenesis of CS-induced lung cancer was not clearly identified, leaving many open questions about risk assessment of CS-containing particle exposure.

At the time of the IARC reviews, most genotoxicity assays with CS had been performed with quartz samples. Some studies gave positive (genotoxic) responses, but most were negative (non-genotoxic). Some quartz samples induced micronuclei (MN) in Syrian hamster embryo cells, Chinese hamster lung V79 cells and human embryonic lung Hel 299 cells, but not chromosomal aberrations (CA) in the same cell types. Two quartz samples induced morphological transformation in Syrian hamster embryo cells in vitro and five quartz samples induced transformation in BALB/c3T3 cells [3]. While quartz did not induce MN in mice in vivo, epithelial cells isolated from the lungs of rats exposed by the intratracheal route to quartz

* Correspondence: borm@nanoconsult.nl
[1]Borm Nanoconsult Holding BV, Proost Willemstraat 1, 6231 CV Meerssen, The Netherlands
Full list of author information is available at the end of the article

showed *hprt* gene mutations [4]. The effect was also seen in rats after administration of low-toxicity particles causing persistent pulmonary inflammation. In addition, inflammatory cells from the quartz-exposed rat lungs caused mutations in epithelial cells in vitro, although direct treatment of epithelial cells in vitro with quartz did not cause *hprt* mutations [4]. Tridymite had been tested in only one study, where it induced sister chromatid exchanges (SCE) in co-cultures of human lymphocytes and monocytes [5]. Only one human study measuring genotoxic endpoints in subjects exposed to dust containing CS, but with no indication of the level of exposure, was available for the IARC reviews; the study showed an increase in the levels of SCE and CA in peripheral blood lymphocytes [2].

The IARC evaluation of the carcinogenicity of RCS was based on sufficient evidence of tumour induction in animals (mainly in rats), and sufficient evidence of tumour induction in humans. In the 2012 review, IARC concluded that the rat lung tumour response to CS exposure was most likely a result of impairment of "alveolar-macrophage-mediated particle clearance thereby increasing persistence of silica in the lungs, which results in macrophage activation and the sustained release of chemokines and cytokines". In rats, this "persistent inflammation is characterized by neutrophils that generate oxidants that induce genotoxicity, injury and proliferation of lung epithelial cells leading to the development of lung cancer" [2]. However, the possibility of CS surface-generated oxidants or a direct genotoxic effect could not be ruled out, and it was not known which of these mechanisms, if any, occur in humans.

In 2011 Borm et al. [6] wrote a comprehensive review to complement the IARC (1997) review [1] including more recent publications. They summarized and evaluated the most relevant publications on the in vitro and in vivo genotoxicity of CS. Borm et al. discussed the genotoxic mode of action (MoA) of CS in relation to its carcinogenic activity, and, consistent with the later IARC (2012) review [2], three possible MoAs were proposed:

- **Direct,** which would require RCS particles to enter the nucleus and interact directly with DNA, release of free radicals that damage DNA, or disruption of chromosome segregation during mitosis.
- **Indirect,** in which RCS depletes antioxidants, thus increasing steady-state endogenous oxidative damage, or increased oxidative damage arising from mitochondrial activity, inhibition of DNA repair etc.
- **Secondary**, in which RCS causes inflammation, and thus genotoxicity is mediated by e.g. phagocyte-derived oxidants.

A series of in vitro studies investigating induction of DNA stand breaks (comet assay) or MN had suggested that quartz induces DNA damage in the absence of cytotoxicity. However, there was no evidence that CS particles can enter the nucleus of target cells, and secondary genotoxicity due to physiological stress induced at high concentrations may explain these findings. Quartz particles have been observed inside A549 human lung epithelial cells [7] but not within the nucleus or mitochondria. In these studies, it appears that fixed cells were embedded in Epon™ (epoxy resin blend) and sectioned with an ultramicrotome before microscopic examination. However, whatever method (light microscopy, EM, confocal microscopy) has been used for such observations, concerns have been raised [8] that when sectioning embedded cells or tissue for microscopic analysis, it is possible that particles on the surface of a cell could be moved by the ultramicrotome and accidentally deposited in the cytoplasm – "drag effects". The uptake of nanoparticles in the nucleus and mitochondria, such as reported for nanosize amorphous silica, is not considered relevant to this discussion, since these particles use either specific receptors or penetrate through very small (< 10 nm) nuclear pores [9], and RCS particles are not nanosized.

More important in this respect is that RCS particles have not been found within epithelial cells after in vivo exposure in either animals or humans despite numerous in vivo studies, with larger numbers of animals, using high doses of different particles. Lifetime exposure or follow-up of rats after inhalation [10] or instillation [11] did not observe such particles upon careful and multiple lung tissue investigations [12].

In the original review of Borm et al. [6] it was noted that at least a 5-fold higher dose of CS was required to reach a threshold for genotoxic effects than for pro-inflammatory effects in vivo. This ratio even increases to 60/120-fold if the deposition in the proximal alveolar region is considered [13]. These data strongly suggested that inflammation is the driving force for genotoxicity observed in vivo, and that primary genotoxicity of deposited CS would play a role only at very high, possibly implausible, exposures and deposited doses. Thus, Borm et al. posed the hypothesis that the overriding mechanism of CS genotoxicity is via inflammation-driven secondary genotoxicity [6].

It is interesting to note how the risk assessment is handled by different countries and committees. The Health Council of the Netherlands (DECOS) concluded that the carcinogenicity of quartz is mediated by a non-stochastic genotoxic mode of action, in which a long-term irritation leads to endogenous lipid peroxidation, which produces tissue damage causing release of reactive molecules [14]. Since the irritation precedes the genotoxicity, a threshold below which cancer risk can be considered nil is implicated, and the OEL for RCS was set later at 0,075 mg/m^3. The UK Health and Safety

Executive [15] confirmed that most standard tests on genotoxicity were negative, but that the process of inflammation may cause genotoxicity as a result of increased production of reactive oxygen species (ROS) leading to oxidative DNA damage. Since the extent of genotoxicity was directly related to the severity of inflammation, HSE concluded that it was most likely that CS was not a direct-acting genotoxic agent but could lead indirectly to genotoxicity as a secondary consequence of inflammation and as such would be associated with a threshold. The workplace exposure limit for RCS was set by HSE at 0.1 mg/m^3. In a draft screening assessment of quartz and cristobalite, Environment Canada and Health Canada [16] concluded that the "vast majority of the positive genotoxicity assay results can be explained by the generation of reactive oxygen species, as demonstrated experimentally, where ROS scavenging prevents the genotoxicity." Along with epidemiological and animal data on carcinogenicity and inflammatory responses they used a threshold approach to reach a limit of 25 μg/m^3 for inhalation exposure to crystallina silica equivalent with the Canada Labour Code with an Occupational Exposure Limit of 25 μg/m^3.

The purpose of the current paper is to review the evidence that has been published since 2011 on the three modes of action [2, 6] and to consider whether this requires modification of the current approach for risk assessment. Comments on silica nanoparticles are only included where they have relevance/meaning for the evaluation of RCS induced genotoxicity mechanisms.

Methods

The terms used for the initial search of different databases, including PubMed, Toxline, CCRIS, NTP and ECHA, included the following:

- Quartz or crystalline silica + genotoxicity;
- Quartz or crystalline silica + mutation;
- Quartz or crystalline silica + chromosome;
- Quartz or crystalline silica + micronucleus;
- Quartz or crystalline silica + DNA repair;
- Quartz or crystalline silica + comet.

In addition, searches were performed on the same combination of these terms but also include inflammation, surface, toxicity and fibrosis to retrieve papers that indirectly discussed genotoxicity of RCS. The latter search strings produced a much larger number of hits consistent with our previous review [6]. For example, the number of hits in PubMed for fibrosis or toxicity or inflammation was 413, whereas the same search terms previously retrieved 376 references [6]. Table 1 shows the results of the searches on PubMed, Toxline and CCRIS, both unsorted (all results) and sorted (excluding what was non-relevant). We also searched NTP and ECHA (general search window), but these databases do not take Boolean search terms. Only one file was detected in the ECHA database, but no registration dossier was identified.

Table 1 The number of references retrieved from different databases for the search between 2011 and 2017 using specific combinations of search items relating to genotoxicity

Search item/Database Quartz or crystalline silica +	PubMed	ToxLine	CCRIS	Total
genotoxicity	18	2	0	20
mutation	32	58	0	90
chromosome	11	13	0	24
Micronucleus	10	1	1	12
DNA repair	2	8	0	10
Comet	12	0	0	12
Total (after exclusion of double hits)	**59**	**81**	**1**	**141**
Inflammation OR fibrosis OR toxicity	413	220	0	633
Surface	2929	392	0	3321

The search strings identified 141 papers published since 2011 (see Table 1). These were then filtered depending on whether the abstract contained any genotoxicity data from established hazard identification assays or mechanistic studies that could help explain the biological processes occurring after exposure to CS. Study quality (i.e. Klimisch score) was not considered relevant as the majority of studies were not performed according to GLP or regulatory guidance (for appropriate study types) but did contain potentially useful data for building a weight of evidence. In many papers CS has been used as a positive control in evaluation of the (geno) toxicity of other particles. These papers were considered relevant, and included in the review, but it is questionable whether the results of a study not specifically directed to the investigation of the substance should be considered with the same level of weight.

Of the papers selected for detailed review, 7 dealt with in vitro genotoxicity, 5 papers contained data on in vivo genotoxicity outcomes (one paper contained both in vitro and in vivo genotoxicity data). Five papers were classified as containing biologically relevant data, which would aid interpretation of the genotoxicity data, thus, of the 141 papers identified by the searches, 17 new publications were considered relevant and the review of the genotoxicity of RCS that follows was based on these.

In vitro genotoxicity

A large portion of the in vitro studies only used RCS (mostly DQ12) as a reference material in their efforts to screen the genotoxicity of other particles. Nevertheless, these were included in the overview, but need to be considered with great care in the final evaluation. An overview of all in vitro studies is shown in Table 2, and a detailed presentation is given in the text below.

Downs et al. [17] studied the induction of MN in vitro and in vivo by amorphous silica and gold nanoparticles, andDQ12 quartz was included as a reference control in both arms of the study. DQ12 was milled to reduce the average size to 410 nm (size range from 100 to 800 nm). Whole human donor blood was cultured in RPMI-1640 medium containing foetal bovine serum (FBS) and antibiotics, and the lymphocytes were stimulated to divide by addition of phytohaemagglutinin. After 44–48 h cells were centrifuged, re-suspended in fresh medium, and treated with a butanol suspension of DQ12 quartz at 4 different concentrations (32, 100, 320 and1000 μg/mL). Since cytochalasin B can interfere with the cellular uptake of nanoparticles, 2 treatment regimens were followed. For the first set of duplicate cultures cytochalasin B was added 4 h after the start of treatment, which then continued for a further 20 h. In the second set of cultures cytochalasin B was present for the full 24 h of DQ12 treatment. Cytotoxicity was determined using the cytokinesis block proliferation index (CBPI), and 1000 binucleate cells per culture (2000 per concentration) were scored for MN. Except for the lack of treatment in the presence of metabolic activation this design complies with OECD Test Guideline 487. Negative control MN frequencies were normal and were significantly increased by treatment with the positive control chemicals, mitomycin C and vinblastine. Following both treatment regimens, MN frequencies in DQ12 quartz-treated cultures were similar to those in vehicle controls and not significantly different. Interestingly, amorphous nanoparticles (15 and 55 nm) also did not induce MN at concentrations up to 1000 μg/mL.

Zhang et al. [18] compared the effects of native and active bentonite particles (containing 6.8 and 6.5% quartz respectively) as well as DQ12 quartz on induction of comets and MN in a cytochalasin B-blocked human B cell line (HM2.CIR). Active bentonite was obtained by treating native bentonite with H_2SO_4 (10–15%) causing a large specific surface area. Cells were exposed to the two samples of bentonite particles (BP) at concentrations ranging from 30 to 240 μg/mL for 3 different time periods, 24, 48 and 72 h. Concentrations were chosen based on absence of toxicity (trypan blue exclusion) from a separate experiment, but there were no concurrent toxicity measurements in the assays themselves and no indication of toxicity levels at tested concentrations. Additionally, 100 μL of supernatant from a formulation of 240 μg/mL was tested to assess genotoxicity of the water-soluble fraction and sampled at all 3 time points. For the MN test the frequencies of mononucleate, binucleate and multinucleate cells were not recorded, and so toxicity based on cell proliferation (e.g. CBPI) could not be established. MN in a total of 1000 binucleate cells per sample were scored, and whilst all slides were scored by the same individual it is unclear whether slides were coded to avoid bias. Treatment of cells with DQ12 quartz only, showed significant induction of both MN and %tail moment at high concentrations (240 μg/mL) and/or longer incubation periods (i.e. 72 h). In addition, the values for DQ12 MN frequencies were lower as compared to an equivalent particle mass of bentonite. MN frequencies at the highest concentration (240 μg/mL) after 72 h exposure were 6.00% MN for quartz and 8.25% MN for active bentonite compared to 1.67% in concurrent controls. Leaching of soluble components was indirectly excluded as a cause for bentonite genotoxicity. A possible explanation is that the difference in MN response is caused by a higher surface area in the BP samples or presence of small amounts of redox metals. However, no experiments were performed to investigate this option.

Guidi et al. [19] examined the genotoxicity of crystalline quartz (pure quartz flour obtained by grinding a very pure Madagascan crystal form in a ball mill), and vitreous (amorphous) silica generated by milling/grinding a very pure silica glass (Suprasil for optical applications), in an alveolar epithelial cell line (A549), and in a mouse macrophage cell line (RAW264.7). The comet assay and MN were used to estimate genotoxic potential, and trypan blue dye exclusion was used as a measure of toxicity at the start and end of treatments. Cultures were treated for 4 and 24 h with 5 different concentrations (plus appropriate controls) of quartz or vitreous silica (VS) ranging between 5 and 80 μg/cm^2. In epithelial A549 cells both quartz and vitreous silica treatment showed little toxicity after 4 and 24-h exposure, with the highest concentration (80 μg/cm^2). RAW264.7 cells were, however, more sensitive to toxicity induced by quartz, with negligible toxicity induced at the 4-h time point but a dose-related decrease in viability observed following 24 h treatment. The comet data showed small but statistically significant increases in % tail DNA in RAW264.7 cultures treated with quartz at all doses, a dose response relationship was not observed. All other combinations of cells and treatments did not increase the % tail DNA above concurrent controls. Quartz also induced reductions in proliferation of both RAW264.7 and A549 cells. On the other hand, VS induced an increase in proliferation in RAW264.7 cells. No increases in MN frequency by quartz or VS were noted inA549 or RAW264.7 cells. The different cellular responses were not explained by the ability to internalise particles since uptake was claimed to occur to the same degree in both cell types. Therefore, the different effect in A549 cells is

Table 2 Overview of in vitro genotoxicity outcomes obtained with crystalline silica of respirable size in in vitro studies

Sample characteristics	Test system	Outcomes	Reference
DQ12 quartz milled to 410 nm average diameter (100–800 nm). Used as positive control	Micronuclei (MN) in human PBL pooled from 2 donors (similar to OECD test guideline 487) after 24 h incubation in the absence of metabolic activation. Dose-response study.	No increase in MN in the concentration range testing at 32, 100, 320 and 1000 μg/ml. Particle number at lowest concentration was 5.32×10^9	[17]
DQ12 quartz as positive control in evaluation bentonite genotoxicity. GSD: 2.0 μm, surface area: 5.7 m^2/g Bentonite particles (BP; 6.8 and 6.5% CS). GSD 2.7 and 2.5 μm. Surface area: 60 and 108 m^2/g	COMET and MN in Human B cell line (HM2.CIR), at concentrations 30–240 μg/ml COMET and MN in Human B cell line (HM2.CIR), at concentrations 30, 60, 180, 240 μg/ml	Slightly NS elevation of MN and COMET in cell line, after 24 h exposure to highest concentration (240 μg/ml). At 72 h of exposure all values are increased. Dose-dependent increase in MN and COMET above concentrations of 60 and 120 μg/ml, respectively; but only at 24 h. At 48 and 72 h all BP samples show increased MN and COMET. Bentonite particles show a stronger effect than DQ12 quartz.	[18]
Pure milled quartz from mineral source (respirable, surface area 4. 2 m^2/g) and vitreous silica (respirable, 5.0 m^2/g). Size range determined with SEM between 0.5 and 5 μm	Macrophage cell line (RAW 264.7) and epithelial cell line (A549) were incubated 4 or 24 h. Concentrations 5–80 μg/cm^2. MN frequency and % tail DNA (comet) were assessed	Only quartz and not vitreous silica caused changes in % tail DNA, but exclusively in RAW cell line and not in A549 cells. The effect was visible both at 4 and 24 h. Particle uptake was assessed and noted to be similar in both cell types, although quantitative data are lacking	[19]
DQ12 (3 μm) as reference particles for fibre study to elucidate effect of mineral composition Quenching all particles with aluminium lactate	Primary rat alveolar macrophages, 2 h incubation with 200 μg/cm^2 Primary rat alveolar macrophages, 2 h incubation with 200 μg/cm^2	Tail intensity in comet assay was induced 20-fold over con trol in the presence of significant cytotoxicity induced by DQ12 Particle toxicity and tail moment induction was reduced to control levels by pre-incubation with aluminium lactate (100 uM)	[20] [20]
DQ12 quartz as positive control in study aiming to investigate metal nanoparticles.	ToxTracker reporter assay in mouse embryonic stem (mES) cells. GFP induction and cell viability were determined with flow cytometry. mES cells were exposed to quartz particles (6.25, 25, 50 and 100 μg/mL) for 24 h	DNA damage reporter (*Bscl2*) and the general stress reporter (*Btg2*) genes were not induced by treatment with any concentration of quartz. Only the anti-oxidant reporter gene was induced in a concentration dependent way. No genotoxicity was observed in mES cells using the comet assay.	[21]
Ground Min-U-Sil (CS) with mean size of 3.7 um and purity of 99.5% CS. Aged versus freshly ground CS	Human bronchial epithelial cells (BEAS-IIB) and lung cancer cells with altered (H460) or deficient (H1299) p53 expression	Freshly fractured or aged silica produced divergent cellular responses in certain downstream cellular events, including ROS production, apoptosis, cell cycle and chromosomal changes, and gene expression. Exposure to freshly fractured silica also resulted in a rise in aneuploidy in cancer cells with a significantly greater increase in p53-deficient cells	[22]
Quartz Q1 with mean size (D_{50}) of 12.1 μm. 0.89 m^2/gram and DQ12 (D_{50}, 3 μm)) with or without different organosilane coatings (PTMO, SIVO 160) and Al-lactate as control inhibitor	Primary rat alveolar macrophages, $1.5–2 \times 10^5$ cells per well, 2 h incubation with 75 μg/cm^2	Both Q1 and DQ12 caused significant DNA damage in comet assay associated to cytotoxicity (LDH leakage). Both toxicity and DNA damage were blocked by pre-treatment of DQ12 with Al-lactate or organosilane compounds. Surface binding was found to be effective up to 168 h after treatment in artificial lysosomal fluid (pH 4.5).	[20]

suggested to be due to elevated antioxidant capacity or DNA repair efficiency [7] in A549 cells.

Ziemann et al. [20] investigated genotoxic effects from fibrous samples of alkaline earth silicate (AES) wools commonly used in furnace linings that under extreme heat generate cristobalite (a form of crystalline silica). DQ12 quartz and aluminium oxide were included as positive and negative particulate controls respectively. The tests were performed in primary rat alveolar macrophages, using a short treatment time of 2 h. The alkaline comet assay was used to evaluate genotoxic potential of all materials at a single concentration (200 μg/cm^2). The comet assay was performed with and without several modifications, including modification with human 8-oxoguanine DNA glycosylase (hOGG1, which enhances breaks due to7,8-dihydro-8-oxoguanine, 8-oxoG) and aluminium lactate (AL; a purported "quencher" of biological effects from crystalline silica). DQ12 quartz induced a 20-fold increase in tail intensity over Al_2O_3 particle controls. Pre-treatment of quartz samples with AL completely inhibited the DNA-damaging potential of DQ12 as observed in the comet assay. The tail intensity of DQ12-treated cells was explained by the induction of oxidative damage by DQ12.

Karlsson et al. [21] used Toxtracker, a reporter based assay performed in mouse embryonic stem cells, using DQ12 as a reference particle in studying the effects of metal nanoparticles on the system. The reporter genes used were *Bscl2* (DNA damage via ATR pathway), *Srxn1* (*Nrf2* antioxidant response pathway for ROS) and *Btg2* (general stress via P53 pathway). Cells were treated with quartz particles for 24 h at concentrations of 6.2, 25, 50 and 100 μg/mL. Cell survival (reduction in cell number) was not affected at any of the tested concentrations. Data from the reporter assay showed that the DNA damage reporter (*Bscl2*) and the general stress reporter (*Btg2*) genes were not induced by treatment with any concentration of quartz. Only the antioxidant response (*Srxn1*) was induced in a concentration-dependent manner up to a maximum of threefold (relative to solvent controls) at the highest tested concentration of DQ12 (100 μg/mL). The advantage of this reporter based assay is the separation of genotoxic pathway responses from the antioxidant response indicative of elevated ROS. In vitro tests such as the micronucleus assay are often conducted in culture medium with low levels of ROS scavengers or antioxidants; as such they will result in positive responses due to ROS that do not occur in vivo due, in part to a far higher level of antioxidants. It is therefore useful to understand the contribution ROS makes to the in vitro response. In these mouse embryonic stem cells there appears to be no induction of DNA damage as measured by ATR pathway. Of course, it is possible that there may have been induction of gene expression at higher concentrations. On the other hand, the elevated ROS response indicates that treatments did produce effects, and reinforces the ROS-related effects seen from other studies.

Gwinn et al. [22] compared various molecular alterations induced by freshly fractured and aged CS (Min--U-Sil) in human immortalized/transformed bronchial epithelial cells (BEAS-IIB) and lung cancer cells with altered (H460) or deficient (H1299) p53 expression. This was of interest because there is strong evidence that fracturing silica results in the generation of increased levels of ROS on the cleavage planes, which can react with water to generate •OH radicals, and exposure to fractured silica produces enhanced lung injury and disease in exposed workers. As well as the molecular alterations, chromosomal aberrations were examined in cells that had been exposed to sieved fractured or aged silica at 500 μg/mL for 6 or 24 h. It appears that only a single experiment was performed, and only 50 cells per treatment were scored for aberrations. Significant increases in the percentage of cells with aberrations were seen at both 6 and 24 h in the H460 and H1299 cells including appearance of dicentric chromosomes. However, these cell lines do not have normal p53 function, although apoptosis was induced in these cells. By contrast, in the BEAS-IIB cells, which have normal p53 function, small increases in the percentage of aberrant cells were not significant. It should however be noted that with such small numbers of cells scored, these results are of questionable biological relevance. Aneuploidy, as measured by flow cytometry, was also induced in the H460 and H1299 cells exposed to both freshly fractured and aged silica, but was not induced in the BEAS-IIB cells. From these data it seems that normal healthy cells with functional p53 are not sensitive to ROS-induced structural or numerical chromosome damage.

Ziemann et al. [23] studied the cytotoxic and genotoxic effects of DQ12 quartz and new pure quartz (Q1) particles from the ceramic industry in primary rat alveolar macrophages. In the study they used several commercially available organosilane coatings to block the highly reactive silanol groups at the quartz surface. Both quartzes were coated with different amounts of hydrophobic DynasylanR PTMO (propyltrimethoxysilane) and hydrophilic DynasylanR SIVO 160 (oligomeric, amino-modified siloxane). Primary alveolar macrophages isolated from female Wistar rats by bronchoalveolar lavage were pre-cultured for 24 h, and then treated for 4 h in the dark. At the end of treatment, samples of culture supernatant were taken for measurement of LDH release (measure of cytotoxicity). For the alkaline comet assay, cells were placed on ice for 10 min to allow detachment from the culture vessel surface without using trypsin, which can cause membrane damage, these detached cells were analysed for DNA strand breaks. Both the test quartz (Q1) and DQ12 caused significant cytotoxicity and DNA damage at the test concentration of 77 μg/cm^2. Both PTMO and SIVO 160 inhibited quartz-induced LDH release in a concentration dependent manner. Both PTMO and SIVO 160 clearly reduced the tail intensity of comets induced by Q1 and by DQ12, and thus reduced DNA damage. These data suggest that reduction in surface reactivity via organosilanes leads to a reduction in DNA damage. However, the chosen target cells are not relevant for fixing DNA damage into mutations (see below), and genotoxicity was not evaluated in the in vivo model reported in this paper which only investigated the effects of CS on lung organ weights and biochemical analysis of BAL fluid from treated male Wistar rats after 3 months intratracheal instillation with Quartz.

Interestingly most studies described above have used classical tests to measure DNA/chromosome damage (comet, MN) in primary or cultured macrophages. These cells play a role in the MoA to produce ROS and growth factors to create an environment for increased DNA damage, proliferation and fixation of damage. However, macrophages are not considered relevant as surrogate target cells to evaluate genotoxic damage to the lung [6]. In addition, MN and comet results do not correlate with particle induced carcinogenicity as demonstrated by Darne et al. [24]. They studied MN and comet induction in Syrian hamster embryo (SHE) cells, and in Chinese hamster lung (V79) cells, to evaluate the genotoxicity of quartz (Min-U-Sil, fully crystallised), commercial cristobalite (Chd, partly crystallised) and chrysotile (asbestos) as known carcinogens, and diatomaceous earth (DE, 100% amorphous) as control. The key data are summarised in Table 3. Reduction in cell number was used to estimate toxicity from both SHE and V79 cultures, and all silica species tested showed statistically significant reduction in cell numbers, with several materials inducing 50% toxicity and above in SHE cells at the highest tested concentration (amorphous, partly crystallized silica, and quartz induced 40–50% toxicity). However, in V79 cells, only amorphous silica induced more than 50% toxicity, whereas quartz and partly crystallised silica induced 35 and 25% toxicity respectively. Chrysotile was highly toxic to both cell types. The cell transformation data showed that amorphous silica (DE) did not induce morphological transformation (except for 3 colonies in one experiment at 15.24 μg/cm^2), while a concentration-dependent increase in transformation frequency was induced by the two other silica samples. It should be noted that Min-U-Sil did not induce any cytotoxicity at concentrations up to 50 μg/cm^2 but did induce morphological transformation in a dose-dependent manner. The partially crystalline commercial cristobalite was slightly cytotoxic and also induced transformation in a dose-dependent manner. Whereas cell transformation correlated well with carcinogenic hazard of the above materials, only the highest concentration of chrysotile showed a statistically significant increase in MN frequency in SHE cells (24 h). In V79 cells, statistically significant increases in MN frequency were caused by amorphous silica (therefore a "false positive" compared to cell transformation) and chrysotile. The comet assay (both at 3 and 24-h exposures) showed no statistically significant increases in % tail DNA except for the highest concentration of chrysotile in SHE cells treated for 24 h without FPG. Interestingly, trypan blue exclusion at both time points showed cellular toxicity of 80% and above in all treatments.

In vivo genotoxicity (animal, human)

An overview of the papers included in this section is given in Table 4, including both animal and human data. As stated before in section A, Downs et al. [17] compared the induction of comets and MN in rats by amorphous silica and gold nanoparticles, and milled DQ12 quartz was used as a control for both parts of the study *(in vitro, in vivo)*. Adult male Wistar rats were dosed intravenously with a suspension of quartz particles (400 nm, 100 mg/kg, 2×10^{11} particles, 3.12 10^9 μm^2) on 3 occasions, 48, 24 and 4 h before sacrifice. The dose of quartz (100 mg/kg) was the maximum tolerated dose (MTD), determined in a preliminary study. At termination, blood was removed from the abdominal *vena cava* for both MN and comet analysis. Whole body perfusion was performed on the animals, and the livers and lungs were separately perfused before standard processing for the alkaline comet assay [25, 26]. Comets (% tail DNA) were measured using an image analysis system from 150 nuclei for blood, liver and lung. For the MN assay in blood, fixed reticulocytes (RETs) were analysed using the Litron Microflow method [27, 28]. Cytotoxicity was determined from the percentage of RETs and the percentage of MN-RETs was determined in at least 10,000 RETs. For the comet assay, small (1.5–1.7-fold) increases in % tail DNA were seen in lungs, liver and blood of animals treated with DQ12 quartz, but none of these were statistically significant. No increases in the frequencies of MN-RETs were seen in quartz-treated animals. The weak genotoxic effects were only seen at the maximum tolerated dose in quartz-treated rats, and were accompanied by effects typically seen following inhalation of RCS such as neutrophilic infiltration, the occurrence of apoptotic cells, an increase in mitotic figures, and the induction of the inflammatory markers (TNF-αand IL-6) in plasma. Therefore, the authors concluded that the particle-induced tissue damage was probably mediated by an inflammatory

Table 3 Morphological transformation versus outcome in genotoxicity assays in Syrian hamster Embryo (SHE) cells treated with different forms of amorphous and crystalline silica

Test material	Dose (μg/cm²)	MN[1] (% of cells) 24 h	Comet[1] (% tail) + FPG, 24 h	Morphological transformation frequency (%)
Control	0	2.3 ± 0.5	13.0 ± 1.0	0.01
Diatomaceous earth (DE) (GSD: 1.35 μm)	3.81			0.02
	7.62			0.02
	11.4		11.0 ± 1.2	
	13.6	2.1 ± 0.8		
	15.24			0.11*
	22.8		18.0 ± 2.0	
	27.2	2.0 ± 0.6		
	30.48			0
	45.7		21.0 ± 2.5 *	
	54.4	1.8 ± 0.6		
Heated DE (see above), containing 47% Cristobalite (GSD: 4.85 μm)	3.81			0.16*
	7.62			0.19*
	11.4		6.5 ± 1.5	
	13.6	3.0 ± 1.0		
	15.24			0.23*
	22.75	2.0 ± 0.6	9.0 ± 1.0	
	30.48			0.4*
	45.7		10.0 ± 4.5	
	54.4	1.8 ± 0.3		
Quartz Min-U-Sil 5 (GSD: 1.33 μm)	3.81			0.24*
	7.62			0.17*
	11.4		9.8 ± 1.2	
	13.6	2.2 ± 1.3		
	15.24			0.71*
	22.8		11.0 ± 2.7	
	27.75	2.2 ± 1.3		
	30.48			0.77*
	45.7		8.0 ± 1.0	
	54.4	1.5 ± 0.3		

[1]Data were estimated from graphical representations in Darne et al [24] (Figures. two A (MN) and Figures. three B (Comet), reproduced with permission). *GSD* Geometric mean diameter
* = statistically significant ($p < 0.05$) compared to control

response. However, the route of administration primarily served to match the purpose of the study, i.e. to study effects of nanoparticles after intravenous administration and therefore the data from this study is not considered appropriate for risk assessment purposes.

Rittinghausen et al. [29] used immunohistochemical methods to quantify various DNA damage markers, including 8-hydroxyguanosine (8-OH-dG) and 8-oxoguanine DNA glycosylase (OGG1), in the lungs of DQ12 exposed rats (intratracheal instillation once per month for 3 months to DQ12 quartz). The dose used induced nominal particle overload and persistent inflammation in the lungs. Nuclei containing 8-OH-dG and cytoplasmic areas containing OGG1 increased > 2-fold in the lungs of DQ12-treated rats. Levels of OGG1 in nuclei increased to a smaller but nonetheless significant amount. Such increases are indicative of oxidative damage to DNA. However, inflammation scores increased by > 6-fold. The levels of 8-OH-dG correlated significantly with the histopathologic inflammation scores,

Table 4 Overview of genotoxicity outcomes obtained with crystalline silica of respirable size in animal or human studies

Sample characteristics	Test system	Outcomes	reference
DQ12 (410 nm) milled to reach this small size	Intravenous injection (tail vein), at a dose of 100 mg/kg to rats as reference to compare to nanosize silicas and gold nanoparticles. Acute effects up to 48 h.	MN and comets were measured in lung, liver and blood after 4 h, 24 h and 48 h. All effects seen were consistent with a secondary genotoxic mechanism: - No increased MN in circulating blood reticulocytes - No increased comets in blood cells - Increased plasma TNF-alpha - Increased apoptosis and liver inflammation after DQ12	[17]
Quartz Q1 with mean size (D_{50}) of 12.1 µm. 0.89 m^2/gram and DQ12 (D_{50}, 3 µm)) with or without different organosilane coatings (PTMO, SIVO 160) and aluminium lactate as control inhibitor	90-day rat study. Particles (total dose 1 mg/animal), administered by intratracheal instillation of two 0.5 mg aliquots in 0.3 ml of PBS on consecutive days. Lavage and histology on day 28 and day 90.	Q1 and DQ12 both induced a persistent inflammatory response at 28 and 90 days. Both toxicity and inflammatory response were reduced to control levels by organosilane coatings of Q1. In vivo genotoxicty responses were not included in this paper.	[23]
DQ12 (respirable), 6 mg total cumulative dose	Instillation (intratracheal) with 3 × 2 mg each month	Poly (ADP-ribose), 8-OH-dG and OGGG 1 induction were assessed in lung tissue using immunohistochemistry (IHC). A good correlation was found between all genotoxicity markers and histopathological inflammation	[29]
DQ12, single dose of 100 mg/kg)	C57BL/6 wild-type (WT) and $p47^{phox-/-}$ mice; DQ12 administered by pharyngeal aspiration	In vivo oxidative DNA damage in lung tissue was not affected by quartz exposure and did not differ between p47phox− /− and WT mice. Neutrophils from the bone marrow of DQ12-treated WT mice, but not from $p47^{phox-/-}$ mice, caused increased oxidative DNA damage when co-cultured with A549 epithelial cells.	[31]
Occupational exposure to respirable silica (< 70% RCS)	Male workers ($n = 50$) exposed to FCS dust in grinding, milling, bagging and sandblasting. Life time exposure by inhalation. Control group ($n = 29$) were office workers.	Both target cells (nasal epithelial cells, NEC) and non-target cells (PBL) were isolated and tested for percentage of MN. Increased MN were found in NEC (3-fold) and PBL (2-fold) of workers versus controls. A multiple regression analysis showed significant contribution of age, smoking and number of years exposure, particularly in workers' target NEC but also in surrogate cells (PBL)	[32]

and the frequencies of OGG1-positive nuclei correlated, but not significantly, with the inflammation scores. As discussed earlier, oxidative damage and other genotoxic effects may well be driven by such inflammatory responses. However, oxidative stress can occur through direct generation of ROS as discussed earlier. Due to the severe particle overload in the lung in this study, secondary mechanisms, that may overwhelm and confuse potentially existing primary genotoxic events, prevented a clear distinction between the different primary and secondary genotoxic mechanisms in terms of the oxidative damage found in the rat lungs. It is interesting, however, that Møller et al. [30], in a review of the literature describing oxidative damage in animals exposed to particles, critically assessed the different ways in which oxidative damage to DNA could be measured as a marker of particle-induced genotoxicity in animal tissues. They considered assays of 8-oxo-7,8-dihydroguanine by antibodies (i.e. immunohistochemical methods), and/or unrealistically high background levels of 8-oxo-7,8-dihydroguanine, as non-optimal since these studies suggested experimental problems due to spurious oxidation of DNA. Such studies reported more induction of DNA damage after exposure to particles than did the publications based on more optimal methods such as the detection of FPG-sensitive sites, or where the number of oxidised guanine nucleobase lesions in control animals were below 10 lesions/10^6 dG. Møller et al. [30] also carefully considered the routes of administration used, stating that studies using intra-tracheal instillation of particles into the airways of animals is a non-physiological procedure. Thus, the data of Rittinghausen et al. [29] would likely be considered non-optimal by Møller et al. [30]

Van Berlo et al. [31] investigated the contribution of phagocyte-derived ROS to inflammation, oxidative stress, and DNA damage responses 24 h after pharyngeal aspiration of DQ12 quartz (100 mg/kg) in the lungs of C57BL/6 wild-type and $p47^{phox-/-}$mice, a mouse model featuring impaired phagocyte ROS generation due to knockout of the $p47^{phox}$ NOX2 enzyme complex. Bone marrow-derived neutrophils were used for parallel in vitro investigations in co-culture with A549 human alveolar epithelial cells. DQ12 quartz induced a marked neutrophil influx in both wild-type and $p47^{phox-/-}$mouse lungs. Significant increases in mRNA expression of the oxidative stress markers haemoxygenase-1 (HO-1) and γ-glutamylcysteine synthetase (γ –GCS) were observed only in quartz-treated wild-type animals. However, oxidative DNA damage, as measured by the FPG-modified comet assay, in lung tissue was not affected byDQ12 quartz exposure and did not differ between $p47^{phox-/-}$ and wild type mice. Differences in mRNA expression of the DNA repair genes OGG1, APE-1, DNA Polβ, and XRCC1 were also absent.DQ12 quartz treatment of co-cultures containing wild-type neutrophils, but not $p47^{phox-/-}$ neutrophils, caused increased oxidative DNA damage in A549 epithelial cells. The authors concluded that neutrophil-derived ROS significantly contribute to pulmonary oxidative stress responses after acute DQ12 quartz exposure, but their role in induction of oxidative DNA damage could be shown only in vitro.

It is important to note that the ATR pathway examined by Karlsson et al. [21] detects single strand breaks is relevant for RCS because these lesions can be indirectly induced by ROS, but other pathways such as XRCC1 (BER) as investigated here [29'are probably not.

Human data

One new paper described genotoxicity in humans exposed to RCS. Demircigil et al. [32] investigated the frequencies of MN in target nasal epithelial cells (NEC) and peripheral blood lymphocytes (PBL; effectively a surrogate tissue) of glass industry workers, sandblasters and stone grinders from 4 locations in Turkey. A total of 50 exposed males were selected, working mainly in grinding, mixing and bagging tasks. Mineralogical and elemental analysis indicated that the workers were exposed to dusts containing 70–100% CS. A control group of 29 males who were not exposed to the dusts were matched for age and smoking status. PBL were cultured using standard methods for 72 h, with cytochalasin B present for the final 28 h. NEC were obtained by scraping the inner nasal turbinate with a cytological brush, smearing the cells on to wet slides and allowing them to dry. Cells were fixed, stained with Feulgen and counterstained with Fast Green. For each individual 3000 nasal epithelial cells were scored for presence of MN.

The MN frequencies (from 1000 binucleate cells/individual) in the control peripheral blood samples (5.59 ± 2.86 MN/1000 binucleate cells) were in the normal range for young men in their thirties [33] According to Knasmueller et al. [34]. The control MN frequencies in nasal epithelial cells (from 3000 cells/individual) reported by Demircigil et al. [32] (2.84 ± 1.61 per 1000 cells) were the highest seen across 16 different published studies in this cell type. The lowest published control frequency was 0.14 MN/1000 cells. However, even considering the high background levels, MN frequencies in nasal epithelial cells were approximately 3-fold higher in workers than in controls, and the difference was statistically significant ($p < 0.001$). Moreover, a multiple linear regression (MLR) analysis of MN in NEC showed that the years of exposure was a highly significant descriptor ($P < 0.001$; B = 5.47) on top of smoking ($P = 0.002$) and age ($P = 0.006$). This clearly indicates a dose-response relationship suggesting direct genotoxicity; however such effects could be mediated by the high number of neutrophils (> 70%) present in nasal lining fluid.

In the peripheral blood lymphocytes, 2-fold increases in MN frequencies were found in workers compared to controls. Given that Fenech and Bonassi [33] report control MN frequencies in healthy young males up to 12/1000 binucleate cells, the levels seen in CS workers (also around 12/1000) may not be outside the normal range. A sophisticated MLR analysis of MN frequency on individuals versus years of exposure, age and smoking showed age and number of exposure years as significant descriptors (both $P < 0.005$), whereas smoking was of borderline ($P = 0.087$) significance.

If the increased MN frequencies in peripheral blood lymphocytes do represent a genotoxic effect, it could not be due to direct genotoxicity since RCS particles would not conceivably enter the blood or blood lymphocytes. Demircigil et al. [32] hypothesize that the MN could be caused by indirect or secondary effects such as reactive oxygen species or pulmonary inflammation as discussed earlier by Borm et al. [6]. An argument to support this mode of action is that levels of MN correlated well between PBL and NEC in the group of workers ($n = 50$).

Other mode of action data

Fazzi et al. [35] investigated the different processes by which ROS are induced following phagocytosis of CS (α-quartz; average size 1.7 μm), by macrophages. Human monocytes, isolated from peripheral blood of normal human subjects, were differentiated into primary human macrophages. These, together with mouse bone marrow macrophages (from C57BL/6 J, BALB/c, and $p47^{phox-/-}$ mice), and the macrophage cell lines RAW 264.7 and IC21, were used to study the contributions of NADPH oxidase (Phox) and mitochondrial ROS (mtROS) to CS-induced lung injury. 1×10^5 macrophages were seeded into 96 well plates 24 h prior to exposure. Treatment was by media replacement with 20 μg/cm^2 silica particles suspended in PBS for periods up to 6 h.

CS induces a rapid and sustained production of superoxide anion by RAW 264.7 (derived from BALB/c mice) macrophages, but the response is greater in IC21 macrophages (derived from C57BL/6 J mice). Consistent with this, in response to CS, $p47^{phox}$ protein expression was decreased in IC21, but not in RAW 264.7 macrophages, even though baseline levels of Phox proteins were similar in the 2 cell lines. This reduced $p47^{phox}$ expression in IC21 macrophages was linked to enhanced generation of mtROS, cardiolipin oxidation, and accumulation of cardiolipin hydrolysis products, culminating in cell death. The effect of CS on $p47^{phox}$ protein expression in primary C57BL/6 J macrophages was similar to that seen in the IC21 macrophages, exhibiting a significantly decreased $p47^{phox}$ protein expression (2–4 h). In contrast, no decrease in $p47^{phox}$ protein expression was observed in BALB/c macrophages after CS exposure. The response to CS exposure in human macrophages was similar to that seen in C57BL/6 J macrophages, although decreased $p47^{phox}$ protein expression was observed at later (4–8 h) times. The authors demonstrated that decreased $p47^{phox}$expression was associated with increased mtROS (mitochondrial superoxide anion) production. This was also demonstrated in vivo in $p47^{phox-/-}$ mice, which exhibit increased inflammation and fibrosis in the lung following CS exposure. CS induces interaction between TNFR1 and Phox in RAW 264.7 macrophages, and TNFR1 expression in mitochondria leads to decreased mtROS production and increased RAW264.7 macrophage survival. These results identify the TNFR1/Phox interaction as a key event in the pathogenesis of silicosis that prevents mtROS formation and reduces macrophage apoptosis. Thus, based on these data, and assuming human macrophages behave in a similar way to those in rodents, human macrophages would be expected to exhibit mtROS formation and apoptosis in response to CS exposure.

Pavan and Fubini [36] proposed an adverse outcome pathway for the induction of silicosis, autoimmune pathologies and lung cancer from inhaled CS. They noted that CS particles are cytotoxic, trigger the production of inflammatory substances, oxidants and growth factors from cells, and can damage membranes. However, when the same test was performed on a variety of silica samples the extent and even the nature of the cellular response varied. Coating of the quartz particles with aluminium, iron, and carbon sometimes led to enhanced effects, but sometimes led to reduced effects. Coating with polymers or other substances mainly led to reduced cellular responses. They discuss evidence [37] that implics the surface silanols are critical in the cellular reactivity of CS particles, and explain the above observations. Thus, they propose a pathway in which silanols available for H-bonding with external molecules lead to engulfment of coated particles by macrophages and a strong interaction of the uncoated particle with the phagolysosomal membrane leading to rupture, macrophage activation and inflammatory response. Whilst the data used in this study came from cells in vitro (fibroblasts and endothelial cells) and are therefore of questionable in vivo relevance, the data may still be useful in determining the molecular pathways initiated by CS exposure.

Several in vitro and *invivo* studies [20, 23] support this pathway since several agents known to bind to the silanol groups (aluminium lactate, organosilanes) were able to block cytotoxicity and inflammatory responses induced by DQ12 and workplace quartzes. Earlier work by Schins et al. [7], reviewed in Borm et al. [6], already showed the same for genotoxic outcomes after intratracheal administration of silicas.

Chan et al. [38] used RNA sequencing to evaluate the inflammatory and fibrotic effects of cultured A549 cells in vitro, exposed to CS up to a limit of 20% cytotoxicity. CS was 99% pure (Sigma, USA) and in the 0.5-10 μm size range. A549 cells were grown in DMEM supplemented with penicillin/streptomycin (1% solution) and 10% FBS. For cell treatments CS was suspended in DMEM with a lower level of FBS (1.25%), the original culture media was removed and replaced with DMEM containing CS. Treatment was for 0.5,2,8,16 and 24 h with a range of concentrations of CS (6.25–100 μg/cm^2). Toxicity was estimated via cell counts (cell counting kit-8, Sigma USA) and a maximum level chosen for subsequent RNA sequencing that induced 20% cytotoxicity (12.5 μg/cm^2 at 24 h exposure). For next generation sequencing (NGS), cells were treated with 12.5 μg/cm^2 for 2,8,16 and 24 h. Cultures were washed and RNA extracted using RNeasy kits (Qiagen, USA), quality was assessed using a 2100 bioanalyser (Agilent, USA). The library was prepared according to the TruSeq RNA sample prep kit (illumina, USA) and quantitated on an Agilent bioanalyser (Agilent, USA). The libraries were then amplified on the cBot system (Illumina, USA) and sequenced on the HiSeq 2000 system (TruSeq SBS KIT-HS V3, Illumina, USA). The database for annotation visualisation and integrated discovery (DAVID, LHRI, USA) was used to generate a summary of enriched annotation terms. Gene network analysis was performed using the search tool for the retrieval of interacting genes (STRING database, ELIXIR data resources).

The authors found that CS induced 22 differentially expressed genes, 2 were up-regulated and 20 downregulated in all samples. The major transcriptional pathways with differential gene expression were well-documented silicosis pathways including oxidative stress and inflammation (data not shown). This further reinforces the MoA being primarily ROS induction as seen from the Toxtracker data of [21].

Gene expression was also investigated by Vuong et al. [39], alongside proteomic analysis, in cultured A549 cells in vitro after exposure to cristobalite and quartz (Min--U-Sil 5). Particles were prepared in buffer (0.19% NaCl, 25 μg/mL Tween-80) at a concentration of 10 mg/mL and diluted in culture media (DMEM) for treatment. 70% confluent flasks of A549 cells had culture media removed and replaced with dilutions of particulates in buffer (60, 140, 200 μg/cm^2) prior to incubation for 24 h at 37 °C. At harvest, total protein and total RNA were extracted from treated and control cultures. For both silica samples, protein was analysed by 2D gel electrophoresis, identifying 49 protein spots, 30 of which had identities confirmed by MALDI-TOF analysis and 15 of these showed a dose related change in protein levels compared to untreated controls. Pathway analysis showed that all of the proteins with differential levels were associated with cell death, inflammation, homeostasis and proliferation pathways. Gene expression changes were evaluated using RT-PCR with a panel of 89 genes selected from previous literature on silica particle exposure as well as focusing on genes up and downstream of the protein pathways identified. They found 37 genes with differential expression post treatment with both particles compared to untreated controls. The majority of the genes with significant changes in expression were subsequently found to be involved with ROS, metabolism, homeostasis and inflammatory pathways (data not shown). Whilst the authors did not report any data from DNA reactivity or genotoxicity, the MoA of both cristobalite and Min-U-Sil appeared to be ROS and inflammation related, adding weight to the primary mechanism of toxicity after silica exposure being ROS related.

Pozzolini et al. [40] evaluated the role of surface radicals on cellular toxicity after exposure to unmodified quartz microcrystals (Min-U-Sil-5) and samples processed with ascorbic acid. Three different cell-lines, i.e. the mouse macrophage cell line RAW 264.7, isolated primary human dermal fibroblasts (neonatal foreskin) and an endothelial cell line (HUVEC) were exposed to modified and unmodified samples at a single, final concentration of 100 μg/mL. For cell viability assays the exposure was for 24 and 72 h at 37 °C, and viability was assessed via the MTT assay. ROS activity was measured in fibroblasts and endothelial cells, which were seeded the day prior to exposure and treated with a fluorescent dye (2,7-dichlor-dihydro-fluorescien diacetate, 10 μM) for 30 min prior to treatment with 100 μg/mL quartz (with and without ascorbic acid) which was present for 4 h before plates were read on a fluorescence plate reader (485 nm ex. 520 nm em.). Lipid peroxidation was measured using a spectrophotometric method (TBARS assay). Cells were prepared and treated as above, and exposure to both quartz samples was for 24 h at which point cells were washed, scraped off the surface of the plates and lysed. TBA solution was added in a 2:1 ratio (0.375% thiobarbituric acid, 15% trichoroacetic acid, 0.25 N HCl) for 45 min at 95 °C. After cooling 1 vol. of N-butanol was added and the organic phase read at 532 nm. At 24 and 72 h, fibroblasts showed no decrease in viability with both quartz varieties. However at 72 h there was a slight statistically significant increase in cell number in the presence of ascorbic acid modified quartz, suggesting stimulation of cell proliferation. Endothelial cells showed significant decreases in viability at 24 and 72 h in the presence of both quartz species. Macrophages did not show a reduction in viability at either time point with quartz but did show reduced cell viability from samples treated with ascorbic acid modified quartz (data not shown). Increases in measured ROS were seen after treatment of fibroblasts and endothelial cells with ascorbic acid modified quartz but not when using unmodified quartz. Fibroblasts showed a significantly higher production of ROS than endothelial cells (data not shown). Significant increases in lipid peroxidation were seen in both fibroblasts and endothelial cells treated with modified and unmodified quartz.

QPCR for a limited number of genes involved in inflammation (for endothelial cells) and anti-apoptotic and fibrotic pathways (for fibroblasts) were evaluated at 2 and 5 days post exposure. Fibroblasts showed increases in several genes with ascorbic acid modified quartz only. Endothelial cells also had upregulation in several genes however there were fewer differences between ascorbic acid modified and unmodified quartz.

The authors conclude that the intensity of cell responses is directly related to surface radicals on the quartz crystal, adding further weight to the evidence that the primary driver for toxicity in CS exposed cells is via ROS generation.

Discussion

Reviews performed by panels in national [14–16] or international context [1, 2] have concluded that inhalation exposure to RCS can lead to lung cancer in humans based on sufficient evidence of tumour induction in animals and humans. In the updated 2012 IARC review, IARC concluded that the rat lung tumour response to CS exposure was most likely a result of impairment of "alveolar-macrophage-mediated particle clearance thereby increasing persistence of silica in the lungs, which results in macrophage activation, and the sustained release of chemokines and cytokines" [2].

At the same time, and consistent with the IARC (2012) review [2], Borm et al. [6] proposed 3 possible MoA; direct, indirect and secondary genotoxicity. However at the time there was insufficient data to make a clearer prediction on the most likely mechanism. Therefore in this paper we selected and reviewed a further 17 additional sources of data on CS genotoxicity, involving 7*in vitro* studies with RCS, 5 in vivo studies, 4 mechanistic investigations and a single human exposure study. These publications contain some novel mechanistic insights further supporting the view that the genotoxic MoA is explained by secondary effects from sustained inflammation, although some interesting new data on direct cell transformation are now available that forward further discussion. Before any quantitative comparisons are made, it is worthwhile to make a qualitative observation.

From the in vitro studies reviewed in this paper (Table 2) 5 out of 7 used (DQ12) quartz as a reference or positive control, and did not always focus on the genotoxicity of CS. When used as a reference material, less specific attention is paid to the concentrations and outcomes of the study. The use of RCS for i.v. injection as a positive control in [17] probably is the best example to what can happen if compounds are copy-pasted into studies simply to be used as positive control to other i.v. relevant agents, and not regarding the mechanisms that were extensively discussed [6].

The in vitro test data with CS particles show many inconsistencies in the number and quality of positive responses. This may be due to variation in concentrations of CS. Whereas some studies have used a wide concentration range [17], others have focussed on low-toxicity ranges [18, 21]. Most studies contained enough technical details to convert test concentrations to μg/cm^2 revealing an average level of 75 μg/cm^2 with 2 μg/cm^2 as lowest [21] and 200 μg/cm^2 [20] as highest concentrations.

As noted previously [6] the lowest level at which genotoxic effects are observed in vivo is around 40 μg/cm^2. At this level most in vitro studies reviewed here showed negative outcomes, whereas only two studies [19, 23] noted DNA damage between 60 and 75 μg/cm^2, in macrophages only. A dose of 40 μg/cm^2 resulting from the inhalation of of 155 mg RCS in the rat, and can be derived from concentration multiplied by the rat alveolar surface (3880 cm^2).Although there is variation with regard to surface with rodent age, far more important is deposition of particles in specific hot-spots. Therefore, we state that this dose (155 mg) is an overestimate and it would be better to use the surface of the proximal alveolar region (PAR). Assuming that the PAR is between 300 and 600 cm^2 and all RCS is deposited in the PAR (worst case) an inhaled dose of 12–24 mg would be sufficient to reach this target concentration. The study by Darne et al. [24], reported morphological transformation in SHE cells around 5 μg/cm^2 (see also Table 3). At this dose and up to 50 μg/cm^2, MN and % DNA in the same cells were unaffected. When using this test and level as a critical endpoint, the calculated in vivo dose needed would be about 20 mg or 2–4 mg when including the PAR as a hot-spot region for deposit. This is still 10–15 times the inhaled doses (200 μg/rat) that were shown to cause persistent inflammation in sub-chronic exposure of rats to RCS [6]. For comparison the calculated concentration to initiate an inflammatory response, using the same estimates and assumptions, is between 0.3 and 0.7 μg/cm^2. The safety margin between the calculated NOEL for lung inflammation (0.3–0.7 μg/cm^2) and cell transformation (> 5 μg/cm^2) is around a factor of 10.

It is well documented that different cell types have varying susceptibility to genotoxic insult, influenced largely by age (passage number), genome stability, p53 status, rodent or human origin etc. [41–43]. The in vitro data reviewed here (Table 2) show positive effects predominantly in macrophages. Macrophages, that are a crucial mediator of the inflammatory MoA, are also considered as a target cell of direct genotoxic outcome. Although their role is crucial (confirmed by Fazzi et al. [35]), utmost care should be taken when interpreting these data regarding mutagenicity and carcinogenic hazard of RCS, since genotoxic damage in macrophages will not lead to mutations in the lung epithelium. As it happens, many of the in vitro studies show no genotoxic effects of CS at all, and in those where increases in DNA/ chromosome damage were seen, the effects were predominantly weak. Freshly fractured and aged silica induced structural chromosomal aberrations and aneuploidy in p53-defective human lung cancer cells but not in p53-efficient BEAS-IIB cells [22]. Quartz (but not amorphous silica) induced comets in mouse macrophages (RAW264.7 cells), where significant toxicity was induced, but not in A549 cells where toxicity was not induced [19], but there were no increases in MN with either cell type. Amorphous silica induced MN in V79 cells, but not in SHE cells, whereas quartz and cristobalite did not induce MN even at concentrations producing at least 40% toxicity. Amorphous silica also induced comets in V79 cells at the highest concentration tested (which induced 60% toxicity) and only after 24 h exposure [24]. Morphological transformation of SHE cells was reported by Darne et al. [24] for partially crystallised cristobalite and fully crystallised quartz (Table 3), in the latter case at cytotoxic doses, but such responses could be due to non-genotoxic effects that can be detected in the SHE cell transformation system (see Corvi et al. [44]). In this respect, the study by Darne et al. [24] is considered very important regarding the predictive value of classic genotoxicity tests (MN, comet) with regard to in vivo carcinogenicity.

Apart from cell types used, it is important to note that the combination of dispersion of particles and cell culture medium determines the number and size of particle (aggregates) to which the cells are exposed. As shown by Hadrup et al. [45] these effects were significant in genotoxicity outcomes for hydrophobic particles (carbon black, carbon nanotubes) but not for TiO_2, which we consider to be more like the quartz with regard to hydrophilic surface. On the other hand, other studies [7, 46, 47] demonstrated that the quartz surface can be shielded or modified by agents in the mineral matrix, method of isolation from the matrix (crushing, grinding) or even presence of cations in the medium such as aluminium and PVNO [7]. Therefore, any quantitative comparison between in vitro genotoxicty outcomes of RCS is limited not only by the source, but also the pre-treatment and addition of the sample to the cell culture medium. This is a major difference to the in vivo studies where only source and dose are important.

The recent in vivo data (overview in Table 4) also support an indirect MoA with regard to genotoxic effects noted in animals and humans. DQ12 induced small increases in comets in blood, livers and lungs of rats dosed intravenously at the maximum tolerable dose. Also using this unusual route of administration (at least for assessment of particle toxicity), the responses were concluded to be due to marked inflammatory responses and there was no induction of MN in blood reticulocytes [17]. DQ12 quartz induced (oxidative) lung damage in several sub-chronic and chronic studies in rats using intratracheal instillation. In all instances a persistent pulmonary inflammation was observed both by lavage and by immunohistochemistry [20, 29]. On the other hand, DQ12 did not induce oxidative damage in the lungs of wild-type and NOX2-deficient mice, even though marked neutrophil influx was observed, and increased expression of oxidative stress markers was seen in wild-type mice [31]. This is in line with earlier reports [48, 49] showing that tumour induction by particles is much less pronounced or absent in mice, hamsters, guinea pigs and rabbits. Part of this may be related to a much more pronounced anti-oxidant response in these species as noted by van Berlo et al. [31].

As discussed previously [6, 7, 46] the role of the quartz surface is demonstrated to be crucial in the response to CS. Both in vitro [7, 22, 23] and in vivo studies [23] confirmed the crucial role of the silica surface. Freshly fractured or aged silica produced divergent cellular responses in certain downstream cellular events, including ROS production, apoptosis, cell cycle and chromosomal changes, and gene expression [22]. Pavan and Fubini [36] also propose an adverse outcome pathway for quartz toxicity based on the surface as a driver for toxicity and inflammation. The primary source of the genetic damage in their model is again from persistent inflammation at the site of exposure rather than the relatively small levels of ROS generated from the quartz itself.

There are also clear differences between toxicological effects depending on the method of isolation of RCS from the mineral matrix itself. Miles et al. [45] showed that naturally occurring quartz with occluded crystal surface resulted in significantly less inflammation then crushed reference quartz (DQ12) from 28 and 90 days after intratracheal instillations in rats. This could partly explain the differences observed between published studies and highlights the importance of careful physiochemical characterisation of CS samples used in experimental studies.

Surface treatment of different quartz species with aluminum lactate or hydrophobic coatings reduced both in vitro and in vivo toxicity, in vitro genotoxicity and in vivo inflammation [23]. This confirms earlier findings by Schins et al. [7] and Scherbarth et al. [12] using similar coatings and in vitro and In vivo models. Interestingly, studies by the same group [50] also suggested a differential effect of surface on cellular uptake. Cellular uptake is important to evaluate the observed DNA damage regarding the MoA of RCS. Silica particles need to be internalised into the cell and reach the nucleus where they can either interact with DNA directly, or even interfere with the mechanics of mitotic segregation leading to chromosome breaks or chromosome loss. Whilst there is evidence of induction of DNA strand breaks and chromosome damage, particularly in vitro as seen from the various comet and MN studies, there are several reasons why these responses are likely to be due to indirect or secondary effects. Several studies in this review have specifically addressed the uptake issue and could not demonstrate uptake of RCS in the nucleus, although uptake in the cytoplasm was noted (e.g. [19]). In vivo data [29] could not demonstrate uptake of RCS in epithelial cells. It was also shown that dose-dependent oxidative DNA damage by quartz (20–100 μg/cm^2) may occur in epithelial cells without entering the nucleus of Type II cells as evidenced by transmission electron microscopy. Moreover, this damage could be blocked by mitochondrial electron transport inhibitors [51]. Many of the studies assessing the genotoxicity of mineral fibres used extended exposure times (up to 72 h) before chromosome damage was seen, and therefore it may take longer than 24 h for the cells to internalise larger particulates, depending on cell type [52]. Doak et al. [53] also discussed the effects cytochalasin B can potentially have on cellular uptake in the MN test. Most of the in vitro studies in this review included wash off of the particle treatment followed by a recovery phase in the presence of cytochalasin B. At the time of cytochalasin B addition, the cells would have sufficiently internalised CS particles. Thus, despite most MN studies not being conducted to current OECD guidelines there is adequate evidence that the test conditions would have resulted in intracellular exposures. Finally, a biomarker study in 50 workers versus 29 controls [32] supports the fact that inhalation of RCS can cause genotoxic effects both in target nasal epithelial cells, and surrogate blood lymphocyte cells. The statistical analysis of MN frequency clearly relationship to occupational exposure, age and smoking in this cohort. However, also here the increased levels are considered to be due to indirect effects such as (nasal) inflammation.

As already indicated above we consider the effects of silica nanoparticles as not relevant for the genotoxic properties of RCS. The main reason is that surface characteristics (e.g. surface area) of these NP are completely different. While amorphous silica's are mostly soluble and uptake mechanisms and intracellular transport are highly different [9] It is recommended to conduct a separate review and risk assessment of nanoparticle induced genotoxicity and to evaluate mechanisms and particle characteristics that are important in NP induced genotoxicity.

Conclusions

Overall, the data in this review confirm earlier findings that RCS can induce weak genotoxic effects in vitro, mostly in macrophages. These in vitro effects are most likely explained by intracellular ROS generation induced during particle uptake in the cell cytoplasm, which has only been observed in vitro. The in vivo studies discussed here, along with previous work, confirm that the organ damage and genotoxic effects are caused by the inflammatory status. Considering the accumulating evidence for a secondary genotoxic mode of action in vivo, and an indirect action in vitro, it is recommended to focus on international harmonisation of occupational exposure limits, accepting a safe threshold limit. For this purpose additional research should focus on the difference between rodent and human mechanisms in RCS induced ROS generation and defence. We also recommend to further explore the use of RCS surface activity as a surrogate metric to rank hazards of the multiplicity of RCS containing samples and products.

Abbreviations

8-oxodG: 8-oxo-7,8-dihydro-2′-deoxyguanosine; 8-oxoG: 7,8-dihydro-8-oxoguanine; BSA: Bovine serum albumin; CA: Chromosomal aberrations; CBPI: Cytokinesis block proliferation index; CS: Crystalline silica; CTA: Cell transformation assay; dG: Deoxyguanosine; DPBS: Dulbecco's phosphate buffered saline; FBS: Foetal bovine serum; FPG: Formamidopyridine glycosylase; i.v.: Intravenous; LDH: Lactate dehydrogenase; MI: Mitotic index; MN: Micronucleus or micronuclei; MoA: Mode of action; MTD: Maximum tolerated dose; OGG1: 8-oxoguanine DNA glycosylase; PHA: Phytohaemagglutinin; RI: Replication index; ROS: Reactive oxygen species; SCE: Sister chromatid exchange

Acknowledgements

All opinions, critical data reviews and conclusions in this review are the authors own and were not influenced, or moderated by the sponsors, EuroSil.
The authors thank Dr. Peter Jenkinson (CEHTRA) for his efforts in documentation of the retrieved references from the databases used.

Funding

The review process was supported by EuroSil (Brussels, Belgium).

Authors' contributions

PF and DK reviewed and interpreted the genetic toxicology studies as well as providing rationale for inclusion and exclusion of data for detailed review. PB provided overview of CS effects on human health, mode of action and context for risk assessments. All authors contributed to the body of the manuscript with overall discussion and interpretation drafted by PB. All authors read and approved the manuscript.

Competing interests

The authors have no competing interests although all engaged in consulting activities but none of these have a conflict of interest with the current subject. PB has published several original papers and reviews on RCS in his previous academic settings. DK and PF are experts on genotoxicity and have also published numerous articles on this matter in previous academic settings.

Author details

[1]Borm Nanoconsult Holding BV, Proost Willemstraat 1, 6231 CV Meerssen, The Netherlands. [2]FSToxconsulting Ltd., Raunds, UK. [3]Kirkland Consulting, Tadcaster, UK.

References

1. IARC. Silica, some silicates, coal dust and Para-aramid fibrils. International Agency for Research on Cancer (IARC) working group on the evaluation of carcinogenic risks to humans, Lyon, France, 15-22 October 1996. IARC Monogr Eval Carcinog Risks Hum. 1997;68:1–475.
2. IARC. Silica dust, crystalline, in the form of quartz or cristobalite. International Agency for Research on Cancer (IARC) working group on the evaluation of carcinogenic risks to humans, Lyon, France, 17-24 March, 2009. IARC Monogr Eval Carcinog Risks Hum. 2012;100C:355–405.
3. Uboldi C, Giudetti G, Broggi F, Gilliland D, Ponti J, Rossi F. Amorphous silica nanoparticles do not induce cytotoxicity, cell transformation or genotoxicity in BALB/3T3 mouse fibroblasts. Mutat Res. 2012;745:11–20.
4. Driscoll KE, Deyo LC, Carter JM, Howard BW, Hassenbein DG, Bertram TA. Effects of particle exposure and particle-elicited inflammatory cells on mutation in rat alveolar epithelial cells. Carcinogenesis. 1997 Feb;18(2):423–30.
5. Battal D, Çelik A, Güler G, Aktaş A, Yildirimcan S, Ocakoglu K, et al. SiO2 Nanoparticule-induced size-dependent genotoxicity - an in vitro study using sister chromatid exchange, micronucleus and comet assay. Drug Chem Toxicol. 2015;38:196–204.
6. Borm PJ, Tran L, Donaldson K. The carcinogenic action of crystalline silica: a review of the evidence supporting secondary inflammation-driven genotoxicity as a principal mechanism. Crit Rev Toxicol. 2011;41:756–70.
7. Schins RP, Duffin R, Höhr D, Knaapen AM, Shi T, Weishaupt C, et al. Surface modification of quartz inhibits toxicity, particle uptake, and oxidative DNA damage in human lung epithelial cells. Chem Res Toxicol. 2002;15:1166–73.
8. Hondow N, Harrington J, Brydson R, Doak SH, Singh N, Manshian B, et al. STEM mode in the SEM: a practical tool for nanotoxicology. Nanotoxicology. 2011;5:215–27.
9. Hemmerich PH, von Mikecz AH. Defining the subcellular interface of nanoparticles by live-cell imaging. PLoS One. 2014;8:4.
10. Muhle H, Kittel B, Ernst H, Mohr U, Mermelstein R. Neoplastic lung lesions in rat after chronic exposure to crystalline silica. Scand J Work Environ Health. 1995;21(Suppl 2):27–9.
11. Borm PJ, Schins RP, Albrecht C. Inhaled particles and lung cancer, part B: paradigms and risk assessment. Int J Cancer. 2004;110(1):3–14. Review
12. Scherbart AM, Langer J, Bushmelev A, van Berlo D, Haberzettl P, van Schooten FJ, et al. Contrasting macrophage activation by fine and ultrafine titanium dioxide particles is associated with different uptake mechanisms. Part Fibre Toxicol. 2011; https://doi.org/10.1186/1743-8977-8-31.
13. Castranova V, Porter D, Millecchia L, Ma JY, Hubbs AF, Teass A. Effect of inhaled crystalline silica in a rat model: time course of pulmonary reactions. Mol Cell Biochem. 2002;234-235:177–84.
14. Health Council of the Netherlands. Health Council of the Netherlands: Dutch Expert Committee on Occupational Standards (DECOS). Committee on the Evaluation of the Carcinogenicity of Chemical Substances. Quartz. Rijswijk: Health Council of the Netherlands, 1998; publication no. 1998/02WGD.
15. HSE. Respirable crystalline silica – Phase 2. Carcinogenicity. United Kingdom Health and Safety Executive. Document EH75/5. 2003.
16. Health Canada. Draft Screening Assessment for the Challenge. Quartz, Chemical Abstracts Service Registry Number 14808-60-7. Cristobalite, Chemical abstracts service registry number 14464-46-1. Environment Canada, Health Canada. 2011.
17. Downs TR, Crosby ME, Hu T, Kumar S, Sullivan A, Sarlo K, et al. Silica nanoparticles administered at the maximum tolerated dose induce genotoxic effects through an inflammatory reaction while gold nanoparticles do not. Mutat Res. 2012;745:38–50.
18. Zhang M, Li X, Lu Y, Fang X, Chen Q, Xing M, et al. Studying the genotoxic effects induced by two kinds of bentonite particles on human B lymphoblast cells in vitro. Mutat Res. 2011;720:62–6.
19. Guidi P, Nigro M, Bernardeschi M, Lucchesi P, Scarcelli V, Frenzilli G. Does the crystal habit modulate the genotoxic potential of silica particles? A cytogenetic evaluation in human and murine cell lines. Mutat Res. 2015;792:46–52.
20. Ziemann C, Harrison PT, Bellmann B, Brown RC, Zoitos BK, Class P. Lack of marked cyto- and genotoxicity of cristobalite in devitrified (heated) alkaline earth silicate wools in short-term assays with cultured primary rat alveolar macrophages. Inhal Toxicol. 2014;26:113–27.
21. Karlsson HL, Gliga AR, Calléja FM, Gonçalves CS, Wallinder IO, Vrieling H, et al. Mechanism-based genotoxicity screening of metal oxide nanoparticles using the ToxTracker panel of reporter cell lines. Part Fibre Toxicol. 2014;11:41.
22. Gwinn MR, Leonard SS, Sargent LM, Lowry DT, McKinstry K, Meighan T, et al. The role of p53 in silica-induced cellular and molecular responses associated with carcinogenesis. J Toxicol Environ Health A. 2009;72:1509–19.
23. Ziemann C, Escrig A, Bonvicini G, Ibáñez MJ, Monfort E, Salomoni A, et al. Organosilane-based coating of quartz species from the traditional ceramics industry: evidence of hazard reduction using in vitro and in vivo tests. Ann Work Expo Health. 2017;61:468–80.
24. Darne C, Coulais C, Terzetti F, Fontana C, Binet S, Gaté L, et al. In vitro comet and micronucleus assays do not predict morphological transforming effects of silica particles in Syrian hamster embryo cells. Mutat Res. 2016;796:23–33.
25. Tice RR, Agurell E, Anderson D, Burlinson B, Hartmann A, Kobayashi H, et al. Single cell gel/comet assay: guidelines for in vitro and in vivo genetic toxicology testing. Environ Mol Mutagen. 2000;35:206–21.
26. Singh NP, McCoy MT, Tice RR, Schneider EL. A simple technique for quantitation of low levels of DNA damage in individual cells. Exp Cell Res. 1988;175:184–91.
27. Dertinger SD, Bishop ME, McNamee JP, Hayashi M, Suzuki T, Asano N, et al. Flow cytometric analysis of micronuclei in peripheral blood reticulocytes. I. Intra- and interlaboratory comparison with microscopic scoring. Toxicol Sci. 2006;94:83–91.
28. Macgregor JT, Bishop ME, McNamee JP, Hayashi M, Asano N, Wakata A, et al. Flow cytometric analysis of micronuclei in peripheral blood reticulocytes. II. An efficient method of monitoring chromosomal damage in the rat. Toxicol Sci. 2006;94:92–107.
29. Rittinghausen S, Bellmann B, Creutzenberg O, Ernst H, Kolling A, Mangelsdorf I, et al. Evaluation of immunohistochemical markers to detect the genotoxic mode of action of fine and ultrafine dusts in rat lungs. Toxicology. 2013;303:177–86.
30. Møller P, Danielsen PH, Jantzen K, Roursgaard M, Loft S. Oxidatively damaged DNA in animals exposed to particles. Crit Rev Toxicol. 2013;43:96–118.
31. van Berlo D, Wessels A, Boots AW, Wilhelmi V, Scherbart AM, Gerloff K, et al. Neutrophil-derived ROS contribute to oxidative DNA damage induction by quartz particles. Free Radic Biol Med. 2010;49:1685–93.
32. Demircigil GC, Coskun E, Vidinli N, Erbay Y, Yilmaz M, Cimrin A, et al. Increased micronucleus frequencies in surrogate and target cells from workers exposed to crystalline silica-containing dust. Mutagenesis. 2010;25:163–9.
33. Fenech M, Bonassi S. The effect of age, gender, diet and lifestyle on DNA damage measured using micronucleus frequency in human peripheral blood lymphocytes. Mutagenesis. 2011;26:43–9.
34. Knasmueller S, Holland N, Wultsch G, Jandl B, Burgaz S, Misík M, et al. Use of nasal cells in micronucleus assays and other genotoxicity studies. Mutagenesis. 2011;26:231–8.
35. Fazzi F, Njah J, Di Giuseppe M, Winnica DE, Go K, Sala E, et al. TNFR1/phox interaction and TNFR1 mitochondrial translocation thwart silica-induced pulmonary fibrosis. J Immunol. 2014;192:3837–46.
36. Pavan C, Fubini B. Unveiling the variability of "quartz hazard" in light of recent toxicological findings. Chem Res Toxicol. 2017;30:469–85.
37. Turci F, Pavan C, Leinardi R, Tomatis M, Pastero L, Garry D, et al. Revisiting the paradigm of silica pathogenicity with synthetic quartz crystals: the role

of crystallinity and surface disorder. Part Fibre Toxicol. 2016;13:32.
38. Chan CWH, Tsui SKW, JYW C, Law PTW, WKW S, DYP L, MMK S. Profiling silica-induced molecular events in human lung cells using the RNA-Seq approach. J Pulm Respir Med. 2017;7(2 (suppl)):50.
39. Vuong NQ, Goegan P, De Rose F, Breznan D, Thomson EM, O'Brien JS, Karthikeyan S, Williams A, Vincent R, Kumarathasan P. Responses of A549 human lung epithelial cellsto cristobalite andα-quartz exposures assessed by toxicoproteomics and gene expression analysis. JApplToxicol. 2016;37: 721–31.
40. Pozzolini M, Vergani L, Ragazzoni M, Delpiano L, Grasselli E, Voci A, Giovine M, Scarfi S. Different reactivity of primaryfibroblasts and endothelial cells towardscrystalline silica: A surface radical matter. Toxicology. 2016;361-362: 12–23.
41. Kirkland D, Pfuhler S, Tweats D, Aardema M, Corvi R, Darroudi F, et al. How to reduce false positive results when undertaking in vitro genotoxicity testing and thus avoid unnecessary follow-up animal tests: report of an ECVAM workshop. Mutat Res. 2007;628:31–55.
42. Fowler P, Smith K, Young J, Jeffrey L, Kirkland D, Pfuhler S, et al. Reduction of misleading ("false") positive results in mammalian cell genotoxicity assays. I. Choice of cell type. Mutat Res. 2012;742:11–25.
43. Whitwell J, Smith R, Jenner K, Lyon H, Wood D, Clements J, et al. Relationship between p53 status, apoptosis and induction of micronuclei in different human and mouse cell lines in vitro: implications for improving existing assays. Mutat Res. 2015;789-790:7–27.
44. Corvi R, Aardema MJ, Gribaldo L, Hayashi M, Hoffmann S, Schechtman L, et al. ECVAM prevalidation study on in vitro cell transformation assays: general outline and conclusions of the study. Mutat Res. 2012;744:12–9.
45. Miles W, Moll WF, Hamilton RD, Brown RK. Physiochemical and mineralogical characterisation of test materials used in 28-day and 90-day Intratracheal instillation toxicology studies in rats. Instillation Toxicology. 2008;20:981–93.
46. Donaldson K, Borm PJ. The quartz hazard: a variable entity. Ann Occup Hyg. 1998;42(5):287–94. Review
47. Hadrup N, Bengtson S, Jacobson N, Jackson P, Nocun M, Saber AT, Jensen KA, Wallin H, Vogel U. Influence of dispersion medium onnanomaterial-induced pulmonary inflammationand DNA strand breaks: investigation of carbonblack, carbon nanotubes and three titaniumdioxide nanoparticles. Mutagenesis. 2017;32:581–97.
48. Driscoll KE, Carter JM, Borm PJ. Antioxidant defense mechanisms and the toxicity of fibrous and nonfibrous particles. Inhal Toxicol. 2002;14(1):101–18. Review
49. International Life Sciences Institute (ILSI) Risk Science Institute Workshop. The relevance of the rat lung response to particle overload for human risk assessment: a workshop consensus report. Inhal Toxicol. 2000;12:1–17.
50. Albrecht C, Höhr D, Haberzettl P, Becker A, Borm PJ, Schins RP. Surface-dependent quartz uptake by macrophages: potential role in pulmonary inflammation and lung clearance. Inhal Toxicol. 2007;19(Suppl 1):39–48.
51. H L, Haberzettl P, Albrecht C, Höhr D, Knaapen AM, Borm PJ, et al. Inhibition of the mitochondrial respiratory chain function abrogates quartz induced DNA damage in lung epithelial cells. Mutat Res. 2007;617(1–2):46–57.
52. Dopp E, Schiffmann D. Analysis of chromosome alterations induced by asbestos and ceramic fibres. Toxicol Lett. 1998;96(97):155–62.
53. Doak SH, Manshian B, Jenkins GJS, Singh N. *In vitro* genotoxicity testing strategy for nanomaterials and the adaptation of current OECD guidelines. Mutat Res. 2012;745:104–11.

3

Ambient air pollution and thrombosis

Sarah Robertson[1*] and Mark R. Miller[2]

Abstract

Air pollution is a growing public health concern of global significance. Acute and chronic exposure is known to impair cardiovascular function, exacerbate disease and increase cardiovascular mortality. Several plausible biological mechanisms have been proposed for these associations, however, at present, the pathways are incomplete. A seminal review by the American Heart Association (2010) concluded that the thrombotic effects of particulate air pollution likely contributed to their effects on cardiovascular mortality and morbidity. The aim of the current review is to appraise the newly accumulated scientific evidence (2009–2016) on contribution of haemostasis and thrombosis towards cardiovascular disease induced by exposure to both particulate and gaseous pollutants. Seventy four publications were reviewed in-depth. The weight of evidence suggests that acute exposure to fine particulate matter ($PM_{2.5}$) induces a shift in the haemostatic balance towards a pro-thrombotic/pro-coagulative state. Insufficient data was available to ascertain if a similar relationship exists for gaseous pollutants, and very few studies have addressed long-term exposure to ambient air pollution. Platelet activation, oxidative stress, interplay between interleukin-6 and tissue factor, all appear to be potentially important mechanisms in pollution-mediated thrombosis, together with an emerging role for circulating microvesicles and epigenetic changes.

Overall, the recent literature supports, and arguably strengthens, the contention that air pollution contributes to cardiovascular morbidity by promoting haemostasis. The volume and diversity of the evidence highlights the complexity of the pathophysiologic mechanisms by which air pollution promotes thrombosis; multiple pathways are plausible and it is most likely they act in concert. Future research should address the role gaseous pollutants play in the cardiovascular effects of air pollution mixture and direct comparison of potentially susceptible groups to healthy individuals.

Keywords: Air pollution, Particulate matter, Ozone, Nitrogen dioxide, Diesel exhaust, Thrombosis, Coagulation

Background

Outdoor air pollution is estimated to be responsible for over 3 million premature deaths worldwide [1], and thus represents one of the leading risk factors for all cause disease [2, 3]. Of these, the vast majority of deaths are attributed to cardiovascular disease (CVD) [1]. Thrombosis is the most common underlying pathology triggering the two major cardiovascular disorders: coronary heart disease and stroke. While many of the biological mechanisms underlying the link between air pollution and CVD remains uncertain, the seminal American Heart Association (AHA) review concluded that thrombotic mechanisms may in part explain the observation that exposure to air pollution is associated with adverse cardiovascular events [4]. The aim of the current review is to examine the newly accumulated scientific evidence (2009–2916) on whether or not mechanisms of haemostasis and thrombosis contributes towards CVD induced by exposure to air pollution. The remit of this review also extends to gaseous pollutants, which had not been previously reviewed by the AHA statement [4]. This work forms part of a larger ongoing piece of work being undertaken by the Committee on the Medical Effects of Air Pollutants on estimating the effect of long-term exposure to ambient air pollution on cardiovascular morbidity in the UK today

Air pollution is a complex heterogeneous mixture of gases and particles, arising from a wide variety of stationary and mobile sources; both directly emitted (primary emissions) or formed within the atmosphere (secondary emissions). From a health perspective, nitrogen oxides (NOx) and particulate matter (PM) currently receive the

* Correspondence: Sarah.Robertson3@phe.gov.uk
[1]Centre for Radiation, Chemical and Environmental Hazards, Public Health England, Harwell Science and Innovation Campus, Didcot, Oxfordshire OX11 0RQ, UK
Full list of author information is available at the end of the article

greatest attention, although ozone (O_3) and sulphur dioxide (SO_2) also have potential to cause harm. PM is itself a complex mixture of airborne particles that differ in size, origin and chemical composition. Particles are classified into three classifications based on aerodynamic diameter; coarse (PM_{10}, 2.5–10 µm) fine ($PM_{2.5}$, <2.5 µm) and ultrafine (UFP, <100 nm). At present only PM_{10} and $PM_{2.5}$ are widely monitored (and regulated) in the environment, with most attention given to $PM_{2.5}$ due to the greater penetration into the lung alveoli and its high reactive surface area for a given mass. On this basis and others (e.g. translocation into the blood, different surface composition), UFPs could represent a greater threat to health, but at present cannot be measured routinely in large numbers of individuals without using surrogates such as particle number count (PNC).

There is persuasive evidence, particularly for PM, on the negative impact of air pollution on cardiovascular events and outcomes, including electrocardiographic changes (e.g. reduced heart rate variability), endothelial dysfunction, atherosclerosis and thrombosis. The biological mechanisms underpinning the effects of air pollution on CVD, however, remain poorly defined. Nonetheless, three main hypothesis have been proposed by which air pollution that is inhaled into the pulmonary system can then instigate remote cardiovascular effects: 1) particle induced inflammatory responses in the lungs, leading to the release of inflammatory and oxidative mediators into the circulation; 2) pollutant-induced activation of airway sensory nerves resulting in autonomic imbalance; and 3) direct entry of pollutants (usually with a focus on particles or chemical constituents) into the pulmonary circulation before being carried into the systemic circulation (Fig. 1).

Haemostasis is a complex, orchestrated series of event events to maintain circulating blood in the liquid state and to prevent blood loss following injury through the formation of a blood clot. Excessive clotting, especially in patients with pre-existing CVD, can block major arteries leading to a loss of downstream blood flow, and potentially leading to clinical events such as heart attack, ischaemic stroke or death. In contrast, a reduction in the ability of blood to clot can lead to uncontrolled bleeding with severe blood loss from injury or escape of blood following aneurysm, e.g. thrombotic stroke. Thus the body maintains an intricate balance to preserve haemostasis; a process that involves the interplay of circulating blood cells, a variety of coagulation factors, platelets and fibrinolytic factors, as well as interactions with the vascular wall and endothelial cell-derived mediators (Fig. 2). Clotting may be initiated by either the intrinsic (contact activation) or extrinsic pathway (tissue factor; TF). These two pathways converge into a final common pathway of thrombin production and fibrin clot formation (Fig. 3). In this review, we use the term "haemostasis" to include the whole process: platelet activation, coagulation and fibrinolysis. Exposure to air pollution has been shown to influence each of these dynamic processes, with increasing evidence suggesting that the overall haemostatic balance is shifted towards a pro-coagulant and anti-fibrinolytic state [4]. The 2010 AHA report [4] concluded that there was evidence, albeit somewhat inconsistent, suggesting that PM may adversely affect haemostasis shifting the balance to a pro-coagulant and anti-fibrinolytic state and that this may, in part, contribute to the effects of air pollution on CVD. The mechanisms underlying such an effect were poorly defined but systemic inflammatory activation and alterations in platelet function are proposed as key processes involved in the alterations in haemostasis [4].

This review provides an overview of the updated literature in the area of air pollution, which has growing increasingly topical, with a specific focus on the thrombotic actions given the contribution that pathway could make to the substantial cardiovascular morbidity of air pollution. In our overview we highlight recent advances and explore mechanistic understanding of the pathways linking air pollution exposure and haemostasis parameters. Improved understanding is needed to provide crucial insight into which pollutants are most harmful, who may be most at risk, and informs future research needs and public health policy in respect of advice and interventions.

Search strategy and review structure

Search strategy

This work uses the 2010 AHA scientific statement [4], as an expert review of the literature between January 2004 to March 2009, as a foundation for reviewing the research in this area in the subsequent years. Literature searches were performed in PubMed from the dates of 1st January 2009 to 28th February 2016, using the following search terms: "air pollution" or "particulate matter" *and* "blood" or "thrombosis" or "clot" or "fibrinolysis" or "coagulation" or "embolism" or "platelet". Terms for gaseous were not included due to the large number of irrelevant references these terms produced. Preliminary checks were performed to ensure that relevant references with gaseous pollutants were captured by the term "air pollution". Other papers were identified from prior knowledge, contact with experts in the field and hand searching of the bibliographies of the papers identified in the electronic search. References were downloaded into the referencing software program Endnote (version X8).

Study selection

A total of 2326 publications were identified following removal of duplicates (Fig. 4). These were screened first at the abstract level, and then at the full article level. To be included in the final analysis studies had to meet the following inclusion criteria:

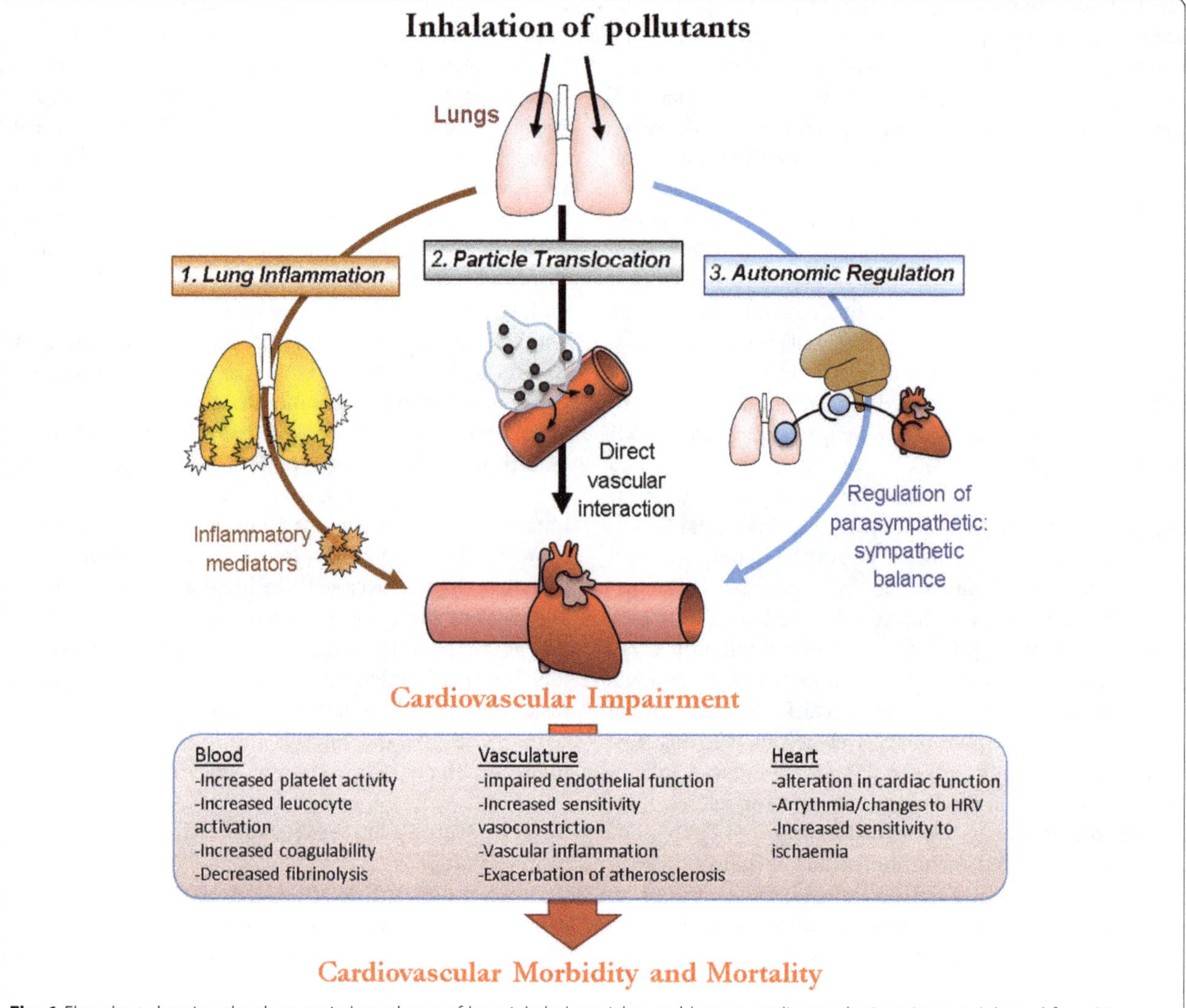

Fig. 1 Flowchart showing the three main hypotheses of how inhaled particles could cause cardiovascular impairment. Adapted from Niemann et al. [78]

- Peer-reviewed articles or published by a recognised institution between 1st January 2009 and 28th February 2016*
- Study type: epidemiological studies, human controlled exposures and intervention studies, in vivo (animal) studies
- Exposure: ambient (outdoor) air pollution – particulate air pollutants**, diesel exhaust (DE), O_3, nitrogen dioxide (NO_2), carbon monoxide (CO), SO_2
- Health outcome: reported on coagulation, fibrinolysis, thrombophilia and platelet profile
- Population: general population (all ages, those with pre-existing health conditions)

* Key earlier publications are discussed for contextual background.

** Included PM size fractions, black carbon (BC), concentrated ambient particles (CAPs) and PM from DE (i.e. diesel exhaust particles (DEP)).

Key exclusion criteria included:

- No original data included (e.g. reviews, editorials and commentaries were excluded). However, reference lists from the identified original articles and reviews were screened to identify any other potentially relevant studies.
- Language: full text not available in the English Language
- Study type: in vitro
- Exposure not relevant to ambient air pollution (e.g. indoor air pollution, occupational exposure***, biomass, cigarette smoke, manufactured nanoparticles)
- Did not provide any mechanistic data beyond mortality or hospital admission

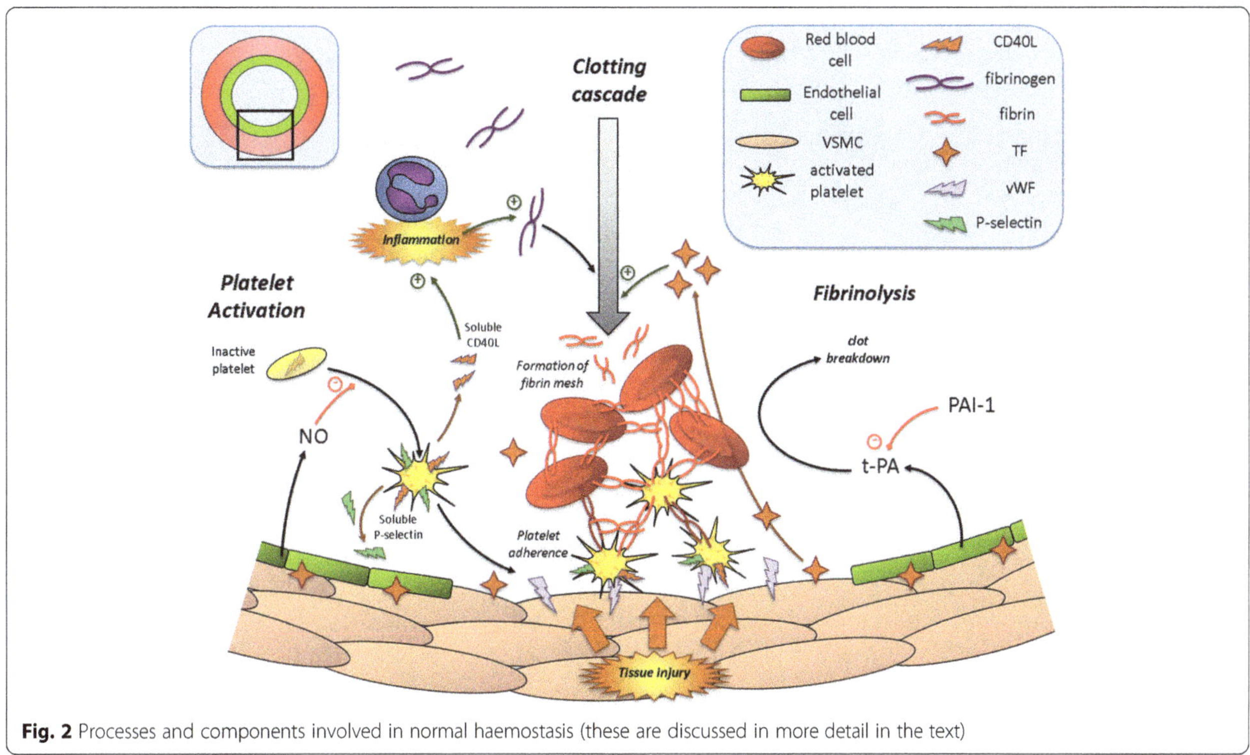

Fig. 2 Processes and components involved in normal haemostasis (these are discussed in more detail in the text)

*** Occupational exposure to manufactured nanoparticles, industrial accidents and environmental events (e.g. volcanic eruptions or wildfires) were not included. Workplace exposures that potentially spill into communities or were representatives of the main aspects of general urban air pollution (e.g. engine emissions from garages, bus depts.) were included.

Review structure

This review provides a narrative summary of the seventy four publications that fulfilled all inclusion criteria. The piece has been structured by study type: epidemiological studies (62%) controlled exposure studies in man (15%) and in vivo animal studies (23%). Epidemiological studies were further subdivided into short-term (7 days of exposure or less) versus long-term (>1 week of exposure). Emphasis has been given as to whether the conclusions of the AHA statement have been strengthened during the 8-year period and where new insight has been made as to possible underlying mechanisms. Of note, we expand the remit from the AHA statement by inclusion of gaseous pollutants (e.g. NO_2, O_3, CO and SO_2).

Epidemiological studies

Short-term exposure to air pollutants

The vast majority of epidemiological studies addressing the haemostatic effects of air pollution have investigated acute exposures (<7 days), with most evaluating alterations in plasma biomarkers of systemic coagulation and fibrinolysis. Fibrinogen, an essential coagulation protein associated with an increased risk of coronary events [5, 6], has been one of the most studied. Hildebrandt and colleagues reported PM to be associated with a 2.4% increase in fibrinogen from 3.1 g/L (baseline) in 38 male patients with chronic obstructive pulmonary disease (COPD) [7]. However, no clear pattern emerged for the other plasma haemostatic biomarkers evaluated. Thus, the increase in fibrinogen in response to exposure may be somewhat artificial, perhaps arising from small sample bias. With a larger sample size ($N = 242$), another study noted no increase plasma fibrinogen levels in patients with COPD per interquartile range (IQR) increase in $PM_{2.5}$ at all lag days (0–10) [8]. Similarly, there were no significant changes in fibrinogen with PM exposure among young and older adults [9–11]. Besides fibrinogen, other biomarkers having pro-coagulant properties or reflecting a pro-thrombotic state have been investigated (including, (plasminogen activator inhibitor type 1 (PAI-1) and tissue-type plasminogen activator (t-PA)) [10, 12, 13]. Earlier studies typically analysed single biomarkers of haemostasis, whereas more recent studies have used a multiple biomarker approach. While most studies have observed pollution-related changes in at least one biomarker, the direction and statistical significance of the pollutant-biomarker association has not been consistent, making it difficult to generalise conclusions. More convincing evidence for associations between exposure to ambient particles and biomarkers of haemostasis comes from studies

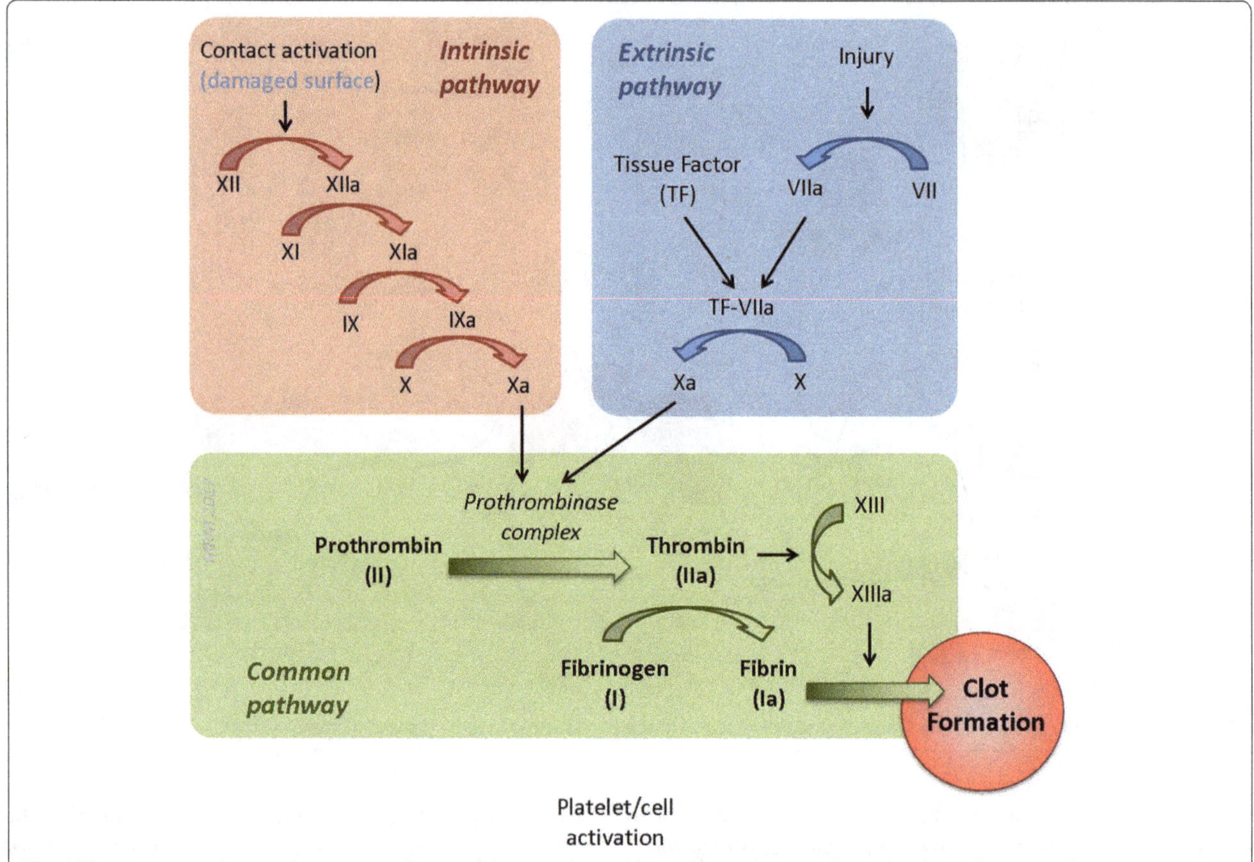

Fig. 3 The intrinsic, extrinsic and common pathways of the coagulation (clotting) cascade. Air pollution has been shown to affect several steps in blood coagulation (these are discussed in more detail in the text)

conducted during the 2008 Beijing Olympics [10, 14]. The air pollution control measures that were put in place in Beijing during the 2008 Olympic Games provided an unprecedented opportunity for quasi-experimental studies to assess the effect on systemic biomarkers of haemostasis and inflammation, among others. The short-term reductions in PM during the Olympic Games was associated with decreases in biomarkers of haemostasis [10, 14]. During the 2008 Beijing Olympic Games, Rich et al. (2012) observed statistically significant improvements in soluble P-selectin (sP-selectin; −34%) and von Willebrand (vWF; −13.1%) among, the 125 healthy young adults studied [14]. An interesting study by Delfino et al. (2009) examined whether medication use modifies the association between particulate air pollution and biomarkers of haemostasis. Here, an association between $PM_{2.5}$ exposure and blood levels of sP-selectin in coronary artery disease (CAD) was only observed in those not taking clopidogrel, providing further evidence for a role of platelets [12]. Further studies are warranted to disentangle the modifying effects of health status and use of different medications, in addition to whether such preventative action of anti-platelet agents are more marked in those with greatest exposure to air pollutants.

Inconsistencies between studies are also likely to reflect the differences in the accuracy of the exposure assessment for individual volunteers. Studies have generally relied on data collected from the nearest fixed-ambient monitoring stations as a surrogate for personal exposure. Unless complex modelling has been performed a key weakness in using fixed-site monitoring data is that it ignores spatial variability. Differences in particle composition across study locations could also be a reason for the inconsistent findings, as physical and chemical characteristics of PM are known to vary widely both with space and time [15, 16]. Very few studies have analysed associations between individual PM constituents and changes in biomarkers of haemostasis. There is limited/suggestive epidemiological evidence that the haemostatic responses are more intrinsically related to chemical composition rather than just particle mass. For example, Wu et al. (2012) demonstrated that certain transition metals (e.g. iron, titanium, cobalt and cadmium) within $PM_{2.5}$, but not PM mass, was associated with increased plasma fibrinogen levels among healthy adults in Beijing. Besides fibrinogen, biomarkers of the fibrinolytic pathway (PAI-1 and t-PA) were also significantly and positively associated with transition metals in $PM_{2.5}$. These epidemiological observations

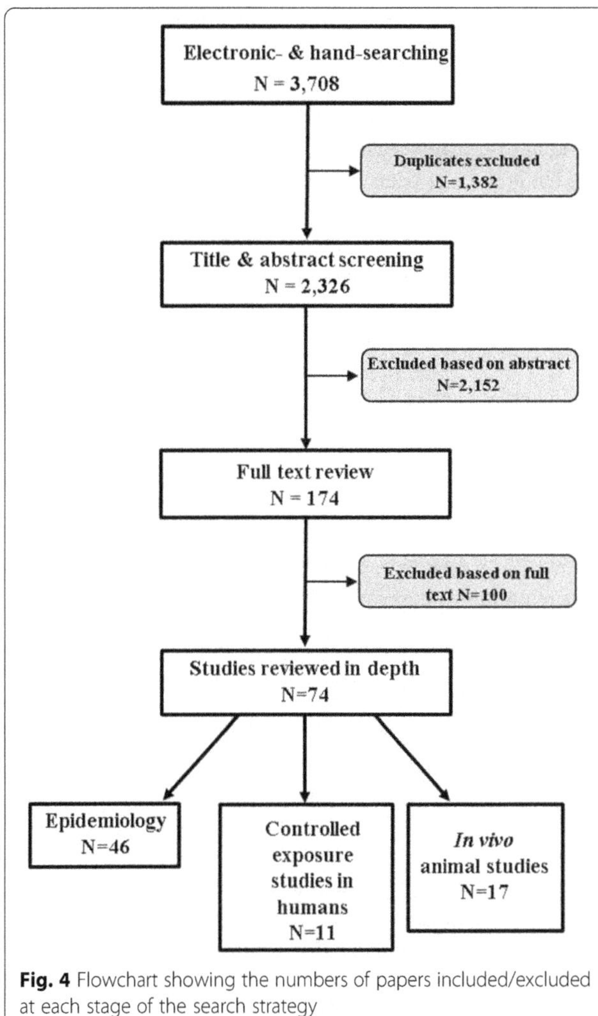

Fig. 4 Flowchart showing the numbers of papers included/excluded at each stage of the search strategy

are consistent with animal and in vitro studies showing a role for transition metals in the PM-induced toxicity [17]. Additionally, studies have shown the administration of chelating agents (chemical compounds that react with metal ions, to decrease their availability for other reactions) can block the effects of air pollution on blood coagulation [18]. Several transition metals have been shown to participate in Fenton and Fenton-like reactions and thus induce oxidative stress. Oxidative stress is a reoccurring mechanism in actions of air pollution [19], and associations between exposure and biomarkers of oxidative stress have been observed in both in vivo and in vitro studies [20]. To the best of our knowledge, only one study that has investigated the effects of genetic polymorphisms related to oxidative stress and particulate pollution exposure on markers of haemostasis [21]. Stronger associations between PM and haemostatic biomarkers were observed among individuals who were genetically predisposed to oxidative damage [21]. However, unexpectedly, exposure was associated with a decrease in the levels of circulating biomarkers of haemostasis, counter intuitively suggesting a potentially protective effect of PM against thrombosis [21]. Besides oxidative-stress related polymorphisms, other epidemiological studies have investigated the effect of polymorphisms in the fibrinogen genes on responses to PM exposure [22]. For example, carriers of the FGB rs1800790 minor allele elicited greater fibrinogen responses to PM than those with a major allele [22]. Such 'unforeseen' functional consequences of genetic polymorphisms may, in part, account for discrepant findings between studies investigating different populations. Further work in this area is clearly warranted.

Size distribution in ambient air may also be important. An increasing body of experimental data (see below) has shown that the ultrafine fraction within PM is more toxic than the fine or coarse fractions, attributed to the larger surface area per unit mass of ultrafine particles (UFPs). The large majority of these studies have focussed on pulmonary responses and as yet, there are too few population studies to conclude whether different particle size fractions have different magnitudes of association with haemostatic outcomes. Only a few studies have specifically investigated the effect of particle size on the haemostatic effects of PM and results have been mixed [10, 12, 21, 23, 24]. This is likely the consequence of limited statistical power of studies together with methodological heterogeneity. Of particular interest is the study by Rückerl et al. (2014) which used a particle counter with a lower particle cut-off size than the more conventional methods. Nevertheless, analysis of the different size fractions of UFP (3–10 nm, 10–30 nm, 30–50 nm, 50-100 nm) did not reveal a certain size range to be more influential than others. Also, associations were stronger for $PM_{2.5}$ than for UFPs; inconsistent with the notion that UFPs have greater biological activity, although it is noteworthy that this study found a reduced thrombus formation in association with PM.

There is some limited evidence that different particle sizes have different intervals of time (lag) between exposure and biomarker changes, suggesting that the mode of action may be different for the various particle sizes [10]. It has been suggested that inhaled UFPs may translocate into the circulation [25–27] with the potential for direct pro-aggregatory effects on platelets. However, particle translocation remains controversial and a recent study showed that the translocated fraction is less than 1% (mass) of the delivered dose to the lung [28]. The exact pathway for the translocation into the circulation also remains unclear. While some studies [10], report associations between haemostatic biomarkers and concentrations of ambient UFPs for time lags representing direct effects (ie. lag 0), the time course of others [29] is more likely to represent indirect effects, with findings very rarely being consistent across studies for the same biomarker-pollutant pair. It is also not clear whether inflammatory processes mediate the exposure-response relationship. It has been shown that exposure to particulate air pollution can induce platelet aggregation and increased thrombin generation without inducing significant levels of inflammation [29]. Others have suggested that an inflammatory response is an essential component in the haematological changes associated with short-term exposure to air pollution [10, 13, 30]. Of note, most studies have looked at a limited number of inflammatory biomarkers and these may not necessary encompass all aspects of the inflammation response.

There has been limited progress in the use of global coagulation tests in epidemiological studies of short-term exposure. Measurement of individual biomarkers provides only 'snapshots' of the overall coagulation process, and global coagulation tests can provide a more complete picture of haemostatic status. The prothrombin time (PT) test (measures activity of the extrinsic and common pathways) and the activated partial thromboplastin time (APTT) test (measures activity of the intrinsic and common pathways) are widely used global screening tests for blood coagulability. To date, efforts have primarily focused on PM. Shortened PT (i.e. greater coagulability of the blood) has been demonstrated in 1218 normal subjects from the Lombardia Region, Italy after short-term exposure to PM_{10} [31]. No changes in APTT were noted, perhaps instead pointing towards TF-dependent changes in thrombin generation. This result is contrary to a more recent study showing prolonged clotting times with increased levels of PM_{10} in a group of 233 patients with diabetes [13]. However, reduced clotting times were associated with increasing PM_{10} concentrations of the subacute exposure windows (day 0 to day 3) [13].

One of the most exciting areas to have developed in recent years, has been increasing interest in uncovering whether environmental exposures can impact on health through epigenetic mechanisms (alterations in gene expression and function without changing the underlying DNA sequence), such as DNA methylation, histone modifications and non-coding RNA expression [32]. Alterations of DNA methylation have been linked to various human diseases, and epidemiological studies have shown distinct DNA methylation abnormalities with exposure to air pollutants [33, 34]. Evidence for associations between (i) air pollution and epigenetic alterations and (ii) between disease states (including CVD) and epigenetic changes, lends biological plausibility for epigenetic change underpinning the effects of air pollution on haemostasis. The most compelling evidence comes from a recent study demonstrating that exposure to black carbon (BC) particles was associated with a decrease in DNA methylation (hypomethylation) of the tissue factor (F3) gene and subsequent increases in fibrinogen protein expression [35]. The specific mechanism of how air pollution exposure may alter DNA methylation has not been elucidated at present.

Unlike PM, there have been relatively few studies evaluating the relationship between gaseous pollutants and biomarkers of haemostasis, and the evidence has been mixed. The evidence has been mixed with some showing positive associations, some showing no association and a few showing inverse associations [7, 8, 11, 12, 14, 24, 29]. The heterogeneity of these studies makes the data difficult to interpret as studies have tended to use different exposures (NO_2, CO), target populations or outcome measures.

Long-term exposure to air pollutants

As with the studies of short-term exposure to PM discussed above, fibrinogen has been the most widely studied biomarker in long-term exposure (>1 week) epidemiological studies. Using data from the Heinz Nixdorf Recall Study (a prospective population-based cohort of 4814 German adults) plasma fibrinogen levels were found to be elevated by 3.9% among men, but not women, for each 3.91 $\mu g/m^3$ increase in annual average $PM_{2.5}$ [36]. This was found to be independent of short-term changes in air pollution. However, a comparative study using a higher spatial resolution (1 km as compared to 5 km) did not confirm this finding [37]. Large population-based cohort studies in the US and UK have also reported no association between fibrinogen and PM [30, 38–40]. Studies also varied in their ability to adjust for potential confounding factors (medication use, co-morbidities, socio-economic status (SES)). Additionally, different exposure patterns and sources are likely to contribute to the inconsistent results among studies. Evidence from a multi-center and meta-analysis found that long-term exposure to zinc within $PM_{2.5}$, but not other constituents (e.g. iron and nickel) increased fibrinogen concentrations [41]. These findings add to the growing evidence that mass alone does not fully capture the toxicity potential of PM.

A few studies have looked at other markers of clotting and fibrinolysis, with considerable differences in the magnitude and direction of responses obtained [30, 37, 42, 43]. Factor VII (FVII) plays a central role in initiating the process of coagulation. A cohort study of 2086 mid-life women found an inverse relationship with FVII (–3.6%; 95% Cl, –7.8 to 0.8%) for each additional 10 $\mu g/m^3$ of annual $PM_{2.5}$ pollution [42], pointing towards a more hypocoagulable state. However, the measurement and analysis of one or more coagulation biomarkers may not provide a complete picture of the balance between thrombosis and lysis. For example, long-term exposure to PM led to enhanced thrombin generation in patients with diabetes, in the absence of pro-coagulant changes in coagulation parameters (FVII, FVIII, FXII) [13]. The evidence has, for the most part, been directed at particulate air pollutants. Differences in the focus and design of investigations addressing gaseous air pollutants make it difficult to draw meaningful conclusions as to the long-term relationship with coagulation markers [8, 30, 40, 42, 44, 45].

A small number of studies have made use of global coagulation tests in long-term epidemiological studies. Reduced clotting times were observed in association with PM_{10} average over one year among healthy controls and patients with deep vein thrombosis [46]. Patients with diabetes showed hypercoagulability, using endogenous thrombin potential (ETP) with PM_{10} for time windows up to 6 months in patients with diabetes [13]. Interestingly, associations between PM_{10} exposure up to one month, but not longer, and thrombin generation were dependent on TF. The authors proposed microvesicles (small membrane-bound structures secreted from different cell types) to be the main source of the TF [13]. Increased levels of TF-positive microvesicles were also detected in the plasma of diabetic patients for mean PM_{10} measurement over 1 year [13].

Induction of systemic inflammation by air pollution could contribute to a pro-thrombotic state. Consistent with this notion, Viehmann et al. (2015), using data from the Heinz Nixdorf Recall Study, observed a positive correlation between C-reactive protein (CRP; a marker of systemic inflammation) and platelet count in relation to air pollution [37]. However, other studies have found no clear patterns of association between markers of haemostasis and markers of inflammation [13, 40, 44]. In the study by Emmerechts et al. (2012), a systemic inflammatory state could not explain the pro-coagulant during the longer time windows (1 month to 1 year) [13]. Only a limited number of studies have examined whether age, gender, and pre-existing co-morbidities influence the haemostatic effects of long-term air pollution exposure and results have been inconsistent. For example, Forbes et al. (2009) found no effect modification by gender for associations for PM and fibrinogen, whereas PM exposure was associated with increasing fibrinogen levels in men, but not women, in the population-based Heinz Nixdorf Recall cohort study [36]. The latter study is of particular interest as it controlled for a large number of confounding variables. Nevertheless, the study produced some unexpected results, showing no effect modification by medication use or co-morbidities on the association between PM and fibrinogen.

In summary, much of the recent epidemiological research has strengthened the evidence of associations between short- and long-term particulate air pollution exposure and changes in haemostasis. Increased use of assays of global coagulation, reflecting events from beginning of clot formation to fibrinolysis, has contributed to strengthening the evidence that particulate pollutants could cause thrombotic events. However, changes have been modest and, at times, inconsistent. Furthermore, it is not clear whether differences in susceptibility exist within populations (for example, age, sex, pre-existing disease). The magnitude of these changes is in general small, and their clinical relevance has yet to be ascertained. It is, however, possible that, if untreated, these haemostatic changes over the long-term could ultimately lead to exacerbation of myocardial ischaemia and other clinical outcomes in response to a triggering factor. The current evidence is too sparse to draw conclusions about the effects of exposure of gaseous pollutants on haemostasis.

Controlled human exposure studies

Controlled human exposure studies provide a means to investigate biological mechanisms for pollutants in isolation with fewer confounding variables. Despite the heterogeneity in study design and the possibility of publication bias against negative findings, it is difficult to deny that particulate air pollution promotes a pro-thrombotic state. In recent years, much of the research has focussed on DE and CAPs. A series of controlled human exposure studies have demonstrated impaired fibrinolysis, by measurement of t-PA (the activator of fibrinolysis) in healthy volunteers after exposure to DE generated under either transient engine speed and load (300 $\mu g/m^3$; 1 h) [47] and idling (250 $\mu g/m^3$; 1 h) conditions [48]. Similar observations have been observed in patients with coronary heart disease (CHD) following DE exposure [49] and in healthy volunteers after exposure to coarse CAPs (89.0 $\mu g/m^3$; 2 h) [50].

In recent years, major advances have been made in supporting thrombus formation following DE exposure. Ex vivo thrombus formation has been assessed, using a Badimon chamber (mimics flow conditions within the coronary circulation of man), after DE exposures (320–350 $\mu g/m^3$) lasting 1 and 2 h in healthy volunteers [51, 52]. Interestingly, DE exposure was associated with increased expression of platelet-leukocyte aggregates, as well as increased circulating levels of soluble forms of CD40L, suggesting that the enhanced thrombus formation was mediated through platelet activation [51, 52]. DE exposures did not have any significant effect on cellular and soluble markers of inflammation [51, 52]. The latter suggest that short-term exposure to DE may lead to a pro-thrombotic state, independent of systematic inflammation. However, these studies have been typically limited to measuring a small number of blood markers of inflammation, and cannot exclude other markers of inflammation. The question as to whether particulate air pollutants affect platelets through direct and/or indirect effects thus remains undetermined.

Significant advancements have been made in recent years as to whether the anti-fibrinolytic, and pro-thrombotic responses are due to diesel PM or the associated DE gaseous components (or both). Acute exposures of healthy volunteers to DE with a particle trap abolished the effects on endogenous fibrinolysis and ex vivo thrombus formation [51]. While the filters were effective in terms of particle removal (reduced particle concentration by 98%), the catalytic oxide coatings led to measurable increases in concentrations of NO_2. Nevertheless, a study by the same investigators found that bradykinin-induced release of tPA into plasma did not change significantly after exposure to NO_2 at 4 ppm for 1 h [53], suggesting that NO_2 does not appear to be a major factor in the anti-fibrinolytic effects of dilute DE inhalation. Strengthening the role of particles, thrombotic effects appear to be relatively consistent in inhalation studies performed using diesel engine emissions at equivalent particle mass concentrations but different gaseous components [52]. However, controlled exposure to O_3 (0.3 ppm for 2 h) reduced plasma PAI-1 within 24 h in healthy volunteers, suggesting a pro-thrombotic effect of O_3 [54].

The source and chemical nature of the particles appears to be important. For example, exposure to CAPs, from non-exhaust traffic related sources, did not significantly affect the fibrinolytic balance in patients with CHD [55]. Furthermore, a pure carbon nanoparticulate exposure alone had no discernible effect on blood coagulation and fibrinolysis in healthy volunteers [56]. However, to date these effects have not been studied extensively and therefore only limited information is available on these issues. Although diesel motor emissions constitute a significant proportion of UFPs in the urban environment, it is as yet unclear which fraction of particulate from DE plays the largest role in the thrombolytic/fibrinolytic effects. Studies using inhaled laboratory generated ultrafine carbon particles (50 $\mu g/m^3$; count medium diameter, 32 nm; 2 h) – as surrogates for ambient UFP- have reported platelet activation and increased vWF (mediates platelet-platelet or platelet-vessel interaction) levels in persons with type 2 diabetes [10, 57, 58].

Gene expression profiling analysis using microarray has demonstrated changes in expression levels of genes involved in the clotting cascade [59]. Expression of the F2R gene (located at chromosome 5q13.3), which encodes the thrombin receptor, were elevated 30-fold in 14 healthy participants after a 1 h exposure to diluted DE (300 $\mu g/m^3$) compared to clean air [59]. In addition, DE exposure decreased expression of the gene encoding the urokinase-type plasminogen activator (PLAU), a secreted serine protease involved in the breakdown of clots [59]. Genes related to oxidative stress pathways have been shown to be differentially regulated in response to exposure to air pollution. In particular, inducible nitric oxide synthase 2A (NOS2A), a biomarker of oxidative stress, was upregulated in healthy volunteers 24 h after DE exposure (300 $\mu g/m^3$, 60 min on 2 separate days) [59]. Further evidence is required to confirm a role for oxidative stress in causing PM-induced pro-coagulant/thrombotic effects. It is also worth noting that the changes in the gene expression level of coagulation markers have not been frequently reflected at the protein level after DE exposure.

Taken as a whole, controlled exposure studies in man support the notion that particulate air pollution exposure favours a pro-thrombotic state. The most common human controlled inhalation studies are to DE. Exposures are acute (1–2 h) and concentrations used are high, but within the range that could occur in the urban environment (for example, during high air pollution episodes or in areas of dense traffic). It has been reported that O_3exposure, but not NO_2, promotes thrombosis, but these are isolated studies. A number of different mechanisms have been postulated to mediate thrombogenic actions of particulate air pollution. Arguably, one of the strongest hypotheses for the enhanced thrombotic profile in response to exposure suggests an increase in platelet activation. Inflammation and oxidative stress continue to be implicated as a mechanism underlying pollution-induced pro-thrombotic and anti-fibrinolytic effects, although findings are inconsistent. Most investigations used young, healthy subjects and there is insufficient data to ascertain whether pre-existing conditions further promote the thrombogenic effects of air pollution.

In vivo studies in animals

Animal models provide greater flexibility to explore the biological mechanisms of air pollutant exposure. In relation to the haemostatic system in particular, in vivo models in which induction of thrombosis can be directly studied, as opposed to relying on surrogates or biomarkers alone, or blood clotting ex vivo in the absence of the vessel wall, can be studied. Together with biomarkers, a detailed assessment of effect and mechanism is possible. In recent years, a variety of biological pathways have been argued persuasively. In terms of environmental sources of air pollution, the focus has remained on PM, through inhalation of urban ambient particles or instillation techniques to deliver particulates in the absence of gases. There is increasing evidence that the association between exposure to PM and alterations in haemostasis is mediated, at least in part, by interleukin-6 (IL-6). Mutlu et al. (2007) first drew our attention to a role of IL-6 in mediating PM-related pro-thrombotic effects [60]. In C57 mice, intratracheal administration of coarse ambient particles (PM_{10}; 10 μg), collected from an urban background site in Düsseldorf, Germany, increased lung production of IL-6, reduced clotting times and enhanced thrombin generated within 24 h compared with saline instillation [60]. Additionally, the role of alveolar macrophages as the critical source of this elevated IL-6 was confirmed by depleting alveolar macrophages using intracheally instilled liposomal clodronate

[60]. IL-6 dependent activation of coagulation has also been suggested in studies using different particle size fractions and other exposure methods [61]. Work by Budinger et al. (2011) demonstrated an IL-6-dependent increase in coagulation activation markers (thrombin-anti-thrombin (TAT)) following inhalation exposure (8 h per day, for 3 days) to fine CAPs ($PM_{2.5}$; 88.5 ± 13.4 μg/m^3) and after the instillation $PM_{2.5}$ (200 μg) [61]. Unfortunately, because studies have used different methods in assessing the haemostatic effects, makes comparisons between studies difficult.

Budinger et al. (2011) also showed a role of IL-6 in the increased levels of TF antigen following PM exposure [61]. IL-6 knockout mice did not display the increased levels of TF following inhalation exposure (8 h per day, for 3 days) to fine CAPs ($PM_{2.5}$; 88.5 ± 13.4 μg/m^3) and after the instillation $PM_{2.5}$ (200 μg) [61]. However, measurements of TF antigen do not necessarily reflect the functional capacity and integrity of TF [62]. Perhaps the most convincing evidence for a role of TF in mediating thrombus formation following exposure to PM comes from the study by Kilinç et al. (2011) [62]. In mice intratracheal administration of UFPs (approx. 0.36 μg) collected near a Dutch roadside tunnel (mainly used by heavy diesel trucks) increased plasma thrombin generation at 4 and 24 h post-exposure [62]. The extrinsic pathway is initiated when TF comes in contact with and activates factor VII (Fig. 3). Kilinç et al. (2011) showed that the increased thrombin generation 4 h after exposure to UFP to be blocked by administration of TF/FVIIa inhibitor [62]. TF-driven thrombin generation was supported by observations that thrombin generation parameters were similar in wildtype and FXII (important protein involved in the initiation of the intrinsic pathway; Fig. 3) deficient mice 4 h after UFP exposure [62]. Of note, this study did not provide evidence for a causal link between IL-6 and TF. The use of FXII knockout mice to study the role of the intrinsic coagulation pathway provided support for the intrinsic pathway in the later phases of thrombin generation (20 h after UFP exposure) [62]. While intratracheal instillation of UFP increased thrombin generation in wildtype mouse plasma at 20 h post-exposure, no effect was seen in FXII knockout mice. Similar results were obtained by pharmacological inhibition of FXII by the inhibitor corn trypsin inhibitor [62]. Overall, these results suggest distinct mechanisms regulate pollution-related haemostatic effects over different timescales. However, more studies are needed with air pollution from different sources and different particle sizes. Inhalation studies are also required. Intratracheal administration is a more artificial route of delivering pollutants to the lungs and does not simulate normal animal inhalation exposure conditions [63]. Nevertheless, intratracheal instillation of particle suspensions has been shown to be a reliable way of producing excellent dispersion of particles throughout the lobes of rodent lungs and across the surface of the alveoli, leading to pulmonary effects that are directly comparable to that of inhalation studies [64, 65].

The study by Kilinç et al. (2011) did not assess whether the initiation of the intrinsic coagulation pathway following exposure was a consequence of an inflammatory response and/or particle translocation processes [62]. Interestingly, Budinger et al. (2011) suggested that IL-6 is significantly associated with PM-induced thrombogenic effects independent of other inflammatory markers [61]. Two studies have been published examining the effect of anti-inflammatory agents on thrombogenic factors in mice following exposure to DEP (15–30 μg) [66, 67]. Both studies demonstrated a critical role for inflammation in mediating DEP-induced thrombotic effects [66, 67]. Interestingly, the Nemmar et al. (2003) found that inflammation and thrombosis were associated events at 18 h, but not at 4 h [68]. Particle translocation could play a role in the early pro-thrombotic effects of DEP, with inflammation playing a greater role at later stages. Indirect evidence for this concept is provided by the finding that intravenous administration of DEP to the blood has the capacity to increase in vivo thrombosis formation at 2 h, without inducing inflammation [69]. The link between inflammation and thrombosis at later time points after pulmonary instillation is possible (6–24 h), but complex [69]. Smyth et al. (2017) showed intratracheally instillation of DEP (25 μg) in mice to induce platelet aggregation independent of lung inflammation [70]. The study also showed that platelet aggregation persisted in endothelial nitric oxide synthase (eNOS) knockout mice [70], suggesting a lesser influence of vascular-derived mediators in actions of DEP on platelets. There is some discrepancy regarding the role of platelets in mediating the pro-thrombotic effects of particulate air pollution [13, 51, 52, 60–62, 69, 70]. This is likely due to differences in study designs, including species, particle types, doses, exposure methods and different measurable indicators of platelet function. An especially noteworthy study is that by Emmerects et al. (2012) suggesting that continuous exposure of mice to traffic-related air pollution, in a real-life setting (mice were placed in a highway tunnel for 25 or 26 days; mean 24.9 μg/m^3 $PM_{2.5}$) may affect platelet function with an increased release of platelet derived pro-coagulant microvesicles [13]. This study also looked at how age modifies the pollution-induced changes in platelet counts and activation but no clear patterns emerged [13]. More studies assessing the potential effect modification by age, as well effects of co-morbidities are clearly needed. One study has examined hypertension and demonstrated enhanced platelet aggregation and thrombin generation 24 h after intratracheal instillation of DEP (15 μg) in mice induced with experimental hypertension compared with wildtype controls [71]. There is limited evidence to support the assertion that exposure to air pollution may have a priming effect that leads to an augmented response to subsequent stimuli [72]. Platelets from CAPs-exposed mice ($PM_{2.5}$; 88.5 μg/m^3; 6 h/day; 5 days/week for 2 weeks) showed a 54% increase in fibrinogen binding in response to the agonist adenosine diphosphate (ADP), compared to saline exposed mice [72].

As discussed above, impairment of endogenous fibrinolysis has been suggested from studies exposing humans to DE by inhalation under controlled experimental conditions [47, 49]. Subsequent studies showed that this effect was directly attributable to the exhaust particles [73]. Increased aorta PAI-1mRNA levels, suggesting the presence of vascular injury and/or fibrinolytic activation were observed in rats exposed to O_3 (0.38 ppm) or DEP (2.2 mg/m^3) alone for 16 weeks (5 h/day, 1 day/week) [73]. Interestingly, aortic thrombodulin (TM) and t-PA mRNA levels also increased, which are opposite to the expected direction of change [73]. Further studies are needed to determine whether these exposures would reflect similar changes in corresponding protein levels or activity. A great advantage of the study design employed by Kodavanti et al. (2011) was that they analysed disparities in exposure to both acute (2 days) and sub-chronic (16 weeks) pollution in the same study. The analysis found that the associations between exposure and mRNA markers of haemostasis to be strongest after a longer series of exposures [73]. This study also showed a synergistic decrease in effects following DE and O_3 (0.5 ppm + 2 mg/m^3 5 h/day; 1 day/week for 16 weeks) co-exposure [73]. Concentrations of PAI-1 mRNA in mouse fat tissue has also been shown to increase following inhalation exposure (8 h per day, for 3 days) to fine CAPs ($PM_{2.5}$; 88.5 ± 13.4 μg/m^3) and after the instillation $PM_{2.5}$ (200 μg) [61]. Notably, studies in IL-6 null mice revealed no significant effect of the loss of IL-6 on the induction of PAI-1 expressions following exposure [61]. Treating wildtype mice with the TNF-α receptor antagonist etanercept (10 mg/kg i.p.) prevented upregulation of PAI-1 expression following exposure [61]. In contrast etanercept had no effect on PM-induced thrombus formation [61]. Another study showed curcumin (45 mg/kg), a compound with anti-inflammatory and anti-oxidant properties, to block the DEP-induced up-regulation of TNF-α and PAI-1 in mice (15 μg DEP via intratracheal instillation, 4 times/week, for 1 week), but to only partially inhibit PM-induced thrombosis [66]. Collectively, these data suggests that PM exposure is associated with both the activation of coagulation and impairment of fibrinolysis, but that these facets are regulated via distinct mechanisms.

Lastly, this review found limited evidence linking oxidative stress to the effects of pollution exposure on thrombosis and fibrinolysis. For example, the pulmonary and systematic inflammation induced by ultrafine carbon particles (180 μg/m^3, 24 h) in aged spontaneously hypertensive rats (SHRs) was associated with increased hemeoxygenase-1 levels (HO-1; a marker of oxidative stress), alongside changes in biomarkers of thrombosis [74]. Additionally, oxidation of the low density lipoprotein (LDL) receptor has an influence on the thrombotic effects of inhaled vehicular emissions [73].

In summary, the majority of animal studies support the notion that particulate air pollution exposure leads to an enhanced thrombogenicity. The use of in vivo *of thrombus formation in blood vessels* in situ *is a strength of animal studies given that clot formation will be heavily influenced by the vascular wall and flow conditions of the blood prior to clot formation. Whilst* in vivo *studies generally use high air pollution exposures, the similarity of many of the mechanistic pathways with those shown in epidemiological and controlled exposure studies in man suggests that these exposures are relevant. Multiple mechanisms have been postulated, including inflammation, oxidative stress, interplay between TF and IL-6 (potentially independently of other inflammation pathways), increases in coagulation factors, and impaired fibrinolysis. A role of platelet activation in the enhanced thrombosis is one of the most consistent observations. The thrombotic effects of gaseous pollutants and the use of models of susceptible populations is an avenue for future research, and one that would provide a useful foundation addressing these matters in human studies, particularly if dose and time responses can be defined.*

Summary and conclusions

In 2015, ambient air pollution was estimated to be the 5th leading risk factor for death globally, with CVD accounting for the majority of these deaths [2]. Given the global commitment to reduce premature non-communicable diseases by 25% by 2025 [75], an improved understanding of the mechanisms underlying the significant detrimental effects of air pollution on CVD will help achieve this target. Specifically, improved knowledge of the mechanistic pathways linking air pollution to negative effects on cardiovascular health has the potential to improve policy, and ultimately improve health and life expectancy of people by allowing target intervention. In 2010, a seminar review of literature suggested a role of the haemostatic system to the overall cardiovascular effects of air pollution, although a great deal of uncertainty remained [4]. This review discusses the growing body of evidence from 2009 to 2016, expanding the remit to include gaseous co-pollutants as well as airborne particulates of different size fractions.

A large body of work (2326 references screened, 74 assessed) has been published on the topic in the last seven years. Overall, examination of this literature supports the contention that exposure to air pollution promotes coagulation and impairs fibrinolysis, leading to an unfavourable imbalance in haemostatic factors that would be expected to increase the risk of thrombotic events in susceptible individuals. As noted in the AHA review, inconsistent findings between studies are commonplace. However, the volume of publications supporting the pro-thrombotic effect of air pollution far outweigh those showing no effect or the opposite effect, even given the assumption that there may be a publication bias towards studies suggesting a health risk of pollutions. Potential reasons for the inconsistencies are many. In general, the investigations assessed were, in our opinion, of high scientific quality – both in their design, implementation and analysis. Instead, a major source of discrepancies most likely reflects the differences in study design and increasing complexity of the endpoints open for investigation. Additionally, the nature of exposure is also likely to play a significant role in the differences between studies, in a manner that will depend on the study type under investigation. For example, distinguishing the effects of individual pollutants remains a challenge for epidemiological studies, especially where there is high correlation between pollutants (e.g. $PM_{2.5}$ and NO_2 from traffic-derived sources). Controlled exposure studies in man and animals are frequently criticised for the high concentrations of their exposures; a criticism that still applies to many of the studies performed in recent years. Indeed, little consensus has been reached in striking a balance between using a realistic dose that models long-term exposure with obtaining suitably high exposure to explore pathogenic mechanisms in short-term studies. However, the number of studies, both epidemiological and experimental, assessing the effects of longer periods of exposure are increasing. Overall, results of these studies are somewhat reassuring in that the direction of effect matches those of short-term studies.

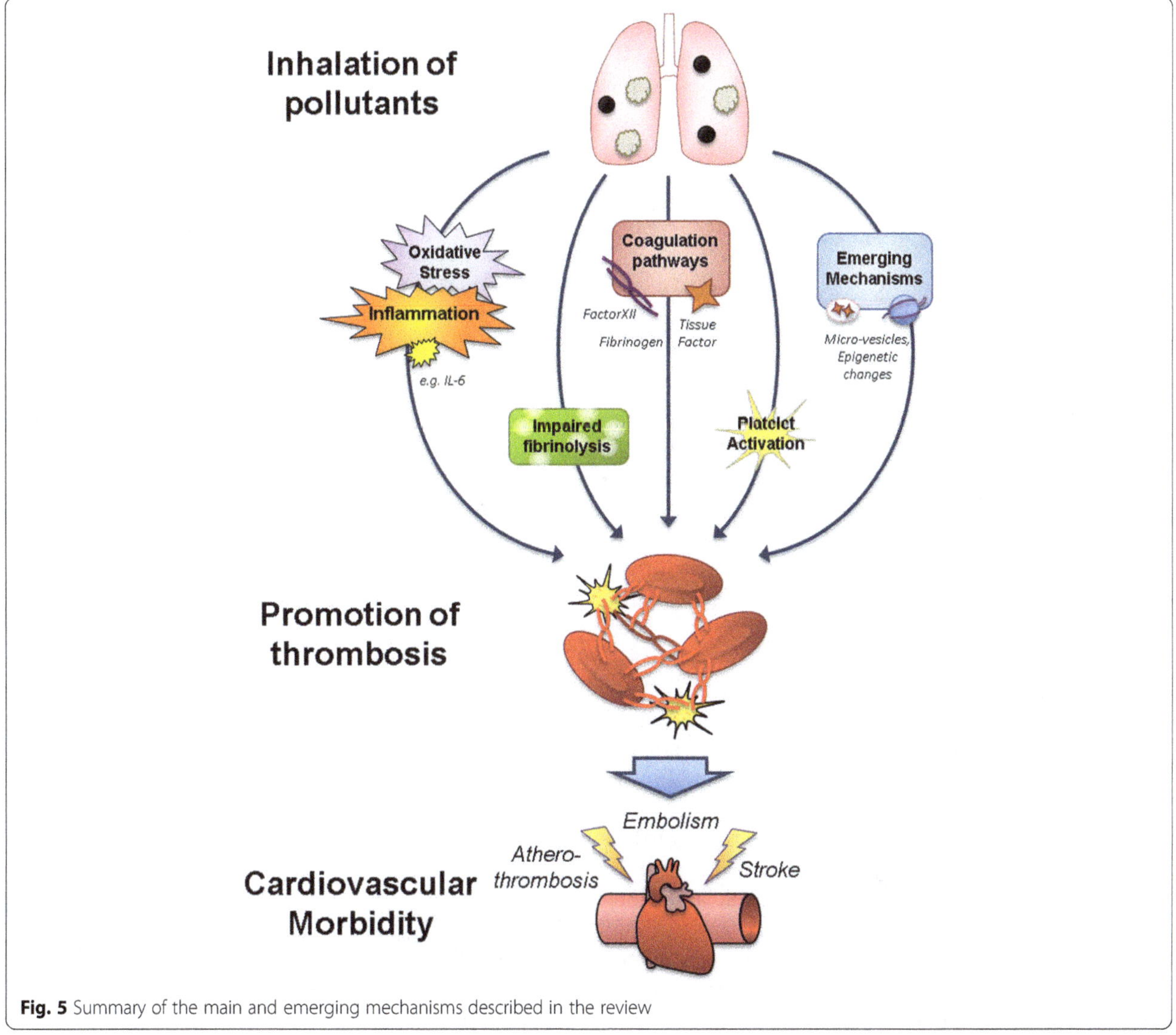

Fig. 5 Summary of the main and emerging mechanisms described in the review

While the remit of this literature review was to address whether gaseous co-pollutants have haemostatic effects, there have been too few studies to make this assumption with any certainty. Epidemiological studies suggest that it is likely that ambient levels of gases such as NOx, O_3, and possibly SO_2, are associated with biomarkers of thrombotic pathways, however, a paucity of experimental studies means it is not possible to draw any conclusions as to the wider functional consequences of such observations, or address more taxing issues such as causality. Of those few studies available, it does appear that gases can alter thrombotic pathways, however, initial indications suggest that inconsistences between studies could be even greater than that of PM; an observation that might not be especially surprising given that our focus is on a physiological system (the blood) some distance from the initial organ of exposure (the lung). Obtaining evidence of a dose-dependency of the effects of gases will again be important for advancing this area.

While our understanding of the pathophysiologic mechanisms by which air pollution promotes thrombosis remains incomplete, significant progress has been made. Similarities in the pattern of biological actions on the haemostatic system suggest that the findings of short-terms studies provide relevant, and valuable, information. Multiple mechanistic pathways are plausible, including platelet activation, oxidative stress, interactions between inflammatory mediators and impaired fibrinolysis. Emerging pathways of interest include the role of circulating microvesicles, epigenetic modifications and alterations in sensitivity to the above caused by genetic polymorphisms. A schematic overview of these pathways is shown in Fig. 5. There is great complexity in the coagulation cascade and its interaction with other pathways leading to thrombosis (see Figs. 2 and 3), with many levels of feedback regulation (positive and negative). Subsequently, it has been difficult to disentangle which points in the pathway are pivotal in driving the haemostatic effects of PM. Increases in circulating fibrinogen are one of the more consistent observations across studies, thus the availability or activation of this mediator could be significant. In the same respect, platelets (and platelet-derived mediators) appear to play an important role in driving the pro-thrombotic effects of air pollution. It is likely that these mechanisms act in concert, and potentially acting synergistically to amplify the overall effect on the blood. The mechanism by which inhaled pollutants cause thrombotic effects in distance vascular beds has not been elucidated further to any great degree in the publications reviewed here (refer to [19, 20, 76, 77] for this), although inflammatory and oxidative mediators remain a possibility, and building evidence for the translocation of nano-sized particles into the circulation offer the potential that these particles could directly interfere with blood factors. Experimental studies using interventions (e.g. pharmacological inhibition, genetic modifications) to inhibit specific pathways will be useful in dissecting out the key pathways of interest. Ultimately reducing the health effects of air pollution will rely on removal of pollutants and a better understanding of these mechanisms will help ascertain which pollutants are most harmful and which populations are most at risk. Additionally, while primary prevention is the main desire in this field, there could be value in identifying medications to prevent specific thrombotic pathways for those individuals who may be especially susceptible (e.g. patients with a prior history of ischaemic stroke or CAD) that have an unavoidable exposure to raised levels of air pollution (e.g. reside close to traffic).

In summary, the recent evidence supports a role for a pro-thrombotic effect of air pollution, through the activation of multiple pathophysiological processes. It is highly likely that these effects will contribute to the overall cardiovascular morbidity associated with air pollution and increase the risk of thrombotic effects in those with pre-existing CVD. A clearer understanding of dose-dependency of effects and of the effects of longer-term exposures, would greatly add to the case for causality of the associations between long-term average ambient concentrations of air pollutants and indices of cardiovascular morbidity. Key area of future research will be to assess the role of gaseous pollutants and studies that directly compare potentially susceptible individuals/models with healthy counterparts.

Abbreviations

ADP: Agonist adenosine diphosphate; AHA: American Heart Association; APTT: Activated partial thromboplastin time; CAD: Coronary artery disease; CAP: Concentrated ambient particles; CB: Carbon black; CHD: Coronary heart disease; CO: Carbon monoxide; COPD: Chronic obstructive pulmonary disease; CRP: C reactive protein; CVD: Cardiovascular disease; DE: Diesel exhaust; DEP: Diesel exhaust particles; eNOS: endothelial nitric oxide synthanse; ETP: Endogenous thrombin potential; FVII: Factor VII; H: hour; HO-1: Hemoxygenase-1; IL-6: Interleukin-6; IQR: Interquartile range; Kg: kilogram; LDL: Low density lipoprotein; mg: milligram; NO_2: Nitrogen dioxide; NOS 2A: Nitric oxide synthase 2A (NOS2A); NOx: Nitric oxides; O_3: ozone; PAI-1: Plasminogen activator inhibitor-1; PLAU: urokinase-type plasminogen activator gene; PNC: Particle number concentration; Ppm: parts per million; PT: Prothrombin time; sCD40L: soluble CD40 ligand; SES: Socio-economic status; SHRs: Spontaneously hypertensive rats; SO_2: sulphur dioxide; sP-selectin: soluble platelet selectin; TAT: Thrombin-anti-thrombin; TF: Tissue factor; TM: Thrombodulin; TNF-α: Tumour necrosis factor-alpha; TPA: Tissue plasminogen activator; UFP: Ultrafine particle; vWF: von Willebrand factor; μg: microgram

Funding

This work was partially supported by the National Institute for Health Research Health Protection Research Unit (NIHR HPRU) in Health Impacts of Environmental Hazards (HPRU-2012-10,030). The views expressed are those of the authors and not necessarily those of the NHS, the NIHR, the Department of Health or Public Health England. MRM is funded by a British Heart Foundation Special Project Grant (SP/15/8/31575).

Authors' contributions
SR and MRM both collected the data, analysed and interpreted the data and wrote the manuscript. Both authors read and approved the final manuscript.

Competing interests
The authors declare that they have no competing interests.

Author details
[1]Centre for Radiation, Chemical and Environmental Hazards, Public Health England, Harwell Science and Innovation Campus, Didcot, Oxfordshire OX11 0RQ, UK. [2]University/BHF Centre of Cardiovascular Science, University of Edinburgh, Edinburgh, UK.

References
1. Lelieveld J, Evans JS, Fnais M, Giannadaki D, Pozzer A. The contribution of outdoor air pollution sources to premature mortality on a global scale. Nature. 2015;525(7569):367–71.
2. Cohen AJ, Brauer M, Burnett R, Anderson HR, Frostad J, Estep K, Balakrishnan K, Brunekreef B, Dandona L, Dandona R, et al. Estimates and 25-year trends of the global burden of disease attributable to ambient air pollution: an analysis of data from the global burden of diseases study 2015. Lancet (London, England). 2017;389(10082):1907–18.
3. Lim SS, Vos T, Flaxman AD, Danaei G, Shibuya K, Adair-Rohani H, Amann M, Anderson HR, Andrews KG, Aryee M, et al. A comparative risk assessment of burden of disease and injury attributable to 67 risk factors and risk factor clusters in 21 regions, 1990-2010: a systematic analysis for the global burden of disease study 2010. Lancet (London, England). 2012;380(9859):2224–60.
4. Brook RD, Rajagopalan S, Pope CA 3rd, Brook JR, Bhatnagar A, Diez-Roux AV, Holguin F, Hong Y, Luepker RV, Mittleman MA, et al. Particulate matter air pollution and cardiovascular disease: an update to the scientific statement from the American Heart Association. Circulation. 2010;121(21):2331–78.
5. van de Loo J. Circulating factors of the haemostatic systems as indicators of increased or reduced coronary risk. Br J Haematol. 1995;91(4):777–82.
6. Danesh J, Lewington S, Thompson SG, Lowe GD, Collins R, Kostis JB, Wilson AC, Folsom AR, Wu K, Benderly M, et al. Plasma fibrinogen level and the risk of major cardiovascular diseases and nonvascular mortality: an individual participant meta-analysis. JAMA. 2005;294(14):1799–809.
7. Hildebrandt K, Ruckerl R, Koenig W, Schneider A, Pitz M, Heinrich J, Marder V, Frampton M, Oberdorster G, Wichmann HE, et al. Short-term effects of air pollution: a panel study of blood markers in patients with chronic pulmonary disease. Particle and fibre toxicology. 2009;6:25.
8. Dadvand P, Nieuwenhuijsen MJ, Agusti A, de Batlle J, Benet M, Beelen R, Cirach M, Martinez D, Hoek G, Basagana X, et al. Air pollution and biomarkers of systemic inflammation and tissue repair in COPD patients. Eur Respir J. 2014;44(3):603–13.
9. Thompson AM, Zanobetti A, Silverman F, Schwartz J, Coull B, Urch B, Speck M, Brook JR, Manno M, Gold DR. Baseline repeated measures from controlled human exposure studies: associations between ambient air pollution exposure and the systemic inflammatory biomarkers IL-6 and fibrinogen. Environ Health Perspect. 2010;118(1):120–4.
10. Gong J, Zhu T, Kipen H, Wang G, Hu M, Guo Q, Ohman-Strickland P, SE L, Wang Y, Zhu P, et al. Comparisons of ultrafine and fine particles in their associations with biomarkers reflecting physiological pathways. Environ Sci Technol. 2014;48(9):5264–73.
11. Wu S, Deng F, Wei H, Huang J, Wang H, Shima M, Wang X, Qin Y, Zheng C, Hao Y, et al. Chemical constituents of ambient particulate air pollution and biomarkers of inflammation, coagulation and homocysteine in healthy adults: a prospective panel study. Part Fibre Toxicol. 2012;9:49.
12. Delfino RJ, Staimer N, Tjoa T, Gillen DL, Polidori A, Arhami M, Kleinman MT, Vaziri ND, Longhurst J, Sioutas C. Air pollution exposures and circulating biomarkers of effect in a susceptible population: clues to potential causal component mixtures and mechanisms. Environ Health Perspect. 2009;117(8): 1232–8.
13. Emmerechts J, Jacobs L, Van Kerckhoven S, Loyen S, Mathieu C, Fierens F, Nemery B, Nawrot TS, Hoylaerts MF. Air pollution-associated procoagulant changes: the role of circulating microvesicles. J Thromb Haemost. 2012; 10(1):96–106.
14. Rich DQ, Kipen HM, Huang W, Wang G, Wang Y, Zhu P, Ohman-Strickland P, Hu M, Philipp C, Diehl SR, et al. Association between changes in air pollution levels during the Beijing Olympics and biomarkers of inflammation and thrombosis in healthy young adults. JAMA. 2012;307(19):2068–78.
15. Son JY, Lee JT, Kim KH, Jung K, Bell ML. Characterization of fine particulate matter and associations between particulate chemical constituents and mortality in Seoul, Korea. Environ Health Perspect. 2012;120(6):872–8.
16. Steenhof M, Gosens I, Strak M, Godri KJ, Hoek G, Cassee FR, Mudway IS, Kelly FJ, Harrison RM, Lebret E, et al. In vitro toxicity of particulate matter (PM) collected at different sites in the Netherlands is associated with PM composition, size fraction and oxidative potential–the RAPTES project. Part Fibre Toxicol. 2011;8:26.
17. Gray DL, Wallace LA, Brinkman MC, Buehler SS, La Londe C. Respiratory and cardiovascular effects of metals in ambient particulate matter: a critical review. Rev Environ Contam Toxicol. 2015;234:135–203.
18. Sangani RG, Soukup JM, Ghio AJ. Metals in air pollution particles decrease whole-blood coagulation time. Inhal Toxicol. 2010;22(8):621–6.
19. Miller MR, Shaw CA, Langrish JP. From particles to patients: oxidative stress and the cardiovascular effects of air pollution. Futur Cardiol. 2012;8(4):577–602.
20. Kelly FJ, Fussell JC. Role of oxidative stress in cardiovascular disease outcomes following exposure to ambient air pollution. Free Radic Biol Med. 2017;110:345–67.
21. Frampton MW, Bausch J, Chalupa D, Hopke PK, Little EL, Oakes D, Stewart JC, Utell MJ. Effects of outdoor air pollutants on platelet activation in people with type 2 diabetes. Inhal Toxicol. 2012;24(12):831–8.
22. Peters A, Greven S, Heid IM, Baldari F, Breitner S, Bellander T, Chrysohoou C, Illig T, Jacquemin B, Koenig W, et al. Fibrinogen genes modify the fibrinogen response to ambient particulate matter. Am J Respir Crit Care Med. 2009;179(6):484–91.
23. Chen R, Zhao Z, Sun Q, Lin Z, Zhao A, Wang C, Xia Y, Xu X, Kan H. Size-fractionated particulate air pollution and circulating biomarkers of inflammation, coagulation, and vasoconstriction in a panel of young adults. Epidemiology. 2015;26(3):328–36.
24. Ruckerl R, Hampel R, Breitner S, Cyrys J, Kraus U, Carter J, Dailey L, Devlin RB, Diaz-Sanchez D, Koenig W, et al. Associations between ambient air pollution and blood markers of inflammation and coagulation/fibrinolysis in susceptible populations. Environ Int. 2014;70:32–49.
25. Oberdorster G, Sharp Z, Atudorei V, Elder A, Gelein R, Lunts A, Kreyling W, Cox C. Extrapulmonary translocation of ultrafine carbon particles following whole-body inhalation exposure of rats. J Toxicol Environ Health A. 2002; 65(20):1531–43.
26. Shimada A, Kawamura N, Okajima M, Kaewamatawong T, Inoue H, Morita T. Translocation pathway of the intratracheally instilled ultrafine particles from the lung into the blood circulation in the mouse. Toxicol Pathol. 2006;34(7):949–57.
27. Miller MR, Raftis JB, Langrish JP, McLean SG, Samutrtai P, Connell SP, Wilson S, Vesey AT, Fokkens PHB, Boere AJF, et al. Inhaled nanoparticles accumulate at sites of vascular disease. ACS Nano. 2017;11(5):4542–52.
28. Buckley A, Warren J, Hodgson A, Marczylo T, Ignatyev K, Guo C, Smith R. Slow lung clearance and limited translocation of four sizes of inhaled iridium nanoparticles. Part Fibre Toxicol. 2017;14(1):5.
29. Rudez G, Janssen NA, Kilinc E, Leebeek FW, Gerlofs-Nijland ME, Spronk HM, ten Cate H, Cassee FR, de Maat MP. Effects of ambient air pollution on hemostasis and inflammation. Environ Health Perspect. 2009;117(6):995–1001.
30. Hajat A, Allison M, Diez-Roux AV, Jenny NS, Jorgensen NW, Szpiro AA, Vedal S, Kaufman JD. Long-term exposure to air pollution and markers of inflammation, coagulation, and endothelial activation: a repeat-measures analysis in the multi-ethnic study of atherosclerosis (MESA). Epidemiology (Cambridge, Mass). 2015;26(3):310–20.
31. Baccarelli A, Zanobetti A, Martinelli I, Grillo P, Hou L, Giacomini S, Bonzini M, Lanzani G, Mannucci PM, Bertazzi PA, et al. Effects of exposure to air pollution on blood coagulation. J Thromb Haemost. 2007;5(2):252–60.
32. Marczylo EL, Jacobs MN, Gant TW. Environmentally induced epigenetic toxicity: potential public health concerns. Crit Rev Toxicol. 2016;46(8):676–700.
33. Baccarelli A, Wright RO, Bollati V, Tarantini L, Litonjua AA, Suh HH, Zanobetti A, Sparrow D, Vokonas PS, Schwartz J. Rapid DNA. Methylation changes after exposure to traffic particles. Am J Respir Crit Care Med. 2009;179(7):572–8.
34. Tarantini L, Bonzini M, Apostoli P, Pegoraro V, Bollati V, Marinelli B, Cantone L, Rizzo G, Hou L, Schwartz J, et al. Effects of particulate matter on genomic DNA methylation content and iNOS promoter methylation. Environ Health Perspect. 2009;117(2):217–22.
35. Bind MA, Lepeule J, Zanobetti A, Gasparrini A, Baccarelli A, Coull BA, Tarantini L, Vokonas PS, Koutrakis P, Schwartz J. Air pollution and gene-

specific methylation in the normative aging study: association, effect modification, and mediation analysis. Epigenetics. 2014;9(3):448–58.
36. Hoffmann B, Moebus S, Dragano N, Stang A, Mohlenkamp S, Schmermund A, Memmesheimer M, Brocker-Preuss M, Mann K, Erbel R, et al. Chronic residential exposure to particulate matter air pollution and systemic inflammatory markers. Environ Health Perspect. 2009;117(8):1302–8.
37. Viehmann A, Hertel S, Fuks K, Eisele L, Moebus S, Mohlenkamp S, Nonnemacher M, Jakobs H, Erbel R, Jockel KH, et al. Long-term residential exposure to urban air pollution, and repeated measures of systemic blood markers of inflammation and coagulation. Occup Environ Med. 2015;72(9): 656–63.
38. Dabass A, Talbott EO, Venkat A, Rager J, Marsh GM, Sharma RK, Holguin F. Association of exposure to particulate matter (PM) air pollution and biomarkers of cardiovascular disease risk in adult NHANES participants (2001-2008). Int J Hyg Environ Health. 2015;219(3):301–10.
39. Forbes LJ, Patel MD, Rudnicka AR, Cook DG, Bush T, Stedman JR, Whincup PH, Strachan DP, Anderson RH. Chronic exposure to outdoor air pollution and markers of systemic inflammation. Epidemiology (Cambridge, Mass). 2009;20(2):245–53.
40. Lanki T, Hampel R, Tiittanen P, Andrich S, Beelen R, Brunekreef B, Dratva J, De Faire U, Fuks KB, Hoffmann B, et al. Air pollution from road traffic and systemic inflammation in adults: a cross-sectional analysis in the European ESCAPE project. Environ Health Perspect. 2015;123(8):785–91.
41. Hampel R, Peters A, Beelen R, Brunekreef B, Cyrys J, de Faire U, de Hoogh K, Fuks K, Hoffmann B, Huls A, et al. Long-term effects of elemental composition of particulate matter on inflammatory blood markers in European cohorts. Environ Int. 2015;82:76–84.
42. Green R, Broadwin R, Malig B, Basu R, Gold EB, Qi L, Sternfeld B, Bromberger JT, Greendale GA, Kravitz HM, et al. Long-and short-term exposure to air pollution and inflammatory/hemostatic markers in midlife women. Epidemiology (Cambridge, Mass). 2015;27(2):211–20.
43. Emmerechts J, Hoylaerts MF. The effect of air pollution on haemostasis. Hamostaseologie. 2012;32(1):5–13.
44. Panasevich S, Leander K, Rosenlund M, Ljungman P, Bellander T, de Faire U, Pershagen G, Nyberg F. Associations of long- and short-term air pollution exposure with markers of inflammation and coagulation in a population sample. Occup Environ Med. 2009;66(11):747–53.
45. Mostafavi N, Vlaanderen J, Chadeau-Hyam M, Beelen R, Modig L, Palli D, Bergdahl IA, Vineis P, Hoek G, Kyrtopoulos S, et al. Inflammatory markers in relation to long-term air pollution. Environ Int. 2015;81:1–7.
46. Baccarelli A, Martinelli I, Zanobetti A, Grillo P, Hou LF, Bertazzi PA, Mannucci PM, Schwartz J. Exposure to particulate air pollution and risk of deep vein thrombosis. Arch Intern Med. 2008;168(9):920–7.
47. Mills NL, Tornqvist H, Robinson SD, Gonzalez M, Darnley K, MacNee W, Boon NA, Donaldson K, Blomberg A, Sandstrom T, et al. Diesel exhaust inhalation causes vascular dysfunction and impaired endogenous fibrinolysis. Circulation. 2005;112(25):3930–6.
48. Barath S, Mills NL, Lundback M, Tornqvist H, Lucking AJ, Langrish JP, Soderberg S, Boman C, Westerholm R, Londahl J, et al. Impaired vascular function after exposure to diesel exhaust generated at urban transient running conditions. Part Fibre Toxicol. 2010;7:19.
49. Mills NL, Tornqvist H, Gonzalez MC, Vink E, Robinson SD, Soderberg S, Boon NA, Donaldson K, Sandstrom T, Blomberg A, et al. Ischemic and thrombotic effects of dilute diesel-exhaust inhalation in men with coronary heart disease. N Engl J Med. 2007;357(11):1075–82.
50. Graff DW, Cascio WE, Rappold A, Zhou H, Huang YC, Devlin RB. Exposure to concentrated coarse air pollution particles causes mild cardiopulmonary effects in healthy young adults. Environ Health Perspect. 2009;117(7):1089–94.
51. Lucking AJ, Lundback M, Barath SL, Mills NL, Sidhu MK, Langrish JP, Boon NA, Pourazar J, Badimon JJ, Gerlofs-Nijland ME, et al. Particle traps prevent adverse vascular and prothrombotic effects of diesel engine exhaust inhalation in men. Circulation. 2011;123(16):1721–8.
52. Lucking AJ, Lundback M, Mills NL, Faratian D, Barath SL, Pourazar J, Cassee FR, Donaldson K, Boon NA, Badimon JJ, et al. Diesel exhaust inhalation increases thrombus formation in man. Eur Heart J. 2008;29(24):3043–51.
53. Langrish JP, Lundback M, Barath S, Soderberg S, Mills NL, Newby DE, Sandstrom T, Blomberg A. Exposure to nitrogen dioxide is not associated with vascular dysfunction in man. Inhal Toxicol. 2010;22(3):192–8.
54. Devlin RB, Duncan KE, Jardim M, Schmitt MT, Rappold AG, Diaz-Sanchez D. Controlled exposure of healthy young volunteers to ozone causes cardiovascular effects. Circulation. 2012;126(1):104–11.
55. Mills NL, Robinson SD, Fokkens PH, Leseman DL, Miller MR, Anderson D, Freney EJ, Heal MR, Donovan RJ, Blomberg A, et al. Exposure to concentrated ambient particles does not affect vascular function in patients with coronary heart disease. Environ Health Perspect. 2008;116(6):709–15.
56. Mills NL, Miller MR, Lucking AJ, Beveridge J, Flint L, Boere AJ, Fokkens PH, Boon NA, Sandstrom T, Blomberg A, et al. Combustion-derived nanoparticulate induces the adverse vascular effects of diesel exhaust inhalation. Eur Heart J. 2011;32(21):2660–71.
57. Stewart JC, Chalupa DC, Devlin RB, Frasier LM, Huang LS, Little EL, Lee SM, Phipps RP, Pietropaoli AP, Taubman MB, et al. Vascular effects of ultrafine particles in persons with type 2 diabetes. Environ Health Perspect. 2010; 118(12):1692–8.
58. Samet JM, Rappold A, Graff D, Cascio WE, Berntsen JH, Huang YC, Herbst M, Bassett M, Montilla T, Hazucha MJ, et al. Concentrated ambient ultrafine particle exposure induces cardiac changes in young healthy volunteers. Am J Respir Crit Care Med. 2009;179(11):1034–42.
59. Pettit AP, Brooks A, Laumbach R, Fiedler N, Wang Q, Strickland PO, Madura K, Zhang J, Kipen HM. Alteration of peripheral blood monocyte gene expression in humans following diesel exhaust inhalation. Inhal Toxicol. 2012;24(3):172–81.
60. Mutlu GM, Green D, Bellmeyer A, Baker CM, Burgess Z, Rajamannan N, Christman JW, Foiles N, Kamp DW, Ghio AJ, et al. Ambient particulate matter accelerates coagulation via an IL-6-dependent pathway. J Clin Invest. 2007;117(10):2952–61.
61. Budinger GR, McKell JL, Urich D, Foiles N, Weiss I, Chiarella SE, Gonzalez A, Soberanes S, Ghio AJ, Nigdelioglu R, et al. Particulate matter-induced lung inflammation increases systemic levels of PAI-1 and activates coagulation through distinct mechanisms. PLoS One. 2011;6(4):e18525.
62. Kilinc E, Van Oerle R, Borissoff JI, Oschatz C, Gerlofs-Nijland ME, Janssen NA, Cassee FR, Sandstrom T, Renne T, Ten Cate H, et al. Factor XII activation is essential to sustain the procoagulant effects of particulate matter. J Thromb Haemost. 2011;9(7):1359–67.
63. Driscoll KE, Costa DL, Hatch G, Henderson R, Oberdorster G, Salem H, Schlesinger RB. Intratracheal instillation as an exposure technique for the evaluation of respiratory tract toxicity: uses and limitations. Toxicol Sci. 2000;55(1):24–35.
64. Henderson RF, Driscoll KE, Harkema JR, Lindenschmidt RC, Chang IY, Maples KR, Barr EB. A comparison of the inflammatory response of the lung to inhaled versus instilled particles in F344 rats. Fundam Appl Toxicol. 1995; 24(2):183–97.
65. Miyabara Y, Ichinose T, Takano H, Sagai M. Diesel exhaust inhalation enhances airway hyperresponsiveness in mice. Int Arch Allergy Immunol. 1998;116(2):124–31.
66. Nemmar A, Subramaniyan D, Ali BH. Protective effect of curcumin on pulmonary and cardiovascular effects induced by repeated exposure to diesel exhaust particles in mice. PLoS One. 2012;7(6):e39554.
67. Ali BH, Al Za'abi M, Shalaby A, Manoj P, Waly MI, Yasin J, Fahim M, Nemmar A. The effect of thymoquinone treatment on the combined renal and pulmonary toxicity of cisplatin and diesel exhaust particles. Exp Biol Med (Maywood). 2015;240(12):1698–707.
68. Nemmar A, Nemery B, Hoet PH, Vermylen J, Hoylaerts MF. Pulmonary inflammation and thrombogenicity caused by diesel particles in hamsters: role of histamine. Am J Respir Crit Care Med. 2003;168(11):1366–72.
69. Tabor CM, Shaw CA, Robertson S, Miller MR, Duffin R, Donaldson K, Newby DE, Hadoke PW. Platelet activation independent of pulmonary inflammation contributes to diesel exhaust particulate-induced promotion of arterial thrombosis. Part Fibre Toxicol. 2016;13:6.
70. Smyth E, Solomon A, Birrell MA, Smallwood MJ, Winyard PG, Tetley TD, Emerson M. Influence of inflammation and nitric oxide upon platelet aggregation following deposition of diesel exhaust particles in the airways. Br J Pharmacol. 2017;174(13):2130–9.
71. Nemmar A, Zia S, Subramaniyan D, Fahim MA, Ali BH. Exacerbation of thrombotic events by diesel exhaust particle in mouse model of hypertension. Toxicology. 2011;285(1–2):39–45.
72. Wilson DW, Aung HH, Lame MW, Plummer L, Pinkerton KE, Ham W, Kleeman M, Norris JW, Tablin F. Exposure of mice to concentrated ambient particulate matter results in platelet and systemic cytokine activation. Inhal Toxicol. 2010;22(4):267–76.
73. Kodavanti UP, Thomas R, Ledbetter AD, Schladweiler MC, Shannahan JH, Wallenborn JG, Lund AK, Campen MJ, Butler EO, Gottipolu RR, et al. Vascular and cardiac impairments in rats inhaling ozone and diesel exhaust particles. Environ Health Perspect. 2011;119(3):312–8.

74. Upadhyay S, Stoeger T, George L, Schladweiler MC, Kodavanti U, Ganguly K, Schulz H. Ultrafine carbon particle mediated cardiovascular impairment of aged spontaneously hypertensive rats. Part Fibre Toxicol. 2014;11:36.
75. Magnusson RS, Patterson D. The role of law and governance reform in the global response to non-communicable diseases. Glob Health. 2014;10:44.
76. Newby DE, Mannucci PM, Tell GS, Baccarelli AA, Brook RD, Donaldson K, Forastiere F, Franchini M, Franco OH, Graham I, et al. Expert position paper on air pollution and cardiovascular disease. Eur Heart J. 2015;36(2):83–93b.
77. Fiordelisi A, Piscitelli P, Trimarco B, Coscioni E, Iaccarino G, Sorriento D. The mechanisms of air pollution and particulate matter in cardiovascular diseases. Heart Fail Rev. 2017;22(3):337–47.
78. Niemann B, Rohrbach S, Miller MR, Newby DE, Fuster V, Kovacic JC. Oxidative stress and cardiovascular risk: obesity, diabetes, smoking, and pollution: part 3 of a 3-part series. J Am Coll Cardiol. 2017;70(2):230–51.

4

Differences in MWCNT- and SWCNT-induced DNA methylation alterations in association with the nuclear deposition

Deniz Öner[1†], Manosij Ghosh[1†], Hannelore Bové[2,3], Matthieu Moisse[4,5], Bram Boeckx[4,5], Radu C. Duca[6], Katrien Poels[6], Katrien Luyts[1], Eveline Putzeys[1,7], Kirsten Van Landuydt[7], Jeroen AJ Vanoirbeek[1,6], Marcel Ameloot[3], Diether Lambrechts[4,5], Lode Godderis[6,8] and Peter HM Hoet[1*]

Abstract

Background: Subtle DNA methylation alterations mediated by carbon nanotubes (CNTs) exposure might contribute to pathogenesis and disease susceptibility. It is known that both multi-walled carbon nanotubes (MWCNTs) and single-walled carbon nanotubes (SWCNTs) interact with nucleus. Such, nuclear-CNT interaction may affect the DNA methylation effects. In order to understand the epigenetic toxicity, in particular DNA methylation alterations, of SWCNTs and short MWCNTs, we performed global/genome-wide, gene-specific DNA methylation and RNA-expression analyses after exposing human bronchial epithelial cells (16HBE14o- cell line). In addition, the presence of CNTs on/in the cell nucleus was evaluated in a label-free way using femtosecond pulsed laser microscopy.

Results: Generally, a higher number of SWCNTs, compared to MWCNTs, was deposited at both the cellular and nuclear level after exposure. Nonetheless, both CNT types were in physical contact with the nuclei. While particle type dependency was noticed for the identified genome-wide and gene-specific alterations, no global DNA methylation alteration on 5-methylcytosine (5-mC) sites was observed for both CNTs. After exposure to MWCNTs, 2398 genes were hypomethylated (at gene promoters), and after exposure to SWCNTs, 589 CpG sites (located on 501 genes) were either hypo- ($N = 493$ CpG sites) or hypermethylated ($N = 96$ CpG sites).

Cells exposed to MWCNTs exhibited a better correlation between gene promoter methylation and gene expression alterations. Differentially methylated and expressed genes induced changes (MWCNTs > SWCNTs) at different cellular pathways, such as p53 signalling, DNA damage repair and cell cycle. On the other hand, SWCNT exposure showed hypermethylation on functionally important genes, such as SKI proto-oncogene (*SKI*), glutathione S-transferase pi 1 (*GTSP1*) and shroom family member 2 (*SHROOM2*) and neurofibromatosis type I (*NF1*), which the latter is both hypermethylated and downregulated.

Conclusion: After exposure to both types of CNTs, epigenetic alterations may contribute to toxic or repair response. Moreover, our results suggest that the observed differences in the epigenetic response depend on particle type and differential CNT-nucleus interactions.

Keywords: Carbon nanotubes, DNA methylation, Gene expression, Nuclear uptake, Toxicity, Epigenetics, Epigenomics, Genotoxicity, Nanoparticles, Nanomaterials, In vitro

* Correspondence: peter.hoet@kuleuven.be
†Equal contributors
[1]Laboratory of Toxicology, Unit of Environment and Health, Department of Public Health and Primary Care, KU Leuven, 3000 Leuven, Belgium
Full list of author information is available at the end of the article

Background

Carbon nanotubes (CNTs) are a class of graphene-based engineered nanomaterials. These have a tubular and fibre structure with a diameter in nanometer (nm). CNTs can be divided into categories by the number of layers of the rolled-up graphene, which will define their diameter size: e.g. single-walled CNTs (SWCNTs) with a diameter between 0.7 and 3 nm and multi-walled CNTs (MWCNTs) with a diameter between 10 and 200 nm [1]. SWCNTs are present in stiff, rope-like bundles due to the increased van der Waals forces caused by their extremely small diameter and high surface area. In contrast, MWCNTs can be present in agglomerated, curly or needle-like structure.

Since CNTs display high electrical and thermal conductivity, mechanical durability and functionalization properties, they are valuable nanomaterials for the use in industry (e.g. surface films and coatings, microelectronics, energy storage, composites) and for biotechnological and biomedical approaches [2]. The market of CNTs is expected to keep on growing in the next five years based on several online market reports.

The increase in the production of CNTs raised concern regarding inhalation toxicity because of their fibre shape that is similar to asbestos fibres. In addition, their nano dimensions might result in unexpected toxic and adverse effects. For instance, It was found that MWCNTs are internalized in cells through both direct penetration and endocytosis [3]. Endosomal leakage has been seen since MWCNTs are able to pierce lysosomes because of their greater diameter, leaving fibres within the cytosol [3]. In particular, this effect might increase the inflammatory response and interaction of MWCNTs with cytosolic materials such as nucleus, proteins, organelles and RNAs. In contrast, bundled SWCNTs are not able to pierce the cell membranes due to their physicochemical properties (e.g. extremely small diameter, appearance in bundles caused by van der Waals forces) but are internalized through endocytosis [4].

Subtle DNA methylation or gene expression alterations mediated by CNT exposure might contribute to disease progression or susceptibility [5–8]. Noteworthy, in cancer cells, typically global hypomethylation occurs with gene-specific hypermethylation. Global hypomethylation (in particular, hypomethylation of centromeric regions), which leads to uncondensed DNA, might be linked with impaired segregation of the chromosomes and increased genotoxicity parameters, such as increased formation rate of micronucleus and chromosomal breaks [7]. In addition, gene expression alterations or mutations on *DNMT1* gene will lead to global hypomethylation after cell divisions (passive DNA demethylation). Gene-specific hypermethylation is linked with gene silencing (downregulation of gene expression). In addition, DNA methylation on cytosine residues 'hot spots' for spontaneous mutations due to impaired DNA repair mechanisms [9]. Gene-specific hypomethylation may up-regulate gene expression, stress-response or pro-oncogenic signalling mechanisms of the cell.

For the case of CNTs, MWCNT-uptake in *Allium cepa* resulted in increase in global DNA methylation and genotoxic response Ghosh et al. [10]. In mammalian cells and in vivo, changes in DNA methylation after CNT-exposure occurred. After intra-tracheal administration of CNTs, the gene promoter region of ATM serine/tyrosine kinase (*ATM*), which functions in DNA damage pathway, was altered in lung tissue of mice Tabish et al. [11]. Gene-specific alterations in the inflammatory response genes [such as interferon-gamma (*IFN-γ*) and tumour necrosis factor alpha (*TNF-α*)] and global DNA hypomethylation in the lung and blood after exposure to MWCNTs were observed and correlated with cytokine production and collagen deposition Brown et al. [12]. It has also been reported that exposure to some carbon-based nanoparticles (carbon black, short MWCNTs and SWCNTs) cause DNA hypermethylation at the global level in adenocarcinoma human alveolar basal epithelial cells (A549 cell line) J. Li et al. [13]. Sierra et al., observed hypomethylation of 755 CpG sites in the human lung epithelial cells (BEAS-2B) exposed to MWCNTs and four weeks of exposure induce more differentially methylated probes than their two weeks of exposure counterparts Sierra et al. [14]. In a recent study, hypermethylation of p16/Ink4a and p19/Arf followed by gene-silencing and loss of p16 and p19 proteins in mesothelioma are noted after intra-peritoneal injection to mesothelioma-inducing CNT and asbestos Chernova et al. [15]. Considering above-mentioned background, epigenetic alterations are important players in the CNT-toxicity and disease outcome.

We previously reported DNA methylation alterations at the gene-specific level in human monocyte cells after 24 h incubation with CNTs (at the concentrations of 25 and 100 μg/ml) [16]. However, CNT-type-specific DNA methylation alterations could not be determined in the monocytes, which play a role in immune response. Bronchial epithelial cells are the first barrier when CNTs reach the lungs after inhalation at occupational settings. Since CNTs are likely to deposit on the lung tissue, studying DNA methylation and subsequent gene expression alterations in these cells will elucidate possible forthcoming adverse effects upon exposure.

The mechanism of CNT-induced epigenetic alterations are currently not known. Epigenetic alterations may be caused by direct CNT-nuclear interactions which might affect the DNA methylation changes. We hypothesized that differential nuclear deposition will affect the epigenome. The following points were assessed considering similarities and differences of MWCNTs and SWCNTs: 1) CNTs localisation in nuclei of 16HBE cells. 2) Identification of global and genome-wide, gene-specific DNA methylation and expression alterations. 3) Identification of aberrant methylation and expression on functionally important genes and cellular networks in order to predict the adverse effects of CNTs.

Results

Characterisation of Cnts

MWCNTs and SWCNTs were obtained from the European Commission Joint Research Centre (JRC, Ispra, Italy) and the National Institute of Technology (NIST, Gaithersburg, Maryland, USA), respectively. The nanomaterials were characterized in detail by the manufacturers [17, 18] and previously summarized in our published study [16]. All characteristics of CNTs are summarized in Additional file 1: Table S1. In brief, the diameters of MWCNTs are approximately 11 nm and the length is on average 846 nm. The diameters of SWCNTs are about 0.8 nm and the pristine length is 8000 nm. The CNTs have a high purity (> 95% carbon) but rare elemental impurities are detected. The dynamic light scattering (DLS) analyses (Fig. 1) revealed that CNT dispersions remained stable at the experimental concentrations and that the average size was approximately 50 nm to 500 nm. The size distribution at high dose SWCNTs (100 µg/ml), showed a large peak between 500 nm to 5000 nm and a minor peak between 50 nm to 500 nm. These results might indicate increased agglomeration of the SWCNTs. We did not detect endotoxin contamination in the MWCNTs and SWCNTs dispersions, measured by an established protocol [19].

Nuclear localisation of CNTs

First of all, we investigated whether fibres can reach the nuclei of the cells. Any physical interaction between CNTs and nuclei might define their epigenetic effects. Label-free detection of CNTs was carried out by imaging their white-light generation under femtosecond pulsed laser illumination as previously described by Bové et al. for carbon black particles [20]. To validate the technique for imaging CNTs, a calibration curve of spiked ultrapure water containing known CNTs concentrations (25 and 100 µg/ml) was made and measured under identical imaging conditions (see supplementary information for a detailed description). A linear relation was observed (R^2 = 0.90) between the amount of added and detected CNTs (Additional file 1: Figure S1). This indicated that the described technique is also applicable for detecting CNTs in solution.

Next, the technique was applied to determine the number and total area of CNTs deposited inside both the cells and their corresponding nuclei. In Fig. 2, representative images are shown of both types of CNTs partially attached to or inside of the nuclei of the cells (for MWCNTs Fig. 2a-b and for SWCNTs Fig. 2c-d, Additional files 2-5: Video S1-S4). CNTs in the nucleus is demonstrated by selected z-stack slice images throughout the nucleus from top to bottom (Fig. 2b for MWCNTs, Fig. 2d for SWCNTs) and representative video of these images (Additional file 2: Video S1 and Additional file 3: Video S2). Quantitative analysis for the measurement of CNT number and total area (total area of aggregates/ cell or nucleus in µm^2) was performed using 2D images. Quantitative analysis (Fig. 3) revealed that: i) Both CNTs were internalized in the cell and in the

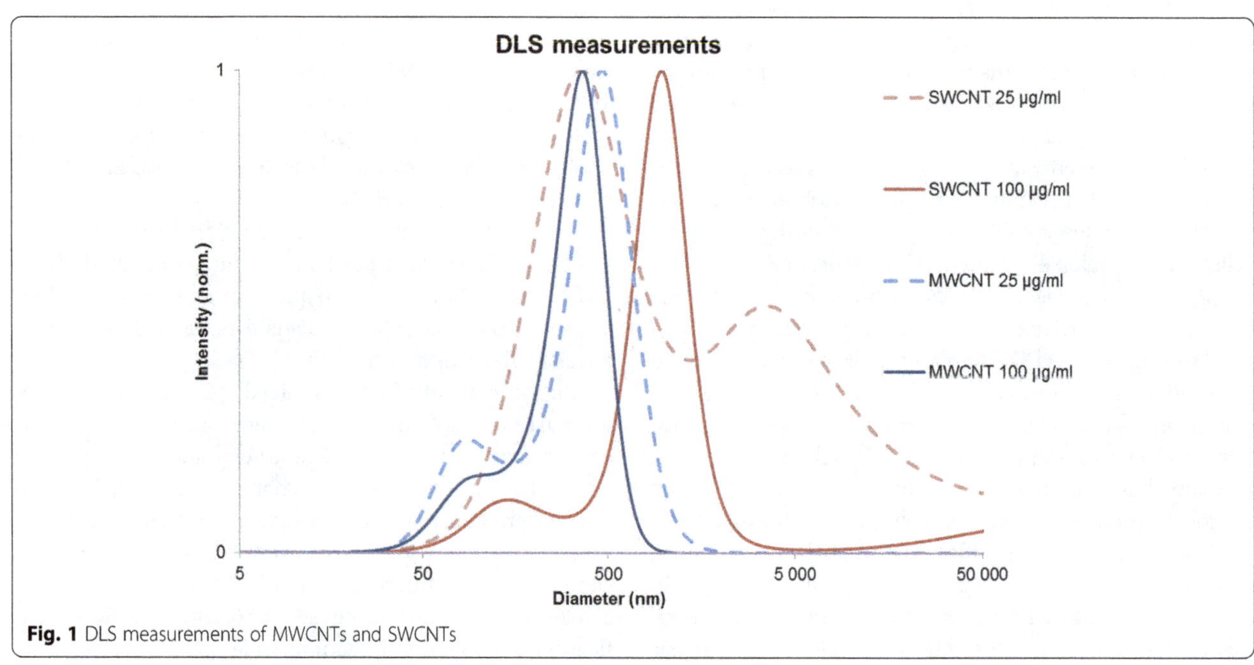

Fig. 1 DLS measurements of MWCNTs and SWCNTs

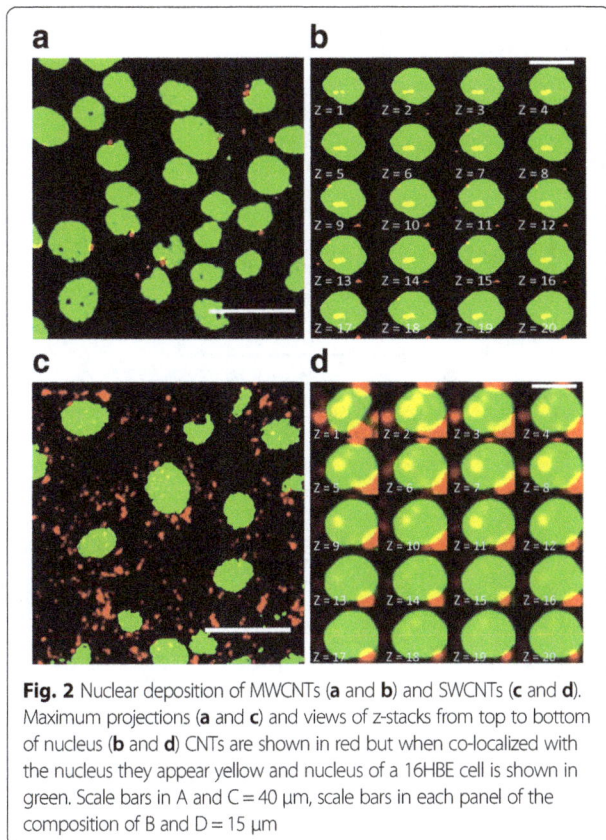

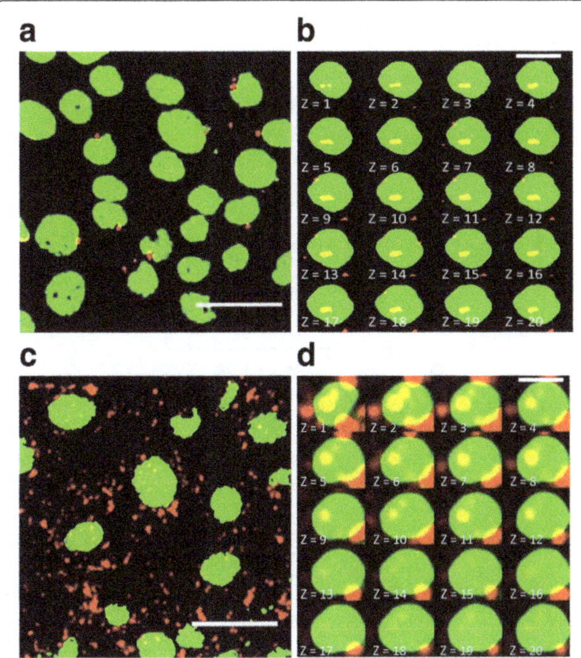

Fig. 2 Nuclear deposition of MWCNTs (**a** and **b**) and SWCNTs (**c** and **d**). Maximum projections (**a** and **c**) and views of z-stacks from top to bottom of nucleus (**b** and **d**) CNTs are shown in red but when co-localized with the nucleus they appear yellow and nucleus of a 16HBE cell is shown in green. Scale bars in A and C = 40 μm, scale bars in each panel of the composition of B and D = 15 μm

nucleus in a dose-dependent way (Fig. 3a-d); ii) There is a significant higher cellular uptake (by means of number and total area of aggregates) for SWCNTs compared to MWCNTs (Fig. 3a-b). iii) There is a significant higher nuclear uptake (by means of number a total area of aggregates) for SWCNTs compared to MWCNTs (Fig. 3c-d). However, the ratio nucleus/cellular uptake (data not shown) is similar for the two types of CNTs.

Representative videos, which show single nuclei with deposited CNTs through z-stack images taken from top to the bottom and turning around their y-axes, also clearly demonstrate the particle type dependent difference in nuclear uptake (see Additional file 2: Video S1 and Additional file 3: Video S2, Additional file 4: Video S3 and Additional file 5: Video S4). In summary, both CNTs were in physical contact with the DNA but SWCNTs were spread in greater amounts over both the nucleus and the cell.

The cytotoxicity and genotoxicity of CNTs

We studied the cytotoxicity and genotoxicity of CNTs in order to understand possible toxic mechanisms that contribute to epigenetic effects [7, 21]. MWCNTs were found to be non-cytotoxic up to a concentration of 256 μg/ml as assessed by both water-soluble tetrazolium salt-1 (WST)-1 and lactate dehydrogenase (LDH) assays (Additional file 1: Figure S2). SWCNTs induced dose-dependent cytotoxicity at doses higher than 64 μg/ml measured by WST-1 assay, despite, no cytotoxicity was observed by LDH assay. Next, induction of DNA strand breaks by CNTs was investigated (after 3 and 24 h exposure). As demonstrated in Additional file 1: Figure S3, no increase in DNA damage was noted after 3 h of exposure. Interestingly, a non-significant increase in DNA damage after 24 h of SWCNTs was observed (mean difference is 0.05 to 0.1% for MWCNTs and − 9.6 to − 9.7% for SWCNTs). As shown in Additional file 1: Figure S4, no dose-dependent increase in micronuclei formation was noted after 24 h of MWCNTs and SWCNTs exposure.

DNA methylation alterations induced by CNTs

The global DNA 5-methylcytosine (5-mC) and 5-hydroxymethylcytosine (5-hmC) alterations at all cytosine residues were analysed using liquid chromatography-mass spectrometry (LC-MS/MS) method, as reported by Godderis et al. [22]. As demonstrated in Fig. 4, exposure to CNTs did not change the global level of 5-mC and 5-hmC in the DNA compared to untreated cells (only cell culture medium and vehicle-treated) after 24 h of exposure. Treatment with 5-aza-2′-deoxycytidine (or known as Decitabine), a hypomethylating agent, induced decreased 5-mdC levels but no overall changes in 5-hmdC.

Although CNTs did not induce alterations at the global level, gene-specific DNA methylation alterations occurred. Whole-genome methylation of CpG sites of the DNA samples (from the cells exposed to CNTs for 24 h) were assessed with the Infinium HumanMethylation450K BeadChip array. The methylation level of the genes was assessed by two different approaches: one based on individual CpG sites across the genomic regions and another based on methylation of the promoter regions. We performed the latter analysis because subtle methylation differences in neighbouring CpG sites, such as those in gene promoters, can also be functional and affect gene expression. Subsequently, next generation RNA-sequencing microarray was performed in order to validate whether certain methylation alterations resulted in differential expression.

The hierarchical cluster analysis

Hierarchical cluster analysis was performed on differential methylation and expression profiles of untreated and MWCNT- and SWCNT-exposed samples, using the top 500 most differentially methylated and expressed genes, ranked by their FDR-corrected p value that referred as q value. As shown in Fig. 5a-b, MWCNT- and SWCNT-exposed cells cluster together in a distinct cluster from untreated samples. Although, some irregularities could be seen among the same exposure groups, this is possibly due to batch effect which was statistically corrected

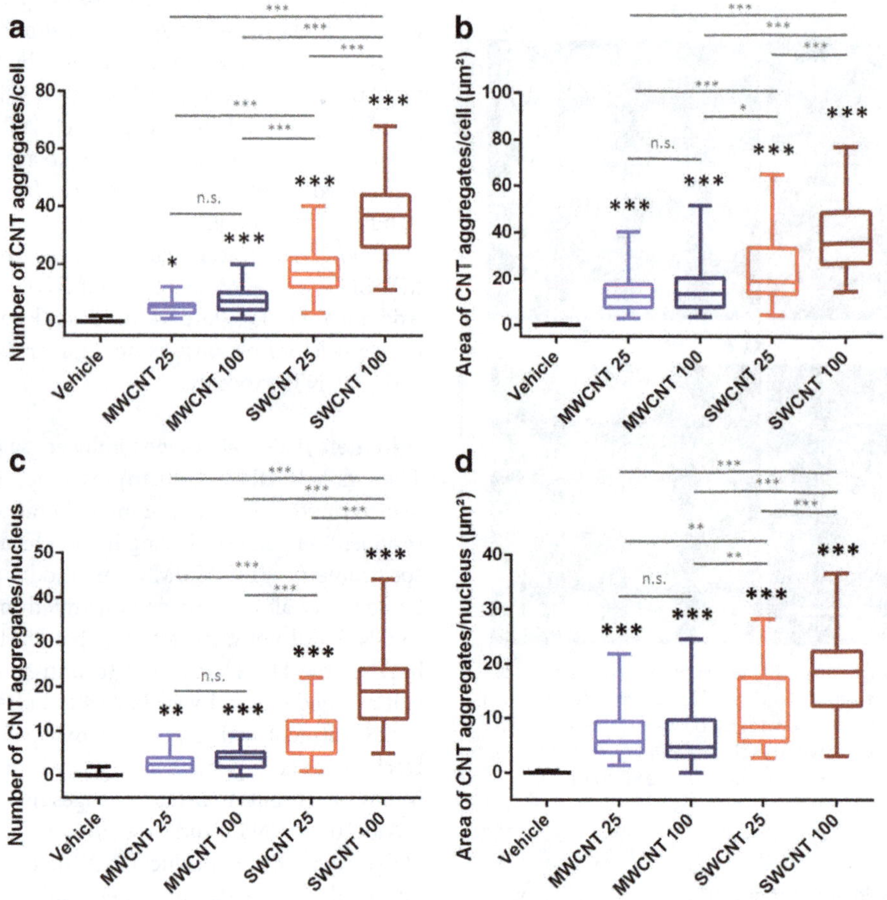

Fig. 3 Quantitative analysis of the cellular and nuclear deposition of MWCNTs and SWCNTs. **a** Number of CNT aggregates per cell; **b** total area of CNT aggregates per cell (μm^2); **c** number of CNT aggregates per nucleus, **d** total area of CNT aggregates per nucleus (μm^2). All conditions were significantly different from the control condition (vehicle) and from each other (one way ANOVA, Tukey multiple comparison) except for the different doses of MWCNTs [not significant (n.s.)]. The box plots represent median and quartiles, and the whiskers represent the 1.5 interquartile range of the lower and upper quartile ($N = 50$ for each condition). 25 and 100 represents exposure concentrations as μg/ml

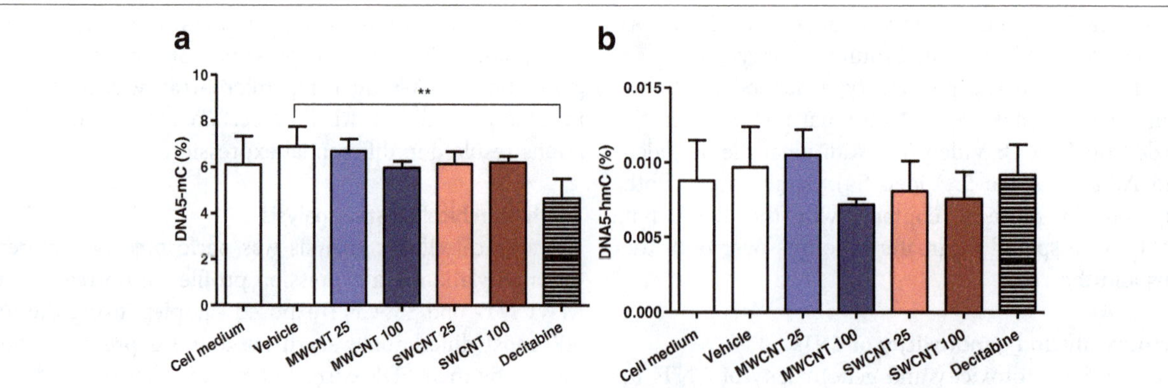

Fig. 4 Global DNA methylation and hydroxymethylation analysis after exposure to MWCNTs and SWCNTs. After exposure to MWCNTs and SWCNTs at the selected doses, the whole genomic DNA within the cells were measured by means of (**a**) DNA methylation (5-mC) and (**b**) hydroxymethylation (5-hmC) using LC-MS/MS technique. No significantly different effects were detected between the various conditions. 25 and 100 represents exposure concentrations as μg/ml. Statistics were performed using one-way ANOVA, Dunnett's multiple comparison test. Only decitabine-exposed cells decreased DNA 5-mC % in comparison to vehicle-exposed cells. ** indicates p value < 0.01

for downstream analyses. As explained in supplementary information (see supplementary information, dose specific analysis of the epigenetic data), dose-dependent difference within each CNT remained vague.

Differentially methylated and expressed genes

After exposure to MWCNTs, 3340 differentially hypomethylated promoter regions were identified, corresponding to 2398 genes (since some genes are characterized by alternative splice variants with same gene promoters). No differential methylation alterations at individual CpG sites were detected. Exposure to SWCNTs resulted in hypomethylated gene promoter regions located at five different genes: A-kinase anchoring protein 8 like (*AKAP8L*), forkhead box K2 (*FOXK2*), eukaryotic translation initiation factor 4E (*EIF4E*), small nucleolar RNA U13 (*snoU13*) and *RP11-223 I10.1*. When assessing individual CpG sites, 589 differentially methylated single CpG sites were identified of which 493 were hypomethylated and 96 hypermethylated. These CpG sites were located on 501 different genes.

Exposure to MWCNTs induced 4028 differentially expressed genes, with 2446 of them upregulated (log_2FC > 0) and 1582 of them downregulated (log_2FC < 0). Exposure to SWCNTs induced 4964 differentially expressed genes with 2751 of them being upregulated and 2213 of them being downregulated.

Correlation between gene methylation and expression

To ascertain whether differential methylation changes of individual CpG sites or gene promoters were aligned with gene expression changes after exposure to MWCNTs and SWCNTs, scatter plots were generated. In Fig. 6a-b the association between methylation and gene expression alterations are depicted using mean $\Delta\beta$ values and mean log_2FC for all differentially methylated genes. Only significant differentially methylated gene promoters [FDR corrected p value (q value) < 0.05] were mapped. The $\Delta\beta$ value of gene promoters in MWCNT-exposed cells ranged between − 0.05 to 0 (indicating only hypomethylation) whereas in SWCNT-exposed cells, they ranged between − 0.10 to 0.10 (indicating hypomethylation and hypermethylation). Although the differential methylation was comparably weaker in comparison to SWCNT-exposed cells, hypomethylation at the gene promoters ($\Delta\beta$ < − 0.01) was strongly associated with increased gene expression (log_2FC > 0.2) for

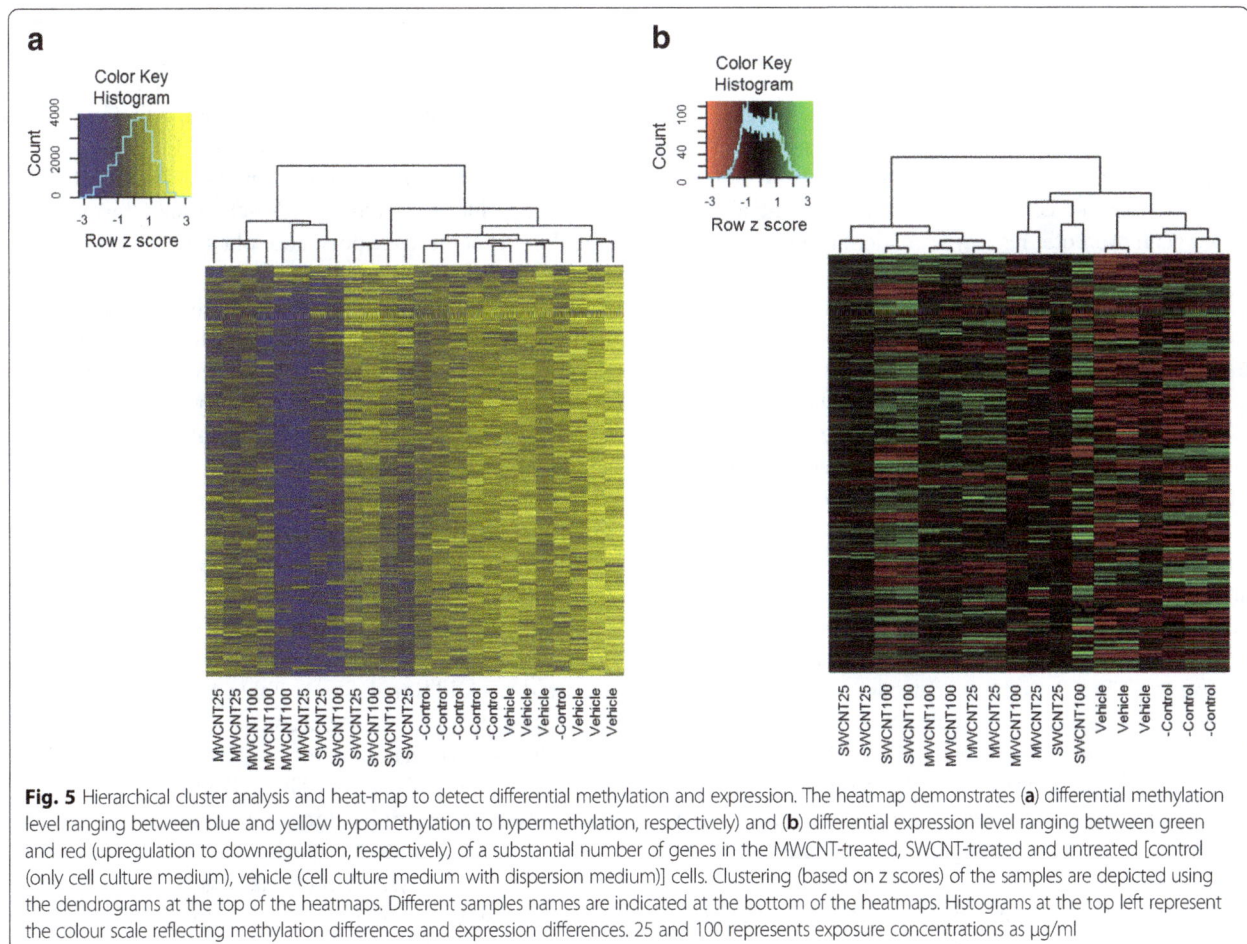

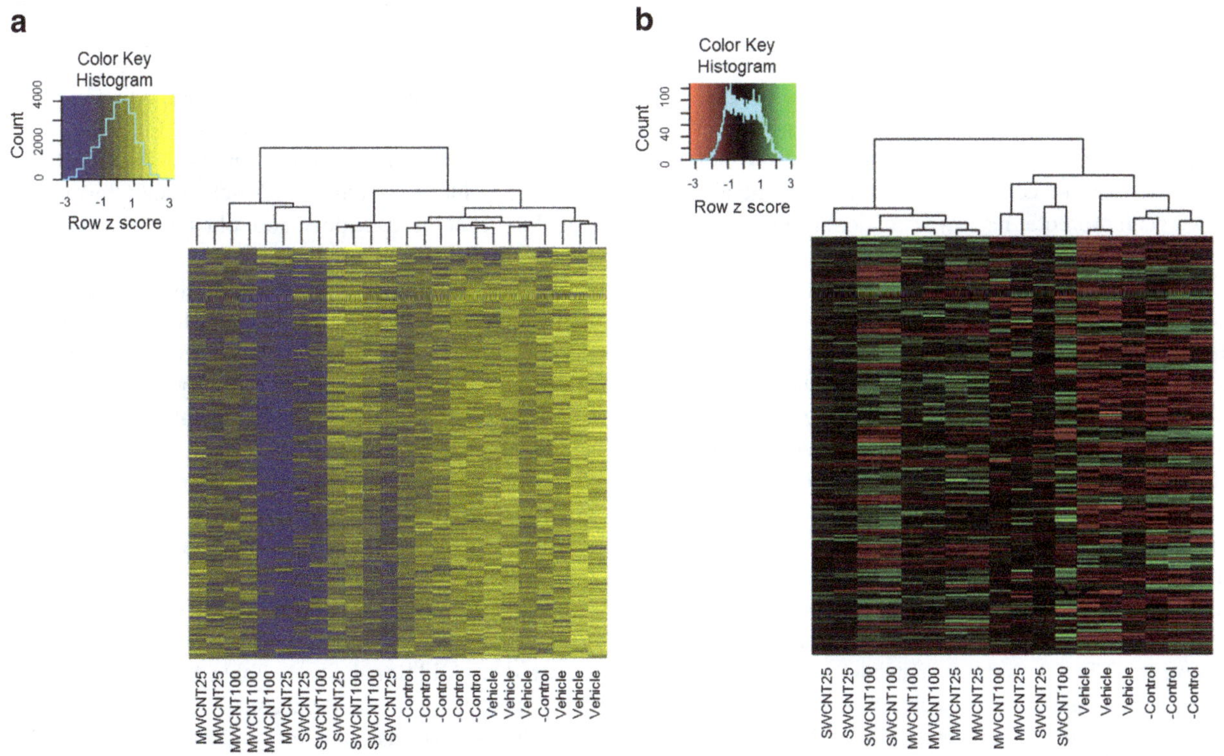

Fig. 5 Hierarchical cluster analysis and heat-map to detect differential methylation and expression. The heatmap demonstrates (**a**) differential methylation level ranging between blue and yellow hypomethylation to hypermethylation, respectively) and (**b**) differential expression level ranging between green and red (upregulation to downregulation, respectively) of a substantial number of genes in the MWCNT-treated, SWCNT-treated and untreated [control (only cell culture medium), vehicle (cell culture medium with dispersion medium)] cells. Clustering (based on z scores) of the samples are depicted using the dendrograms at the top of the heatmaps. Different samples names are indicated at the bottom of the heatmaps. Histograms at the top left represent the colour scale reflecting methylation differences and expression differences. 25 and 100 represents exposure concentrations as μg/ml

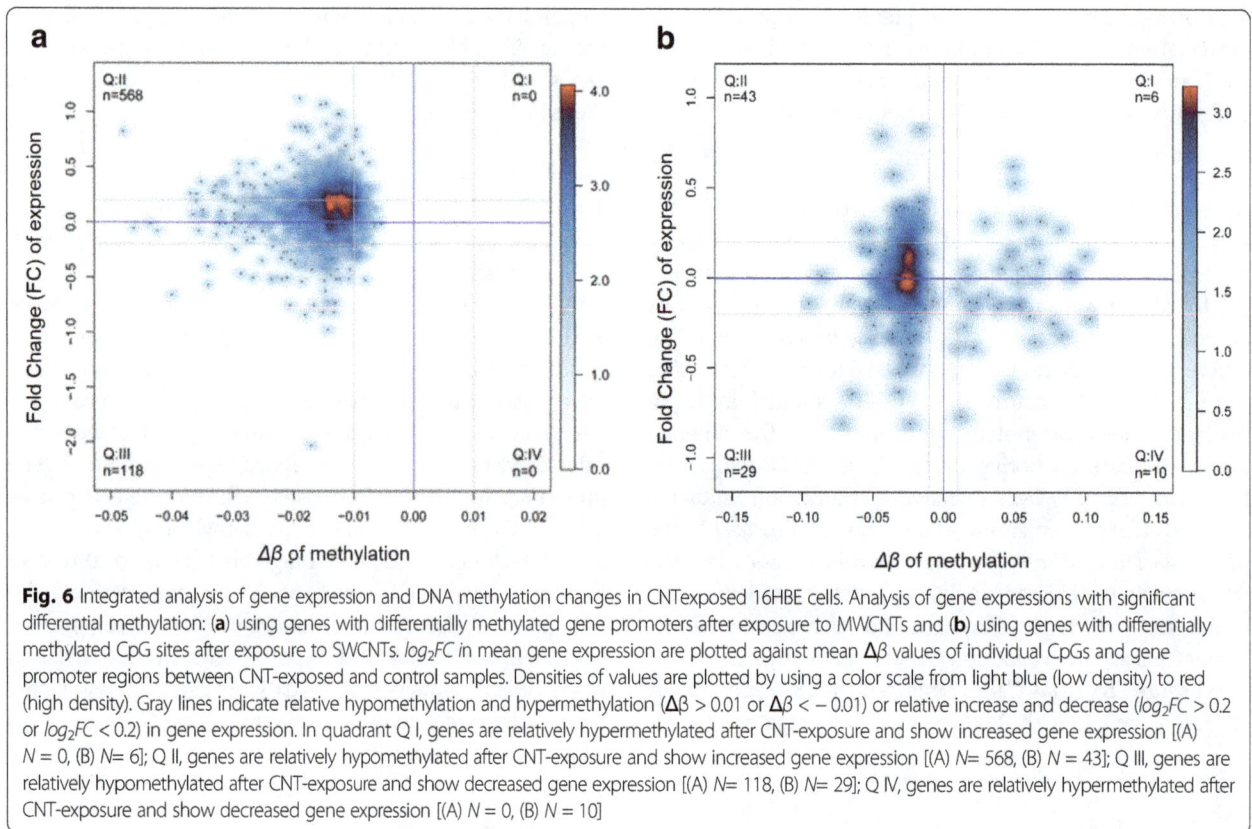

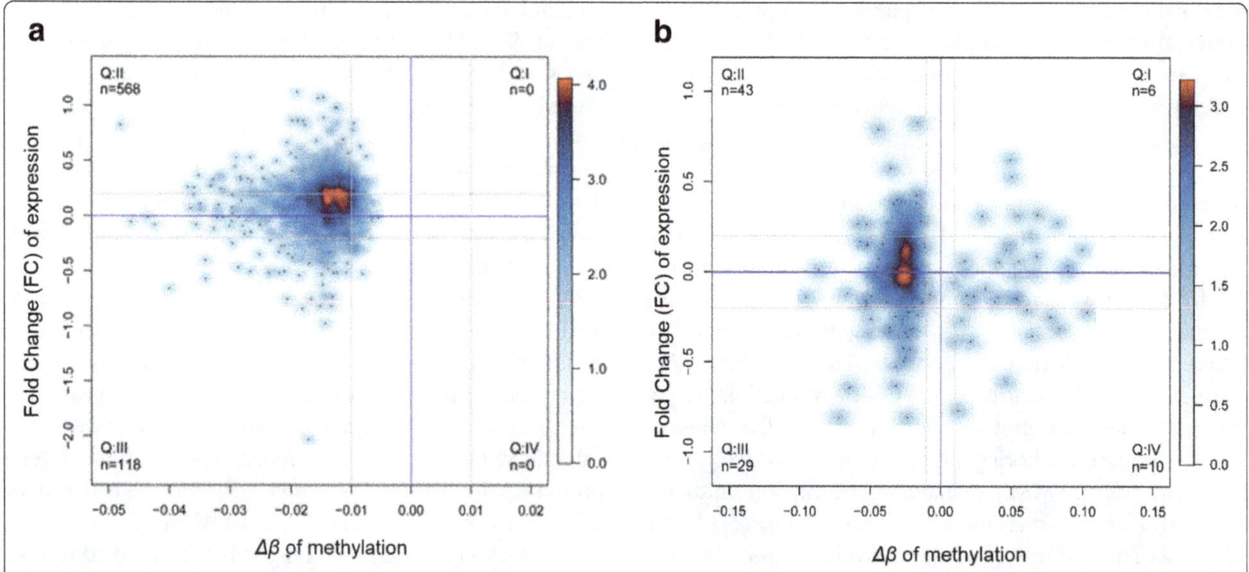

Fig. 6 Integrated analysis of gene expression and DNA methylation changes in CNTexposed 16HBE cells. Analysis of gene expressions with significant differential methylation: (**a**) using genes with differentially methylated gene promoters after exposure to MWCNTs and (**b**) using genes with differentially methylated CpG sites after exposure to SWCNTs. log_2FC in mean gene expression are plotted against mean $\Delta\beta$ values of individual CpGs and gene promoter regions between CNT-exposed and control samples. Densities of values are plotted by using a color scale from light blue (low density) to red (high density). Gray lines indicate relative hypomethylation and hypermethylation ($\Delta\beta > 0.01$ or $\Delta\beta < -0.01$) or relative increase and decrease ($log_2FC > 0.2$ or $log_2FC < 0.2$) in gene expression. In quadrant Q I, genes are relatively hypermethylated after CNT-exposure and show increased gene expression [(A) $N = 0$, (B) $N = 6$]; Q II, genes are relatively hypomethylated after CNT-exposure and show increased gene expression [(A) $N = 568$, (B) $N = 43$]; Q III, genes are relatively hypomethylated after CNT-exposure and show decreased gene expression [(A) $N = 118$, (B) $N = 29$]; Q IV, genes are relatively hypermethylated after CNT-exposure and show decreased gene expression [(A) $N = 0$, (B) $N = 10$]

MWCNTs-exposed cells using another technique: RNA sequencing. Smaller associations between single CpG site methylation and gene expression changes were noted for SWCNTs-exposed cells. Since only five differentially methylated gene promoter regions were identified after SWCNT exposure no profound analysis could be performed.

Gene-function analyses

1. MWCNTs: Using differentially methylated genes after exposure to MWCNT (total 2398 genes), functional – Gene Ontology (GO) analysis is reported in Additional file 1: Table S2 and Gene functional classification is reported in Additional file 1: Table S3. GO enrichments were involved in multicellular organism development and regulation of small Guanosine-5′-triphosphate (GTP)ase mediated signal transduction pathways whereas no enrichment using Kyoto Encyclopedia of Genes and Genomes (KEGG) pathway database was noted. Functional gene classification analyses resulted in following gene groups (top 5 clusters): pleckstrin homology-like domain, GTPase activator activity, positive regulation of GTPase activity/metal binding/zinc finger, nucleus/DNA binding and protein binding groups, in consistency with the GO analysis.

Using differentially expressed genes after exposure to MWCNT (in total 4028 genes), functional – GO analysis is reported in Additional file 1: Table S4, KEGG pathway analysis is reported in Additional file 1: Table S5 and gene functional classification analysis is reported in Additional file 1: Table S6. Enriched GO terms were noted in protein transport and phosphorylation ontologies, which play a crucial role in nearly all cellular signalling, enabling activation or deactivation of the proteins. Enriched KEGG pathways were noted in metabolic pathways, Human t-lymphotropic virus-1 (HTLV-I) infection and with close proximity of significance tumour protein 53 (TP53) signalling pathway. Functional gene classification analyses resulted in the following top five clusters: phosphoproteins/transcription, transcriptional regulation DNA-templated, zinc finger/metal binding, chromosome/phosphoproteins, and WD repeat domain groups.

2. SWCNTs. Using differentially methylated genes after exposure to SWCNTs, functional –GO analysis is reported in Additional file 1: Table S7, KEGG pathway analysis is reported in Additional file 1: Table S8 and gene functional classification analysis is reported in Additional file 1: Table S9. The GO analysis resulted in enrichment of multiple glucuronidation processes. The KEGG analysis resulted in enrichment of wide-range of metabolic pathways. Functional gene classification analyses resulted in following gene groups (4 clusters): Uridine 5′-diphospho-glucuronosyltransferase (UDP

glucuronosyltransferases), transmembrane proteins, zinc-finger C2H2 like, immunoglobulin subtype/signal peptides.

Using differentially expressed genes after exposure to SWCNTs (in total 4964 genes), functional – GO analysis is reported in Additional file 1: Table S10, KEGG pathway analysis is reported in Additional file 1: Table S11 and gene functional classification analysis is reported in Additional file 1: Table S12. Enriched GO terms were noted in protein transport, DNA damage response, cell cycle and cell migration and adhesion ontologies. KEGG analysis metabolic, endocytosis, cell cycle and p53 signalling.

Functional gene classification analyses resulted in following top five clusters: nucleic acid binding, sister chromatid cohesion, ankyrin repeats, transcriptional regulation, ATP-binding groups.

Since CpG specific hypermethylation was only noted by SWCNTs and hypermethylation was generally linked with gene silencing in tumorigenesis, we further investigated this set of differentially hypermethylated genes [23, 24]. As demonstrated in Fig. 7, genes in developmental and cellular proliferation pathways were identified as follows: SKI proto oncogene (*SKI, gene body and 3'UTR*), neurofibromin 1 (*NF, gene body*), shroom family member 2 (*SHROOM2, 5'UTR*), glutathione s-transferase pi 1 (*GSTP1, 1st exon and 5'UTR*), kruppel like factor 2 (*KLF2, gene body*), von hippel-lindau tumor suppressor (*VHL, TSS200*), discoidin domain receptor tyrosine kinase 1 (DDR1, TSS1500 and 5'UTR), mixed lineage kinase domain like (*MLKL, TSS1500*), dimethylarginine dimethylaminohydrolase 2 (*DDAH2, TSS1500*), nitric oxide synthase trafficking (*NOSTRIN, 5'UTR and 1st exon*), ERG ETS transcription factor (*ERG, gene body*), ecdysoneless cell cycle regulator (*ECD, TSS200*), kinesin family member 15 (*KIF15, TSS200*). Using the network analysis, regulation of fibroblast proliferation by alterations on *GSTP1, SKI, NF1* genes and eye morphogenesis by alterations on *NF1, SKI* and *SHROOM2* genes were identified. By checking expression values of these three differentially methylated genes only NF1 showed hypermethylation and downregulation. Of note, aberrations on NF1 gene have been noted in lung adenocarcinoma and *NF1* mutations are observed with TP53 alterations [25–27].

RT-PCR analysis of the selected genes

Following our analyses, we used RT-PCR to validate our data analysis according to the pathways that are proposed by our data mining analysis. We focused on lowest dose of exposure (25 μg/ml) in order to identify early contributor of potentially altered pathways such as p53 signalling, DNA damage response and cell cycle, by investigating the alterations of the hub-genes (i.e. ATM, P53 and AKT1) and downstream products (i.e. NF1, BCL2L11 and BAX). Demonstrated in Fig. 8, we noted downregulation of the expression of ATM gene for both CNTs, upregulation of the expression of BCL2L11 for SWCNTs and downregulation of the expression of NF1 for SWCNT genes, as expected. Consequently, it can be concluded that ATM, BCL2L11 and NF1 genes which are involved in up- and downstream pathways of tp53, DNA damage response, apoptosis and cell cycle signalling are differentially methylated and expressed after CNT exposure and may potentially contribute alteration of proposed signalling pathways.

Discussion

In this study, we observed greater aggregation and particle deposition of the cell nucleus after exposure to SWCNTs. Comparably, MWCNTs were relatively smaller in size and localized over the nucleus less than SWCNTs. In addition, increasing concentrations of MWCNTs did not lead to significantly different values in the area and aggregates of the MWCNTs near the nucleus. As a matter of fact, SWCNTs are more in contact with the cell nucleus compared to MWCNTs regardless of the increasing concentrations. Although, such nuclear-CNT interactions will have an on various aspects of nucleus, here, we first aimed to identify, how nuclear deposition will have an impact on the genetic and epigenetic toxicity of the CNTs.

In the literature, more DNA methylation alterations on CpG sites were noted after four weeks of exposure in comparison to two weeks of exposure Sierra et al., [14]. This observation of low number of DNA methylation changes after short period of exposure is in correlation with our study, since, we detected vague response on dose-specific analysis. Therefore, we improved the power of the statistics by combining two different doses, however more replicates may be necessary in future studies. In addition, Sierra et al. observed that most of the hypomethylated genes after two weeks exposure became hypermethylated after four weeks of exposure Sierra et al., [14]. This may indicate that possible DNA demethylation and gene-silencing mechanisms occurred during the prolonged exposure. Of note, in cancer cells, global loss of DNA methylation and increased gene-specific methylation have been noted (Baylin and Ohm, [28]; Esteller, [29]). Gene-silencing through increased methylation increase the risk of spontaneous mutation (Li and Zhang, [9]). Regarding the loss of DNA methylation, currently two main processes are known: active and passive DNA demethylation processes in the development (Li and Zhang, [9]). Active DNA demethylation refers to removal of methylation from the 5-mC by enzymatic processes. Alternatively, passive DNA demethylation refers to alterations or inhibition of DNA maintenance genes, such as DNMT1, leading the loss of DNA methylation on cytosine residues. DNA demethylation may also occur via TET-mediated 5-mC oxidation leading to formation of 5-hmC. However, in this study, we did not

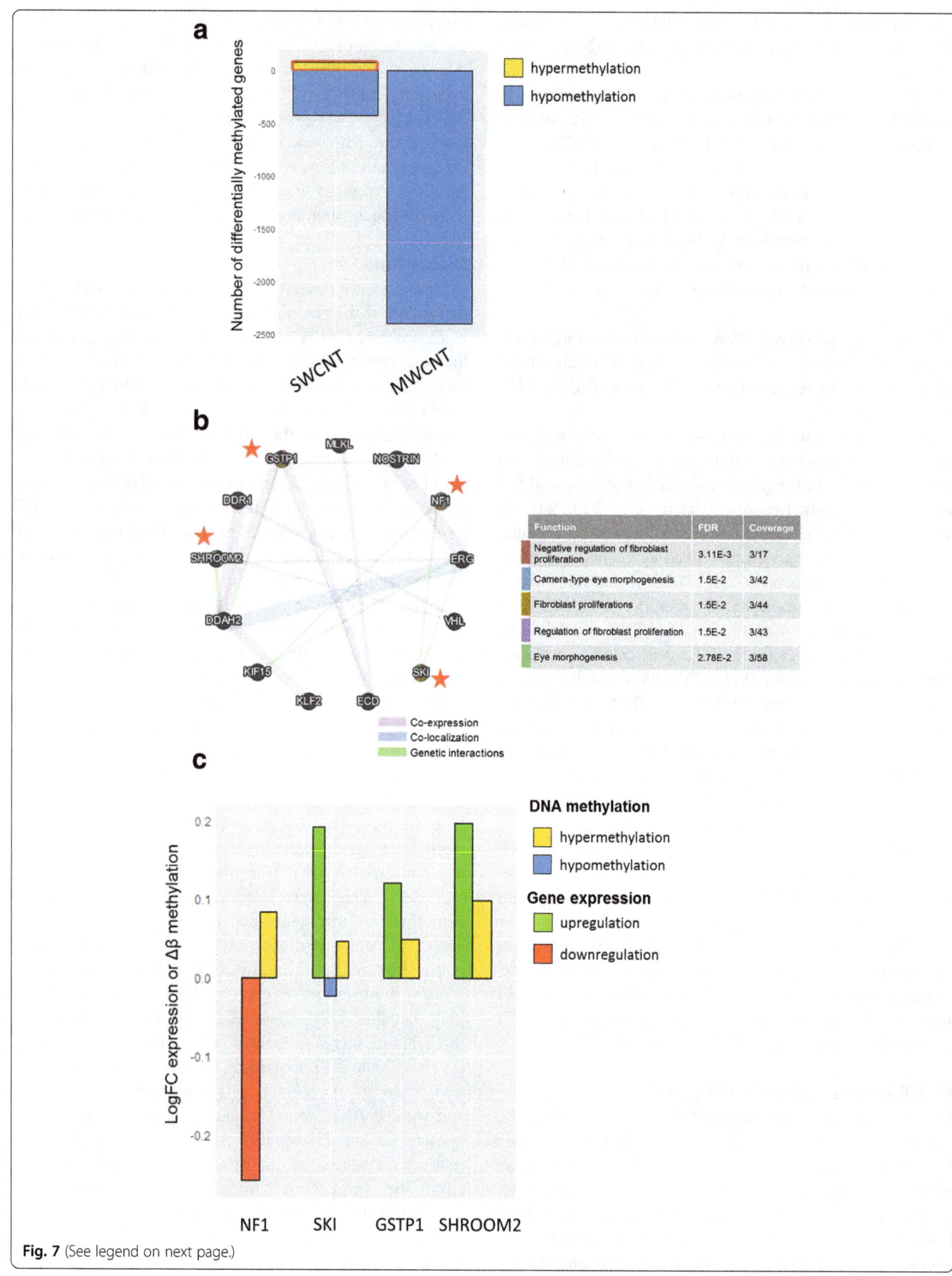

Function	FDR	Coverage
Negative regulation of fibroblast proliferation	3.11E-3	3/17
Camera-type eye morphogenesis	1.5E-2	3/42
Fibroblast proliferations	1.5E-2	3/44
Regulation of fibroblast proliferation	1.5E-2	3/43
Eye morphogenesis	2.78E-2	3/58

Fig. 7 (See legend on next page.)

(See figure on previous page.)

Fig. 7 Differentially hypermethylated genes by their CpG site after exposure to SWCNTs. **a** set of differentially hypermethylated genes (by CpG sites) were selected. **b** Selected set of genes were proceeded for functional analysis using web-based GeneMania tool (http://www.genemania.org). The genes, which involve in the enriched networks are indicated with a red star and were further investigated for gene expression status (**c**)

detect any alterations on DNMT1 and TET genes (based on our RNA sequencing data) nor in global 5-hmC methylation levels. Other mechanisms which may induce changes in DNA methylation machinery may require further investigation such as histone modifications, miRNA mechanisms, genotoxicity, oxidative stress or inflammation. For instance, early stress response on key genes such as ATM may initiate epigenetic machinery through alterations on DNA damage response. Of note, we observed downregulation of ATM gene at the lowest dose of exposure, which may result in impaired cell cycle and DNA damage response mechanism in the cell, resulting in increased genotoxicity, leading to changes in methylation. Importantly, here, we show CNTs localized in the cellular nucleus, which could lead to loss/gain of DNA methylation by mechanical interference.

Considering genotoxic endpoint, we observed more pronounced cyto- and genotoxicity by SWCNTs compared to MWCNTs. The same type of SWCNTs have been already associated with DNA damage and alterations on cellular signalling pathways Pacurari et al., [30]. In agreement with our findings, non-cytotoxic and non-genotoxic effects of this type of MWCNTs have been reported in an OECD project Hannu Norppa [31].

From literature, we know that DNA damage and epigenetic factors are in association. For instance, it is noted that knock down of the DNA methyl transferase 1 (*DNMT1*) gene, a major regulator of DNA methylation maintenance, activates wide-range of genotoxic check point genes [32, 33]. DNA hypomethylation on genes such as DNMT1 and stress response might trigger activation of DNA repair pathways. On the other hand, gene silencing on tumour suppressor genes may lead to toxic responses in the cell. The specific interaction between genotoxicity and epigenetic alterations require further mechanistic research.

From the DNA methylation/gene expression point of view, the differences in DNA methylation after exposure to MWCNTs and SWCNTs can be summarised via three main points.

First, DNA methylation alterations on gene promoter regions were observed after exposure to MWCNTs, while methylation changes at the single CpG sites (and some gene promoters) were observed after exposure to SWCNTs. Methylation alterations on gene promoter regions can be a result of indirect interactions of MWCNTs with the cytosolic proteins and RNAs that in turn affect the epigenetic machinery within the DNA level. Our analysis shows that SWCNTs have significantly more physical contact with nuclei compared to MWCNTs. Since SWCNTs are likely to be endocytosed into cellular vesicles, they may not be in contact with the cytosolic proteins or RNAs but rather directly in touch with the nucleus. This might be a valid explanation for the high number of CpG site methylation (alterations) after SWCNTs exposure and gene promoter hypomethylation after exposure to MWCNTs.

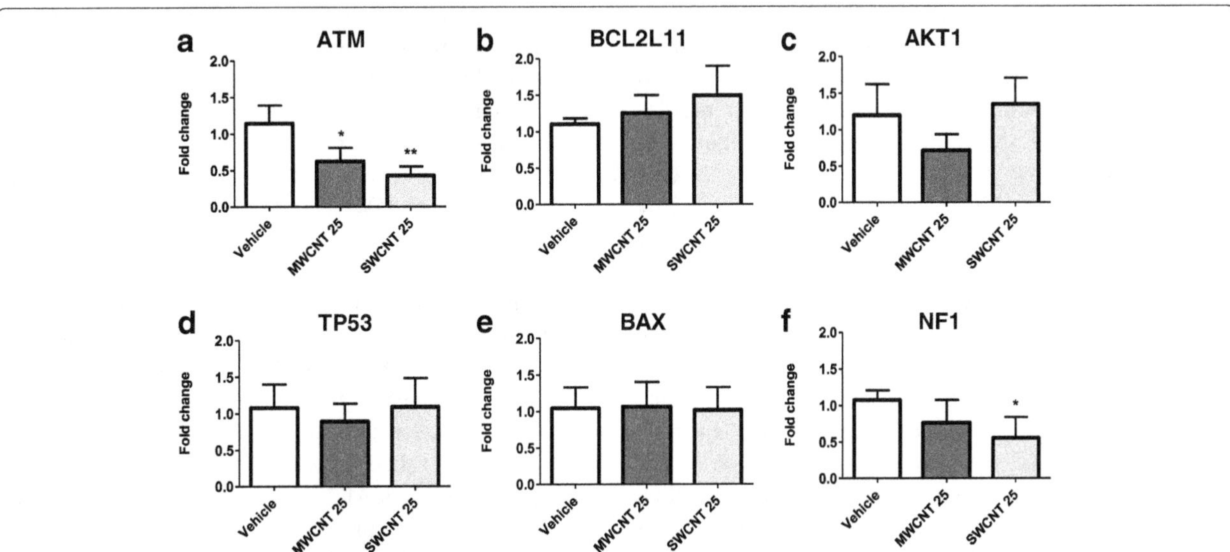

Fig. 8 RT-PCR analysis of the selected genes, **a**) ATM, **b**) BCL2L11, **c**) AKT1, **d**) TP53, **e**) BAX, **f**) NF1, after low dose (25 μg/ml) exposure of MWCNTs and SWCNTs. * indicates $p < 0.05$, using t-test, two-tailed (95%confidence)

As expected, methylation changes of gene promoters have a different (stronger) effect on the expression profile compared to the methylation of the CpG sites. This is due to the fact that hypomethylation on gene promoter regions will foster the binding of transcription factor and activate the gene transcription.

Second, only hypomethylation was seen after exposure to MWCNTs whereas both hypomethylation and hypermethylation (to a smaller extent than hypomethylation) was seen after exposure to SWCNTs. Hypomethylation may lead to the activation of a cellular response that may trigger damage repair within the cell. Therefore, hypomethylation might serve as a buffer response of the cell toward toxic exposures such as nanoparticles. It might also be related with the increased inflammation that may trigger an activation of the cellular response. On the other hand, hypermethylation is associated with the gene silencing. The gene silencing has been typically observed in diseased tissues such as tumours [34]. We observed that a functionally important gene such as NF1 (a gene which serves as a tumour suppressor and acts in fibroblast proliferation) was both hypermethylated and downregulated. However, it is important to note that the study addresses the in vitro conditions when the exposure is limited to 24 h. The nuclear deposition of CNTs may alter in prolonged exposure or in in vivo conditions where the active clearance of the particles are present.

Third, both CNTs altered similar pathways by means of gene expression and methylation alterations. When only methylation alterations were concerned, overrepresentation at GTPase mediated signal transduction, multicellular organism development and inflammatory pathways were seen after exposure to MWCNTs, whereas overrepresentation on glucuronidation, metabolic and endocytosis processes were seen by SWCNTs exposure.

It has been shown that differences in physicochemical structure of CNTs affect their toxic properties and potential disease outcome. For instance, long, needle-like MWCNTs are shown to induce mesothelioma in rodents, like asbestos fibres, through asbestos-like toxicity mechanisms [15, 35]. This was not observed by their shorter counterparts. Therefore, it is crucial to note that differences observed by different types of CNTs might well be related to their size and shape. For instance, SWCNTs are long fibres with an extremely small diameter. Although, they do not have a needle-like shape, they keep their fibre structure and high surface area, which makes them more reactive. In contrast, MWCNTs that have been used in this study, are relatively short with an average diameter of 11 nm, allow them to be easily internalized and cleared out in/from the cells. This explains the greater amount of SWCNTs localised in the nucleus and the hypermethylation observed by SWCNTs only.

Nevertheless, common pathway alterations in MWCNT- and SWCNT-treated cells were noted and summarised. In Fig. 9, an overview of the most altered cell survival pathways such as p53, DNA damage response, cell cycle, phosphatidylinositide 3 kinases-protein kinase B (PI3K-AKT) pathway, mitogen-activated protein kinase (MAPK) signalling, by differentially methylated and/or expressed genes were visualized. This analysis are performed in order to give a better visualization of functionally altered pathways after exposure to MWCNTs and SWCNTs.

P53 is a critical tumour suppressor gene that orchestrates cellular stress response such as cell cycle, DNA repair, and apoptosis. The classical alteration of p53 signalling includes alterations of ATM gene, which phosphorylates checkpoint kinase 2 (CHK2) and phosphorylation of p53 from several sites, after exposure to DNA damaging agents. Activated (phosphorylated) P53 stimulates downstream cellular responses such as cell cycle. The cell cycle signalling involves cyclin dependent kinase inhibitor 1A [CDKN1A (p21)] and cyclin dependent kinases (CDKs) such as cyclin dependent kinase 4 (CDK4) and cyclin dependent kinase 6 (CDK6) and DNA damage repair. The cell cycle signalling is crucial for the cell to maintain normal rate of proliferation. Therefore, the cell cycle deregulation in the cell increases the risk of cancer initiation by altering the proliferation rate. The studies on the relevance of cell cycle in cancer point out deregulation of p21 and CDKs (CDK4 and CDK6) [36, 37]. The potential role of p53 in malignant transformation of lung epithelial cells after continuous SWCNT exposure and activation of pAkt/p53/Bcl-2 signalling axis was noted by whole genome gene expression analysis [38, 39]. In our analysis we noted alterations on TP53, DNA damage response and cell cycle signalling induced by CNTs. Genes such as fas cell surface death receptor (FAS), BCL2 associated x, apoptosis regulator (BAX), NADPH oxidase activator 1 (NOXA1), tumour protein P53 inducible protein 3 (TP53I3), shisa family member 5 (SHISA5), PERP TP53 apoptosis effector (PERP), TP53 were differentially expressed by both type of CNT-exposure. Differential methylation and expression on ATM, p21 and CDK4 genes were noted in the cells exposed to MWCNTs. For SWCNTs, only differential gene expression of ATM and CDK4 genes were noted.

In addition, PI3K-AKT signalling can contribute to the alterations in p53 signalling. PI3K group of genes including phosphoinositide-3-kinase regulatory subunit 2 (PIK3R2) gene, were activated by receptor tyrosine kinases (RTKs) such as fibroblast growth factor receptor 1 (FGFR1), platelet-derived growth factor receptor beta (PDGFR), insulin-like growth factor 1 Receptor (IGFR). PI3K phosphorylates AKT genes, which stands upstream or various cellular processes such as p53 signalling, cellular differentiation and apoptosis. Upon activation of the The forkhead box O (FOXO) transcription factors, BCL2 like 11 (BCL2L11, also known as BIM) acts as a

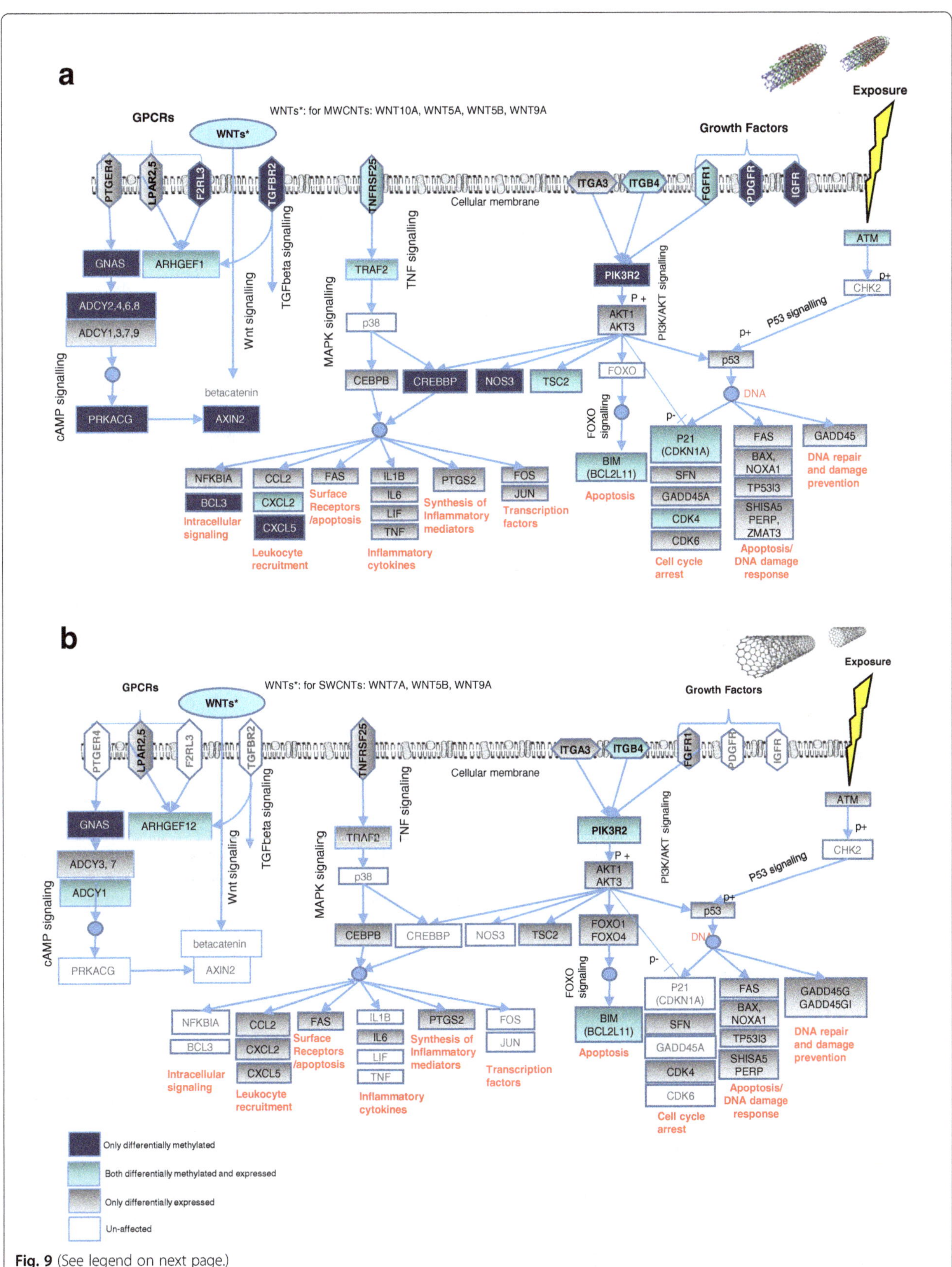

Fig. 9 (See legend on next page.)

(See figure on previous page.)
Fig. 9 An overview of functionally altered pathways. The diagram demonstrates the functionally altered cell signalling pathways after exposure to **a** MWCNTs and **b** SWCNTs. The grey coloured boxes which consist the differentially expressed genes, the dark blue colour indicates only differentially methylated genes, turquoise blue colour indicates both differentially methylated and expressed genes within the mentioned pathways. Genes that are written in white boxes are unaffected. Blue circles indicate DNA. 'p+' and 'p-' indicate phosphorylation and de-phosphorylation, respectively

regulator of apoptosis. Exposure to SWCNTs induced differential methylation and expression on PIK3R2 gene and both types of CNTs altered methylation and expression state of BCL2L11 gene. Exposure to MWCNTs induced differential methylation on *IGFR, PDGFR* and methylation/expression changes on FGFR1 genes.

Concerning MWCNTs, increased inflammatory response was evident. For instance, the KEGG pathway 'HTLV infection' was noted for MWCNT-exposed cells. In addition, alterations on tumor necrosis factor receptor superfamily member 25 (TNFRSF25) and tumor necrosis factor receptor associated factor 2 (TRAF2), which mediate signal transduction and activate inflammatory response through MAPK and nuclear factor-kappa B (NF-κB) pathways, were noted to be both differentially methylated and expressed. In addition, differential expression of inflammatory cytokines such as interleukin 1-beta (IL1-β), interleukin 6 (IL6), leukemia inhibitory factor (LIF) and tumour necrosis factor (TNF) was induced by MWCNTs whereas only differential expression of IL6 was induced by SWCNTs. Differential expression on nuclear factor-kappa B inhibitor alpha (NFKBIA) and differential methylation on B cell lymphoma 3 (BCL3) gene was induced by MWCNTs. Likewise, differential methylation and expression on chemokine (C-X-C motif) ligand 2 (CXCL2) gene was induced by MWCNTs whereas exposure to SWCNTs caused only differential expression.

These results might also explain epigenetic contribution to in vivo CNT-mediated adverse effects. For instance, exposure to SWCNTs caused fibrogenic pulmonary responses in rodents [40–43]. MWCNTs (NM400) showed adverse pulmonary effects in mice, summarized as increased cytokine formation such as IL1-β, IL6, TNF, Chemokine (C-X-C motif) ligand 1 (CXCL1), C-C Motif Chemokine Ligand 2 (CCL2), C-C Motif Chemokine Ligand 4 (CCL4), and C-C Motif Chemokine Ligand 5 (CCL5) and increase in the genes related to cellular adhesion, inflammation, oxidative stress and DNA damage repair [44, 45].

In this study, we used two different microarrays and generated tremendous data which can be used to elucidate and speculate alterations in important pathways. Variances and irregularities between samples could be seen due to many reasons and these changes might affect the observed results. These reasons include experimental protocols, aging of the cells, and the batch effects that occurs during microarray processing. In order to overcome these issues, the cells were harvested at the same passage number (passage 4) and batch correction was applied during the bioinformatics analyses.

Collectively, we demonstrate localisation of CNTs (SWCNT > MWCNT) in cellular nucleus in a label-free way and CNT induce subtle epigenetic and gene expression alterations in vitro at the acute phase. Although differences between two CNTs were noted, similar pathways altered by two types of CNTs. Our results are consistent with previous studies in which we noted DNA methylation alterations on ATM gene in mouse lungs after intra-tracheal CNT administration and in blood samples of the workers who have exposed to MWCNTs [11, 46]. Downregulation of ATM gene may regulate DNA damage response, DNA damage checkpoints, cell cycle, and p53 signalling and these signalling are enriched in our data analyses. Overall, our data provide possible pathways and gene sets which may alter by CNT exposure at the acute phase. Importantly, there is a need to investigate epigenetic and functional outcomes of the proposed mechanisms after a longer exposure period.

Conclusions

In the current study we have shown that SWCNTs are engulfed and distributed superiorly compared to MWCNTs, at both the cellular and nuclear level. Accordingly, increased cytotoxicity and genotoxicity for SWCNTs were found. Although, no global DNA methylation nor hydroxymethylation alterations were seen for both types of CNTs, whole-genome DNA methylation alterations were particle type dependent. Transcriptomic profiles of CNTs show differential regulation of a diverse set of genes but alterations in similar pathways (i.e. DNA damage, DNA damage repair, tp53, cell cycle, protein phosphorylation). In particular, exposure to SWCNTs induced fibroblast proliferation and exposure to MWCNTs induced alterations in the genes responsible for inflammation.

It can be postulated that epigenetic mechanisms serve in repair or toxic response to the exposure and might increase the disease susceptibility by hypomethylation or hypermethylation. In particular, specific DNA hypermethylation and gene silencing should be taken in caution hence it might lead to gene silencing at tumour suppressor genes. These differences elucidate cellular epigenetic behaviour of the cells is dependent on type of CNTs and CNT-nuclear interactions. Overall, DNA methylation alterations might result in adverse effects in rodents and human after the inhalation exposure.

Methods

Cell cultures and particle preparation

Dulbecco's Modified Eagle Medium (DMEM), Dulbecco's Modified Eagle Medium: Nutrient Mixture F12 (DMEM/F12), Hank's Balanced Salt Solution without $CaCl_2$ and $MgCl_2$ (HBSS-), phosphate buffered saline without $CaCl_2$ and $MgCl_2$ (PBS-), penicillin-streptomycin, amphothericin-B, L-glutamine, fetal calf serum (FCS), 0.5% Trypsin-EDTA were purchased from Invitrogen (Merelbeke, Belgium).

16HBE human bronchial epithelial cell lines (16HBE14o-) were provided by Dr. Gruenert (University of California, San Francisco). The cells were cultured in DMEM/F12 supplemented with 5% of FCS and 1% of Penicillin-Streptomycin (10,000 U/ml), L-glutamine (200 mM) and, Amphotericin-B (250 μg/ml), incubated at 37 °C in a 100% humidified atmosphere containing 5% CO_2. Culture medium was renewed every 2 or 3 days and 2.5×10^5 confluent cells were sub-cultured in a new cell culture T25 flasks. To do this, the cells were enzymatically released by 0.05% trypsin-EDTA solution (diluted in HBSS-).

Stock of cells was generated from the same passage number (passage number 4) and kept in liquid nitrogen to avoid the effect of aging in epi-genotoxicity analysis. Cells from the same stock were grown until passage 4 for epigenetic experiments. When the desired passage number was reached and the cells became confluent, 16HBE14o- cells were seeded in wells of plates at 2×10^5 cells/cm^2 of density and allowed to attach for 24 h to reach 80% confluence.

CNT suspensions were prepared as described in the European project of Engineered Nanoparticle Risk Assessment (ENPRA) [47]. In brief, CNTs were diluted in Baxter sterile water containing 2% serum to reach a final concentration of 2.56 mg/ml. The suspension was sonicated for 16 min using probe sonication at frequency 22.5 kHz, watt 7.35 W with 50% amplitude (MICROSON XL 2000). Final concentrations were by diluting 1/10 of the intermediate concentrations. Fresh CNT suspensions were prepared before each experiment to avoid aggregation of CNTs. While exposing CNTs, no serum was added in the cell culture medium and each concentration involved 0.02% of serum.

Physicochemical assessment of CNTs

Two different reference materials of CNT were used, NM400 MWCNTs were obtained from the European Commission Joint Research Centre (JRC, Ispra, Italy) and SRM:2483 SWCNTs were from National Institute of Technology (NIST, Maryland, USA) [17, 18].

Endotoxin determination was performed using ENDOSAFE PTS cartridges (Charles River laboratories, Massachusetts, USA). 1/1000 dispersion from the master solution of CNTs in ENDOSAFE LAL reagent (Charles River laboratories, Massachusetts, USA) water was used.

DLS analysis was performed to gain information about the suspension and aggregation state of the nanomaterials in the cell medium at 25 and 100 μg/ml of concentration.

Transmission Electron Microscopy (TEM) images of the MWCNTs and SWCNTs were previously demonstrated [16].

Nuclear deposition

Nuclear deposition of MWCNTs and SWCNTs was imaged according to the method that has been reported previously by Bové et al. [20]. The method detects CNTs in a label-free and biocompatible fashion in cellular compartments of interest using femtosecond pulsed laser microscopy. First, before executing cellular experiments, the method was validated for CNTs by measuring spiked ultrapure water with known concentrations of the different nanomaterials using identical imaging conditions as later used for the cellular experiments.

The cells were exposed to MWCNTs and SWCNTs (25 and 100 μg/mL of doses) in 8 well chamber slides for 24 h (Invitrogen, Merelbeke, Belgium) in cell culture medium. Slides were washed five times (to avoid CNTs residuals) with HBSS- and the cells were fixed with 4% paraformaldehyde. Staining was performed by 5 min treatment of SYBERgold (Invitrogen, Merelbeke, Belgium) diluted 1/20000 times in HBSS-. After the cells were washed three times using HBSS-.

Images were acquired using a Zeiss LSM510 META NLO scan head mounted on an inverted laser-scanning microscope (Zeiss Axiovert 200 M; Zeiss, Germany) and a 40×/1.1 water immersion objective. For imaging the stained nuclei, a 30 mW air-cooled Argon ion laser (LASOS Lasertechnik GmbH, Germany) emitting at 488 nm (~ 3 μW maximum radiant power at the sample) was used as excitation source and a band-pass filter 500–530 nm was used for filtering the emission light. A fixed pinhole size of 100 μm was used. CNTs were visualized by femtosecond pulsed laser excitation (~ 4 mW average laser power at the sample, 810 nm, 150 fs, 80 MHz, MaiTai DeepSee, Spectra Physics, USA) and filtering of the emission signal by a 400–410 nm band-pass filter in the non-descanned mode. The pinhole was opened completely. The resulting 512 × 512 images with a pixel size of 0.44 μm were recorded at a pixel dwell time of 3.2 μs. In addition, three-dimensional z-stacks were acquired throughout the cells every 25 - 30 μm to confirm nuclear deposition (~ 225 × 225 × 30 μm image volume). Images were captured using the AIM 4.2 software (Carl Zeiss).

Images were processed with the image-processing program Fiji (ImageJ v1.47, open source software, http://fiji.sc/Fiji). Prior to the analysis, the cell of interest was cropped in a way that non-engulfed CNTs were excluded from the analysis. A threshold was set to the estimated background value and the number and total area of CNT aggregates inside the cell were measured. Next, the corresponding nucleus was cropped and the number and area of deposited CNT aggregates were determined. In total, 50 cells for each exposure conditions including negative controls were analysed.

Cytotoxicity

The cell viabilities were analyzed by two different assays, namely WST-1, LDH assays. Two independent assays (with three replicates) were performed according to optimized protocols. For both experiments, cells (2×10^5 cells/cm^2) were exposed to 4, 8, 16, 32, 64, 128 and 256 μg/ml of MWCNTs and SWCNTs for 24 h and untreated cells were included as negative controls.

In brief, following protocol was applied for WST-1 assay. After the exposure in the 96-well plate, cells were rinsed one time with cell culture medium without phenol red (DMEM). WST-1 solution (Sigma Aldrich, Brussels, Belgium) was diluted 1/20 in DMEM medium and the cells were incubated with this solution for 2 h at 37 °C. Subsequently, the supernatant was transferred to another well plate for absorption measurement of the formazan product at 450 nm optical wavelength. Relative viability was calculated in comparison to untreated (cell medium without serum) cells.

In brief, following protocol was applied for LDH assay. After the exposure, the supernatant was transferred to another plate. The cells were lysed (using 200 μl 0.2% Triton X-100 in PBS+) and incubated for 30 min. The measurement was taken with the addition of the reaction mixture (18.32 mg pyruvate, 21.28 mg NADH, 31.76 mg HCO_3Na dissolved in 40 ml PBS+) was added on the cells. The results were obtained using a spectrometer, 340 nm wavelength every 15 s for 3 min after 5 s of mixing.

Data analysis was calculated according to the absorbance curve and relative viability was calculated according to untreated controls.

Comet assay

Induction of DNA strand breaks after 3 h and 24 h exposure to CNTs was assessed using alkaline comet assay [48]. The assay was performed using Trevigen Comet assay kits (Gentaur, Kampenhout, Belgium) according to the manufacturer's protocol. Due to nanomaterial interference and as well as cell-specific conditions, necessary adjustments were performed. In brief, cells were trypsinized and suspended at $1x10^5$ cells/ml HBSS-. 5 μl of cells were mixed with freshly prepared low melting point agarose and immobilized on Trevigen comet assay slides (Gentaur, Kampenhout, Belgium). After cooling, the slides were immersed in lysis solution for 30 min. Subsequently, the slides were immersed in alkaline solution for 15 min to unwind the DNA. Finally, the slides were electrophoresed for 30 min. SYBERgold staining (1/10000 diluted in distilled water) was applied after cell fixation with 70% of ethanol.

The results were analyzed using a fluorescence microscope. 50 comets in the cells from each 2 replicates were measured for DNA damage by means of the % DNA Tail metric using the CaspLab program (casplab 1.2.3b2) according to the following formula:

$$\text{DNA Tail } (\%) = \frac{\text{Tail}}{\text{Head} + \text{Tail}} \times 100$$

The means of the two medians for each exposure type were represented.

Micronucleus assay

The micronucleus assay was adapted according to the OECD guidelines [49, 50]. Untreated cells were used as negative control and 0.6 mM mitomycin (Sigma Aldrich, Brussels, Belgium) was used as positive control. Mitomycin increased the number of micronuclei (mean 48.5, sd: 21.8, in 500 cells). No Cytochalasin B (CytB) was used. After exposure, the cells were further incubated with cell culture medium for 48 h (corresponding 1.5 doubling time). The number of micronuclei (MNs) in 500 mononucleated cells were counted for each three independent replicates 'blindly' using a light microscope. The means of the three counts were represented.

DNA extraction for epigenetic studies

DNA extraction involved use of the Qiagen DNA/RNA extraction mini kit (QIAGEN, Antwerp, Belgium) following the instructions. The experiment was carried out with three replicates. Untreated and vehicle (dispersion medium)-treated cells were used as a negative control, and 5-Aza-2′-deoxycytidine or in other name, Decitabine (Sigma Aldrich, Brussels, Belgium), a DNA hypomethylation agent, –treated cells (0.1 μM) were used as a positive control. DNA quantification involved use of Nano-drop (Thermo Scientific, 2000c).

Non-specific DNA methylation and hydroxymethylation analysis by LC-MS/MS

A validated protocol of LC-MS/MS (Waters) was used for identifying and quantifying DNA methylation and hydroxymethylation [22]. In total, 1 μg DNA was spiked with the internal standard mixture and dried. The DNA was enzymatically hydrolyzed to individual deoxyribonucleosides with 10 μl digestion mixture containing phosphodiesteraseI, alkaline phosphatase and benzonase nuclease in Tris-HCl buffer at 37 °C for 12 h. Diluted acetonitrile (Fischer Scientific, UK) was added to each sample. During the procedure, direct light was avoided to minimize potential deamination of target compounds.

Gene-specific whole-genome DNA methylation microarray and RNA sequencing

An amount of 200 ng genomic DNA was bisulfite-treated with use of the EZ DNA mini kit (Zymo Research, Orange, CA) following the instructions. Genome-wide assessment of DNA methylation involved the Infinium HumanMethylation450 BeadChip Array.

To analyze the effect of methylation on the transcriptome, RNA sequencing was performed. TruSeq RNA access Library Prep Kit (Illumina) was used to prepare the libraries. The resulting libraries were quantified by qPCR with KAPA Library Quantification for Illumina (Kapa Biosystems) and sequenced on a HiSeq2500 (Illumina) by using a V4 flowcell generating 1 × 50 bp reads.

Data preprocessing and bioinformatics/biostatistical analysis

The Illumina Infinium methylation microarray and RNA-Seq data were processed using Bioconductor R-packages [51].

The 'minfi' package was used for quality check and Type I and II probe normalization by the SWAN method [52]. The 'IMA' package was used for data annotation and further filtering [53]. After data preprocessing, differentially methylated CpG sites were found by using the 'limma' package with a linear modeling approach and empirical Bayes statistics while correcting for batch effect [53, 54]. Gene promoter methylation was defined as the mean methylation level of all CpGs located in a CpG island or shore, between 2000 bp upstream and 500 bp downstream of the gene start site as defined by Ensemble gene annotation v75. Individual CpG sites were linked to genes on the basis of the annotation provided by Illumina. Data were converted into M values because they are preferred over β values for small sample sizes (e.g., < 10) [55] by the following equation:

$$M = \log_2\{\beta/(1-\beta)\}$$

All analyses were performed with correction for batch effect. Finally, all p values were corrected for False Discovery Rate (FDR) [56]. Results were deemed significant with the FDR adjusted $p < 0.05$ ($q < 0.05$).

RNA sequencing reads were processed as previously described [57]. Briefly, the trimmed reads were mapped to the human transcriptome and reference genome (GRCh37.65/hg19) by using TopHat 2.0 [58] and Bowtie 2.0 [59]. Reads were assigned to ensemble gene IDs by using the HTSeq software package. On average, 32,031,451 (+ – 3,819,051) reads were assigned to genes. Differential expression between the different exposure methods was calculated by using EdgeR [60].

Heatmap and correlation analyses

For DNA methylation and for gene expression dataset the genes were ranked by their FDR corrected p values. Z scores for the most significant 500 genes for both type of CNTs were plotted on a heat-map. The clustering analysis involved use of Recursively Partitioned Mixture Model in R (RPMM/R) [61]. Representation of the correlation between RNA expression and DNA methylation data was performed using R, smoothscatter function [51].

Functional GO, pathway and network analysis

Differentially methylated genes that may affect the transcription of genes were proceeded for Gene Ontology (GO, The Gene Ontology Consortium 2000, http://geneontology.org/) analysis, Kyoto Encyclopedia of Genes and Genomes (KEGG, http://www.genome.jp/kegg/) pathway analysis and gene functional classification analysis (for top 3000 genes if data set is > 3000 genes) [62–65]. The web-tool DAVID 6.8 (updated in May 2016) was used in contrast to *Homo sapiens* background [66, 67] at EASE 0.1. When FDR corrected p value was smaller than 0.05, the GO annotation or KEGG pathway were considered significant. For gene functional classification analysis highest stringency was used and top five cluster was selected for interpretation. GeneMania web-tool was used for functional network analysis (http://www.genemania.org) [68].

Gene expression analysis by RT-PCR

Primer sequences were designed according to online bioinformatics tool, primer bank (https://pga.mgh.harvard.edu/primerbank/index.html) [69–71]. The primers were further justified in the NCBI primer designing tool (https://www.ncbi.nlm.nih.gov/tools/primer-blast/) Ye et al., [72]. The forward and reverse primers of the corresponding gene were listed in Table 1.

For the validation assay, we performed four replicates ($N = 4$). The exposures were performed from two different stock solutions on four different T25 vials. RNA is extracted immediately by AllPrep DNA/RNA mini kit (QIAGEN, Belgium) and quality and quantity was obtained using Nano-drop (Thermo Scientific, 2000c). 1 μg of RNA is converted to complementary DNA (cDNA) using SuperScript III First strand kit (Invitrogen, Belgium) according to manual of the kit. After cDNA conversion, gene of interest were amplified using Platinum® SYBR® Green qPCR SuperMix-UDG (Invitrogen, Belgium) according to the kits manual. Westburg Eco 48 well custom reaction plates (Westburg, The Netherlands) and Westburg Eco Adhesive seals (Westburg, The Netherlands) were used to carry out the reverse transcription-PCR (RT-PCR) experiment. GAPDH gene is included as a

Table 1 The primer sequences of the tested genes

Primers	
Name	Sequence
BAX forward	CCC GAG AGG TCT TTT TCC GAG
BAX reverse	CCA GCC CAT GAT GGT TCT GAT
TP53 forward	CAG CAC ATG ACG GAG GTT GT
TP53 reverse	TCA TCC AAA TAC TCC ACA CGC
AKT1 forward	GTC ATC GAA CGC ACC TTC CAT
AKT1 reverse	AGC TTC AGG TAC TCA AAC TCG T
NF1 forward	AGA TGA AAC GAT GCT GGT CAA A
NF1 reverse	CCT GTA ACC TGG TAG AAA TGC GA
ATM forward	GGC TAT TCA GTG TGC GAG ACA
ATM reverse	TGG CTC CTT TCG GAT GAT GGA
BCL2L11 forward	TAA GTT CTG AGT GTG ACC GAG A
BCL2L11 reverse	GCT CTG TCT GTA GGG AGG TAG G
GAPDH forward	TGG TAT CGT GGA AGG ACT CA
GAPDH reverse	CCA GTA GAG GCA GGG ATG AT

housekeeping gene. Log fold changes were calculated in relative to the results obtained from vehicle-treated cells. The data was analysed in relative to the vehicle-treated control cells. $2^{-\Delta\Delta Ct}$ values were calculated to show the relative fold change of the expression.

Statistical analysis

Statistical analyses concerning cytotoxicity and genotoxicity involved the use of one way ANOVA with Dunnett's multiple comparison. The statistics concerning nuclear deposition measurements is conducted using one way ANOVA with Tukey's multiple comparison. These statistics were performed using graphpad Prism 5 for Windows (GraphPad Software, La Jolla, CA, https://www.graphpad.com/). The statistics for RT-PCR is conducted using two-tailed t-test (interval 95%). Data are represented as mean ± SD. The bioinformatics and statistics for the microarray data were performed by using R explained in the section Data preprocessing and bioinformatics/biostatistics analyses.

Additional files

Additional file 1: Figure S1. Validation of the label-free imaging of CNTs. **Figure S2.** Cytotoxicity assessment of MWCNTs and SWCNTs at a variety of doses. **Figure S3.** DNA damaging effects of MWCNTs and SWCNTs. **Figure S4.** Micronuclei formation in the cells after exposure to MWCNTs and SWCNTs. **Table S1.** Physicochemical characterization of MWCNTs and SWCNTs. **Table S2.** Enriched GO terms by differentially methylated genes (by gene promoter regions) after exposure to MWCNTs. **Table S3.** Gene functional classification analysis using differentially methylated genes (by gene promoter regions) after exposure to MWCNTs. **Table S4.** Enriched GO terms by differentially expressed genes (by gene promoter regions) after exposure to MWCNTs. **Table S5.** Enriched KEGG terms by differentially expressed genes (by gene promoter regions) after exposure to MWCNTs. P53 signalling was noted in italic since its close proximity to significance. **Table S6.** Gene functional classification analysis using differentially expressed genes after exposure to MWCNTs. **Table S7.** Enriched GO terms by differentially methylated genes (by single CpG sites on the genomic regions) after exposure to SWCNTs. **Table S8.** Enriched KEGG terms by differentially methylated genes (by single CpG sites on the genomic regions) after exposure to SWCNTs. **Table S9.** Gene functional classification analysis using differentially methylation CpG sites after exposure to SWCNTs. **Table S10.** Enriched GO terms by differentially expressed genes (by single CpG sites) after exposure to SWCNTs. **Table S11.** Enriched KEGG terms by differentially expressed genes (by single CpG sites) after exposure to SWCNTs. **Table S12.** Gene functional classification analysis using differentially expressed genes after exposure to SWCNTs. (DOCX 596 kb)

Additional file 2: Video S1. 3D video of z-stacks images (top to bottom) of MWCNTs in the nucleus. (AVI 42 kb)

Additional file 3: Video S2. 3D video of z-stacks images (top to bottom) of SWCNTs in the nucleus. (AVI 28 kb)

Additional file 4: Video S3. 3D video of MWCNTs around the nucleus. (AVI 54 kb)

Additional file 5: Video S4. 3D video of SWCNTs around the nucleus. (AVI 49 kb)

Abbreviations

[BCL2L11 (BIM)]: BCL2 like 11; [CDKN1A (p21)]: Cyclin dependent kinase inhibitor 1A; AKAP8L: A-kinase anchoring protein 8 like; ATM: ATM serine/tyrosine kinase; BAX: BCL2 associated x, apoptosis regulator; BCL3: B cell lymphoma 3; CCL2: C-C motif chemokine ligand 2; CCL4: C-C motif chemokine ligand 4; CCL5: C-C motif chemokine ligand 5; CDK4: Cyclin dependent kinase 4; CDK6: Cyclin dependent kinase 6; CDKs: Cyclin dependent kinases; CHK2: Checkpoint kinase 2; CNTs: Carbon nanotubes; CpG: Cytosine-phosphate-guanine; CXCL1: Chemokine (C-X-C motif) ligand 1; CXCL2: Chemokine (C-X-C motif) ligand 2; CytB: Cytochalasin B; DDAH2: Dimethylarginine dimethylaminohydrolase 2; DDR1: Discoidin domain receptor tyrosine kinase 1; DLS: Dynamic light scattering; DMEM: Dulbecco's Modified Eagle Medium; DMEM/F12: Dulbecco's Modified Eagle Medium: Nutrient Mixture F12; DNMT1: DNA methyl transferase 1; ECD: Ecdysoneless cell cycle regulator; EIF4E: Eukaryotic translation initiation factor 4E; ENPRA: Engineered Nanoparticle Risk Assessment; ERG: ERG ETS transcription factor; FAS: Fas cell surface death receptor; FCS: Fetal calf serum; FGFR1: Fibroblast growth factor receptor 1; FOXK2: Forkhead box K2; FOXO: Forkhead box O; GO: Gene Ontology; GTP: Guanosine-5'-triphosphate; GTSP1: Glutathione s-transferase pi 1; HBSS: Hank's Balanced Salt Solution; HTLV-I: Human t-lymphotropic virus-1; IFN-γ: Interferon-gamma; IGFR: Insulin-like growth factor 1 receptor; IL1-β: Interleukin 1 beta; IL6: Interleukin 6; KEGG: Kyoto Encyclopedia of Genes and Genomes; KIF15: Kinesin family member 15; KLF2: Kruppel like factor 2; LC-MS/MS: Liquid chromatography-mass spectrometry; LDH: Lactate dehydrogenase; LIF: Leukemia inhibitory factor; MAPK: Mitogen-activated protein kinase; MLKL: Mixed lineage kinase domain like; MNs: Micronuclei; MWCNTs: Multi-walled CNTs; NF1: Neurofibromatosis type I; Nm: Nanometer; NOSTRIN: Nitric oxide synthase trafficking; NOXA1: NADPH oxidase activator 1; NF-κB: Nuclear factor-kappa B; NFKBIA: Nuclear factor-kappa B inhibitor alpha; PBS: Phosphate buffered saline; PDGFR: Platelet-derived growth factor receptor beta; PERP: PERP TP53 apoptosis effector; PI3K-AKT: Phosphatidylinositide 3 kinases-protein kinase B; PIK3R2: Phosphoinositide-3-kinase regulatory subunit 2; RTKs: Receptor tyrosine kinases; SHISA5: Shisa family member 5; SHROOM2: Shroom family member 2; SKI: SKI proto-oncogene; snoU13: Small nucleolar RNA U13; SWCNTs: Single-walled CNTs; TEM: Transmission electron microscopy; TNF: Tumour necrosis factor; TNF-α: Tumour necrosis factor alpha; TNFRSF25: Tumour necrosis factor receptor superfamily member 25; TP53: Tumour protein 53; TP53I3: Tumour protein P53 inducible protein 3; TRAF2: Tumour necrosis factor receptor associated factor 2; UDP: Uridine 5'-diphospho-glucuronosyltransferase; VHL: Von hippel-lindau tumor suppressor; WST-1: Water-soluble tetrazolium salt-1; 5-mC: 5-methylcytosine; 5-hmC: 5-hydroxymethylcytosine

Acknowledgements

The authors thank Thomas van Brussels for technical microarray assistance.

Funding
This work was granted by Stichting Tegen Kanker (Foundation Against Cancer), grant agreement no: 2012–218, Project No: 3 M150270. Manosij Ghosh is a postdoctoral fellow of European Respiratory Society RESPIRE (RESPIRE2) grant agreement no: 2014–7310.

Authors' contributions
DÖ and MG performed the experiments, generated the data and discussed the findings. DÖ prepared the draft manuscript and MG further improved the manuscript on results and discussion section. HB measured the nuclear uptake of the particles in cells and the nucleus and MA provided the technical assistance for nuclear deposition imaging using light microscopy. MM, BB pre-processed the DNA methylation and gene expression microarray using bioinformatics techniques and DL involved in the study design. RCD, JV and KP provided their technical assistance for LC-MS/MS measurements and involved in establishing the protocol. EP, KL and KVL helped for establishing study design, cell culture methods. PH and LG designed, supervised the project and the revised manuscript, PH established the manuscript in final form. All authors read and revised the manuscript and agreed on publication.

Competing interests
The authors declare that there is no competing of interest.

Author details
[1]Laboratory of Toxicology, Unit of Environment and Health, Department of Public Health and Primary Care, KU Leuven, 3000 Leuven, Belgium. [2]Centre for Surface Chemistry and Catalysis, KU Leuven, Celestijnenlaan 200F, 3001 Leuven, Belgium. [3]Biomedical Research Institute, Agoralaan Building C, Hasselt University, 3590 Diepenbeek, Belgium. [4]Laboratory for Translational Genetics, Department of Human Genetics, KU Leuven, 3000 Leuven, Belgium. [5]Laboratory for Translational Genetics, VIB Centre for Cancer Biology, VIB, 3000 Leuven, Belgium. [6]Laboratory for Occupational and Environmental Hygiene, Unit of Environment and Health, Department of Public Health and Primary Care, KU Leuven, 3000 Leuven, Belgium. [7]Department of Oral Health Sciences, Unit of Biomaterials (BIOMAT), KU Leuven, 3000 Leuven, Belgium. [8]External Service for Prevention and Protection at Work, IDEWE, B-3001, Leuven, Belgium.

References
1. Donaldson K, Aitken R, Tran L, Stone V, Duffin R, Forrest G, et al. Carbon Nanotubes: A review of their properties in relation to pulmonary toxicology and workplace safety. Toxicol Sci. 2006;92:5–22.
2. Volder MFLD, Tawfick SH, Baughman RH, Hart AJ. Carbon Nanotubes: Present and future commercial applications. Science. 2013;339:535–9.
3. Mu Q, Broughton DL, Yan B. Endosomal leakage and nuclear translocation of multiwalled carbon Nanotubes: Developing a model for cell uptake. Nano Lett. 2009;9:4370–5.
4. Yaron PN, Holt BD, Short PA, Lösche M, Islam MF, Dahl KN. Single wall carbon nanotubes enter cells by endocytosis and not membrane penetration. J Nanobiotechnol. 2011;9:45.
5. Herceg Z. Epigenetic mechanisms as an Interface between the environment and genome. In: Roach RC, Hackett PH, Wagner PD, editors. Hypoxia: Springer US; 2016. p. 3–15. [cited 2017 Feb 25] Available from: http://link.springer.com/chapter/10.1007/978-1-4899-7678-9_1
6. Jirtle RL, Skinner MK. Environmental epigenomics and disease susceptibility. Nat Rev Genet. 2007;8:253–62.
7. Luzhna L, Kathiria P, Kovalchuk O. Micronuclei in genotoxicity assessment: From genetics to epigenetics and beyond. Front Genet. 2013;4 [cited 2017 Apr 10] Available from: http://www.ncbi.nlm.nih.gov/pmc/articles/PMC3708156/
8. Sharma S, Kelly TK, Jones PA. Epigenetics in cancer. Carcinogenesis. 2010;31:27–36.
9. Li E, Zhang Y. DNA methylation in mammals. Cold Spring Harb Perspect Biol. 2014;6:a019133.
10. Ghosh M, Bhadra S, Adegoke A, Bandyopadhyay M, Mukherjee A. MWCNT uptake in Allium Cepa root cells induces cytotoxic and genotoxic responses and results in DNA hyper-methylation. Mutat Res. 2015;774:49–58.
11. Tabish AM, Poels K, Byun H-M, Luyts K, Baccarelli AA, Martens J, et al. Changes in DNA Methylation in mouse lungs after a single intra-tracheal Administration of Nanomaterials. PLoS One. 2017;12:e0169886.
12. Brown TA, Lee JW, Holian A, Porter V, Fredriksen H, Kim M, et al. Alterations in DNA methylation corresponding with lung inflammation and as a biomarker for disease development after MWCNT exposure. Nanotoxicology. 2016;10:453–61.
13. Li J, Tian M, Cui L, Dwyer J, Fullwood NJ, Shen H, et al. Low-dose carbon-based nanoparticle-induced effects in A549 lung cells determined by biospectroscopy are associated with increases in genomic methylation. Sci Rep. 2016;6:20207.
14. Sierra MI, Rubio L, Bayón GF, Cobo I, Menendez P, Morales P, et al. DNA methylation changes in human lung epithelia cells exposed to multi-walled carbon nanotubes. Nanotoxicology. 2017;11:857–70.
15. Chernova T, Murphy FA, Galavotti S, Sun X-M, Powley IR, Grosso S, et al. Long-fiber carbon Nanotubes replicate asbestos-induced Mesothelioma with disruption of the tumor suppressor gene Cdkn2a (Ink4a/Arf). Curr Biol CB. 2017;27:3302–3314.e6.
16. Öner D, Moisse M, Ghosh M, Duca RC, Poels K, Luyts K, et al. Epigenetic effects of carbon nanotubes in human monocytic cells. Mutagenesis. 2016;32:181.
17. NIST. Certificate of Analysis Standard Reference Material 2483. National Institute of Standards and Technology; 2011. Available from: https://www-s.nist.gov/srmors/certificates/2483.pdf. Accessed 28 Jan 2018.
18. Rasmussen K, Mast J, De Temmerman P-J, Verleysen E, Waegeneers N, Van Steen F, et al: Multi-walled Carbon Nanotubes, NM-400, NM-401, NM-402, NM-403: Characterisation and Physico-Chemical Properties. European commission; 2014. Report No.: 26796. Available from: https://ec.europa.eu/jrc/sites/default/files/mwcnt-online.pdf. Accessed 28 Jan 2018.
19. Smulders S, Kaiser J-P, Zuin S, Van Landuyt KL, Golanski L, Vanoirbeek J, et al. Contamination of nanoparticles by endotoxin: Evaluation of different test methods. Part. Fibre Toxicol. 2012;9:41.
20. Bové H, Steuwe C, Fron E, Slenders E, D'Haen J, Fujita Y, et al. Biocompatible label-free detection of carbon black particles by Femtosecond pulsed laser microscopy. Nano Lett. 2016;16:3173–8.
21. Ramírez T, Stopper H, Hock R, Herrera LA. Prevention of aneuploidy by S-adenosyl-methionine in human cells treated with sodium arsenite. Mutat Res Mol Mech Mutagen. 2007;617:16–22.
22. Godderis L, Schouteden C, Tabish A, Poels K, Hoet P, Baccarelli AA, et al. Global Methylation and Hydroxymethylation in DNA from blood and saliva in healthy volunteers. Biomed Res Int. 2015;2015:e845041.
23. Baylin SB, Herman JG. DNA hypermethylation in tumorigenesis: Epigenetics joins genetics. Trends Genet TIG. 2000;16:168–74.
24. Helman E, Naxerova K, Kohane IS. DNA hypermethylation in lung cancer is targeted at differentiation-associated genes. Oncogene. 2012;31:1181–8.
25. Cancer Genome Atlas Research Network. Comprehensive molecular profiling of lung adenocarcinoma. Nature. 2014;511:543–50.
26. Redig AJ, Capelletti M, Dahlberg SE, Sholl LM, Mach S, Fontes C, et al. Clinical and molecular characteristics of NF1-mutant lung cancer. Clin Cancer Res Off J Am Assoc Cancer Res. 2016;22:3148–56.
27. Saito M, Shiraishi K, Kunitoh H, Takenoshita S, Yokota J, Kohno T. Gene aberrations for precision medicine against lung adenocarcinoma. Cancer Sci. 2016;107:713–20.
28. Baylin SB, Ohm JE. Epigenetic gene silencing in cancer – A mechanism for early oncogenic pathway addiction? Nat Rev Cancer. 2006;6:107–16.
29. Esteller M. Epigenetics in cancer. N Engl J Med. 2008;358:1148–59.
30. Pacurari M, Yin XJ, Zhao J, Ding M, Leonard SS, Schwegler-Berry D, et al. Raw single-wall carbon nanotubes induce oxidative stress and activate MAPKs, AP-1, NF-kappaB, and Akt in normal and malignant human mesothelial cells. Env Health Perspect. 2008;116:1211–7.
31. Hannu Norppa. In vitro testing strategy for nanomaterials including database. Finnish Institute of Occupational Health; 2015. Available from: http://www.oecd.org/officialdocuments/publicdisplaydocumentpdf/?cote=env/jm/mono(2015)17/ann9&doclanguage=en
32. Szyf M. The role of dna hypermethylation and demethylation in cancer and cancer therapy. Curr Oncol. 2008;15:72–5.
33. Unterberger A, Andrews SD, Weaver ICG, Szyf M. DNA methyltransferase 1 knockdown activates a replication stress checkpoint. Mol Cell Biol. 2006;26:7575–86.
34. Herman JG, Baylin SB. Gene silencing in cancer in association with promoter Hypermethylation. N Engl J Med. 2003;349:2042–54.

35. Huaux F, de Bousies VD, Parent M-A, Orsi M, Uwambayinema F, Devosse R, et al. Mesothelioma response to carbon nanotubes is associated with an early and selective accumulation of immunosuppressive monocytic cells. Part Fibre Toxicol. 2016;13 [cited 2017 Dec 9] Available from: https://www.ncbi.nlm.nih.gov/pmc/articles/PMC4994252/
36. Kastan MB, Bartek J. Cell-cycle checkpoints and cancer. Nature. 2004; 432:316–23.
37. Malumbres M, Barbacid M. Cell cycle, CDKs and cancer: A changing paradigm. Nat Rev Cancer. 2009;9:153–66.
38. Chen D, Stueckle TA, Luanpitpong S, Rojanasakul Y, Lu Y, Wang L. Gene expression profile of human lung epithelial cells chronically exposed to single-walled carbon nanotubes. Nanoscale Res Lett. 2015;10:1–12.
39. Wang L, Luanpitpong S, Castranova V, Tse W, Lu Y, Pongrakhananon V, et al. Carbon NANOTUBES induce malignant transformation and tumorigenesis of human lung epithelial cells. Nano Lett. 2011;11:2796–803.
40. Chou C-C, Hsiao H-Y, Hong Q-S, Chen C-H, Peng Y-W, Chen H-W, et al. Single-walled carbon Nanotubes can induce pulmonary injury in mouse model. Nano Lett. 2008;8:437–45.
41. Mangum JB, Turpin EA, Antao-Menezes A, Cesta MF, Bermudez E, Bonner JC. Single-walled carbon Nanotube (SWCNT)-induced interstitial fibrosis in the lungs of rats is associated with increased levels of PDGF mRNA and the formation of unique intercellular carbon structures that bridge alveolar macrophages in situ. Part Fibre Toxicol. 2006;3:15.
42. Shvedova AA, Kisin ER, Mercer R, Murray AR, Johnson VJ, Potapovich AI, et al. Unusual inflammatory and fibrogenic pulmonary responses to single-walled carbon nanotubes in mice. Am J Physiol-Lung Cell Mol Physiol. 2005; 289:L698–708.
43. Shvedova AA, Kisin E, Murray AR, Johnson VJ, Gorelik O, Arepalli S, et al. Inhalation vs. aspiration of single-walled carbon nanotubes in C57BL/6 mice: Inflammation, fibrosis, oxidative stress, and mutagenesis. Am. J. Physiol.-Lung Cell. Mol. Physiol. 2008;295:L552–65.
44. Cao Y, Jacobsen NR, Danielsen PH, Lenz AG, Stoeger T, Loft S, et al. Vascular effects of multiwalled carbon nanotubes in dyslipidemic ApoE−/− mice and cultured endothelial cells. Toxicol Sci Off J Soc Toxicol. 2014;138:104–16.
45. Kermanizadeh A, Gosens I, MacCalman L, Johnston H, Danielsen PH, Jacobsen NR, et al. A multilaboratory toxicological assessment of a panel of 10 engineered Nanomaterials to human health—ENPRA project—The highlights, limitations, and current and future challenges. J Toxicol Environ Health Part B. 2016;19:1–28.
46. Ghosh M, Öner D, Poels K, Tabish AM, Vlaanderen J, Pronk A, et al. Changes in DNA methylation induced by multi-walled carbon nanotube exposure in the workplace. Nanotoxicology. 2017;11:1195–210.
47. Jacobsen N, Pojano G, Wallin H, Jensen K. Nanomaterial dispersion protocol for toxicological studies in ENPRA. Intern ENPRA Proj Rep. 2010;6. http://www.nanotechia.org/sites/default/files/files/PROSPECT_Dispersion_Protocol.pdf. Accessed 28 Jan 2018.
48. Collins AR. The comet assay for DNA damage and repair. Mol Biotechnol. 2004;26:249–61.
49. Doak S, Manshian B, Jenkins G, Singh N. In vitro genotoxicity testing strategy for nanomaterials and the adaptation of current OECD guidelines. Mutat Res Toxicol Environ Mutagen. 2012;745:104–11.
50. OECD. Test no. 487: In vitro mammalian cell micronucleus test. Paris: Organisation for Economic Co-operation and Development; 2014. [cited 2016 Jun 15] Available from: http://www.oecd-ilibrary.org/content/book/9789264224438-en
51. R Core Team. R: A language and environment for statistical computing: R Proj. Stat. Comput; 2017. [cited 2016 Mar 14]. Available from: http://www.gbif.org/resource/81287
52. Aryee MJ, Jaffe AE, Corrada-Bravo H, Ladd-Acosta C, Feinberg AP, Hansen KD, et al. Minfi: A flexible and comprehensive bioconductor package for the analysis of Infinium DNA methylation microarrays. Bioinformatics. 2014;30:1363–9.
53. Wang D, Yan L, Hu Q, Sucheston LE, Higgins MJ, Ambrosone CB, et al. IMA: An R package for high-throughput analysis of Illumina's 450K Infinium methylation data. Bioinformatics. 2012;28:729–30.
54. Smyth GK. Limma: Linear models for microarray data. Bioinforma. Comput. Biol. Solut. Using R bioconductor. New York: Springer; 2005. p. 397–420.
55. Zhuang J, Widschwendter M, Teschendorff AE. A comparison of feature selection and classification methods in DNA methylation studies using the Illumina Infinium platform. BMC Bioinformatics. 2012;13:59.
56. Benjamini Y, Hochberg Y. Controlling the false discovery rate: A practical and powerful approach to multiple testing. J R Stat Soc Ser B Methodol. 1995;57:289–300.
57. Nassar D, Latil M, Boeckx B, Lambrechts D, Blanpain C. Genomic landscape of carcinogen-induced and genetically induced mouse skin squamous cell carcinoma. Nat Med. 2015;21:946–54.
58. Kim D, Pertea G, Trapnell C, Pimentel H, Kelley R, Salzberg SL. TopHat2: Accurate alignment of transcriptomes in the presence of insertions, deletions and gene fusions. Genome Biol. 2013;14:R36.
59. Langmead B, Salzberg SL. Fast gapped-read alignment with bowtie 2. Nat Methods. 2012;9:357–9.
60. Robinson MD, McCarthy DJ, Smyth GK. edgeR: A bioconductor package for differential expression analysis of digital gene expression data. Bioinformatics. 2010;26:139–40.
61. Houseman EA, Koestler DC. RPMM.pdf. 2015 [cited 2016 Jun 15]; Available from: https://cran.r-project.org/web/packages/RPMM/RPMM.pdf. Accessed on 28 Jan 2018.
62. Ashburner M, Ball CA, Blake JA, Botstein D, Butler H, Cherry JM, et al. Gene ontology: Tool for the unification of biology. Nat Genet. 2000;25:25–9.
63. Consortium TGO. Gene ontology consortium: Going forward. Nucleic Acids Res. 2015;43:D1049–56.
64. Ogata H, Goto S, Sato K, Fujibuchi W, Bono H, Kanehisa M. KEGG: Kyoto encyclopedia of genes and genomes. Nucleic Acids Res. 1999;27:29–34.
65. Kanehisa M, Goto S. KEGG: kyoto encyclopedia of genes and genomes. Nucleic Acids Res. 2000;28:27–30.
66. Huang DW, Sherman BT, Lempicki RA. Systematic and integrative analysis of large gene lists using DAVID bioinformatics resources. Nat Protoc. 2009;4:44–57.
67. Huang DW, Sherman BT, Lempicki RA. Bioinformatics enrichment tools: Paths toward the comprehensive functional analysis of large gene lists. Nucleic Acids Res. 2009;37:1–13.
68. Warde-Farley D, Donaldson SL, Comes O, Zuberi K, Badrawi R, Chao P, et al. The GeneMANIA prediction server: Biological network integration for gene prioritization and predicting gene function. Nucleic Acids Res. 2010;38:W214–20.
69. Spandidos A, Wang X, Wang H, Seed B. PrimerBank: A resource of human and mouse PCR primer pairs for gene expression detection and quantification. Nucleic Acids Res. 2010;38:D792–9.
70. Wang X, Seed B. A PCR primer bank for quantitative gene expression analysis. Nucleic Acids Res. 2003;31:e154.
71. Spandidos A, Wang X, Wang H, Dragnev S, Thurber T, Seed B. A comprehensive collection of experimentally validated primers for polymerase chain reaction quantitation of murine transcript abundance. BMC Genomics. 2008;9:633.
72. Ye J, Coulouris G, Zaretskaya I, Cutcutache I, Rozen S, Madden TL. Primer-BLAST: A tool to design target-specific primers for polymerase chain reaction. BMC Bioinformatics. 2012;13:134.

5

Multi-cellular human bronchial models exposed to diesel exhaust particles: assessment of inflammation, oxidative stress and macrophage polarization

Jie Ji[1*†], Swapna Upadhyay[1*†], Xiaomiao Xiong[1], Maria Malmlöf[1,2], Thomas Sandström[3], Per Gerde[1,2] and Lena Palmberg[1]

Abstract

Background: Diesel exhaust particles (DEP) are a major component of outdoor air pollution. DEP mediated pulmonary effects are plausibly linked to inflammatory and oxidative stress response in which macrophages (MQ), epithelial cells and their cell-cell interaction plays a crucial role. Therefore, in this study we aimed at studying the cellular crosstalk between airway epithelial cells with MQ and MQ polarization following exposure to aerosolized DEP by assessing inflammation, oxidative stress, and MQ polarization response markers.

Method: Lung mucosa models including primary bronchial epithelial cells (PBEC) cultured at air-liquid interface (ALI) were co-cultured without (PBEC-ALI) and with MQ (PBEC-ALI/MQ). Cells were exposed to 12.7 μg/cm^2 aerosolized DEP using Xpose*ALI*®. Control (sham) models were exposed to clean air. Cell viability was assessed. CXCL8 and IL-6 were measured in the basal medium by ELISA. The mRNA expression of inflammatory markers (*CXCL8, IL6, TNFα*), oxidative stress (*NFKB, HMOX1, GPx*) and MQ polarization markers (*IL10, IL4, IL13, MRC1, MRC2 RETNLA, IL12* and*IL23*) were measured by qRT-PCR. The surface/mRNA expression of TLR2/TLR4 was detected by FACS and qRT-PCR.

Results: In PBEC-ALI exposure to DEP significantly increased the secretion of CXCL8, mRNA expression of inflammatory markers (*CXCL8, TNFα*) and oxidative stress markers (*NFKB, HMOX1, GPx*). However, mRNA expressions of these markers (*CXCL8, IL6, NFKB,* and *HMOX1*) were reduced in PBEC-ALI/MQ models after DEP exposure. TLR2 and TLR4 mRNA expression increased after DEP exposure in PBEC-ALI. The surface expression of TLR2 and TLR4 on PBEC was significantly reduced in sham-exposed PBEC-ALI/MQ compared to PBEC-ALI. After DEP exposure surface expression of TLR2 was increased on PBEC of PBEC-ALI/MQ, while TLR4 was decreased in both models. DEP exposure resulted in similar expression pattern of TLR2/TLR4 on MQ as in PBEC. In PBEC-ALI/MQ, DEP exposure increased the mRNA expression of anti-inflammatory M2 macrophage markers (*IL10, IL4, IL13, MRC1, MRC2*).

(Continued on next page)

* Correspondence: jie.ji@ki.se; swapna.upadhyay@ki.se
†Equal contributors
[1]Institute of Environmental Medicine, Karolinska Institute, Box 210, SE-171 77 Stockholm, Sweden
Full list of author information is available at the end of the article

(Continued from previous page)

Conclusion: The cellular interaction of PBEC with MQ in response to DEP plays a pivotal role for MQ phenotypic alteration towards M2-subtypes, thereby promoting an efficient resolution of the inflammation. Furthermore, this study highlighted the fact that cell–cell interaction using multicellular ALI-models combined with an in vivo-like inhalation exposure system is critical in better mimicking the airway physiology compared with traditional cell culture systems.

Keywords: Diesel exhaust particles, Air-liquid interface multicellular model, Inflammation, Macrophage polarization, Oxidative stress

Background

Automobile exhaust mediated air pollution continues to be an unavoidable respiratory health hazard throughout the world. Acute air pollution episodes with high concentrations of particulate matter have been associated with increased emergency room visits and hospitalization due to exacerbation of respiratory diseases like asthma and chronic obstructive pulmonary disease (COPD) [1, 2]. Diesel engines, by virtue of their high efficiency, robustness and low running costs are of wide-usage globally. Diesel exhaust particles (DEP) are the products of incomplete combustion of diesel engine fuel. DEP constitute a complex mixture of particles (< 1.0 μm in diameter) and combustion gases with a carbon core surrounded by trace metals, salts and organic hydrocarbons.

Upon exposure, DEP can deposit on the human airway mucosa. They may cross the epithelium and cell membranes of resident macrophages, subsequently binding to different cytosolic receptors which may lead to cell growth and differentiation [3]. Acute exposure to DEP in humans results in extensive bronchial and alveolar inflammation with influx of phagocytic cells [2, 4]. Long-term exposure to DEP has been associated with greater incidence of cough and chronic bronchitis [5]. Exposure to DEP has also been associated with a number of long-term adverse effects, such as exacerbation of pre-existing lung disease (asthma and COPD), respiratory infections and worsening of cardiovascular disease, as well as increased mortality [6–8].Similarly, many animal studies have examined the effects of DEP and reported alterations in oxidative stress and inflammatory endpoints [9, 10]. Even though animal studies still serve as a major method of mechanistic investigation, current literature underlines several limitations in the study designs particularly related to dosimetry. Large differences in sensitivity between species and within different strains of the same species have also been observed. The response to DEP exposure has been examined in in vitro studies employing airway epithelial cells, nasal epithelial cells, alveolar macrophages, mast cells, and cell lines [11–13]. These studies have shown that DEP can generate reactive oxygen species (ROS), which in turn trigger a variety of cellular consequences, such as DNA damage, apoptosis and inflammatory responses [14, 15]. These potentially injurious effects of ROS can be neutralized by a variety of antioxidants, including Heme oxygenase 1(HMOX1), glutathione peroxidase (GPx), and superoxide dismutase(SOD) [16].

Human airway epithelium acts as the first line of defense between external environment and internal milieu, thus playing a central role in the response to DEP exposure. Airway macrophages (MQ) and epithelial cells are the two most abundant cell types present in both the conducting- and lower airways, thereby serving as the crucial first responders to airborne particles deposited in the lung [17, 18]. Additionally, the airway epithelium acts both as a physical barrier against the inhaled stimulant (DEP) and as an orchestrator of the innate immune response [17, 19].

The classically activated macrophages (M1) arise in response to the T helper type 1 (Th1) cytokine interferon gamma (IFN-γ) and lipopolysaccharide (LPS). M1-MQs possess bactericidal and tumoricidal activity; generate reactive oxygen species (ROS) and nitric oxide; promote Th1 responses; and produce high levels of pro-inflammatory cytokines like tumor necrosis factor alpha (TNF-α) and interleukin (IL-6) etc. [20, 21]. On the other hand, the alternative activated macrophages (M2), generated by the T helper type 2 (Th2) cytokines IL-4 or IL-13, play a central role in tissue repair, tissue remodeling, matrix deposition and healing, and promote Th2 responses [20, 21]. M2-MQ express high levels of scavenger mannose and galactose receptors, and produce high levels of IL-10 and IL-1 receptor antagonist [22, 23]. Macrophage polarization have been studied in certain scenarios like bacterial infection, cancer, and asthma [22, 23] and is considered to be an evolving topic of interest. In humans, phenotypic alteration of MQ is considered to play a pivotal role in the onset of airway disease and has potential implications for the treatment of chronic respiratory disease like asthma and COPD.

Byrne et al. [24] reported that M1 associated cytokines; IL-12 and IFN-γ are increased in response to exposure to particulate matter in air pollutants. On the other hand, exposure to cigarette smoke has been shown to alter macrophages towards M2 phenotype [25]. Different nanoparticles can perturb polarization and reprogramming of the macrophages, which is dependent on their chemical composition [26], size [27] and surface coating [28]. According to Miao et al. [29], many nanoparticle types like Ag-NP, Au-NP, ZnO-NP, TiO-NP, and SiO-NP can induce a M1 phenotype polarization and there are a few reports on NP-induced M2-MQ polarizations. The knowledge on DEP exposure related macrophage polarization is still lacking. Based on a study conducted by Jaguin et al. [30] it was shown that by treating human blood monocyte-derived MQ with DEP, the expression of several M1 and M2 markers which are involved in MQ activation was impaired, but without inhibiting the overall polarization process. DEP exposure also attenuated the LPS-induced M1-MQs effects. Because DEP can activate the oxidative stress pathways [31], this may suggest that the alteration of M1/ M2 markers upon DEP exposure is Aryl Hydrocarbon Receptor (AhR)- and Nrf2-dependent. Bauer et al. [24] showed that in co-cultures of human primary alveolar macrophages with epithelial cells, ozone exposure lead to a modified macrophage response inducing M2 activation status with a reduced phagocytic activity. In vivo studies in rats suggest that inhalation of ozone is associated with accumulation of both classically- and alternatively activated MQ in the lungs [32]. It has been well established that close cellular cross talk between airway epithelial cells and MQ in the presence of different stimuli (environmental- or intentional exposure) regulate the inflammatory response in association with macrophage polarization. The lung microenvironment has been shown to influence MQ phenotype- and function [33]. However, most in vitro studies [11, 34] investigating the cellular inflammatory response to air pollutants have used mono-culture systems, which do not address the interaction between different cell types present in the airways, and have limited applicability to in vivo situations. The cross talk between MQ and epithelial cells are essential as they both function within the first line of defense against inhaled toxic agents in both upper- and lower airways.

Previously, we reported that the toll-like receptors (TLR), including TLR2 and TLR4 on the surface of both macrophages [35] and epithelial cells [36], are very critical in recognizing a wide spectrum of inhaled pathogens. Although the involvement of TLR2/4 in the innate immune response to DEP are well known [37], there is still no consensus on how DEP modulate TLR2/4 expression, and especially the interaction of the different cell types involved.

Therefore, in this study we performed DEP exposure with precise dosimetry using air liquid interface (ALI) co-culture models of human primary bronchial epithelial cells (PBEC) with macrophages (THP-1 derived macrophages) to mimic cell-cell interaction of in vivo condition. Further the interaction between epithelial cells and MQ in response to DEP exposure for the alteration of MQ polarization was investigated using both mono- (PBEC-ALI or MQ) and co-cultured (PBEC-ALI/MQ) models.

Methods

Cell cultures

Bronchial mucosa models with PBEC cultured at ALI (PBEC-ALI)

The PBEC were harvested from healthy bronchial tissues obtained from 10 donors in connection with lobectomy following their informed and written consent. All procedures performed in the study were in accordance to the approval of the Ethical Committee of Karolinska Institutet, Stockholm. The cells used in this study are well characterized and have been used in other studies [36, 38, 39].

The airlifted PBEC models were developed as previously described [39]. Briefly, PBEC were seeded (1×10^5 cell/cm^2) and cultured on transwell inserts (0.4 μM pore size, BD Falcon™) in twelve-well plates under standard conditions (5% CO_2 at 37 °C). One ml PneumaCult™-Ex medium (Stemcell technologies, Cambridge, UK) supplemented with 96 μg/ml hydrocortisone (Stemcell technologies, Cambridge, UK) and penicillin streptomycin antibiotics (PEST, 1%, Bio Whittaker, Lonza, Basel, Switzerland) was added to the basal and apical chamber of the insert. In the following 7 days, expand medium was replaced every second day. At confluence (95%), the models were airlifted by aspirating all the PneumaCult™-Ex expand medium and adding 1 ml PneumaCult™-ALI maintenance medium (Stemcell technologies, Cambridge, UK) supplemented with 96 μg/ml hydrocortisone, 2 mg/ml heparin (Stemcell technologies, Cambridge, UK) and 1% PEST to the basal chamber only. Maintenance medium was changed every second day. After 3 weeks of culturing at ALI, the number of PBEC reached 1.5×10^6 cells/insert and the cells were observed in a well differentiated state including ciliated cells and mucus producing cells.

THP-1 derived macrophage (MQ)

Human monocyte cell line (THP-1) was purchased from the American Type Culture Collection (TIB-202™, ATCC, Rockville, MD, USA), and grown in T75 flasks using RPMI-1640 cell medium (Gibco Life technologies, Paisley, UK) supplemented with 1% PEST and 10% heat-inactivated fetal bovine serum (FBS; Gibco Life technologies, Paisley, UK) and maintained in 5% CO_2 at 37 ° C. The cell culture medium was replaced every second day. On attainment of the cell concentration 8 × 105 cells/mL, the THP-1 cells were sub-cultured in Petri dishes at a concentration of 1×10^6 cells/ml. To differentiate THP-1 cells into macrophage-like cells [40], 5 ng/ml phorbolmyristate acetate (PMA) (Sigma,

Germany) was added in RPMI-1640 cell medium (Gibco Life technologies, Paisley, UK) [41]. After 48 h of incubation, the medium was collected, and the plates were washed three times with PBS. The non-adherent cells were washed away and counted to calculate the adherence rate. In this study, about 70% of the cells were attached and had spread out. The adherent cells were then trypsinized and collected for further analysis. Trypan blue was used to detect the effects of trypsinization. Viability of more than 95% was acceptable. Non-differentiated THP-1 cells and differentiated THP-1 cells were documented using BX50 light microscope (Olympus Optical Co., Tokyo, Japan). Anti-CD68-PE-Cy7 (BD Pharmingen, San Diego, CA, United States) was used as a marker to detect the purity of the MQ by flow cytometry (LSR Fortessa™, BD Bioscience, United States). The determined purity was more than 80% in all cases.

Co-culture of PBEC-ALI and MQ (PBEC-ALI/MQ)

In the pilot study, we co-cultured MQ placed underneath the PBEC-ALI models (PBEC-ALI/MQ_{sub}), but low effects of the addition of MQ after DEP exposure were seen (Additional file 1: Figure S1, S2). Therefore, in the following studies, PBEC-ALI was co-cultured with MQ on top of the epithelial layer (PBEC-ALI/MQ).

Two hundred μl THP-1 culture medium containing 1. 5×10^5 MQ was added to the apical side of the differentiated PBEC models, giving an estimated ratio of MQ: PBEC = 1:10 [42], and was incubated in 5% CO_2 at 37 °C for 2 h. As a control, mono-culture of MQ were performed by adding 200 μl THP-1 culture medium containing 1.5×10^5 MQ to all inserts. One ml PneumaCult™-ALI maintenance medium with all the supplements was added to the basal chamber of the insert, and incubated in 5% CO_2 at 37 °C for 2 h. Prior to exposure, after adhesion of MQ, THP-1 culture medium from the apical chamber was aspirated.

DEP generation and characterization

DEP were generated and collected from a three cylinder, 3.8 l tractor engine (Model 1113 TR; Bolinder-Munktell) at the Swedish Engine Test Center, Uppsala. The engine was run at 1600 rpm on diesel fuel (Swedish environment class MK 3) working at 80% of its rated 41.2 kW output. The exhaust, which was diluted 11-fold with air, was passed through a Tepcon electrostatic filter (Model 2200; Act Air, Cardiff, UK) at a total flow rate of 1600 kg/h and was precipitated on the filter at 44 °C. The DEP soot was scraped from the Teflon-coated electrodes and stored in the dark at – 20 °C.

The aerodynamic particle size distribution of re-aerosolized DEP was analyzed by using a 9-stage Marple Cascade Impactor (MCI, MSP Corp). One mg DEP was loaded to the PreciseInhale™ platform (Inhalation Sciences, Stockholm, Sweden) and generated as aerosols at 100 bar pressure. DEP aerosols were pumped through the MCI at an airflow rate of 2 L/min. Particles were captured by impaction on the MCI stages based on their size. The aerodynamic size distribution of the DEP was then calculated from the amount of particles captured on each stage of the impactor. The experiment was repeated in triplicate.

To characterize the DEP, the particles were deposited on glass cover slips using PreciseInhale exposure system with a cylindrical 1 L holding chamber. The particle deposition flow rate was 120 mL/min. The specimens were mounted on an aluminum stub and sputter coated with 10 nm Platinum (Q150T ES, West Sussex, UK) and analyzed in an Ultra 55 field emission scanning electron microscope (SEM) (Zeiss, Oberkochen, Germany) at 5 kV using the secondary electron detector.

Endotoxin level in the DEP samples was determined using the Limulus amebocyte lysate assay (LAL; Endosafe® Endochrome-K™ U.S. Lisence No.1197, Charles River Laboratories, Wilmington, Massachusetts, USA). According to the manufacturer's instruction, the particles were diluted in endotoxin specific buffer and *Escherichia coli* 0111: B4 was used as standard.

Exposure of PBEC-ALI, PBEC-ALI/MQ and MQ to DEP

In order to mimic the in vivo exposure situation of the lung, the model was exposed to clean air (sham) or to aerosolized DEP using the Xpose*ALI* exposure system as previously described [39]. The models including only PBEC (PBEC-ALI), models co-cultured with MQ (PBEC-ALI/MQ) and mono-cultures of MQ were then placed inside the exposure modules. Compressed air of 100 bars was used to aerosolize the DEP into the 300 ml holding chamber. The DEP aerosol was then pulled from holding chamber at a main flow rate of 120 ml/min and diverted into triplicate exposure branches at a flow rate of 10 ml/min. DEP exposures were carried out for 3 mins (the exposure time period was chosen according to pilot study described in Additional file 1). In the corresponding controls, sham exposures were performed with identical flow rate settings- and exposure duration using clean air and a clean system. The inside of the aerosol holding chamber was covered with wet filter papers to maintain the humidity which increased the viability of the cells substantially. In addition, in the exposure module the inserts including bronchial models were always in contact with the basal medium during the exposures.

Following exposure, cells were removed from the exposure modules and placed in 12-well plates with fresh basal medium, and incubated for 24 h in 5% CO_2 and 37 °C.

DEP exposure dose and uptake

To calculate the DEP exposure dose and uptake, the models ($n = 3$/time point) were exposed to DEP for 15 s, 45 s and 3mins respectively, corresponding to low-, medium- and high-exposure doses (Additional file 1). After each exposure, DEP were collected from all 3 inserts separately by rinsing them with 200 μL 99% ethanol. The deposited DEP dose in each insert was quantified by measuring the absorbance using spectrophotometric technique (Cary 60 UV-Vis, Agilent Technologies, Palo Alto, CA, United States) [43] and calculating the deposited dose of DEP using a standard curve.

After exposure, a spectrophotometric analysis was performed to quantify the actual exposure dose of DEP in each insert (DI), using the following formula:

$$DD(DEP\ dose) = \frac{\mathrm{DI}}{\mathrm{IS\ (insert\ surface)}}$$

To investigate the DEP uptake, a commercial QuadriWave Lateral Shearing Interferometry (QWLSI) (SID4-Bio, Phasics SA, Saint Aubin, France) was directly plugged onto the microscope (Labphot-2, Nikon FX-35DX) to detect distribution of mass across the model.

Cell viability assay

The cell viability of both PBEC-ALI and PBEC-ALI/MQ were determined after 24 h (DEP versus sham) using three different methods:

Trypan blue assay: The samples were stained by trypan blue (diluted with PBS in 1:5 ratio) following a 24 h exposure. The viable cell fraction was assessed using conventional light microscopy (Motic, AE2000 Inverted Microscope, Motic Deutschland GmbH, Wetzlar, Germany) using a 20× magnification. Four fields of the insert were selected and in each field 200 cells were counted. The viability of more than 95% was accepted. This assay was repeated twice on separate inserts from each donor.

Lactate dehydrogenase release (LDH) assay: Cell viability of both PBEC-ALI and PBEC-ALI/MQ were determined by measuring the level of released LDH in the basal media. The assay was carried out according to the manufacturer's instruction (Thermo Fisher Scientific, Pittsburgh, United States). 50 μl basal medium from sham, DEP exposed cells and LDH positive control (0.2% Triton 100X treated) were transferred to a clear 96-well plate (Nunc, Thermo Fisher Scientific). 50 μl LDH reaction mixture was then added to each sample well and mixed by gentle tapping. After 30 min of incubation at room temperature, the reaction was stopped by adding 50 μl of stop solution. LDH release was quantified by measuring absorbance at 490 nm (A490) and 680 nm (A680) using a plate reader. Data were normalized to sham exposure.

Annexin V Assay via fluorescence automated cell sorting (FACS): To detect the early and late cellular apoptosis rate of the models after exposure, both PBEC-ALI and PBEC-ALI/MQ after 24 h of incubation post exposure (DEP and sham) were trypsinized and treated with annexin V–PE/7-AAD according to the manufacturer's instructions (BD Pharmingen, San Diego, CA, United States) [39]. Apoptotic cells were detected by collecting 2000 cells using FACS (LSR Fortessa™, BD Bioscience, United States).

Quantitative real time polymerase chain reaction (qRT- PCR)

Transcript expression of genes involved in oxidative stress (*NFKB, HMOX1, GPx*), pro-inflammation (*CXCL8, IL6, TNF*), tissue injury/repair (*MMP9* and *TIMP1*) *TLR2/TLR4*and macrophage polarization (M1; *IL23, IL12*, M2; *IL10, IL4, IL13, MRC1, MRC2, RETNLA*) were analyzed using the qRT-PCR technique. The list of genes assessed, and corresponding primer pairs are provided in Additional file 1: Table S1. Total mRNA from both PBEC-ALI and PBEC-ALI/MQ and MQ only were isolated following 24 h exposure (DEP and sham) using the RNeasy Mini Kit (Qiagen; $n = 6$) as described previously [44]. Concentration of RNA was measured using the Nano drop (ND1000 Technology). 1 μg mRNA was reverse transcribed to generate complementary DNA (cDNA) using the high capacity RNA to cDNA kit (Life technologies, Paisley, UK) and a thermal cycler (Mycycler™, Biorad). qRT-PCR was performed using the AB 7500 System. The 20 μl qRT-PCR reaction mix consisted of 10 μl Fast SYBR® Green Master Mix (Life technologies, Paisley, UK), 200 nmol of each primer, 5 ng cDNA, and nuclease free water. Beta actin (*ACTB*) was used as the reference control. Expression of each target gene was quantified as a fold change following normalization with *ACTB* and sham. The results were calculated as $2^{-\Delta Ct}$ (ΔCt = Ct (gene of interest) - Ct (beta actin).

ELISA

Concentrations of IL-6 and CXCL-8 in basal medium were measured using the in-house ELISA method described previously [45]. Commercially available antibody pairs MAB206-15, MAF206-15 and MAB208-15, MAF208-15 (R&D SYSTEMS®, UK) were used to measure IL-6 and CXCL-8 respectively. The detection range was 3-375 pg/ml and 12.5-6400 pg/ml for IL-6 and CXCL-8 respectively. MMP-9, TIMP-1, CC-10, TGF-β, IL-13 and IL-10 in basal medium were measured using purchased DouSet ELISA Kit (DY911, DY970, DY4218, DY240, DY213, DY217B; R&D SYSTEMS®, UK). The measurements of TNF-α in basal medium were performed by purchased HS quantikine ELISA Kit

(HSTA00E; R&D SYSTEMS®, UK). All the analyses of MMP-9, TIMP-1, TNF-α, CC-10, TGF-β, IL-13 and IL-10 were performed according to the manufacturer. For all the duplicated samples, an intra-assay variation < 10% was accepted.

FACS

To distinguish between PBEC and MQ in PBEC-ALI/MQ, cells were trypsinized and washed twice with PBS, and incubated with monoclonal antibody (anti-CD68-PE-Cy7; Cat No.25-0689-42, eBioscience, Thermo Fisher Scientific, Pittsburgh, United States). The CD68 $^+$ cells were MQ and CD68 $^-$ cells were PBEC. To analyze the expression of TLR2 and TLR4, the trypsinized cells were incubated with monoclonal antibodies (anti-TLR2-APC, Cat No.558319, BD Pharmingen, San Diego, CA, United States; anti-TLR4-PE, Cat No.12-9917-42, eBioscience, Thermo Fisher Scientific, Pittsburgh, United States) for 30 mins in dark. The cells were then washed 3 times and re-suspended in PBS. For PBEC-ALI, the TLR2/TLR4 were detected directly. For PBEC-ALI/MQ, the cells were gated by anti-CD68 antibody first followed by TLR2/TLR4 detection in both CD68 $^+$ cell populations (MQ) and CD68 $^-$ cell populations (PBEC). For all analysis, unstained cells were used to provide the gating controls for determining positivity [46]. Analyses were performed using the flow cytometer (LSR Fortessa™, BD Bioscienc, United States) and calculated as median fluorescence intensity (MFI).

Statistics

The results are expressed as medians and interquartile ranges (25th-75th percentiles). All the comparisons between groups were performed by Wilcoxon signed rank t test. A p-value $< 0.05$was considered as significant. All the data were analyzed using the STATISTICA9 (StatSoft, Inc. Uppsala, Sweden) software.

Results

DEP characterization

The re-suspended DEP aerosols used in this study had a particle size distribution as shown in Fig. 1A. The mass median aerodynamic diameter (MMAD, P50) was calculated to be 0.57 μm, which may represent a slight overestimation of the actual MMAD because the major fraction of particles was deposited on the cascade impactor end filter without further size separation. Figure 1b indicated SEM analysis of DEP at different magnifications. Figure 1B (a) showed that DEP were evenly distributed over the surface area of exposure with Xpose*ALI* exposure system. Figure 1B (d), high resolution SEM image elucidates the agglomerated structure of DEP, which is in agreement with a previous report by Kireeva et al. [47]. According to the LAL test, the DEP are free from LPS contamination (data not shown).

DEP exposure: Dose and uptake

According to spectrophotometric analysis the dose per surface area was:

$$DD = \frac{57.17\mu g/ml \times 0.2ml}{0.9\ cm2} = 12.7\mu g/cm^2$$

Based on Fig. 1C, the MQ appeared more contrasted, which made them easy to be distinguished among the epithelial cells after DEP exposure. Some parts of MQ were very dense which may indicate the engulfment of DEP particles. Also MQ can be segmented in order to measure the mass of each of them. Based on these measurement (data not shown), MQ mass were higher than the surface mass of epithelial area, which may confirm phagocytosis of DEP particles.

Effects of DEP on cell viability

Based on the trypan blue staining procedure a cell viability more than 95% was accepted. The results of the colorimetric LDH assay on both PBEC-ALI and PBEC-ALI/MQ models are shown in Additional file 1: Figure S3A. The early apoptosis rate was between 4% and 22.5%; the late apoptosis rate was between 0.2% and 8.5%, and the total apoptosis rate was between 5.5% and 25%, when assessed with annexin V–PE/7-AAD 24 h, following exposure to DEP (Additional file 1: Figure S3B). Trypan blue staining, LDH activity assay and apoptosis assay did not exhibit any alteration before and after exposure to DEP. Thus, none of the DEP doses used in this study were cytotoxic.

Effects of DEP exposures in mono-culture models compared with co-cultured models

Pro-inflammatory, oxidative stress and tissue injury/repair responses

One of the key features of DEP-associated health effects is inflammation; Secretion and mRNA expression of CXCL-8 (Fig. 2a, b) and IL-6 (Fig. 2c, d) as well as mRNA expression of *TNFα* (Fig. 2e) were detected. We also found that the secretion of CXCL-8 was significantly induced by the DEP exposure in PBEC-ALI (Fig. 2a). An increased mRNA expression of *CXCL8* (Fig. 2b: 3-fold,) and *TNFα* (Fig. 2e: 2.5-fold) was detected. Both CXCL-8 and IL-6 secretion were significantly increased after sham exposure in PBEC-ALI/MQ compared to the PBEC-ALI (Fig. 2a, c). Interestingly, *IL6* and *TNFα* transcript after sham exposure (Fig. 2d, e) as well as *CXCL8* and *TNFα* transcript after DEP exposure (Fig. 2b, e) were significantly decreased in PBEC-ALI/MQ compared to PBEC-ALI.

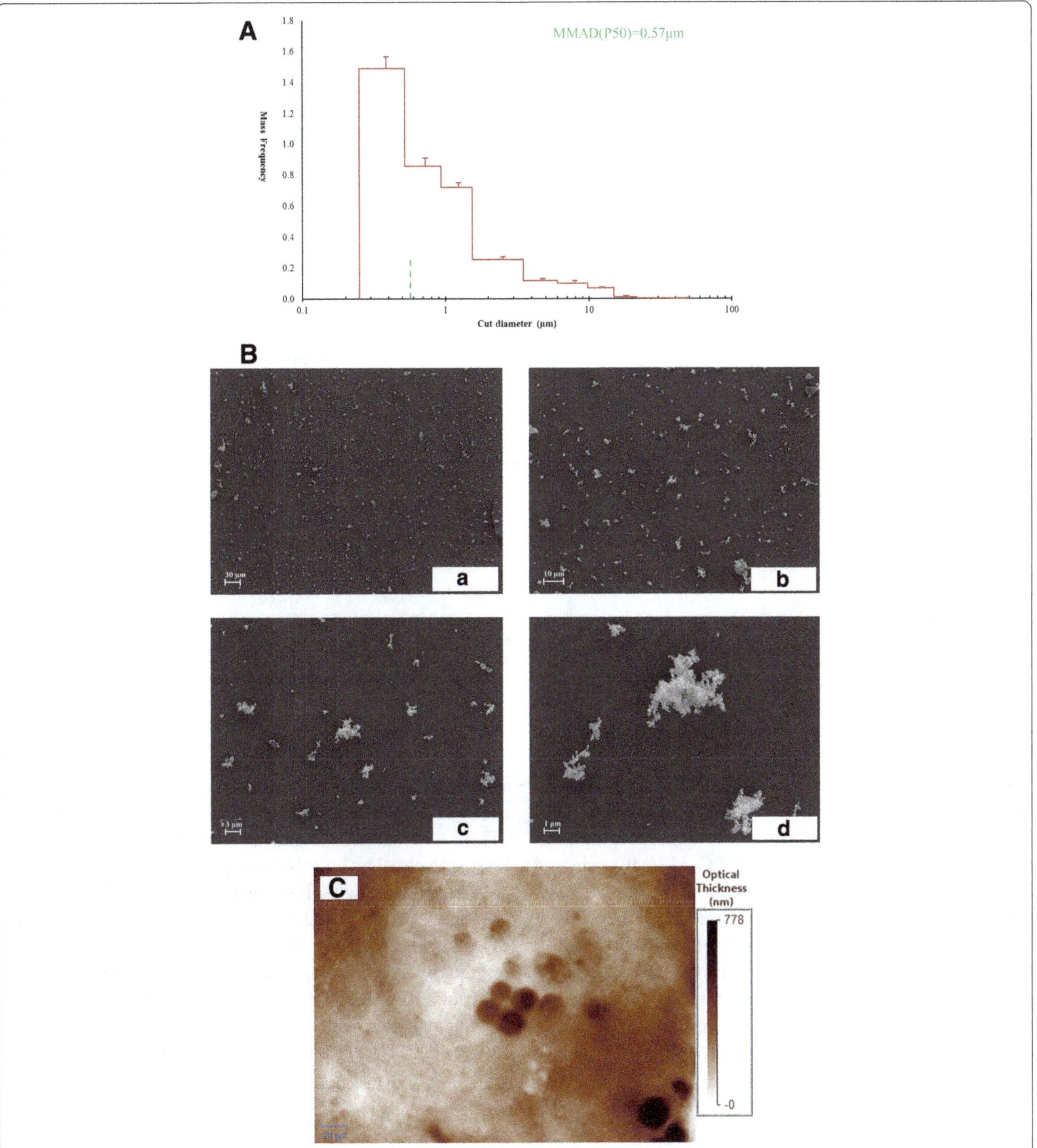

Fig. 1 Characterization and uptake of diesel exhaust particles (DEP) (**A-C**). **A**: Mass distribution of DEP in different size ranges measured by the 9-stage Marple Cascade Impactor; MMAD (P50): Mass Median Aerodynamic Diameter; The MMAD (P50) of DEP was estimated to be 0.57 μm. 1B: SEM image of DEP with different magnifications; **B** (a): 500X, bar: 30 μm; **B** (b): 2000X, bar: 10 μm; **B** (c): 5000X, bar: 3 μm; **B** (d): 15000X, bar: 1 μm. **C**: Quantitative phase image of the apical side of PBEC-ALI/MQ, which reflects the distribution of mass across the field; Bar: 20 μm

Oxidative stress is also considered as a main effect of DEP-induced toxicity. Redox sensitive transcription factors like *NFKB*, antioxidant enzymes like *HMOX1* and *GPx* are considered to play important roles in this process. In PBEC-ALI, exposure to DEP increased the mRNA expression of *NFKB* (> 6-fold) (Fig. 3a), *HMOX1* (4-fold) (Fig. 3b) and *GPx* (1.5-fold) (Fig. 3c). However, compared to sham exposure, DEP exposure significantly reduced *GPx* mRNA expression in PBEC-ALI/MQ (Fig. 3c). In sham exposed models, *HMOX1* (Fig. 3b) and *GPx* (Fig. 3c) mRNA expressions were twice as high in PBEC-ALI/MQ than in PBEC-ALI. However,

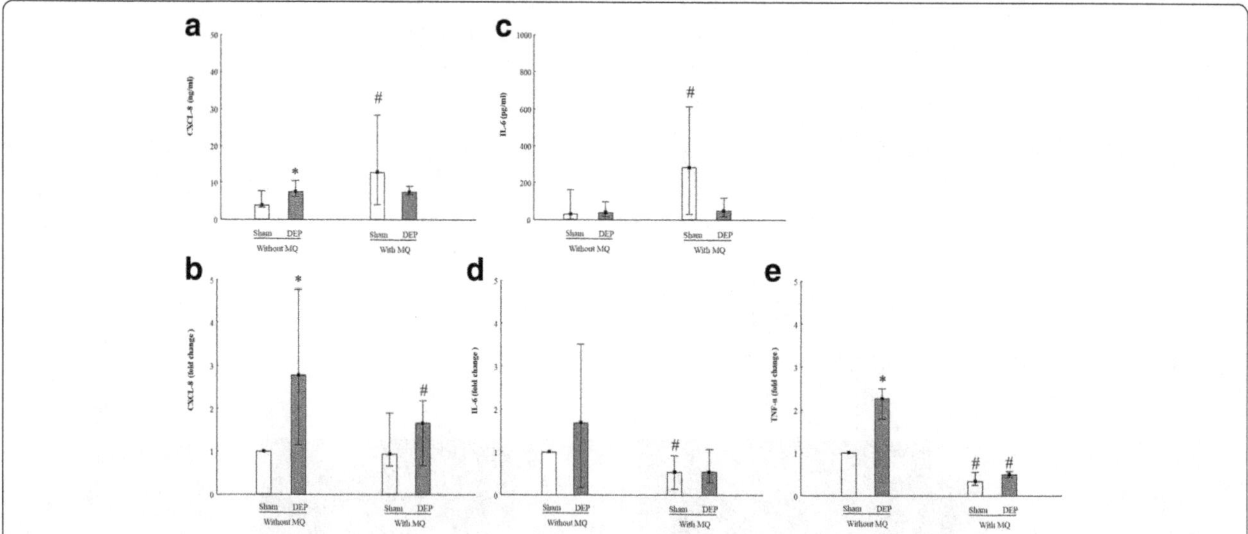

Fig. 2 Release and mRNA expression of inflammatory biomarkers in models after exposure to diesel exhaust particles (DEP). Levels of CXCL-8 (**a**) and IL-6 (**c**) secretion in basal medium in PBEC-ALI and PBEC-AL/MQ ($N = 9$) after exposure to DEP and incubated for 24 h; Fold change of *CXCL8* (**b**), *IL6* (**d**) and *TNFα* (**e**) expression in PBEC-ALI and PBEC-AL/MQ($N = 6$) after exposure to DEP and incubated for 24 h; Exposure: sham: clean air; DEP: 12.7 μg/cm^2; Data presented as median and 25th -75thpercentiles, fold change =$2^{-\Delta Ct}$ of models / $2^{-\Delta Ct}$ of sham exposed PBEC-ALI; *: $P < 0.05$ VS Sham exposure; #: $P < 0.05$ VS PBEC-ALI

after DEP exposure, *NFKB* (Fig. 3a) and *HMOX1* (Fig. 3b) mRNA expressions were significantly lower in PBEC-ALI/MQ than in PBEC-ALI.

Pro-inflammatory cytokines and oxidative stress induced by macrophages or epithelial cells may contribute to DEP-induced epithelial damage. In the present study, both MMP-9 and TIMP-1 were detected at both protein- and mRNA levels (Fig. 4a-d). We found that DEP exposure increased TIMP-1 secretion in both models (Fig. 4b). After DEP exposure, PBEC-ALI/MQ released lower levels of TIMP-1 than PBEC-ALI (Fig. 4b). The secretion of MMP-9 was not altered in PBEC-ALI or PBEC-ALI/MQ, but an increased secretion of MMP-9 from DEP exposure when culturing MQ only was observed ($P = 0.027$, data not shown). No effect on expression of MMP-9 and TIMP-1 were detected in either PBEC-ALI or PBEC-ALI/MQ models. In regard to TNF-α, TGF-β and IL-13 secretions, most of the samples were below detection limit, and for CC-10 and IL-10, no significant difference was found (data not shown).

TLR expression

To clarify the impact of DEP exposure on TLRs expression within mono- and co-culture settings, we detected both mRNA expression and cell surface expression of *TLR2* and *TLR4* by using qRT-PCR and FACS analysis, respectively. The mRNA expression of *TLR2* and *TLR4* were increased by DEP exposure in PBEC-ALI, while unchanged in PBEC-ALI/MQ (Fig. 5). For PBEC-ALI, TLR2 and TLR4, surface expression on PBEC were detected by FACS using anti-TLR2/4 antibodies directly. But for PBEC-ALI/MQ, anti-CD68 antibody was used to distinguish between PBEC (CD68 $^-$) and MQ (CD68 $^+$) using FACS (Additional file 1: Figure S4). The ratio of

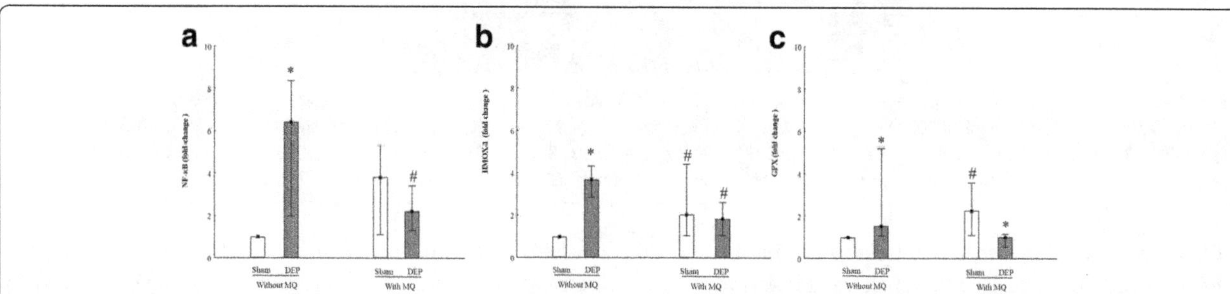

Fig. 3 mRNA expression of oxidative stress related markers in models after exposure to diesel exhaust particles (DEP). Fold change of *NFKB* (**a**), *HMOX1* (**b**) and *GPx* (**c**) expression in PBEC-ALI and PBEC-AL/MQ (N = 6) after exposure to DEP and incubated for 24 h; Exposure: sham: clean air; DEP: 12.7 μg/cm^2; Data presented as median and 25th -75thpercentiles, fold change =$2^{-\Delta Ct}$ of models / $2^{-\Delta Ct}$ of sham exposed PBEC-ALI; *: $P < 0.05$ VS Sham exposure; #: $P < 0.05$ VS PBEC-ALI

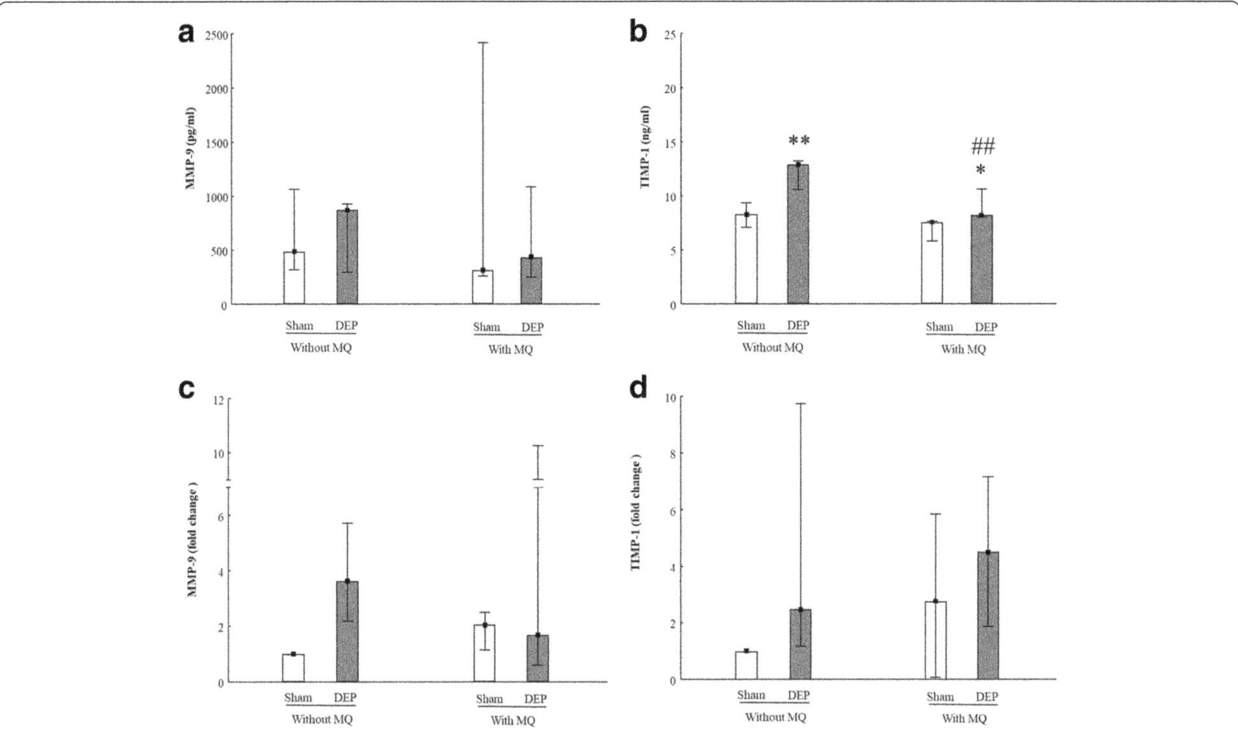

Fig. 4 Release and mRNA expression of extra-cellular markers in models after exposure to diesel exhaust particles (DEP). Levels of MMP-9 (**a**) and TIMP-1 (**b**) secretion in basal medium in PBEC-ALI and PBEC-AL/MQ (N = 9) after exposure to DEP and incubated for 24 h; Fold change of MMP-9 (**c**) and TIMP-1 (**d**) expression in PBEC-ALI and PBEC-ALI/MQ (N = 6) after exposure to DEP and incubated for 24 h; Exposure: sham: clean air; DEP: 12.7 μg/cm^2; Data presented as median and 25th -75thpercentiles,fold change =$2^{-\Delta Ct}$ of models / $2^{-\Delta Ct}$ of sham exposed PBEC-ALI; *,**: $P < 0.05$, 0.01 VS Sham exposure; ##: $P < 0.01$ VS PBEC-ALI

CD68$^+$ and CD68$^-$ cells was 1:10, indicating that the ratio between MQ and PBEC was 1:10, which in turn matched the ratio we seeded (MQ: PBEC = 1:10). After CD68 gating, the TLR2/4 surface expression on PBEC or MQ could be detected separately. After sham exposure, the expression of both TLR2 and TLR4 on PBEC in PBEC-ALI/MQ was significantly attenuated compared to PBEC-ALI (Fig. 6A (c, d)). Figure 6A (c) revealed that following DEP exposure, an increase of TLR2 expression on PBEC surface in PBEC-ALI/MQ was detected. However, DEP exposure significantly reduced the surface expression of TLR4 on PBEC in both PBEC-ALI and PBEC-ALI/MQ (Fig. 6A (d)). DEP exposure resulted in a similar surface expression pattern with increased TLR2 and decreased TLR4 expression on MQ in PBEC-ALI/MQ (Fig. 6B (c, d)). For MQ mono-culture, there was no

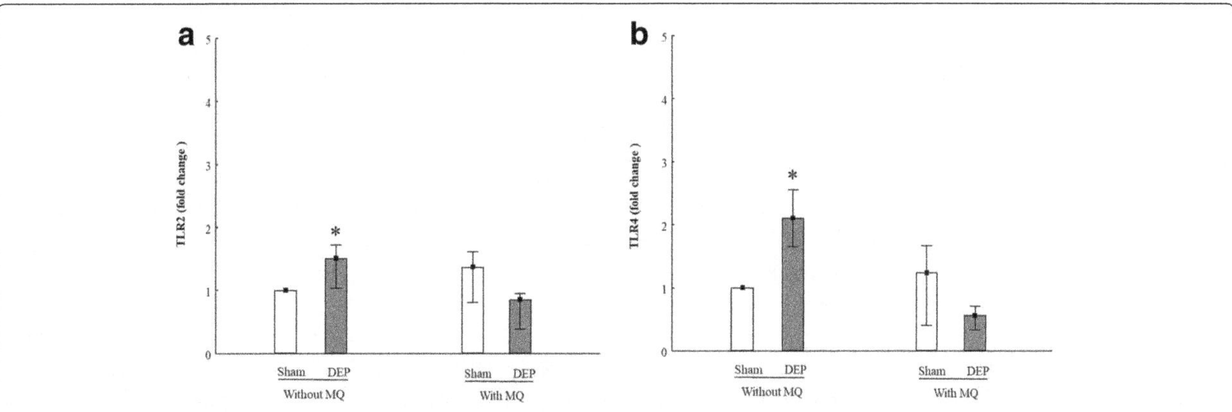

Fig. 5 mRNA expression of Toll-like receptors in models after exposure to diesel exhaust particles (DEP). Fold change of TLR2 (**a**) and TLR4 (**b**) expression in PBEC-ALI and PBEC-AL/MQ (N = 6) after exposure to DEP and incubated for 24 h; Exposure: sham: clean air; DEP: 12.7 μg/cm^2; Data presented as median and 25th -75th percentiles, fold change =$2^{-\Delta Ct}$ of models / $2^{-\Delta Ct}$ of sham exposed PBEC-ALI; *: $P < 0.05$ VS Sham exposure

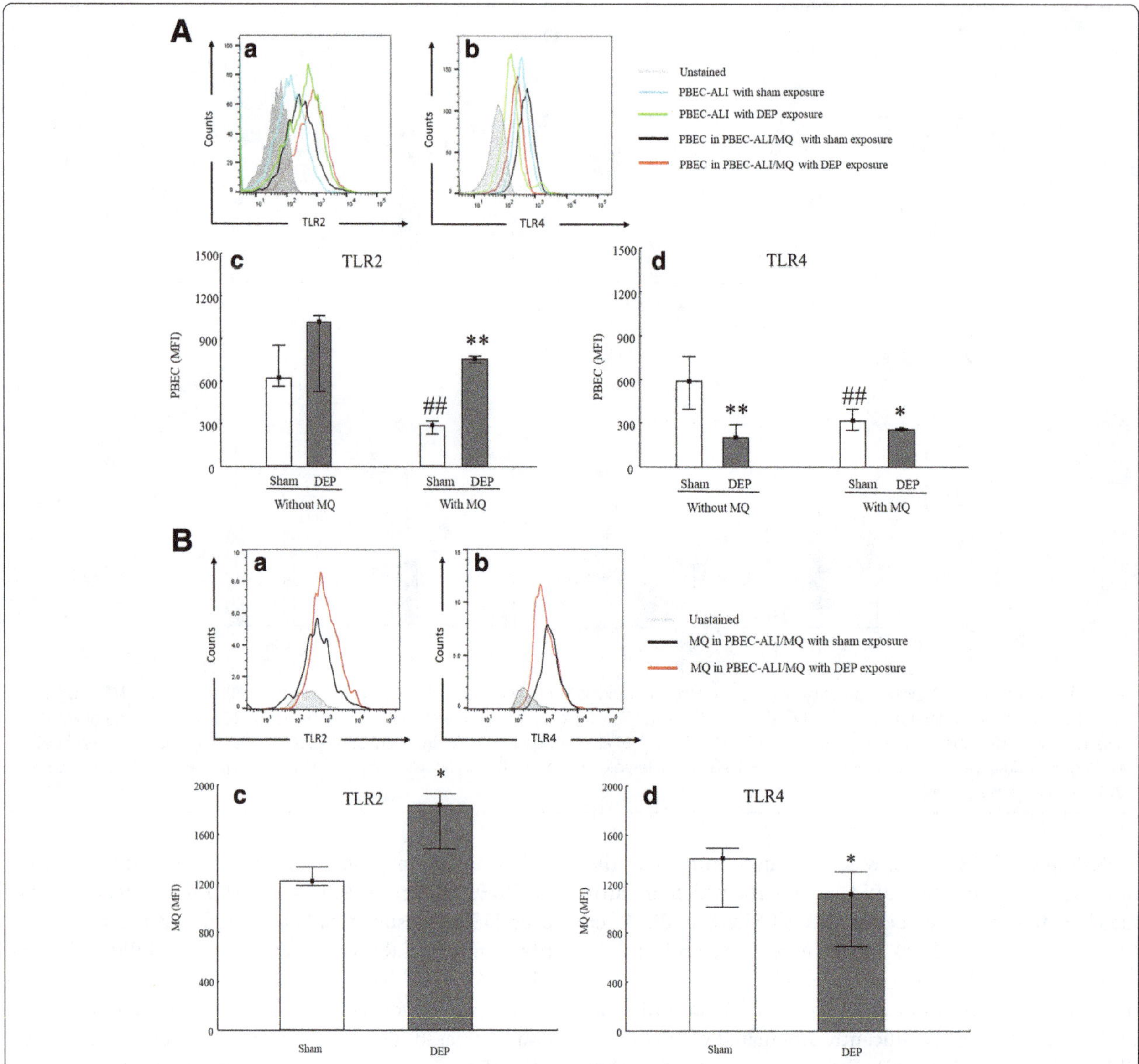

Fig. 6 TLR2 and TLR4 expression on the surface of primary bronchial epithelial cells (PBEC) and macrophages (MQ) after exposure to diesel exhaust particles (DEP). PBEC (**A**) and MQ (**B**) were identified by anti-CD 68-PE-Cy7. A representative mean fluorescence intensity (MFI) of 9 experiments is shown (**A** (a&b), **B** (a&b)); the expression of TLR2 (**A** (c)) and TLR4 (**A** (d)) on surface of PBEC in PBEC-ALI and PBEC-AL/MQ was presented as median and 25th -75th percentiles (N = 9); *, **: $P < 0.05$, 0.01 VS Sham exposure; ##: $P < 0.01$ VS PBEC-ALI. The expression of TLR2 (**B** (c)) and TLR4 (**B** (d)) on surface of MQ which have been co-cultured with PBEC was presented as median and 25th -75th percentiles (N = 9); *: $P < 0.05$ VS Sham exposure; Exposure: sham: clean air; DEP: 12.7 μg/cm^2

difference between sham and DEP exposure regarding TLR2/TLR4 surface expression (data not shown). Further, there was no difference of TLR2/TLR4 surface expression between MQ mono-culture and MQ in PBEC-ALI/MQ (data not shown).

MQ polarization

As polarization is a critical step in macrophage activation, we detected the mRNA expression of specific M1 (*IL23* and *IL12*) and M2 (*IL10, IL4, IL13, MRC1, MRC2* and *RETNLA*) macrophage markers in both models to elucidate the effects of both DEP exposure and co-culturing of MQ with PBEC and its effects on polarization. DEP exposure increased all M2 macrophage transcription markers in PBEC-ALI/MQ, except *RETNLA* (Fig. 7f). However, with PBEC-ALI, there was no induction by DEP exposure on M2 macrophage markers or even a reduced effect by DEP on *IL13* (Fig. 7c) and *RETNLA* (Fig. 7f) mRNA expression. After DEP exposure, *IL4* (Fig. 7b), *MCR1* (Fig. 7d), *MRC2* (Fig. 7e), and *RETNLA* (Fig. 7f) mRNA expression were all increased in PBEC-ALI/MQ models compared to PBEC-ALI. There was no such

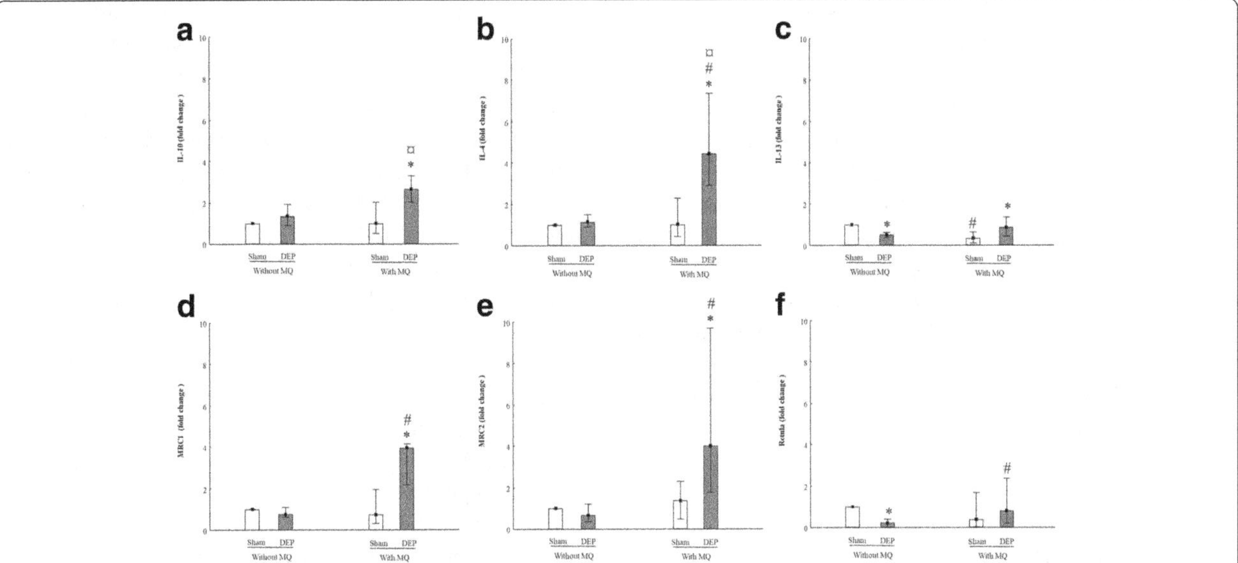

Fig. 7 mRNA expression of M2 macrophage markers after exposure to diesel exhaust particles (DEP). Fold change of *IL10* (**a**), *IL4* (**b**), *IL13* (**c**), *MRC1* (**d**), *MRC2* (**e**) and *RETLNA* (**f**) expression in PBEC-ALI and PBEC-AL/MQ (N = 6) after exposure to DEP and incubated for 24 h; Exposure: sham: clean air; DEP: 12.7 μg/cm^2; Data presented as median and 25th -75th percentiles, fold change =$2^{-\Delta Ct}$ of models / $2^{-\Delta Ct}$ of sham exposed PBEC-ALI; *: $P < 0.05$ VS Sham exposure; #: $P < 0.05$ VS PBEC-ALI; ¤: $P < 0.05$ VS Sham exposed PBEC-ALI

increase observed after sham exposure. As for M1 macrophage markers, there was no statistically significant change between the different models tested (Additional file 1: Figure S5). Interestingly, when mono-culture with MQ only were exposed to DEP, there was no significant influence on either M1 or M2 macrophages markers (data not shown).

Discussion

Our experimental set up to assess the pulmonary toxicity of DEP using co-cultured models consisting of both PBEC and MQ under ALI condition (PBEC-ALI/MQ), and delivery of dry aerosolized particles using the Xpo*seALI*® system with precise dosimetry, offers several unique advantages over the existing models and particle delivery systems. Most of the reported studies have used the conventional mono-culture or co-culture models with lung cells (cell lines or primary cells) under submerged conditions, where the particles have been added directly to the cell culture medium [12–14]. Submerged cell culture conditions and addition of stimulants directly to the cell culture media does not reflect the physiology of airway mucosa (consisting of more than 40 cell types [48]) and inhalation exposure conditions [49, 50]. Moreover, it has been well established that the addition of particles directly to the cell culture medium increases the possibility of particle agglomeration which often leads to unreliable outcomes and therefore limit the reproducibility of the system [51, 52]. We have previously demonstrated that our PBEC-ALI model contains ciliated cells, goblet cells, basal cells and club cells, thereby efficiently mimicking the human bronchial mucosa [7]. THP-1 derived macrophages, identified using the FACS methodology, were then added to the apical side of PBEC-ALI to study cell-cell cross talk and corresponding molecular signaling. Realistic inhalation exposure scenarios were achieved through portion by portion aerosolization of DEP from dry powder formulation using compressed air [15, 16]. The use of high-pressure energy resulted in a high degree of deagglomeration into finer aerosols. The preheated Xpose*ALI*® system and humidified fine aerosols then reached the cell surface with homogenous distribution, thereby mimicking a real-life inhalation exposure. The multi-cellular bronchial mucosa models with PBEC and THP-1 derived macrophages cultured at ALI, in combination with advanced Xpose*ALI*® system used in this study, therefore offers a more realistic and physiologically relevant inhalation exposure scenario with a reliable dose delivery system.

Inflammatory and oxidative stress response following exposure of PBEC-ALI to DEP is evident from the increased secretion of *CXCL8* and *TIMP1*, and increased mRNA expression of *CXCL8, TNFα, NFKB, HMOX1* and *GPx*. Some of these effects were attenuated in the presence of MQ in PBEC-ALI/MQ. *TIMP1* is an inhibitor of Matrix metallopeptidase 9 (*MMP9*), which plays an important role for variety of homeostatic functions and elicit repair responses as balance mechanisms in many chronic lung diseases like COPD [53]. Hence, increased *TIMP1* secretion indicated effects on ECM regulation. Previous studies [12, 54, 55], reported that following exposure to DEP there was an increased release of pro-inflammatory markers, like CXCL-8, IL-6 and TNF-α, both in an ALI model containing human alveolar epithelial tissue models and in submerged models of epithelial cell lines. Our findings are consistent with previous reports. It has been shown by many researchers that exposure to DEP may induce ROS production [56]. Increased ROS may cause the translocation of *NFR2* into the nucleus [57] and binding to antioxidant response elements. Subsequently, antioxidant genes like *HMOX1* or *GPx* [58] can be activated. In line with those studies [54, 59], DEP exposure induced an increased expression of *NFKB*, *HMOX1* and *GPx* in PBEC-ALI models. Interestingly, in PBEC-ALI/MQ, which are PBEC-ALI models co-cultured with THP-1 derived macrophages, the expression of inflammatory genes (*CXCL8* and *TNFα*), antioxidant gene (*HMOX1*) and *NFKB*, as well as TIMP-1 secretion were reduced compared with PBEC-ALI. In contrast, Ishii *et el* [60] reported an increased inflammatory response in submerged co-culture models consisting of PBEC and alveolar macrophages after exposure to ambient particulate matters (PM). Similarly, *TIMP1* expression remained unaltered in A549 and 16HBE cells following exposure to DEP under submerged conditions [61, 62]. This observed difference in inflammatory- and oxidative stress response between our study and those of others [60–62] may be caused not only by the use of different in vitro models (ALI versus submerged culture conditions) or different cell type, but also by the chosen exposure model, where the PBEC-ALI/MQ models were exposed to aerosolized DEP using the Xpose*ALI* system. The exposure of PBEC-ALI/MQ models to aerosolized DEP allows the direct study of cell-particle interaction in contrast to particle exposures performed under submerged conditions, which may lead to the excessive agglomeration of the study particles [50, 51]. Further, the direct interaction of aerosolized particle with cells (DEP with PBEC-ALI/MQ) may initiate faster phagocytosis of particles by MQ, and subsequent release of various pro-inflammatory and anti-inflammatory mediators/cytokines, which in turn may play a crucial role in both innate and adaptive immunity to prevent unnecessary inflammatory response to stimulants [63].

To investigate the possible modulation of TLR signaling by DEP exposure, we analyzed both cell surface and mRNA expression of TLR2 and TLR4. CD68 antibody was used to distinguish between the cell surface expression on PBEC and MQ in PBEC-ALI/MQ models. In this study, both PBEC and MQ in PBEC–ALI/MQ showed an increased surface expression of TLR2, while TLR4 was decreased after DEP exposure. These changes after DEP exposure were not observed in either monoculture models of PBEC or MQ, with exception of TLR4 in PBEC-ALI. On the other hand, exposure to DEP increased mRNA expression of both TLR2 and TLR4 in PBEC-ALI. No significant change was observed in PBEC-ALI/MQ regarding TLR2 or TLR4. In contrast to results detected using FACS, where surface expression on PBEC and MQ could be separated, the mRNA expression in PBEC-ALI/MQ included total expression of both PBEC and MQ. To our knowledge, this is the first study using FACS analysis showing the difference in cell surface expression of TLR2 and TLR4 among multicellular models including both PBEC and MQ after exposure to DEP. According to a previous study [64], alveolar macrophages treated with PM containing low levels of endotoxin induced a TLR2-dependent pathway, which led to the upregulation of TLR2 but a downregulation of TLR4 mRNA expression. As a comparison, exposure to PM with high levels of endotoxin, a TLR4-dependent pathway was activated. However, in contrast to this study with alveolar macrophages, another study using epithelial cells [65] showed contrasting results, where TLR2 expression was not altered after exposure to PM while TLR4 expression increased by PM exposure. Williams et al. [66] demonstrated a downregulation of both TLR2 and TLR4 expression in human myeloid DCs exposed to PM. Therefore, it seems that different cell types and the interaction between them may influence the surface expression of TLR2 and TLR4. Moreover, since endotoxin levels were below detection limit in the DEP used, it is reasonable to assume that, under co-culture condition, DEP mainly activated and modulated TLR2 signaling, which induced an increased cell surface expression of TLR2.

We found that after sham exposure, the surface expressions of TLR2 and TLR4 on PBEC were decreased when co-cultured with MQ, while there were no such alternations after DEP exposure. Interestingly, regardless of DEP exposure there was no difference between surface expression of TLR2/TLR4 on MQ in PBEC-ALI/MQ and MQ mono-culture. Since macrophages have been demonstrated to express at least 10 times more TLR4 than epithelial cells [65], it is possible that during co-culture, MQ take the place of PBEC regarding host defense and decrease the sensitivity of PBEC by inducing a down-regulated expression of TLRs on PBEC. But this protection effect may be masked by strong stimuli like DEP. As a response to particles different cell types expressed different TLRs and the expression level of each TLRs varies a lot between cell types. DEP exposure induced mRNA expressions of both TLR2 and TLR4 in PBEC-ALI, while there was no such increase in PBEC-ALI/MQ. When ligands such as DEP are bound to TLR2 and TLR4, MyD88- or TRIF, pathways may be activated which may lead to *NFKB*- or activator protein (*AP1*) activation [67]. After translocation into the nucleus, these transcription factors subsequently induce the expression of inflammatory genes. Therefore, this may also explain why DEP exposure increased CXCL-8 secretion/mRNA expression and *TNFα* mRNA expression in PBEC-ALI, but not in PBEC-ALI/MQ. But in order to clarify the mechanisms and reveal the implications of DEP exposure regarding TLR pathways, more detailed studies are needed.

It has been shown that through TLRs signaling, bronchial epithelial cells can regulate the inflammatory response of immune cells like macrophages [68]. Polarization is a key feature of macrophages as a result of stimulation, and two major polarization states have been described. Classically active type1 (M1) macrophages exert pro-inflammatory activities by releasing cytokines like TNF-α and IL-6 [69], and alternatively activated type 2 (M2) macrophages secrete anti-inflammatory cytokines like IL-10 with limited production of pro- inflammatory cytokines [70]. Therefore, the reduced expression of pro-inflammatory markers in PBEC-ALI/MQ models compared with PEBC-ALI, may be due to the polarization of macrophages to M2 phenotype, leading to increased secretion of anti-inflammatory mediators. To confirm our hypothesis, we analyzed markers of both M1 and M2 phenotypes and detected the expression of inflammatory (*TNFα, IL6, CXCL8)* anti-inflammatory genes (*IL10, IL4* and *IL13*) as well as typical M2 genes (*MRC1, MRC2* and *RETNLA*) [69, 71]. In PBEC-ALI/MQ, the transcription of anti-inflammatory genes or M2 genes like *MRC1* and *MRC2* expression were increased after DEP exposure compared with sham exposure. DEP-induced effects on MRC1 and MRC2 were not detected in PBEC-ALI models. Moreover, DEP exposure led to an up-regulation of other M2 genes (*IL10, IL4, IL13, RETNL*) in PBEC-ALI/MQ compared to PBEC-ALI. In sham exposed models no such up-regulation were observed, either in co-cultured models or in mono- culture, or whether these cultures included PBEC or MQ. However, in PBEC-ALI models, DEP exposure did not increase *IL10* or *IL4* expression, and even decreased *IL13* expression. Therefore, the anti-inflammatory effects of DEP exposure that only existed in co-culture models depended on a cross-talk between PBEC and MQ, which is also evident from several other studies [17, 63].

Further, the polarization process of macrophage has been shown to be closely associated with different levels of TLR expression on its surface. According to Sauer et al. and Orr et al. [72, 73], the ratio of TLR4 and TLR2 was higher in M1-MQs than in M2-MQs, and the TLR4 deficiency can promote the activation of M2-MQs. These findings were in line with our results that the TLR4 surface expression were downregulated in MQ of PBEC-ALI/MQ after DEP exposure. NF-κB which is an end point and key master of TLR pathways can also regulate the MQ polarization [74]. Similarly, we showed that in PBEC-ALI, DEP exposure induced NF-κB activation and promoted inflammatory effects by upregulation of *CXCL8* and *TNFα*. However, in PBEC-ALI/MQ, macrophages were polarized to an anti-inflammatory M2 phenotype displaying an impaired NF-κB activation, which may increase immunosuppressive capacity. Both IFN-γ or LPS can stimulate the classical pathway of M1 activation [71], but in our present study M1-related genes did not change significantly in PBEC-ALI/MQ models. Therefore, LPS contamination of the DEP used in the current study is an unlikely contributing factor, which was confirmed by the endotoxin levels measured using LAL-assay. These were all below detection limit. Interestingly, in co-cultured models, there were a high variability in cytokine/chemokine secretion after sham exposures, while after DEP exposures, the variation was smaller. Also, these phenomena were only observed in PBEC-ALI/MQ models. Because different phenotypes of the MQ release different cytokines, which may confirm that the proportions of different phenotypes of MQ were changed after DEP exposure compared to sham exposure. We assume that in sham exposure, the MQ in PBEC-ALI/MQ constituted a mixture of M0, M1 and M2 phenotypes with different proportions in each model. However, DEP exposure induced the MQ polarization to M2 phenotype, which induced a different secretion pattern with smaller variations in the MQ phenotypes of each individual model, and subsequently reduced the variability in the cytokine secretion.

One may speculate that the observed stimulation of M2-MQs related genes after an acute exposure to DEP could be a normal defense response following such exposures. Chronic exposure to DEP in contrast, may induce a M1-MQ response leading to a persistent inflammation, which may warrant further investigation.

Conclusion

Taken together, we have demonstrated that DEP induced an inflammatory and oxidative stress response in the PBEC-ALI model, which were reduced in presence of MQ. This cell–cell interaction in the multicellular ALI-model (PBEC-ALI/MQ), in association with exposure to aerosolized ambient particles (DEP), allowed the direct interaction of particles with cell surfaces in a manner that better represented the in vivo situation. This cellular interaction of pulmonary epithelial cells with MQ in response to ambient particles played a pivotal role for MQ phenotypic alteration towards M2-subtypes, resulting in efficient resolution of the inflammatory response. This study also highlighted the fact that even mono-cell models cultured at ALI may be insufficient to investigate the detailed molecular responses, since cell-cell crosstalk is an important factor for the effects of air pollutant exposure. Finally, our physiologically relevant multicellular in vitro models in combination with the advanced exposure system (Xpose*ALI*®) has been shown to be effective in exposing ALI-models to dry aerosolized particles, mimicking the in vivo exposure situation to airborne pollutants.

Additional file

Additional file 1: Supplement. **Table S1**. Primer Used for Quantitative Real-Time PCR (qPCR). **Figure S1**. Positive controls for inflammation, oxidative stress and M1/M2 polarization. **Figure S2**. Release and mRNA expression of inflammatory biomarkers after exposures to diesel exhaust particulates (DEPs). **Figure S3**. Cytotoxicity and cell viability assays to assess the effect of diesel exhaust particles (DEP) exposure in air-liquid interface models using lactate dehydrogenase assay (LDH) and apoptotic cell rate. **Figure S4**. The ratios of primary bronchial epithelial cells (PBEC) and THP-1 cell derived macrophages (MQ) in PBEC-ALI/MQ after exposure to diesel exhaust particulates (DEPs). **Figure S5**. mRNA expression of M1 macrophage markers after exposure to diesel exhaust particles (DEP). (ZIP 1014 kb)

Acknowledgements
Thanks to Phasics SA, Saint Aubin, France for their technical support to capture the image showing uptake and distribution of DEP in multi-cellular ALI-model.

Funding
This study was supported by the Swedish Fund for Research without Animal Experiments (22/10, 40/11, F35/12, F25/13, F34-14 and F36/15), the Swedish Research Council (VR 521 2010-2801 and 2014-02767), the Swedish Heart-lung foundation (20100180, 20120376, 20120818, 20150328, 20150329 and 20150330) European Respiratory Society (ERS: ERS LTRF 2014 - 3567) and by the Karolinska Institutet, Sweden. All these funding sources have support on collection, analysis and interpretation of the data included in the manuscript.

Authors' contributions
JJ, SU, and LP conceived and designed the project; JJ, SU, XX, MM performed the experiments; JJ, SU, and XX, analyzed the data; JJ, SU, TS, PG, LP wrote the manuscript. All authors read and approved the final manuscript.

Competing interests
The authors declare that they have no competing interests.

Author details
[1]Institute of Environmental Medicine, Karolinska Institute, Box 210, SE-171 77 Stockholm, Sweden. [2]Inhalation Sciences Sweden AB, Stockholm, Sweden. [3]Department of Public Health and Clinical Medicine, University Hospital, Umeå, Sweden.

References
1. Paulin L, Hansel N. Particulate air pollution and impaired lung function. F1000Res. 2016;5. PMID:26962445
2. Salvi S, Blomberg A, Rudell B, Kelly F, Sandstrom T, Holgate ST, Frew A. Acute inflammatory responses in the airways and peripheral blood after short-term exposure to diesel exhaust in healthy human volunteers. Am J Respir Crit Care Med. 1999;159:702–9.
3. Mazzarella G, Ferraraccio F, Prati MV, Annunziata S, Bianco A, Mezzogiorno A, Liguori G, Angelillo IF, Cazzola M. Effects of diesel exhaust particles on human lung epithelial cells: an in vitro study. Respir Med. 2007;101:1155–62.
4. Sehlstedt M, Behndig AF, Boman C, Blomberg A, Sandstrom T, Pourazar J. Airway inflammatory response to diesel exhaust generated at urban cycle running conditions. Inhal Toxicol. 2010;22:1144–50.
5. Pronk A, Coble J, Stewart PA. Occupational exposure to diesel engine exhaust: a literature review. J Expo Sci Environ Epidemiol. 2009;19:443–57.
6. Schwarze PE, Totlandsdal AI, Lag M, Refsnes M, Holme JA, Ovrevik J. Inflammation-related effects of diesel engine exhaust particles: studies on lung cells in vitro. Biomed Res Int. 2013;2013:685142.
7. Silverman DT, Samanic CM, Lubin JH, Blair AE, Stewart PA, Vermeulen R, Coble JB, Rothman N, Schleiff PL, Travis WD, et al. The diesel exhaust in miners study: a nested case-control study of lung cancer and diesel exhaust. J Natl Cancer Inst. 2012;104:855–68.
8. Thurston GD, Kipen H, Annesi-Maesano I, Balmes J, Brook RD, Cromar K, De Matteis S, Forastiere F, Forsberg B, Frampton MW, et al. A joint ERS/ATS policy statement: what constitutes an adverse health effect of air pollution? An analytical framework. Eur Respir J. 2017;49. PMID:28077473
9. Yoshizaki K, Brito JM, Moriya HT, Toledo AC, Ferzilan S, Ligeiro de Oliveira AP, Machado ID, Farsky SH, Silva LF, Martins MA, et al. Chronic exposure of diesel exhaust particles induces alveolar enlargement in mice. Respir Res. 2015;16:18.
10. Shvedova AA, Yanamala N, Murray AR, Kisin ER, Khaliullin T, Hatfield MK, Tkach AV, Krantz QT, Nash D, King C, et al. Oxidative stress, inflammatory biomarkers, and toxicity in mouse lung and liver after inhalation exposure to 100% biodiesel or petroleum diesel emissions. J Toxicol Environ Health A. 2013;76:907–21.
11. Labranche N, Khattabi CE, Berkenboom G, Pochet S. Effects of diesel exhaust particles on macrophage polarization. Hum Exp Toxicol. 2017;36:412–20.
12. Tomasek I, Horwell CJ, Damby DE, Barosova H, Geers C, Petri-Fink A, Rothen-Rutishauser B, Clift MJ. Combined exposure of diesel exhaust particles and respirable Soufriere Hills volcanic ash causes a (pro-)inflammatory response in an in vitro multicellular epithelial tissue barrier model. Part Fibre Toxicol. 2016;13:67.
13. Chaudhuri N, Paiva C, Donaldson K, Duffin R, Parker LC, Sabroe I. Diesel exhaust particles override natural injury-limiting pathways in the lung. Am J Physiol Lung Cell Mol Physiol. 2010;299:L263–71.
14. Risom L, Moller P, Loft S. Oxidative stress-induced DNA damage by particulate air pollution. Mutat Res. 2005;592:119–37.
15. Kaimul Ahsan M, Nakamura H, Tanito M, Yamada K, Utsumi H, Yodoi J. Thioredoxin-1 suppresses lung injury and apoptosis induced by diesel exhaust particles (DEP) by scavenging reactive oxygen species and by inhibiting DEP-induced downregulation of Akt. Free Radic Biol Med. 2005; 39:1549–59.
16. Poljsak B, Suput D, Milisav I. Achieving the balance between ROS and antioxidants: when to use the synthetic antioxidants. Oxidative Med Cell Longev. 2013;2013:956792.
17. Bauer RN, Muller L, Brighton LE, Duncan KE, Jaspers I. Interaction with epithelial cells modifies airway macrophage response to ozone. Am J Respir Cell Mol Biol. 2015;52:285–94.
18. Lohmann-Matthes ML, Steinmuller C, Franke-Ullmann G. Pulmonary macrophages. Eur Respir J. 1994;7:1678–89.
19. Proud D, Leigh R. Epithelial cells and airway diseases. Immunol Rev. 2011; 242:186–204.
20. Biswas SK, Mantovani A. Macrophage plasticity and interaction with lymphocyte subsets: cancer as a paradigm. Nat Immunol. 2010;11:889–96.
21. Mosser DM, Edwards JP. Exploring the full spectrum of macrophage activation. Nat Rev Immunol. 2008;8:958–69.
22. Boorsma CE, Draijer C, Melgert BN. Macrophage heterogeneity in respiratory diseases. Mediat Inflamm. 2013;2013:769214.
23. Martinez FO, Helming L, Milde R, Varin A, Melgert BN, Draijer C, Thomas B, Fabbri M, Crawshaw A, Ho LP, et al. Genetic programs expressed in resting and IL-4 alternatively activated mouse and human macrophages: similarities and differences. Blood. 2013;121:e57–69.
24. Byrne AJ, Mathie SA, Gregory LG, Lloyd CM. Pulmonary macrophages: key players in the innate defence of the airways. Thorax. 2015;70:1189–96.
25. Shaykhiev R, Krause A, Salit J, Strulovici-Barel Y, Harvey BG, O'Connor TP, Crystal RG. Smoking-dependent reprogramming of alveolar macrophage polarization: implication for pathogenesis of chronic obstructive pulmonary disease. J Immunol. 2009;183:2867–83.

26. Lucarelli M, Gatti AM, Savarino G, Quattroni P, Martinelli L, Monari E, Boraschi D. Innate defence functions of macrophages can be biased by nano-sized ceramic and metallic particles. Eur Cytokine Netw. 2004;15:339–46.
27. Yen HJ, Hsu SH, Tsai CL. Cytotoxicity and immunological response of gold and silver nanoparticles of different sizes. Small. 2009;5:1553–61.
28. Tran TH, Rastogi R, Shelke J, Amiji MM. Modulation of macrophage functional polarity towards anti-inflammatory phenotype with plasmid DNA delivery in CD44 targeting hyaluronic acid nanoparticles. Sci Rep. 2015;5:16632.
29. Miao X, Leng X, Zhang Q. The current state of nanoparticle-induced macrophage polarization and reprogramming research. Int J Mol Sci. 2017;18. PMID:28178185
30. Jaguin M, Fardel O, Lecureur V. Exposure to diesel exhaust particle extracts (DEPe) impairs some polarization markers and functions of human macrophages through activation of AhR and Nrf2. PLoS One. 2015;10:e0116560.
31. Sawyer K, Mundandhara S, Ghio AJ, Madden MC. The effects of ambient particulate matter on human alveolar macrophage oxidative and inflammatory responses. J Toxicol Environ Health A. 2010;73:41–57.
32. Sunil VR, Patel-Vayas K, Shen J, Laskin JD, Laskin DL. Classical and alternative macrophage activation in the lung following ozone-induced oxidative stress. Toxicol Appl Pharmacol. 2012;263:195–202.
33. Guth AM, Janssen WJ, Bosio CM, Crouch EC, Henson PM, Dow SW. Lung environment determines unique phenotype of alveolar macrophages. Am J Physiol Lung Cell Mol Physiol. 2009;296:L936–46.
34. Miyata R, van Eeden SF. The innate and adaptive immune response induced by alveolar macrophages exposed to ambient particulate matter. Toxicol Appl Pharmacol. 2011;257:209–26.
35. Ji J, von Scheele I, Billing B, Dahlen B, Lantz AS, Larsson K, Palmberg L. Effects of budesonide on toll-like receptor expression in alveolar macrophages from smokers with and without COPD. Int J Chron Obstruct Pulmon Dis. 2016;11:1035–43.
36. von Scheele I, Larsson K, Palmberg L. Budesonide enhances toll-like receptor 2 expression in activated bronchial epithelial cells. Inhal Toxicol. 2010;22:493–9.
37. Mundandhara SD, Becker S, Madden MC. Effects of diesel exhaust particles on human alveolar macrophage ability to secrete inflammatory mediators in response to lipopolysaccharide. Toxicol in Vitro. 2006;20:614–24.
38. Strandberg K, Palmberg L, Larsson K. Effect of budesonide and formoterol on IL-6 and IL-8 release from primary bronchial epithelial cells. J Asthma. 2008;45:201–3.
39. Ji J, Hedelin A, Malmlof M, Kessler V, Seisenbaeva G, Gerde P, Palmberg L. Development of combining of human bronchial mucosa models with XposeALI(R) for exposure of air pollution nanoparticles. PLoS One. 2017; 12:e0170428.
40. Auwerx J. The human leukemia cell line, THP-1: a multifacetted model for the study of monocyte-macrophage differentiation. Experientia. 1991;47:22–31.
41. Park EK, Jung HS, Yang HI, Yoo MC, Kim C, Kim KS. Optimized THP-1 differentiation is required for the detection of responses to weak stimuli. Inflamm Res. 2007;56:45–50.
42. Wottrich R, Diabate S, Krug HF. Biological effects of ultrafine model particles in human macrophages and epithelial cells in mono- and co-culture. Int J Hyg Environ Health. 2004;207:353–61.
43. Rudd CJ, Strom KA. A spectrophotometric method for the quantitation of diesel exhaust particles in Guinea pig lung. J Appl Toxicol. 1981;1:83–7.
44. Dwivedi AM, Upadhyay S, Johanson G, Ernstgard L, Palmberg L. Inflammatory effects of acrolein, crotonaldehyde and hexanal vapors on human primary bronchial epithelial cells cultured at air-liquid interface. Toxicol in Vitro. 2018;46:219–28.
45. Larsson K, Tornling G, Gavhed D, Muller-Suur C, Palmberg L. Inhalation of cold air increases the number of inflammatory cells in the lungs in healthy subjects. Eur Respir J. 1998;12:825–30.
46. Maecker HT, Trotter J. Flow cytometry controls, instrument setup, and the determination of positivity. Cytometry A. 2006;69:1037–42.
47. Kireeva ED, Popovicheva OB, Persiantseva NM, Timofeyev MA, Shonija NK. Fractionation analysis of transport engine-generated soot particles with respect to hygroscopicity. J Atmos Chem. 2009;64:129–47.
48. Franks TJ, Colby TV, Travis WD, Tuder RM, Reynolds HY, Brody AR, Cardoso WV, Crystal RG, Drake CJ, Engelhardt J, et al. Resident cellular components of the human lung: current knowledge and goals for research on cell phenotyping and function. Proc Am Thorac Soc. 2008;5:763–6.
49. Joris F, Manshian BB, Peynshaert K, De Smedt SC, Braeckmans K, Soenen SJ. Assessing nanoparticle toxicity in cell-based assays: influence of cell culture parameters and optimized models for bridging the in vitro-in vivo gap. Chem Soc Rev. 2013;42:8339–59.
50. Paur HR, Cassee FR, Teeguarden J, Fissan H, Diabate S, Aufderheide M, Kreyling WG, Hanninen O, Kasper G, Riediker M, et al. In-vitro cell exposure studies for the assessment of nanoparticle toxicity in the lung-a dialog between aerosol science and biology. J Aerosol Sci. 2011;42:668–92.
51. Lenz AG, Karg E, Brendel E, Hinze-Heyn H, Maier KL, Eickelberg O, Stoeger T, Schmid O. Inflammatory and oxidative stress responses of an alveolar epithelial cell line to airborne zinc oxide nanoparticles at the air-liquid interface: a comparison with conventional, submerged cell-culture conditions. Biomed Res Int. 2013;2013:652632.
52. Limbach LK, Li Y, Grass RN, Brunner TJ, Hintermann MA, Muller M, Gunther D, Stark WJ. Oxide nanoparticle uptake in human lung fibroblasts: effects of particle size, agglomeration, and diffusion at low concentrations. Environ Sci Technol. 2005;39:9370–6.
53. Ji J, von Scheele I, Bergstrom J, Billing B, Dahlen B, Lantz AS, Larsson K, Palmberg L. Compartment differences of inflammatory activity in chronic obstructive pulmonary disease. Respir Res. 2014;15:104.
54. Takizawa H, Ohtoshi T, Kawasaki S, Kohyama T, Desaki M, Kasama T, Kobayashi K, Nakahara K, Yamamoto K, Matsushima K, Kudoh S. Diesel exhaust particles induce NF-kappa B activation in human bronchial epithelial cells in vitro: importance in cytokine transcription. J Immunol. 1999;162:4705–11.
55. Steerenberg PA, Zonnenberg JA, Dormans JA, Joon PN, Wouters IM, van Bree L, Scheepers PT, Van Loveren H. Diesel exhaust particles induced release of interleukin 6 and 8 by (primed) human bronchial epithelial cells (BEAS 2B) in vitro. Exp Lung Res. 1998;24:85–100.
56. Ball JC, Straccia AM, Young WC, Aust AE. The formation of reactive oxygen species catalyzed by neutral, aqueous extracts of NIST ambient particulate matter and diesel engine particles. J Air Waste Manag Assoc. 2000;50:1897–903.
57. Kaspar JW, Niture SK, Jaiswal AK. Nrf2:INrf2 (Keap1) signaling in oxidative stress. Free Radic Biol Med. 2009;47:1304–9.
58. Motohashi H, Yamamoto M. Nrf2-Keap1 defines a physiologically important stress response mechanism. Trends Mol Med. 2004;10:549–57.
59. Zarcone MC, van Schadewijk A, Duistermaat E, Hiemstra PS, Kooter IM. Diesel exhaust alters the response of cultured primary bronchial epithelial cells from patients with chronic obstructive pulmonary disease (COPD) to non-typeable Haemophilus influenzae. Respir Res. 2017;18:27.
60. Ishii H, Hayashi S, Hogg JC, Fujii T, Goto Y, Sakamoto N, Mukae H, Vincent R, van Eeden SF. Alveolar macrophage-epithelial cell interaction following exposure to atmospheric particles induces the release of mediators involved in monocyte mobilization and recruitment. Respir Res. 2005;6:87.
61. Doornaert B, Leblond V, Galiacy S, Gras G, Planus E, Laurent V, Isabey D, Lafuma C. Negative impact of DEP exposure on human airway epithelial cell adhesion, stiffness, and repair. Am J Physiol Lung Cell Mol Physiol. 2003;284:L119–32.
62. Amara N, Bachoual R, Desmard M, Golda S, Guichard C, Lanone S, Aubier M, Ogier-Denis E, Boczkowski J. Diesel exhaust particles induce matrix metalloprotease-1 in human lung epithelial cells via a NADP(H) oxidase/NOX4 redox-dependent mechanism. Am J Physiol Lung Cell Mol Physiol. 2007;293:L170–81.
63. Leema G, Swapna U, Koustav G, Tobias S. Macrophage Polarization in Lung Biology and Diseases. In Lung Inflammation. Edited by (Ed.) DK-CO. London: InTech; 2014.
64. Becker S, Fenton MJ, Soukup JM. Involvement of microbial components and toll-like receptors 2 and 4 in cytokine responses to air pollution particles. Am J Respir Cell Mol Biol. 2002;27:611–8.
65. Becker S, Dailey L, Soukup JM, Silbajoris R, Devlin RB. TLR-2 is involved in airway epithelial cell response to air pollution particles. Toxicol Appl Pharmacol. 2005;203:45–52.
66. Williams MA, Porter M, Horton M, Guo J, Roman J, Williams D, Breysse P, Georas SN. Ambient particulate matter directs nonclassic dendritic cell activation and a mixed TH1/TH2-like cytokine response by naive CD4+ T cells. J Allergy Clin Immunol. 2007;119:488–97.
67. Kawasaki T, Kawai T. Toll-like receptor signaling pathways. Front Immunol. 2014;5:461.
68. Mayer AK, Bartz H, Fey F, Schmidt LM, Dalpke AH. Airway epithelial cells modify immune responses by inducing an anti-inflammatory microenvironment. Eur J Immunol. 2008;38:1689–99.

69. Martinez FO, Gordon S. The M1 and M2 paradigm of macrophage activation: time for reassessment. F1000Prime Rep. 2014;6:13.
70. Mantovani A, Sica A, Sozzani S, Allavena P, Vecchi A, Locati M. The chemokine system in diverse forms of macrophage activation and polarization. Trends Immunol. 2004;25:677–86.
71. Wang N, Liang H, Zen K. Molecular mechanisms that influence the macrophage m1-m2 polarization balance. Front Immunol. 2014;5:614.
72. Sauer RS, Hackel D, Morschel L, Sahlbach H, Wang Y, Mousa SA, Roewer N, Brack A, Rittner HL. Toll like receptor (TLR)-4 as a regulator of peripheral endogenous opioid-mediated analgesia in inflammation. Mol Pain. 2014;10:10.
73. Orr JS, Puglisi MJ, Ellacott KL, Lumeng CN, Wasserman DH, Hasty AH. Toll-like receptor 4 deficiency promotes the alternative activation of adipose tissue macrophages. Diabetes. 2012;61:2718–27.
74. Schlaepfer E, Rochat MA, Duo L, Speck RF. Triggering TLR2, −3, −4, −5, and −8 reinforces the restrictive nature of M1- and M2-polarized macrophages to HIV. J Virol. 2014;88:9769–81.

6

In vitro toxicoproteomic analysis of A549 human lung epithelial cells exposed to urban air particulate matter and its water-soluble and insoluble fractions

Ngoc Q. Vuong[1,4], Dalibor Breznan[1], Patrick Goegan[1], Julie S. O'Brien[1], Andrew Williams[3], Subramanian Karthikeyan[1], Premkumari Kumarathasan[2*] and Renaud Vincent[1,4*]

Abstract

Background: Toxicity of airborne particulate matter (PM) is difficult to assess because PM composition is complex and variable due to source contribution and atmospheric transformation. In this study, we used an in vitro toxicoproteomic approach to identify the toxicity mechanisms associated with different subfractions of Ottawa urban dust (EHC-93).

Methods: A549 human lung epithelial cells were exposed to 0, 60, 140 and 200 μg/cm^2 doses of EHC-93 (total), its insoluble and soluble fractions for 24 h. Multiple cytotoxicity assays and proteomic analyses were used to assess particle toxicity in the exposed cells.

Results: The cytotoxicity data based on cellular ATP, BrdU incorporation and LDH leakage indicated that the insoluble, but not the soluble, fraction is responsible for the toxicity of EHC-93 in A549 cells. Two-dimensional gel electrophoresis results revealed that the expressions of 206 protein spots were significantly altered after particle exposures, where 154 were identified by MALDI-TOF-TOF-MS/MS. The results from cytotoxicity assays and proteomic analyses converged to a similar finding that the effects of the total and insoluble fraction may be alike, but their effects were distinguishable, and their effects were significantly different from the soluble fraction. Furthermore, the toxic potency of EHC-93 total is not equal to the sum of its insoluble and soluble fractions, implying inter-component interactions between insoluble and soluble materials resulting in synergistic or antagonistic cytotoxic effects. Pathway analysis based on the low toxicity dose (60 μg/cm^2) indicated that the two subfractions can alter the expression of those proteins involved in pathways including cell death, cell proliferation and inflammatory response in a distinguishable manner. For example, the insoluble and soluble fractions differentially affected the secretion of pro-inflammatory cytokines such as MCP-1 and IL-8 and distinctly altered the expression of those proteins (e.g., TREM1, PDIA3 and ENO1) involved in an inflammatory response pathway in A549 cells.

Conclusions: This study demonstrated the impact of different fractions of urban air particles constituted of various chemical species on different mechanistic pathways and thus on cytotoxicity effects. In vitro toxicoproteomics can be a valuable tool in mapping these differences in air pollutant exposure-related toxicity mechanisms.

Keywords: Particulate matter (PM), EHC-93, Soluble fraction, Insoluble fraction, A549, Cytotoxicity, Toxicoproteomics, Two-dimensional gel electrophoresis (2D–GE), Mass spectrometry (MS)

* Correspondence: premkumari.kumarathasan@canada.ca; renaud.vincent@canada.ca; renaud.vincent@sympatico.ca
[2]Analytical Biochemistry and Proteomics, Environmental Health Science and Research Bureau, Health Canada, Ottawa, ON K1A 0K9, Canada
[1]Inhalation Toxicology Laboratory, Environmental Health Science and Research Bureau, Health Canada, Ottawa, ON K1A 0K9, Canada
Full list of author information is available at the end of the article

Background

Airborne particulate matter (PM) is a complex mixture of particles with a wide range of sizes and physicochemical properties. Inhalation of airborne PM is linked to the development or exacerbation of respiratory illnesses such as bronchitis [26, 42, 46], asthma [11, 27, 47] and lung cancer [28, 33, 44]; and it is also associated with decline in cognitive function [3, 21, 23, 54] and increased risk of developing diabetes mellitus [9, 36, 60] and cardiovascular disease [15, 20, 32, 41, 58]. A number of epidemiological studies have reported that there is an association between particle composition and health impacts of ambient air particles [5, 10, 30, 66]. However, composition of the respirable particles can vary in different geographical locations depending on the local sources of release [10]. Thus, identifying the drivers of toxic potency and determining their mechanism of effects in airborne PM should be important and useful in the development of regulatory measures to reduce the negative health effects of air pollution.

There are several approaches to the identification of toxic components of ambient air PM. Some studies examined or regressed the toxic effect of the total particles to its water-soluble and/or insoluble components [19, 45, 55, 65], whereas others investigated the effects of particles with defined aerodynamic size range (e.g., <10 μm (PM10), <2.5 μm (PM2.5) and/or <0.1 μm ultrafine particles) in vitro or in vivo [4, 18, 52]. The limitation to most studies assessing the toxicity of PM is the ability to collect sufficient materials for physical and chemical characterization of the particles, and for in vitro and in vivo toxicological investigations. Thus, it is rare to find a single report that could provide all the important details regarding the physicochemical properties, relative cytotoxicities and mechanisms of particle toxicity of the total PM and its constituent components or sub-fractions.

In 1993, a large quantity of ambient air particles from the Environmental Health Centre in Ottawa (EHC-93) was collected to serve the purpose of a reference outdoor urban dust sample to use in different toxicological studies [56, 57]. Since then, EHC-93 has been used extensively in numerous in vivo and in vitro studies. EHC-93 has been partially characterized for the presence of various particle components such as endotoxin, polycyclic aromatic hydrocarbons and metal contents in its total particles [8, 57]. The potency of EHC-93 in causing oxidative/nitrative stress, inflammation and cardiovascular stress in animals has been well documented [2, 7, 24, 51, 56, 58]. EHC-93 was also reported to alter the expression of several genes and cytokines in animals and cells in the respiratory tract [8, 12, 14, 39, 51, 53]. However, a detailed proteomic investigation to assess the molecular mechanisms delineating the toxic effects of EHC-93 as a whole (total) or separated fractions (i.e., insoluble and soluble) has not been conducted. In our recent studies, we demonstrated that in vitro toxicoproteomics is an approach that is capable of distinguishing the pathways associated with cytotoxic effects of respirable particles that are different in physicochemical properties such as carbon black and titanium dioxide [62, 63]. Furthermore, we also showed that our in vitro toxicoproteomic approach was capable of differentiating the effects of particles that were identical in chemical formula (SiO_2) but differed in physical properties such as cristobalite and α-quartz [61]. In this study, we used in vitro toxicoproteomics to dissect the effects of insoluble and soluble components of EHC-93 on A549 human lung epithelial cells. The results from this study showed that cytotoxicity assays, cytokine assays and proteomic analyses (based on two-dimensional gel electrophoresis and mass spectrometry) can differentiate the subtle differences in toxicity between EHC-93 total and its insoluble fraction as well as the drastic difference in toxicity between the soluble fraction and the total or insoluble fraction in A549 cells. To our knowledge, this is the first study that is able to provide extensive details on the physicochemical characteristics of an urban air PM and its sub-fractions, followed by comparing their cytotoxic potencies with multiple assays and comparing their associated cellular mechanisms of effects with proteomic analyses.

Methods

Materials

Culture flasks (T-25 and T-75), 96-well plates and plastic cell scraper were obtained from Corning Inc. (Corning, NY, USA). Dulbecco's Modified Eagle's Medium (DMEM) and fetal bovine serum (FBS) were purchased from Hyclone (Logan, UT, USA). Gentamicin, trifluoroacetic acid, α-cyano-4-hydroxy-cinnamic acid, Tris-HCl, NaCl, Tween-20 and Tween-80 were obtained from Sigma-Aldrich (Oakville, ON, Canada). Iodoacetamide, bis-acrylamide, ammonium persulfate, glycerol, immobilized pH gradient strips, Criterion Cassette (13.3 × 8.7 cm W x L), Tris/Glycine/SDS buffer, and BioSafeCoomassie Blue were purchased from Bio-Rad (Mississauga, ON, Canada). Trypsin, resazurin reduction (CellTiter-Blue®) and lactate dehydrogenase (LDH) cytotoxicity assay kits (CytoTox-96®) were from Promega Corporation (Madison, WI, USA), ATP assay kit (ViaLight™ Plus) was from Lonza Corporation (Rockland, ME, USA), and 5-bromo-2′-deoxyuridine (BrdU) cell proliferation ELISA (chemiluminescent) assay kit was obtained from Roche Diagnostics (Laval, QC, Canada). All materials were analyzed for endotoxin using the chromogenic Limulus amebocyte lysate assay (Lonza, Walkersville, MD, USA). All water used was deionized/demineralized (>16 MΩ resistivity). Water bath Branson 1510 sonicator was from Bransonic (Danbury, CT, USA), which provides an output of 70 watts and 42 kHz was used for all particle preparations and protein extraction purposes.

Particle preparation

The urban dust EHC-93 was collected from baghouse air filters from the Environmental Health Centre in Ottawa, Ontario, Canada in 1993 and its preparation for toxicological studies has been described previously [57]. The water-soluble and water-insoluble fractions of EHC-93 were prepared as follows; a sample of EHC-93 was removed from a – 80 °C freezer and was warmed up to room temperature, 1 g of EHC-93 was placed in a clean 15 mL Falcon tube, re-suspended in 5 mL of sterile water and sonicated in a pre-chilled water bath for 20 min. The tube was then centrifuged (500×g, 10 min), and the aqueous supernatant was collected into another clean 15 mL Falcon tube. The pellet (insoluble) was re-suspended in 5 mL of water, and this process was carried out three times to collect a total volume of 15 mL of aqueous supernatant. The pooled supernatant was further centrifuged (900×g, 3.5 h), the supernatant was collected and the remaining pellet was pooled with the insoluble materials. The aqueous supernatant was then filtered through a 0.2 μm nylon syringe-tip filter into a clean 50 mL Falcon tube. This filter was then washed with 5 mL of methanol and pooled with the aqueous suspension. The pooled aqueous suspension and the pooled pellet were then lyophylized and stored frozen at -80 °C. The final mass percentage recoveries of the particle fractions were 17% water-soluble (soluble) and 83% water-insoluble (insoluble).

To prepare the particles for dosing, the dried particulate materials from the total, insoluble and soluble fractions each were resuspended in particle preparation buffer (NaCl: 1.9 mg/mL or 32.5 mM; Tween-80: 25.0 μg/mL or 19.1 μM) in a Dounce glass-glass micro-homogenizer. The final concentrations of the total, insoluble and soluble fractions were prepared according to their mass percentages (i.e., 10.0, 8.3 and 1.7 mg/mL, respectively). In this manner, the cytotoxicities of the insoluble and soluble fractions relative to the total can be directly assessed. The suspensions were sonicated on ice for 20 min and then dispersed as much as possible by 25 strokes of the homogenizer piston. Particle suspensions were then aliquotted into sterile, O-ring seal microcentrifuge tubes, heated to 56 °C in a water bath for 30 min, and were subsequently frozen at -80 °C until use. All materials were analyzed for endotoxin using the chromogenic Limulus amebocyte lysate assay (Lonza, Walkersville, MD, USA).

Scanning electron microscopy (SEM)

The size and morphology of EHC-93 was characterized by SEM. Images were collected on a JSM-7500F FESEM (JEOL) instrument equipped with a Field Emission Gun (FEG) under the following parameters: beam acceleration voltage, 2 KV; working distance, between 7 and 9 mm; imaging mode, Lower Secondary Electron Image (LEI). Magnification and sizing bar are as indicated in the figure captions for each individual image. Samples were prepared by dropping a small amount of powder onto an aluminum stage painted with carbon paint (Electron Microscope Sciences, (EMS)). The paint was allowed to dry for 20 min, and the excess powder was then removed by blowing the surface with compressed, dry air.

Energy dispersive X-ray spectroscopy (EDX)

EDX spectra were collected using a JSM-7500F FESEM (JEOL) instrument with the following parameters: beam acceleration voltage, 20 KV; acceleration current, 10 mA; working distance, between 8 and 9 mm. Since this instrument is attached to the SEM purchased from JSM, sample analysis was run concomitantly with SEM imaging, and thus, sample preparation for the collection of EDX spectra is identical to that for SEM. It should be noted that the carbon content in the sample cannot be determined because the stage is coated with carbon paint. The weight percent and atomic percent results were produced automatically from the instrument software analysis package.

Inductively coupled plasma–mass spectrometry (ICP-MS)

Elemental analysis on EHC-93 total and its insoluble and soluble fraction were analyzed by ICP-MS in a previous report [58]. The results that are pertinent to this manuscript were summarized in Additional file 1: Table S1.

Powder X-ray diffraction (pXRD)

The powder X-ray diffraction plot was obtained with a Rigaku Ultima IV instrument, equipped with a Cu tube. The powder sample was pressed by hand into a custom sample holder, such that a flat powder sample with a specified surface height would be presented to the X-ray beam. The pXRD plot was then collected in the 2 to 70 2theta degree range in continuous-scan mode, with a sample width of 0.02 degrees, and a scan speed of 0.25 deg./min. Percent distribution was measured following identification and integration of the peak areas for each crystal phase observed in the spectrum.

Cell culture and particle exposure

The A549 cell line (American Type Culture Collection - CCL-185; human, epithelial, lung carcinoma) was subcultured in DMEM supplemented with 50 μg/mL gentamicin and 10% FBS. It should be noted that final FBS concentration the cells are exposed to is 5% after dosing with particles (particle preparations that were used to dose the cells were in serum-free media, then they were added to the 10% FBS culture media that contained the cells). The cells were maintained and subcultured in T-75 flasks in a humidified atmosphere containing 5% CO_2 and 95% air at 37 °C. For exposure experiments, the cells were seeded at 1.5 × 10^6 cells/T-25 flask (for proteomics) or 2.0 × 10^4 cells/well in 96-well plate (for cytotoxicity assays), incubated for 24 h, resulting in approximately 75% confluence prior to dosing with particles. The final volume of culture medium was 5 mL (T-25), 15 mL (T-75) or 200 μL/well (96-well plate). Solutions of particles were prepared from frozen stocks, which were thawed to room temperature, sonicated on ice (20 min), then diluted in the culture medium to generate dosing concentrations that are equivalent to 0, 60, 140 and 200 μg/cm^2 of the total (i.e., 0, 50, 116 and 166 μg/cm^2 for the insoluble fraction and 0, 10, 24 and 34 μg/cm^2 for the soluble fraction). The exposures were performed in this proportional manner so that the contributions of the insoluble and soluble components in EHC-93 total can be directly compared. However, the concentrations for both insoluble and soluble fractions were expressed in equivalent concentrations to the total in all the tables and figures in this study in order to assess the relative impacts of the two fractions. The cells were exposed to the particles by replacing the existing culture medium with the particle-containing medium, and the flasks/plates were returned to the incubator for a 24 h exposure to the particles. To harvest the exposed cells, the medium in each flask was removed and the cells were detached from the flasks using a plastic scraper. The cell suspension was collected in cell culture medium and centrifuged at 350 x g for 5 min, and the supernatant was discarded. The cell pellet was then washed twice with phosphate buffer saline (PBS). The final cell pellet was aspirated dry and stored at −80 °C until further use for proteomic analysis. This experiment was conducted in triplicate (n = 3) for all treatments.

Integrated cytotoxicity assays

The integrated cytotoxicity bioassays which combined endpoints of cell viability (resazurin reduction assay), cellular membrane integrity (intracellular LDH release), and energy metabolism (ATP assay) were conducted in a single 96-well plate as described in a previous study [25]. The assays were carried out in the following sequence; after 24 h of exposure to particles, 100 μL of cell culture supernatant was transferred in a clear 96-well plate and clarified at 300 x g for 5 min (room temperature); 25 μL was used for LDH assay, 75 μL was frozen for other assays such as cytokine assays. Then, 50 μL of resazurin reduction reagent, prepared in culture medium (40% v/v), was added to the remaining 100 μL of culture medium and the cells were incubated (5% CO_2, 37 °C) for 2 h. Aliquots (20 μL) were taken for measurement of resazurin reduction at 10 min and 120 min as described below. The cell culture supernatant was discarded by aspiration and the cells were lysed with 200 μL of lysis buffer (100 mM $MgCl_2$ and 0.025% Triton X-100 in PBS) at room temperature, for 10 min. The lysate was recovered in clean plates and clarified by centrifugation as above; 25 μL of lysate was used for LDH measurement, 50 μL was used for ATP measurement, and 100 μL was frozen for additional analyses. The cell proliferation (BrdU incorporation) assay was performed in a separate 96-well plate. For all assays, supernatants and cell lysates were clarified by centrifugation to prevent interference of particles in the assays. All cytotoxicity assays were conducted in quadruplicate (n = 4) for all treatments.

In the resazurin reduction assay, viable cells reduce a non-fluorescent redox dye resazurin (dark blue in color) to a fluorescent reaction product resorufin (pink in color), and nonviable cells lose metabolic capacity to convert the indicator dye. Mitochondrial, cytosolic and microsomal enzymes have been implicated in the reduction of resazurin [16]. For measurement of resazurin reduction, 20 μL of supernatant aliquots at 10 and 120 min were transferred into clean plates containing 80 μL of serum-free medium per well, shaken at 350 rpm for 30 s on a circular plate shaker, and clarified by centrifugation at 300 x g for 5 min. Fluorescence of the diluted supernatants was measured by top reading at λ_{Ex} = 540 and λ_{Em} = 600 nm (Synergy 2, BioTek, Winooski, VT, USA). Resazurin reduction is calculated by fluorescence at 120 min minus fluorescence at 10 min.

The CytoTox 96® colorimetric assay quantitates the activity of cytosolic LDH released extracellularly during cell membrane damage (an indicator of cell death). The enzymatic activity released in the cell culture supernatants and recovered in the lysis buffer was measured with a coupled enzymatic reaction. LDH catalyzes the oxidation of lactate to pyruvate that is accompanied with the reduction of NAD^+ to NADH, which in turn is consumed simultaneously in a diaphorase-catalysed reduction of tetrazolium salt, generating a soluble red formazan that can be detected by absorbance at 490 nm. For the assay of released LDH, 25 μL of the cell supernatants were combined with 25 μL of cell culture medium and 50 μL of LDH substrate from the assay kit. Absorbance at 490 nm (Synergy 2) was measured after 20 and 40 min of incubation in the dark. For the assay of cellular LDH, 25 μL aliquots of the cell lysates was combined with 25 μL of lysis buffer and 50 μL of substrate from the LDH assay kit. Absorbance at 490 nm was measured immediately and after 10 min of incubation in dark. The relative cellular LDH was calculated as a fraction of total LDH, that is LDH activity in cell lysate was divided by total LDH activity recovered in supernatant and cell lysate.

The ViaLight Plus is a bioluminescent assay for measurement of cellular ATP. Cell injury leading to mitochondrial perturbation results in a decrease of cellular ATP. In the presence of ATP and oxygen, the luciferase enzyme oxidises luciferin to oxyluciferin that accompany with photons emission. Chemiluminescence in the assay is proportional to the concentration of ATP in the cell lysate. The ATP working reagent was prepared 15 min prior to conducting the assay by mixing ATP monitoring reagent and the assay buffer provided in the kit, where 50 μL of the cell lysate was added to 100 μL of freshly prepared ATP reagent in a white-walled 96 well plate. Luminescence was measured (Synergy 2, Biotek) following 2 min incubation in the dark.

The BrdU Cell Proliferation ELISA is an enzyme immunoassay based on the incorporation of the thymidine analog BrdU during DNA synthesis in proliferating cells. Cells were grown in black-walled 96-well plates and exposed to particles for 24 h as described above. The BrdU labelling medium (10 μM BrdU) was added to each well, followed by a 4 h incubation (5% CO_2, 37 °C). The medium was discarded and the plates were dried at 60 °C for 1 h, and stored at −40 °C until use. The cell monolayers were fixed with 200 μL of the fixation-denaturation reagent for 30 min and then incubated with anti-BrdU antibody for 2 h at room temperature. The wells were washed three times with 150 μL of PBS containing 0.01% Tween-80, and the substrate provided in the BrdU ELISA kit was added. The plates were covered with black tape and were shaken for 4 min. Chemiluminescence was measured (Synergy 2) with 1 s integrated readings per well.

ELISA-based secretory cytokine assays

Levels of cytokines from the supernatant were measured by a Millipore MAP 8-plex human cytokine panel (EMD Millipore, Billerica, MA). The simultaneous quantification of cytokine levels was carried out according to Millipore recommended procedure, where a panel of 11 cytokines were assessed (GM-CSF, IL-1β, IL-1RA, IL-6, IL-8, IL-9, IL-10, IL-12p70, MCP-1, TNFα and VEGF), where the procedure was carried out in a Bio-Rad Bio-plex 200 array reader instrument (Bio-Rad Laboratories, Mississauga, ON). Briefly, cell supernatants were thawed on ice and centrifuged at 956 x g for 5 min, at 4 °C. Next, 25 μl of samples were incubated with 25 μl of microbeads labeled with antibodies to the specific cytokines in a 96-well flat-bottom plate overnight at 4 °C. After the incubation the samples were washed twice using Bio-Rad Bioplex Pro II wash system, followed by incubation with the 25 μl of detection antibody cocktail for 1 h at room temperature (RT). The beads were then incubated with 25 μl of streptavidin-phycoerythrin for 30 min at RT, washed twice, and suspended in 150 μl of sheath fluid. The data were analyzed using the Bio-Rad Bio-Plex ManagerTM version 6.0 software, with 5PL curve fit and background fluorescence subtraction. The analysis was conducted in pooled samples of 3 wells per sample within each experiment, in quadruplicate experiments (n = 4). Cytokine levels in cell supernatants were determined from cytokine standard curves included on each plate. Only those cytokines that were detected at a concentration > 5 pg/ml in all data points would be used to filter out noises in the data. The final levels of cytokines for each treatment was adjusted to the viability of cells based on cellular LDH, BrdU incorporation and cellular ATP assays as previously described [8]. Data were expressed as normalized fold-change (FC) relative to the control (0 μg/cm^2).

Protein extraction and two-dimensional gel electrophoresis (2D–GE)

Total protein from the A549 cells (control & particle-exposed) was extracted and subjected to 2D–GE as previously described [62, 63]. Following electrophoresis, the gel was washed for 30 min in water, stained in BioSafeCoomassie Blue (Bio-Rad) overnight (16–20 h), destained twice in water (20 min), and then imaged with a standard scanner. To overcome the typical warping and distortion issues from gel to gel especially near the extremities of the pH range and the molecular weight, a common area across all experimental gels that clearly shows the protein spots was selected to assess the proteome differences among the treatments, where proteins in the window of pH 5.1–7.8 and 100–20 kDa were analyzed [62, 63]. A total of 543 well-resolved protein spots in this common area were compared across all experimental gels, and the identities of 333 of these protein spots were determined using MALDI-TOF-TOF-MS [62, 63]. The protein spots within the gels were matched and quantified with PDQuest™ Advance V8.0.1 (Bio-Rad), where spot volume was quantified using the available "Local regression model (LOESS)" algorithm in PDQuest. The reported spot volume for each protein was used to compare its level of expression across the treatments. In order to calculate the fold change for a protein spot from a treatment group, the treatment/control ratio (n = 3) was first determined. If the treatment/control ratio is between 0 and 1.0, a decreased expression (e.g., 0.5), then the fold-change is calculated by dividing "− 1.0" by the treatment/control ratio (e.g., − 1.0 / 0.5 = − 2.0). If the treatment/control ratio is >1.0, corresponding to increased expression (e.g., 1.5), then this serves as the fold-change by itself (https://www.qiagen.com/). Such fold-change values are used for bioinformatic analyses (e.g. IPA) as reported in Additional file 2: Table S2 and Figs. 4, 5, 6, 7. It should be noted that there is no value between "− 1.0 and 1.0" when the fold-changes are expressed in this manner. For hierarchical cluster analysis, however, fold-changes were calculated based on Log_2(treatment/control) so that the data is continuous (i.e., there is no gap between – 1.0 and 1.0) for the appropriate analysis.

Statistics

Hierarchical cluster analysis was conducted using GenePattern [37], and the resulting heatmap was generated with Java TreeView (https://sourceforge.net/projects/jtreeview/). Two-way analysis of variance (ANOVA) was performed on 2D–GE (n = 3), cytotoxicity assays (n = 4) and cytokine releases (n = 4) data with treatment and dose as factors, using R [35]. When the assumptions of equal variance or normality were not met, the data were rank transformed. Holm-Sidak was the *post-hoc* method used for all pairwise comparison procedures, which is a step-down procedure on a sorted set of null hypotheses. The reported p-values have been adjusted for the family-wise error rate (FWER) which is the probability of making at least one type I error (incorrect rejection of a true null hypothesis) in the set or family of null hypotheses. A protein was considered as having a significant effect if the Holm-Sidak adjusted p-value was less than 0.05. If the *Treatment* x *Dose* interaction was significant for a protein spot, its change in expression for a given treatment and dose that was found significant by Holm-Sidak analysis was reported as it is, as presented in Additional file 2: Table S2. The same applied for those proteins that were found to have significant *Treatment* and *Dose* main effects. If a protein was found to have significant *Treatment* main effect, fold changes were estimated using least square mean [17, 43]. In the case where the *Dose* main effect was significant, the average FC estimate was reported for each significant dose group.

Bioinformatics

It should be noted that multiple protein spots with the same protein ID may have a p-value <0.05, which suggests different isoforms of the same protein were significantly altered (Additional file 2: Table S2). When this was the case, selection for pathway analysis was based on the following order: best matching MW, largest spot volume, highest MOWSE score (molecular weight search) and then greatest FC. Furthermore, protein spots that were deemed as small peptides/fragments (based on MW and unique peptide sequences) of their native proteins were excluded from pathway analysis, unless functional data can be found for such peptides based on UniProt (www.uniprot.org) and PubMed (http://www.ncbi.nlm.nih.gov/pubmed) searches. It should be mentioned that a few cleaved protein products were included in pathway analysis in this study because they are known to serve functional purposes. For example, the precursor of HTRA2 is a 50 kDa mitochondrial membrane protein that became a mature serine protease of 36 kDa (SSP6208, see Additional file 2: Table S2) in the cytosol after 133 of its N-terminal amino acids has been proteolytically cleaved [50], where the mature peptide serves as an inhibitor of XIAP and IAPs [50]. Furthermore, an arbitrary ±1.10 FC cut-off was also applied on all significant proteins (adjusted p-value <0.05) when conducting pathway and network analyses. Protein interaction network and pathway analyses were conducted using Ingenuity Pathway Analysis (www.ingenuity.com).

Results

Physicochemical characterization of the EHC-93 particles

The electron micrographs in Fig. 1 show that the EHC-93 Ottawa urban dust is a complex mixture of particles with a broad range of size, shape, crystallinity, aggregation, porosity and surface structure. Majority of the materials appear to be crystalline particles with a wide range of sizes, where most particles possess flat non-porous plains and sharp edges. Some particles found in small quantities appeared as long thin rods (Fig. 1d), and as spherical non-porous, spherical porous and spherical ordered porous (biological origin) (Fig. 1c) materials. X-ray diffraction data in Table 1 showed that calcite ($CaCO_3$), α-quartz (SiO_2), gypsum ($CaSO_4$) and dolomite ($CaMg(CO_3)_2$) were the major crystalline particles in EHC-93, which constituted of 41, 18, 13 and 13% of the crystalline particles, respectively. The EDX analysis revealed that Ca (31.9% by mass), Si (23.2% by mass) and S (11.4% by mass) are the three dominant elements in EHC-93 (Table 2). This EDX result is similar to that of the IPC-MS result from a previous study which also showed that Ca and Si are major elements in EHC-93 total (Additional file 1: Table S1) [58]. The combined results suggested that majority of the insoluble components in EHC-93 are calcite followed by α-quartz and gypsum.

The results in Table 3 showed that EHC-93 total particles contain a very small amount of endotoxin (100.0 EU/kg material). Almost all of the endotoxin was found in the insoluble fraction of EHC-93 (91.6 ± 1.4 EU/kg equivalent mass to the total). Only a trace quantity of endotoxin can be found in the soluble fraction of EHC-93 (2.5 ± 1.0 EU/kg equivalent mass to the total).

Cytotoxic effects of EHC-93, and its insoluble and soluble components in A549 cells

The cytotoxicity assays in Fig. 2 indicated that EHC-93 Ottawa urban air particles (total) had mild cytotoxic effect on A549 cells at low level of exposure (60 μg/cm^2). However, EHC-93 total were cytotoxic to A549 cells at higher doses (140 and 200 μg/cm^2), where they were capable of causing significant damage to the cell membrane based on LDH release assay (Fig. 2a), reducing cell proliferation based on BrdU incorporation assay (Fig. 2b) and decreasing metabolic energy content based on cellular ATP assay (Fig. 2c). Resazurin reduction assay did not

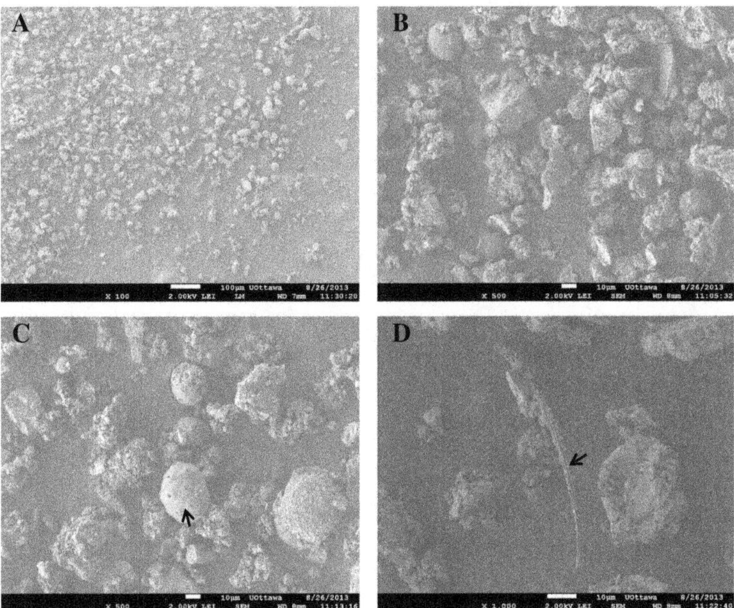

Fig. 1 The particles in the EHC-93 sample observed by scanning electron microscopy at various magnifications to show the contents in the particulate matter. **a** is a 100X magnification image of the particles (scale bar is 100 μm). **b** and **c** are 500X magnification images of the particles (scale bars are 10 μm) that shows the majority of the particles have the appearance of mineral particles, where the arrow in **c** points to a spherical ordered particle (biological origin). **d** is a 1,000X magnification image (scale bar is μm), and it shows a thin rod (arrow) in the middle of the image

detect any significant effect by EHC-93 total or its subfractions (Fig. 2d). It was observed that the trend of cytotoxicity of the insoluble fraction was remarkably similar to that of total PM, suggesting that the insoluble components drove most of the toxic effects of EHC-93 in A549 cells. Nevertheless, subtle cytotoxicity differences between the insoluble fraction and total PM can be observed in most assays, where the insoluble components appeared even more potent than EHC-93 total, and a significant difference between the two exposures was observed in the level of cellular ATP at the highest dose (two-way ANOVA: *Treatment x Dose* interaction at 200 μg/cm^2, $p < 0.05$) (Fig. 2c). The soluble materials were relatively non-toxic to A549 cells, and their effects were significantly different than the total and insoluble components in most assays.

Table 1 The percentage distribution of the major mineral crystals in the EHC-93 Ottawa urban dust detected by X-ray diffraction

Mineral crystal	% Distribution
Calcite ($CaCO_3$)	41
α-quartz (SiO_2)	18
Gypsum ($CaSO_4$)	13
Dolomite ($CaMg(CO_3)_2$)	13
Albite ($NaAlSi_3O_8$)	10
Halite (NaCl)	5

Changes in the expression of proteins in A549 cells following exposures to EHC-93 and its insoluble and soluble fractions

Two-way ANOVA results in Additional file 2: Table S2 indicated that 206 protein spots were differentially altered significantly by the treatments (adjusted *p*-value <0.05), and 154 of these protein spots have been identified via MALDI-TOF-TOF-MS. The effects of particle treatments on most of these protein spots (i.e., 126 out of 154 identified proteins) were particle-specific (i.e., *Treatment* main effect, *Treatment* & *Dose* main effects, and *Treatment X Dose* interaction). It should be kept in mind that two-way ANOVA results are meant to identify

Table 2 The percentage distribution of the major elements in the EHC-93 Ottawa urban dust detected by energy dispersive X-ray spectroscopy

Element	Weight %	Atomic %
Na	6.99	9.96
Mg	2.72	3.66
Al	6.46	7.84
Si	23.17	27.04
S	11.41	11.66
Cl	7.74	7.16
K	3.70	3.10
Ca	31.89	26.08
Fe	5.94	3.49

Table 3 Endotoxin levels in EHC-93 total and its water-insoluble and soluble fractions

PM	Endotoxin (EU/kg material[a])
Total[b]	100.0 ± 1.0
Insoluble	91.6 ± 1.4
Soluble	2.5 ± 1.0

[a]The quantity of endotoxin unit (EU) was expressed relative to EHC-93 total for direct comparison (i.e., 91.6 and 2.5 EU can be detected from 0.83 and 0.17 kg of materials from the insoluble and soluble fractions, respectively)
[b]Data has been published [8]

significant differential changes in protein expression among the treatments, and these changes are not always significantly different from the control. For example, all of the *Treatment* main effects in Additional file 2: Table S2 were not due to significant difference from the control after particle exposures. Rather, most of the *Treatment* main effects were significant differences between the soluble fraction and the total and/or insoluble fraction based on Holm-Sidak multiple pair-wise comparison tests (adjusted *p*-values were not shown), and some were due to differences between the total and insoluble fraction. On the other hand, significant differences from the control as well as among the treatments can be identified by *Treatment* & *Dose* main effect and *Treatment X Dose* interaction as demonstrated in Additional file 2: Table S2. Holm-Sidak multiple pair-wise comparison tests showed that EHC-93 total and its insoluble fraction affected the expression of most protein spots similarly (e.g., same direction of expression), and that their effects were different from the soluble materials (e.g., opposite directions of expression) (Additional file 2: Table S2). Despite their similarity, differences between the total and insoluble fraction can be identified based on their FCs and adjusted *p*-values (not shown) following Holm-Sidak analysis. It should be noted that the two-way ANOVA results in Additional file 2: Table S2 revealed multiple significant protein spots with the same protein ID, an indication of different isoforms of the same protein and/or post-translational modification of the native protein. A large portion of the significant protein spots were small fragments of their native proteins (based on MW and unique peptide sequences).

Hierarchical cluster analysis was conducted to visually compare changes in the proteome of A549 cells following 24 h of exposure to EHC-93 and its insoluble and soluble fractions. The results based on all 543 protein spots examined by 2D–GE (Additional file 3: Figure S1)

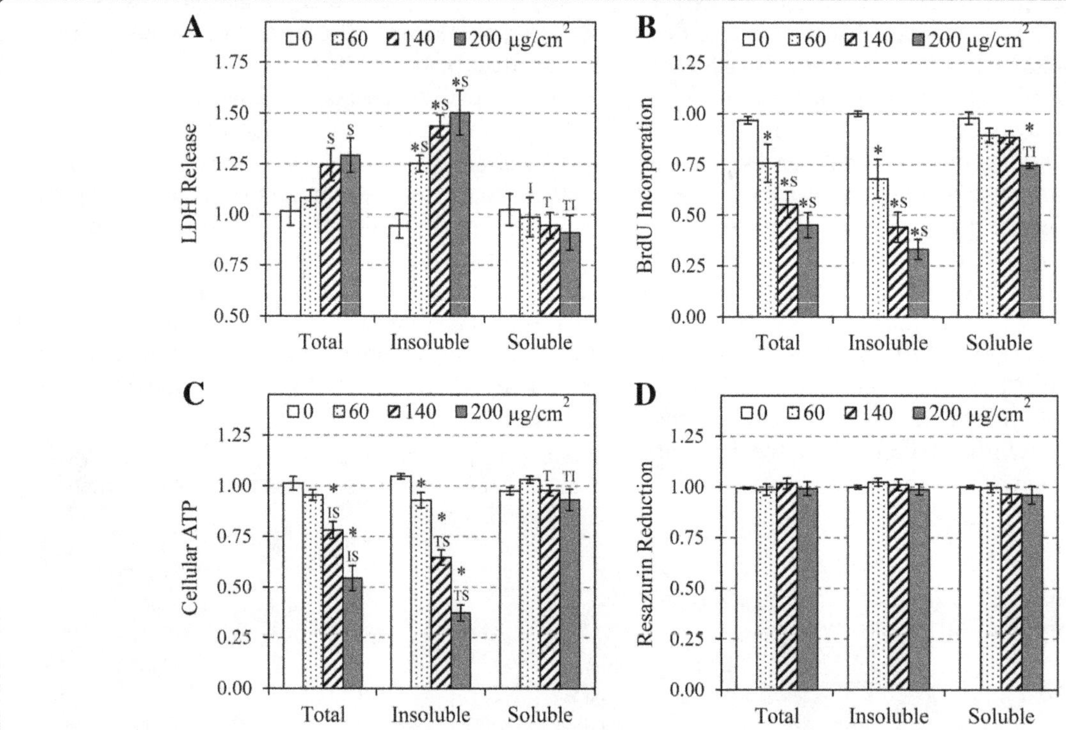

Fig. 2 The cytotoxicities of EHC-93 total and its water-insoluble (insoluble) and water-soluble (soluble) fractions in A549 cells after 24 h of exposure were assessed by LDH release (**a**), BrdU incorporation (**b**), cellular ATP (**c**) and resazurin reduction(**d**) assays. Data are expressed as mean fold effect +/− standard error, relative to the control (0 μg/cm^2), $n = 4$. Two-way ANOVA was used to determine significant effects of the particles, where Holm-Sidak was the post-hoc method used for all pairwise comparison procedures. * indicates significant difference compared to control. [T] indicates significant difference compared to EHC-93 total. [I] indicates significant difference compared to the insoluble fraction. [S] indicates significant difference compared to the soluble fraction

or only the significantly altered protein spots (Fig. 3) showed that the insoluble fraction and EHC-93 total formed a cluster that is separate from the soluble fraction. Such observations indicated that the total EHC-93 mixture and its insoluble components affected the proteome of A549 cells similarly, and that their effects differed from those of the soluble materials. It should be noted that the effects of the total PM and the insoluble were different enough that the two treatments formed two separate sub-clusters (Additional file 3: Figure S1 and Fig. 3). The significantly altered protein spots in Fig. 3 appeared to form five interesting clusters (I – V).

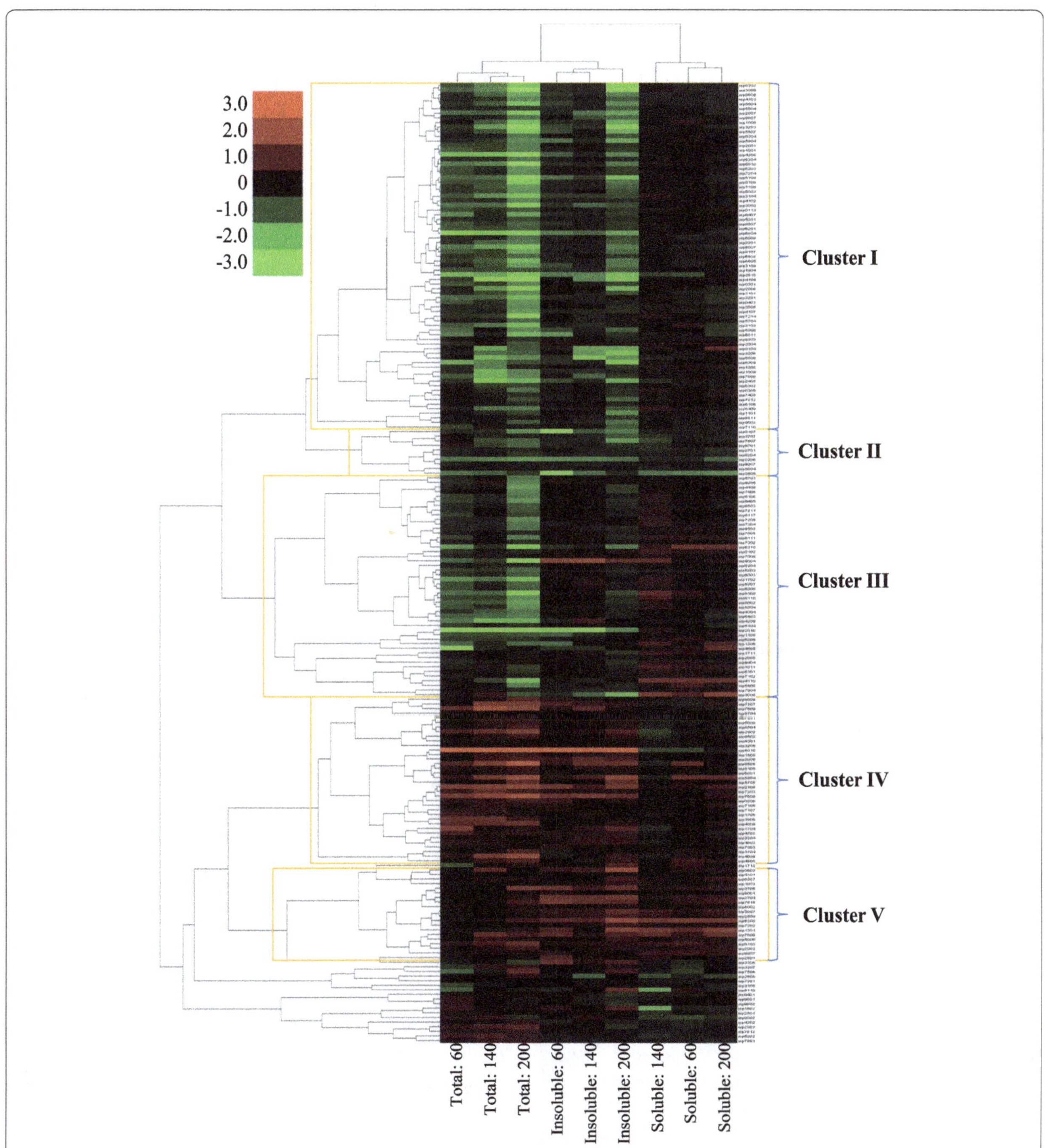

Fig. 3 Unsupervised hierarchical cluster analysis of the protein spots that were significantly affected due to particle exposures (Two-way ANOVA: $p < 0.05$). The expression of each protein spot was calculated by Log_2(Treatment/Control), $n = 3$. Red is coded for increased expression and green is coded for decreased expression. The number indicates the dose in μg/cm^2. The involvment of the proteins in different clusters in various cellular functions is listed in Additional file 4: Table S3

Cluster I was dominated by those protein spots that were down regulated by the total and insoluble fraction; and these proteins were found to be involved in cellular movement, cell growth and proliferation, cell death and survival, molecular transport and small molecule biochemistry pathways (Additional file 4: Table S3). Cluster II was a small group of protein spots that were decreased in expression by all treatments, but the number of protein in this cluster was not large enough to conduct a reliable bioinformatics analysis. Cluster III displayed the protein spots that the total and insoluble fraction treatments generally decreased their expressions, while the soluble fraction generally increased their expressions; these proteins were involved predominantly in cellular movement, carbohydrate metabolism, cell growth and proliferation, cell death and survival, and cell morphology pathways (Additional file 4: Table S3). Cluster IV consisted of those protein spots that were strongly increased by most total and insoluble exposures but were weakly increased or decreased by the soluble treatments. The proteins in this cluster were found to be in the lipid metabolism, small molecule biochemistry, and cell growth and proliferation pathways. Cluster V showed the protein spots that were increased in expression by all treatments; these proteins are involved in cellular morphology, cellular function and maintenance, cellular assembly and organization, and cell death and survival.

Effects of EHC-93 and its insoluble and soluble components on various pathways and networks in A549 cells

Ingenuity Pathway Analysis results in Table 4 revealed that EHC-93 and its insoluble and soluble fractions can affect the expression of the proteins involved in a number of biological functions including cell death, cell proliferation, cell differentiation, cellular movement, inflammatory response, protein metabolism and reactive oxygen species (ROS) metabolism. In these pathways, the patterns of protein expression in A549 cells influenced by the soluble fraction were noticeably different from the total and insoluble fraction, and the differences between the latter two are more subtle but distinguishable (Additional file 5: Figure S2). Generally, most of these proteins were altered by the total and insoluble fraction treatments in the same direction but varying in magnitude, whereas the soluble fraction exposure may cause no effect or opposite effects to that of the total and insoluble fraction treatments. For example, the networks of cell death and proliferation in Fig. 4 showed that the expressions of proteins such as YWHAE, SRSF1, PKM, HSPA9 and ENO1 were down-regulated in the total and insoluble fraction but were up-regulated or unaffected by the soluble fraction. The expression of proteins such as VCP, TREM1 and BUB3 were up-regulated in the total and insoluble fraction but down-regulated or unaffected in the soluble fraction. All these proteins were affected by the total and insoluble fraction in the same direction but varying magnitude. Similarly, the network of protein metabolism in Fig. 5 showed that the expression of PDIA3, HSPA8 and EIF3I were down-regulated due to the soluble fraction exposure, but these proteins were either up-regulated or unaffected by the total and insoluble fraction exposures to varying magnitude. The expression of UFD1L was up-regulated by the soluble fraction, but it was down-regulated by the total and insoluble fraction to different degrees. Of all the networks examined, the network of organ inflammation in Fig. 6 showed the most contrasting effect between the total or insoluble fraction against the soluble fraction, where 10/11 and 9/11 proteins in the network were distinctly altered, respectively. In this network, the total and insoluble fraction significantly increased the expression of PDIA3, TREM1, TUBA1C and VCP to various degrees in A549 cells, whereas exposure to the soluble fraction either did not affect or decreased the expression of these proteins. On the other hand, the expression of ACTB, ENO1 and PKM were significantly decreased in A549 cells to varying magnitude following exposure to the total and insoluble fraction, but these proteins were either unaffected or increased after exposing to the soluble fraction.

Secretion levels of IL-8, MCP-1 and VEGF from A549 cells due to exposures to EHC-93 and its insoluble and soluble fractions

From a panel of 11 cytokines assessed, only 3 cytokines (IL-8, MCP-1 and VEGF) were found to secrete at a reliable detection level (> 5 pg/ml) and were significantly altered due to particle exposures (Fig. 7). It was found that EHC-93 total and its insoluble fraction displayed a similar trend in stimulating the secretion of IL-8, MCP-1 and VEGF from A549 cells that is different from the soluble fraction. The insoluble fraction is significantly more potent than the soluble fraction in stimulating the releases of the pro-inflammatory cytokines interleukin-8 (IL-8) and monocyte chemoattractant protein-1 (MCP-1) from A549 cells (Fig. 7a and b). The insoluble fraction appeared more potent than the total in inducing the secretion of IL-8 and MCP-1 from A549 cells, and it reached statistical significant for MCP-1 at the highest dose (Fig. 7b). Contrarily, the soluble fraction is significantly more potent than the insoluble fraction in causing the release of vascular endothelial growth factor (VEGF) from A549 cells (Fig. 7c). The total and insoluble fraction can stimulate significant release of VEGF from A549 cells, but their potencies were not significantly different.

Discussion

Understanding the mechanisms of particle toxicity of urban air particulate matter (PM) is a challenge, because airborne PM is a complex mixture of particles with a

Table 4 Biological functions indicated by Ingenuity Pathway Analysis (IPA) that were likely impacted by the particles based on the proteins that were significantly affected

	Total		Insoluble		Soluble	
Biological Function	#	*p*-value	#	*p*-value	#	*p*-value
Cell Death and Survival	22	1.51×10^{-05}	24	4.39×10^{-09}	19	4.29×10^{-05}
Cell Growth and Proliferation	21	2.42×10^{-04}	22	6.91×10^{-05}	18	5.85×10^{-04}
Cellular Movement	17	1.83×10^{-05}	18	3.89×10^{-06}	16	6.56×10^{-06}
Acute Inflammation	10	1.45×10^{-03}	9	5.30×10^{-03}	8	6.33×10^{-03}
Chronic Inflammation	10	1.62×10^{-04}	8	3.39×10^{-03}	9	2.15×10^{-04}
Cytoplasm Organization	9	2.03×10^{-02}	10	6.95×10^{-03}	9	6.90×10^{-03}
Protein Metabolism	7	1.07×10^{-02}	10	1.24×10^{-04}	11	3.80×10^{-06}
ROS Metabolism	6	1.40×10^{-03}	8	2.74×10^{-05}	5	3.83×10^{-03}
Allergic Response	7	5.18×10^{-05}	6	4.31×10^{-04}	6	1.71×10^{-04}
Nucleic Acid Metabolism	6	1.62×10^{-03}	7	8.05×10^{-05}	5	1.95×10^{-03}
Mitochondrial Transmembrane Potential	5	1.22×10^{-04}	6	8.52×10^{-06}	5	5.47×10^{-05}

It should be noted that about half of the proteins used in pathway analysis derived from *Treatment* main effect, where the effect of the soluble fraction on these protein spots were typically opposite that of the total and insoluble fraction. The directions of protein expressions of several selected functions were demonstrated as heatmaps in Additional file 5: Figure S2. The # indicate the number of proteins that were significantly affected by each treatment (EHC-93 total, insoluble and soluble at 60 μg/cm^2), and the *p*-value indicate the significance of the biological function based on IPA's calculations. Only the significant functions that were influenced by more than 5 proteins in any particle treatment group are presented

wide range of physicochemical properties. In an attempt to assess the in vitro toxicity of urban air particles, we previously fractionated EHC-93 (Ottawa urban air particles) into water-insoluble and soluble fractions, and used A549 cells to examine the PM exposure-related effects on a few selected genes and secretory proteins in the endothelin system [12]. The current study focuses on integration of multiple cytotoxicity assay and untargeted proteomic analysis results to gain insight into toxicity mechanisms underlying total and fractionated PM exposure-related changes in A549 cells.

This is the first time that multiple cytotoxicity assays were used to investigate the cytotoxic effects of EHC-93 and its insoluble and soluble fraction in the same in vitro study. The results from LDH release, cellular ATP and BrdU incorporation assays indicated that EHC-93 total and its insoluble fraction were both similarly cytotoxic to A549 cells, while the soluble fraction caused very little toxic effect to the cells (Fig. 2). It could be argued that the cells were actually dosed with low concentrations of soluble materials (0, 10, 24 and 34 μg/cm^2), which were 17% mass equivalent to the dosing concentrations of the total (0, 60, 140 and 200 μg/cm^2), and thus such low quantities of the soluble materials were not high enough to exhibit a significant effect. However, this is the actual proportion of the soluble materials present in EHC-93 total, and the present study focused on comparing the cytotoxic effects of the insoluble and soluble fractions in the mass proportion as they were found in the environment. Similarly, A549 cells were dosed with 0, 50, 116 and 166 μg/cm^2 insoluble materials, which are 83% mass equivalent to EHC-93 total concentrations. Nevertheless, the insoluble fraction appeared even more toxic than the total in every equivalent dose of every cytotoxicity assay, and reached statistical significance at the highest dose in ATP assay (two-way ANOVA: *Treatment x Dose* interaction at 200 μg/cm^2, $p < 0.05$) (Fig. 2c). Evidently, the toxic potency of EHC-93 total is not equal to the sum of its insoluble and soluble fractions, suggesting that there were interactions between the insoluble and soluble materials. It is possible that the soluble materials coated the surface of the insoluble components and reduced some of their cytotoxic effects. Such inhibitory coating effect has been previously reported in nano-silica particles [48]. Alternatively, biological effects caused by the soluble materials in A549 cells may be antagonistic to some of those effects elicited by the insoluble materials.

The effects of EHC-93 and its insoluble and soluble fractions on the proteome of A549 cells were examined via 2D–GE and mass spectrometry as previously described [62, 63]. Two-way ANOVA and Holm-Sidak (post-hoc) were the statistical methods used to determine significant effects of particles across treatments. The results in Additional file 2: Table S2 indicated that there was a significant *Treatment* main effect for BUB3 (SSP9301), where the total and insoluble components of EHC-93 affected the expression of BUB3 similarly but their effects were different from the soluble materials. On average, the expression of BUB3 in A549 cells due to EHC-93 total, insoluble and soluble materials exposures were listed as 1.32, 1.11 and −1.12, respectively. It is important to understand that such FCs were relative to the control. More importantly, it must be recognized that

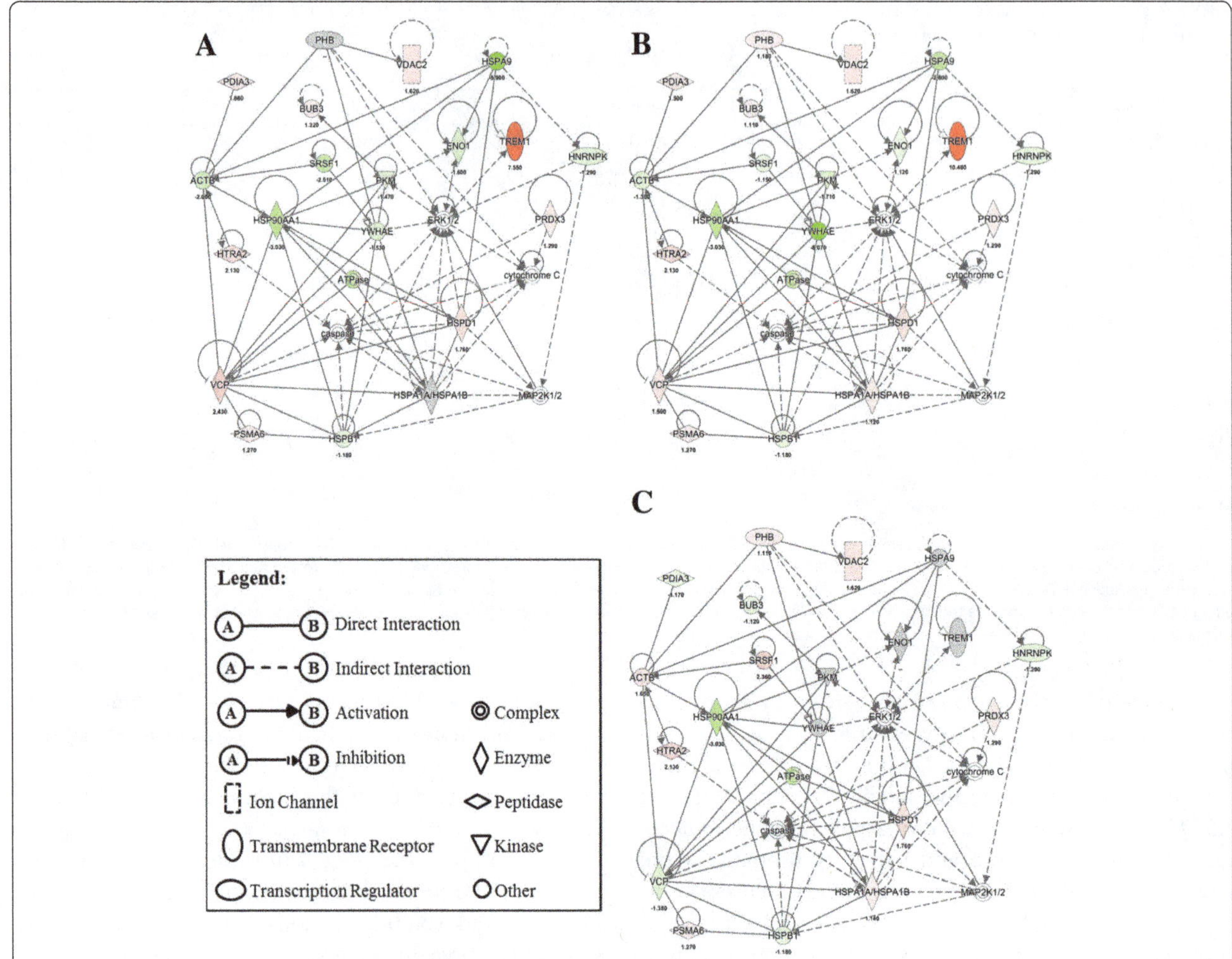

Fig. 4 Protein profiles in the network of cell death and cell proliferation pathway in A549 cells following EHC-93 total (**a**) and its insoluble (**b**) and soluble (**c**) fractions treatments at 60 μg/cm^2. Red indicates increased expression, green stands for decreased expression, grey implies non-significant change and white indicates the protein was not examined in this study. The color scale, representing fold-change, was set at a maximum and minimum of 8 (deepest red) and –6 (darkest green)

the net difference between the effects of the total and soluble fraction was 44% (from 1.32 to −1.12) and the net difference between the effects of the insoluble and soluble fractions was 23% (from 1.11 to −1.12). Thus, such magnitudes of changes between treatments should not be overlooked, particularly when the adjusted *p*-value is very small (adjusted p = 0.003), and especially the goal of this study is to identify the differential responses of A549 cells to EHC-93 particles and its insoluble and soluble components. When conducting pathway and network analyses, a ± 1.10 FC cut-off on all significant proteins (adjusted *p*-value <0.05) should be sufficient to remove nuanced expressions that may not contribute to any biological impact.

Two-way ANOVA results in Additional file 2: Table S2 identified 206 protein spots were significantly altered by the treatments (adjusted *p*-value <0.05), and 154 of these protein spots have been identified via MALDI-TOF-TOF-MS, which can potentially be used for pathway analysis. Unsupervised hierarchical cluster analysis based on all the significantly altered protein spots showed that the total and insoluble fraction treatments clustered together (Fig. 3), suggesting that these two treatments had similar effects on the proteome of A549 cells. Such result holds true regardless if cluster analysis was conducted based both non-significantly and significantly altered protein spots (Additional file 3: Figure S1). In addition, the total and insoluble fraction treatments formed separate sub-clusters, implying that their effects on the proteome of A549 cells were distinguishable (Fig. 3 and Additional file 3: Figure S1). These findings were similar to those in an earlier study in our laboratory that demonstrated that the expression of a selected set of genes (e.g., *MMP2*, *ECE1* and *EDN1*) and secretory proteins (e.g., IL-8 and VEGF) in A549 cells were similarly affected by the total and insoluble components of EHC-93, and that their

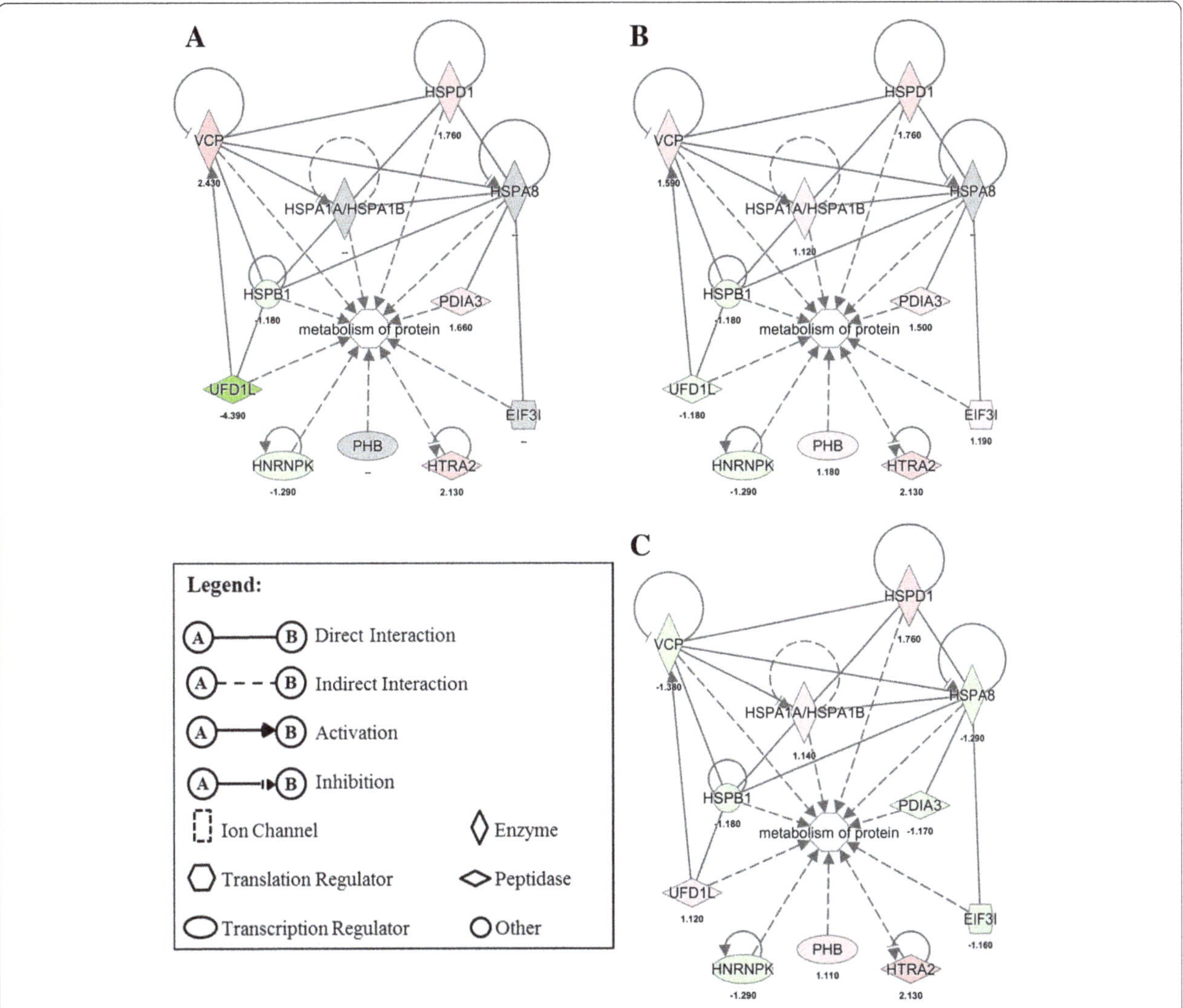

Fig. 5 Protein profiles in the network of protein metabolism pathway in A549 cells following EHC-93 total (**a**) and its insoluble (**b**) and soluble (**c**) fractions treatments at 60 μg/cm^2. Red indicates increased expression, green stands for decreased expression and grey implies non-significant change. The color scale, representing fold-change, was set at a maximum and minimum of 8 (deepest red) and −6 (darkest green)

effects differed from those of the soluble materials [12]. Results from two-way ANOVA and Holm-Sidak multiple comparisons analyses in Additional file 2: Table S2 were in line with the above observations. The total and insoluble fraction PM exposures were observed to alter the proteome of A549 cells more than the soluble fraction, and these changes were not additive. In brief, all proteomic and cytotoxicity assay results in this study unanimously pointed out that the toxic effects of EHC-93 in A549 cells were mainly driven by its insoluble components.

Unsupervised hierarchical cluster analysis revealed that all the doses of the same treatment clustered together, and the highest dose of the total and insoluble fraction exposures induced the greatest change to most protein spots (Fig. 3). These findings suggested that the effects of the total and insoluble fraction would eventually converge to the same outcome as the dose increases. Interestingly, majority of these significantly altered protein spots were not full length native proteins or isoforms based on their molecular weights and unique peptide sequences (Additional file 2: Table S2). These peptides (e.g., SSP2010, 8302, 3104, 4108, 305 and 8109) were possibly cleavage or degradation products of their native proteins, and they may be derived from dying or dead cells that have undergone or have committed to apoptosis or necrosis. This is plausible because functional annotation for the proteins in different clusters in Fig. 3 revealed that cell death and survival and cell growth and proliferation were the two dominant cellular functions affected by particle exposures (Additional file 4: Table S3). In addition, the LDH release, cellular ATP and BrdU incorporation assays indicated that A549 cells were adversely impacted at the higher doses (Fig. 2). Altogether, these results suggested that the A549 cells

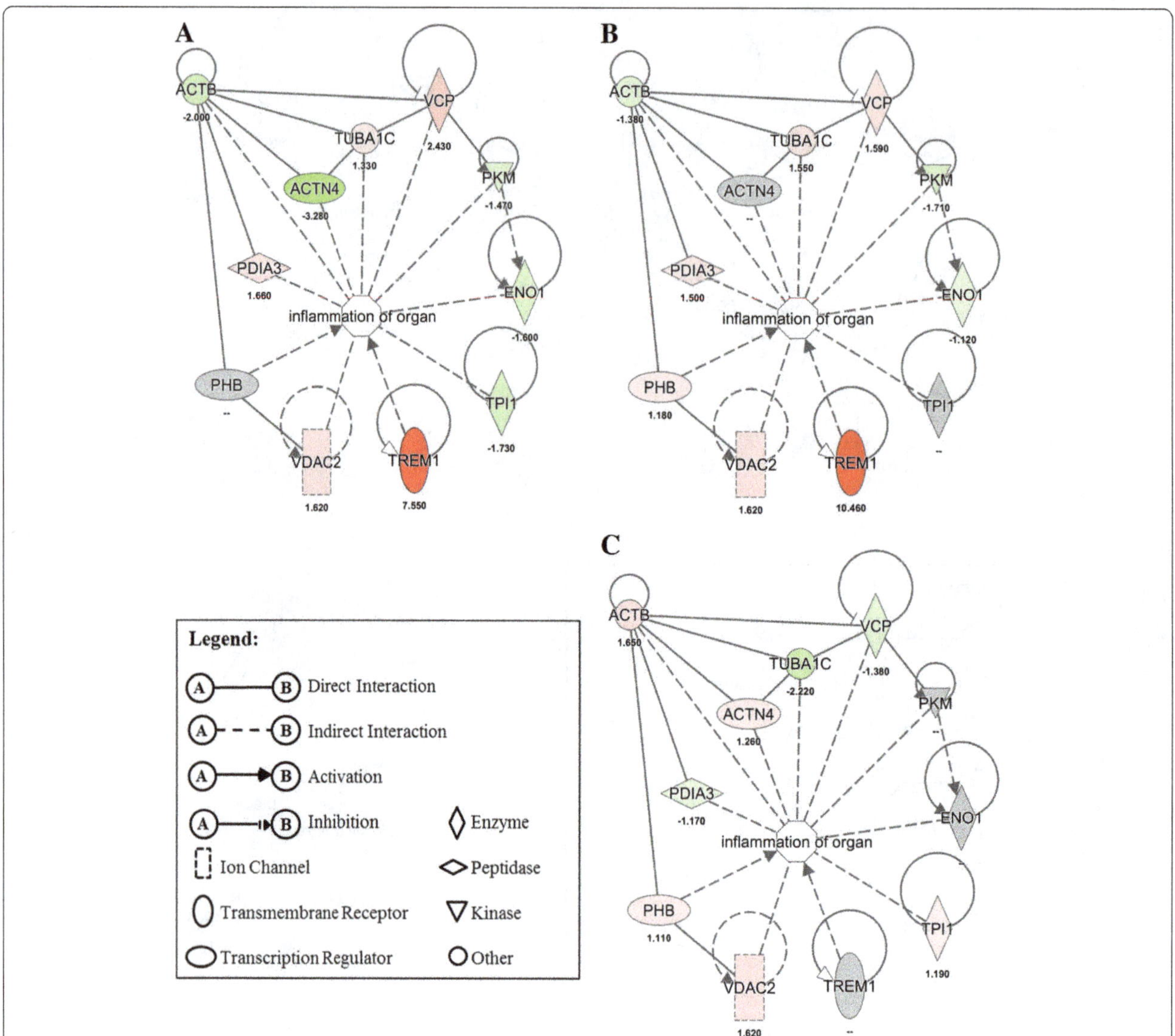

Fig. 6 Protein profiles in the network of organ inflammation pathway in A549 cells following EHC-93 total (**a**) and its insoluble (**b**) and soluble (**c**) fractions treatments at 60 μg/cm^2. Red indicates increased expression, green stands for decreased expression and grey implies non-significant. The color scale, representing fold-change, was set at a maximum and minimum of 8 (deepest red) and −6 (darkest green)

exposed to the higher doses of PM (140 and 200 μg/cm^2) had undergone terminal stage of particle toxicity (i.e., dead or dying cells), while the lowest dose (60 μg/cm^2) revealing an early stage of particle toxicity (i.e., live cells). It should be noted that the chosen exposure doses for most in vitro toxicology studies, including the current study, are well beyond the actual environmental levels in order to obtain measurable responses. Therefore, there is more value to examine the effect of the particles on A549 cells at the low toxicity dose to capture the early signs of particle toxicity.

Pathway analysis revealed that the significantly altered proteins in A549 cells following exposure to the particles at 60 μg/cm^2 dose were involved in pathways such as ROS metabolism, inflammatory response, cytoplasm organization, cellular movement, cell growth and proliferation, and cell death and survival (Table 4). These pathways were likely the mechanisms employed by A549 cells to handle the effects of the exposed particles at a low toxicity level. It should be noted that about half of the significantly altered proteins in these pathways were derived from *Treatment* main effect, where their expressions were not necessarily different from the control significantly. Rather, their expression were mostly opposite in direction between the soluble fraction and the total or insoluble fraction (Additional file 5: Figure S2). It should be clarified that the proteomic results based on 2D–GE data did not have sufficient power to confidently determine if any of the pathways in Table 4 was actually activated or

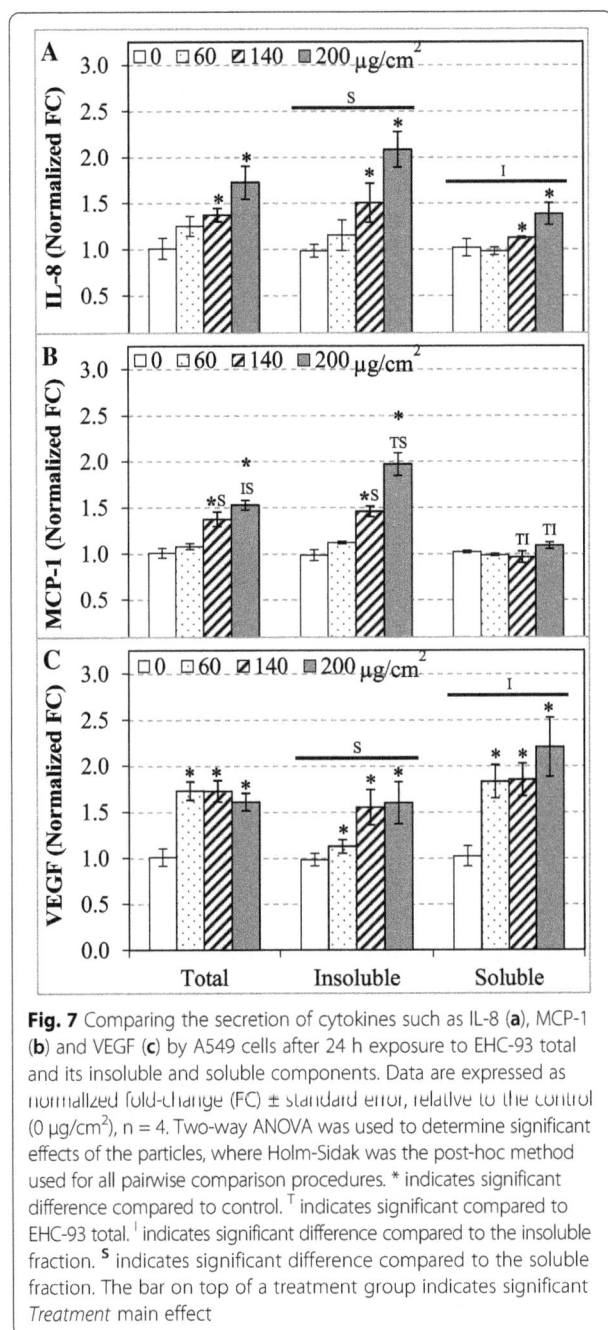

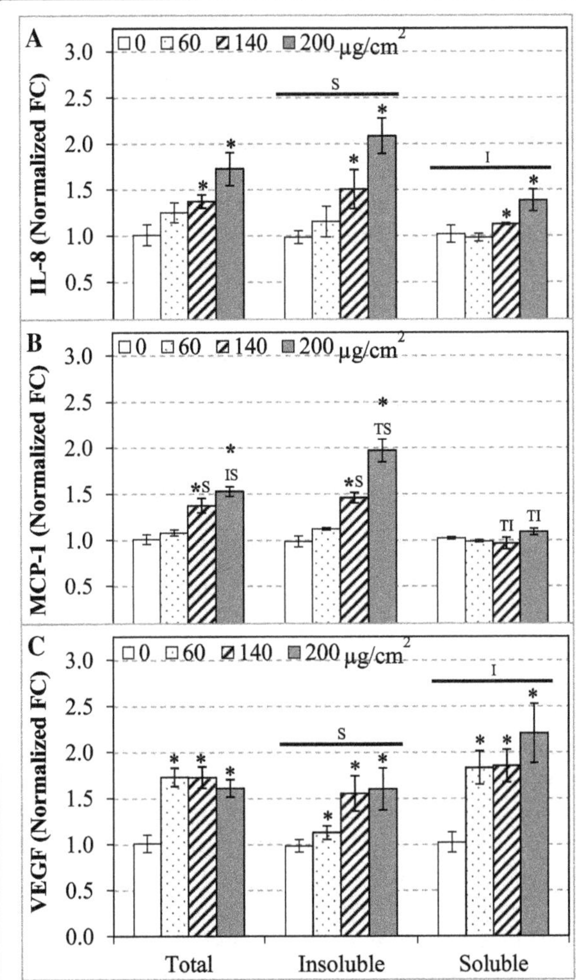

Fig. 7 Comparing the secretion of cytokines such as IL-8 (**a**), MCP-1 (**b**) and VEGF (**c**) by A549 cells after 24 h exposure to EHC-93 total and its insoluble and soluble components. Data are expressed as normalized fold-change (FC) ± standard error, relative to the control (0 μg/cm²), n = 4. Two-way ANOVA was used to determine significant effects of the particles, where Holm-Sidak was the post-hoc method used for all pairwise comparison procedures. * indicates significant difference compared to control. T indicates significant compared to EHC-93 total. I indicates significant difference compared to the insoluble fraction. S indicates significant difference compared to the soluble fraction. The bar on top of a treatment group indicates significant *Treatment* main effect

inactivated. Rather, we relied on the cytokine release (Fig. 7) and cytotoxicity assays (Fig. 2) data to determine the phenotypic effects of the particles.

It is interesting to note that a large number of significantly altered proteins were involved in the cell death and survival pathways (Additional file 5: Figure S2), suggesting that this dose (60 μg/cm²) was sufficient to cause such effects. This is consistent with the cytotoxicity assay results (Fig 2a–c). Examining the pattern of proteins expressed in the networks of cell death and cell proliferation pathways in Fig. 4 may provide insights to the molecular mechanisms that dictate the contrasting effects of the insoluble and soluble fractions. In this network, the extracellular signal-regulated kinase 1/2 (ERK1/2) was found in one of the main nodes, where this protein is known to modulate a broad biological functions in cells, including cell death and cell proliferation [38]. It was noticeable that the soluble fraction treatment did not significantly alter the expression of a number of proteins up- and down-stream of ERK1/2. For example, only the total and insoluble treatments significantly decreased the expression of 14–3-3 protein epsilon (YWHAE), pyruvate kinase (PKM) and enolase-1 (ENO1) and significantly increased the expression of triggering receptor expressed on myloid cells 1 (TREM1). Down regulation of ENO1 and PKM may explain the decreased ATP levels in A549 cells follow the total and insoluble fraction exposures in Fig. 2c (significant only in the insoluble fraction treatment at dose 60 μg/cm²) as these two proteins are known to serve distinct enzymatic functions in the last two steps of glycolysis [59]. Interestingly, these proteins are known to serve several other biological functions such as cell death, cell proliferation and stress response, and their expressions can be modulated in response to various stimuli [64, 68]. ENO1 has been reported to regulate the kinase activity of ERK1/2 in A549 cells [68], and ERK1/2 can modulate the nuclear translocation of PKM in U251 human glioblastoma cells that is necessary for PKM's auto-regulation of expression [64]. Knockdown of PKM expression (via siRNA) has been shown to decrease the production of ATP and induce apoptosis and autophagy in A549 cells [13, 49], which is consistent with the LDH release and BrdU incorporation trends (Fig. 2a and b). These findings were similar to the proteomic results observed for the total and insoluble fraction exposures and were also consistent with the cytotoxicity data (Fig. 2c) in this study. Furthermore, PKM has been shown to phosphorylate the mitotic checkpoint protein BUB3, which is essential for the BUB3-BUB1 complex to be recruited to the kinetochore spindle during mitosis [22]. The expression of BUB3 in A549 cells was increased by the total and insoluble fraction treatments, but its expression was decreased by the soluble fraction (Fig. 4). It is evident that the cytotoxicity assay and proteomic results were mutually complementary in explaining the toxic effects of the particles, extensive investigations would be required to better understand the PM-driven mechanisms of particle toxicity in the cell death and cell proliferation pathways.

Of all the networks examined, the network related to inflammatory process in Fig. 6 showed the most contrasting effect between the total or insoluble fraction against the soluble fraction, where 10/11 and 9/11 proteins in the network were distinctly altered, respectively. It should be cautioned that the relationships of the proteins involved in this network are not straight forward to interpret because inflammation is a process that involves multiple cell types such as epithelial cells, neutrophils and macrophages. Interestingly, inflammatory stimuli are known to increase the expression of triggering receptor expressed on myeloid cells 1 (TREM1) on neutrophils, monocytes and macrophages, where this receptor is known to amplify the secretion of pro-inflammatory mediators such as IL-1β, IL-6, IL-8, MCP-1 and TNFα from these cells [6, 40]. Furthermore, TREM1 has been reported to be expressed in lung cancer epithelial cells. For instance, A549 cells exposed to silica nano-particles have been associated TREM1 signaling [31]. Increased expression of this receptor in the cells exposed to the total and insoluble fraction is a possible mechanism for the release of IL-8 and MCP-1 in A549 cells (Fig. 7). In addition, a recent mouse lung injury model demonstrated that increased expressions of protein disulfide-isomerase associated 3 (PDIA3) and ENO1 were important for alveolar epithelial type II (AT-II) cells to repair bleomycin-induced injury in the lung of mice [29]. Over-expression of PDIA3 in murine embryonic fibroblast cells is known to exacerbate apoptosis via Bak signaling [67]. Mutze et al. [29] and Zhao et al. [67] hinted that increased level of PDIA3 in injured cells may determine whether the cells would commit to injury repair or apoptosis. As increased level of PDIA3 (Fig. 6) in A549 cells in the present study coincided with increased LDH release and decreased BrdU incorporation and cellular ATP levels (Fig. 2) after exposure to the total and insoluble fraction at the 60 $\mu g/cm^2$ dose, the results point perhaps to an inflammatory process directed-apoptosis. EHC-93 is known to contain inflammatogenic constituents such as silica (Table 1) and endotoxins (Table 3). Moreover, previous studies have shown that EHC-93 was capable of stimulating the release of pro-inflammatory cytokines such as IL-8 [8, 12, 14, 39] and MCP-1 [8] from bronchial or lung epithelial cells. Sakamoto et al. [39] demonstrated that the secretion of IL-8 from human epithelial bronchial cells by EHC-93 total was induced by the influx of calcium from the extracellular media, where the signalling was suspected to be mediated by a membrane receptor and/or ion channel [39]. Whether EHC-93 total or its insoluble components induced secretion of IL-8 and MCP-1 from A549 epithelial cells were mediated by calcium influx, and the involvement of a membrane receptor/ion channel, will be explored in future studies.

It should be noted that correlating the in vitro results in this study to those in vivo results from previous studies is not straight forward. When EHC-93 total particles were inhaled by rats, the inhalation did not result in lung injury but it elicited inflammatory responses and cardiovascular effects [7, 51, 56, 58]. These results suggested that the efficient clearance mechanism in the respiratory tract of healthy animals and humans would make the inhaled particles only mildly toxic. Intriguingly, the data based on in vitro and intratracheal instillation studies suggested that the particles can be toxic if they were deposited and retained in the lungs. For example, the in vitro results in the present study demonstrated that A549 human type II lung epithelial cells were sensitive to the cytotoxic effects of EHC-93 and its water-insoluble components upon exposure, where the particles are potent in stimulating proteins involved in inflammatory responses and cell death, while decreasing cellular ATP and cell proliferation. On the other hand, direct injection of either EHC-93, its soluble or insoluble fractions into the lungs of rats via intratracheal instillation triggered inflammation based on the number of cells and protein levels in lavaged lung fluid [2]. However, exposure to EHC-93 and its soluble, but not insoluble, fraction caused mild lung injury in rats based on the observed necrosis to type I alveolar cells and the subsequent ^{3}H–thymidine uptake by type II alveolar cells [2], which would proliferate and differentiate to replace type I cells. It is not clear why the instilled insoluble fraction did not induce lung injury even when it contains varying amount of insoluble minerals (Table 1), endotoxins (Table 3), PAHs and metals [57]. It is possible that the insoluble particles were cleared from the lung. As for the instilled soluble materials, they can be readily absorbed by the cardiovascular system and affect various cell types, where the observed lung injury was attributed to the presence of soluble zinc and copper [1, 34]. In addition, the immunoassay results in this study showed that the soluble materials had greater potency than the insoluble materials in stimulating the secretion of a potent vasculogenic/angiogenic signaling protein vascular endothelial growth factor (VEGF) from A549 cells (Fig. 7c), which are type II alveolar cells. In this point of view, the effects of the soluble materials could be mediated by type II alveolar cells via paracrine signalling.

In summary, most of the results in this study and previous in vitro study [12] consistently showed that the cytotoxic effects of EHC-93(total) and its insoluble fraction in A549 cells were similar to each other and their effects were differed from the soluble fraction. These results indicated that the insoluble materials in EHC-93 are the drivers of toxic potency in A549 human lung epithelial cells. The culminated physicochemical characterizations from the previous [57, 58] and present studies have built a repertoire of identified insoluble components in EHC-93 including metals (e.g., iron, lead, magnesium and zinc), minerals (e.g., calcite, silica and gypsum), carbonaceous materials (e.g., phenanthrene, pyrene, fluoranthene and benzo[b]fluoranthene) and endotoxins at defined quantities or relative quantities. This repertoire would allow present and future studies to better assess the contribution of toxic potency and assess the pathways of effects of one or a combination of particles. The majority of the insoluble components are mineral crystal particles such as calcite ($CaCO_3$), α-quartz (SiO_2), gypsum ($CaSO_4$) and dolomite ($CaMg(CO_3)_2$) (Table 1). As these insoluble mineral particles can contribute to the total cytotoxic effects of EHC-93, other minor insoluble components such as endotoxins (Table 3), metals (e.g., Fe, Al, Pb, Mg, Sn and Ti) (Additional file 1: Table S1) and PAHs [57] may also add significant cytotoxicity to A549 cells. The insoluble materials in EHC-93 affected markers of inflammatory responses (Figs. 6 & 7) as well as cell death and proliferation in A549 cells (Figs. 2 & 4 and Table 4). Importantly, the proteomic results in this study provided molecular details associated with the toxicity of EHC-93 and its insoluble fraction.

Conclusions

To our knowledge, this is the first study that used in tandem multiple cytotoxicity assays and proteomic analyses to assess the phenotypic outcomes and molecular mechanisms of particle toxicity of an urban air PM (i.e., EHC-93) and its insoluble and soluble fractions on human lung epithelial cells (A549). Both cytotoxicity assays and proteomic results consistently indicated that the insoluble materials explained most of the toxic effects of the total PM. Furthermore, the toxic potency of EHC-93 total is not equal to the sum of its insoluble and soluble fractions, implying inter-component interactions between insoluble and soluble materials that may be reflected through synergistic or antagonistic in vitro responses. Finally, this study demonstrated that in vitro toxicoproteomics is a valuable tool in delineating the toxicity mechanisms of environmental air particles.

Additional files

Additional file 1: Table S1. Elemental content of EHC-93 and its water-insoluble and soluble fractions were examined by IPC-MS [58]. Foot Note: It should be noted that the mass of each element presented did not take into account that the insoluble and soluble fractions corresponded to 83 and 17 mass % of the total. (DOCX 15 kb)

Additional file 2: Table S2. Two-way ANOVA results for the A549 protein spots that changed significantly due to particle exposures ($n = 3$). The SSP number corresponds to the identifier number that PDQuest used to identify the spot based on its coordinate in the gel. The number below *Treatment* main effect (Trt), *Dose* main effect (Dose) or interaction between *Treatment and Dose* (T x D) corresponds to the *p*-value, where the bolded number emphasized *p*-value < 0.05. Only the protein spots identified by MALDI-TOF-TOF-MS/MS are provided here ([61]; [62]). The proteins indicated in red (likely degradation product of the native protein) and fold-change indicated in blue (cut-off at ±1.10) were excluded from pathway analysis. Orange colored spots were used for pathway analysis in the 60 μg/cm^2 dose. The yellow highlight shows multiple protein spots with the same protein ID. See the Materials and Methods section for more information on the protein spot selection criteria for pathway analysis. Foot Note: [§] Spot volume intensity normalized to the control (n = 3). [†]Significant change in protein expression identified by multiple comparison based on Holm-Sidak method (see Materials and Methods), which was used for pathway analysis, and the blank entries imply non-significant changes as compared to the control (i.e., fold-change = 1.0). Those protein spots with *p*-value <0.05 (based on Two-way ANOVA) but did not pass Holm-Sidak test were excluded. (DOCX 1799 kb)

Additional file 3: Figure S1. Unsupervised hierarchical cluster analysis demonstrating the effect of all the tested particles on the proteome of A549 cells. The expressions of all the well-defined protein spots in the 2D gels were examined. The expression of each protein spot was calculated by Log_2(Treatment/Control), $n = 3$. Red is coded for increased expression and green is coded for decreased expression. The number indicates the dose in μg/cm^2. (DOCX 196 kb)

Additional file 4: Table S3. Top cellular functions in which the proteins in various clusters (in Fig. 3) were involved based on IPA. Only those functions that were significantly ($p < 0.05$) influenced by more than 5 proteins were presented. (DOCX 12 kb)

Additional file 5: Figure S2. Changes in the expression of proteins in various pathways in A549 cells that were exposed to EHC-93 total and its insoluble and soluble fractions (at 60 μg/cm^2) examined by hierarchical cluster analysis. These selected pathways were based on the top biological functions identified by Ingenuity Pathway Analysis (in Table 4). The color scales that show fold-changes, Log_2(Treatment/Control), were set between −3 to 3 in panels A - C and −2 to 2 in panels D - F. (DOCX 259 kb)

Abbreviations

2D–GE: Two-dimensional gel electrophoresis; ANOVA: Analysis of variance; BrdU: 5-bromo-2′-deoxyuridine; DMEM: Dulbecco's modified Eagle's medium; EDX: Energy dispersive X-Ray spectroscopy; EHC-93: Ottawa urban air particles collected from the Environmental Health Centre in 1993; EU: Enzymatic unit; FBS: Fetal bovine serum; FC: Fold-change; FWER: Familywise error rate; ICP-MS: Inductively coupled plasma^{-mass} spectrometry; LDH: Lactate dehydrogenase; MALDI-TOF-MS: Matrix-assisted laser desorption ionization-time of flight-mass spectrometry; MOWSE: Molecular weight search; MS: Mass spectrometry; MW: Molecular weight; PBS: Phosphate buffer saline; pI: Isoelectric point; PM: Particulate matter; pXRD: Powder X-ray diffraction; ROS: Reactive oxygen species; RT: Room temperature; SEM: Scanning electron microscopy

Acknowledgements

We would like to thank Drs. Vinita Chauhan and Pahdi Bhaja Krushna for their helpful comments.

Funding

This work was supported by the Clean Air Regulatory Agenda at Health Canada (Grant # 4340565) and Ontario Graduate Scholarship in Science and Technology and Ontario Graduate Scholarship (funding for Ngoc Vuong).

Authors' contributions

NQV: Wrote the manuscript, analyzed all data, prepared all tables and figures, and conducted most of the experimental work (e.g., cell culture, particle exposures, cytotoxicity assays, 2D–GE, MS, statistical analysis, bioinformatic analysis, pathway analysis). DB: Assisted in conducting cytotoxicity assays, conducted endotoxin analysis and contributed to the writing of manuscript. PG: Assisted in the preparation of 2D gels from exposed cells. JSO'B: Conducted physical analyses of the EHC-93 particles. AW: Assisted in statistical analysis. SK: Assisted in statistical analysis. PK: Designed experiments, supported data interpretation and contributed to the writing of manuscript. RV: Designed experiments, contributed to the writing of manuscript and supported data interpretation. All authors read and approved the final manuscript.

Competing interests

The authors declare that they have no competing interests.

Author details

[1]Inhalation Toxicology Laboratory, Environmental Health Science and Research Bureau, Health Canada, Ottawa, ON K1A 0K9, Canada. [2]Analytical Biochemistry and Proteomics, Environmental Health Science and Research Bureau, Health Canada, Ottawa, ON K1A 0K9, Canada. [3]Biostatistics Section, Population Studies Division, Environmental Health Science and Research Bureau, Health Canada, Ottawa, ON K1A 0K9, Canada. [4]Department of Biochemistry, Faculty of Science, University of Ottawa, Ottawa, ON K1H 8M5, Canada.

References

1. Adamson IY, Prieditis H, Hedgecock C, Vincent R. Zinc is the toxic factor in the lung response to an atmospheric particulate sample. Toxicol Appl Pharmacol. 2000;166:111–9.
2. Adamson IY, Vincent R, Bjarnason SG. Cell injury and interstitial inflammation in rat lung after inhalation of ozone and urban particulates. Am J Respir Cell Mol Biol. 1999;20:1067–72.
3. Ailshire JA, Crimmins EM. Fine particulate matter air pollution and cognitive function among older US adults. Am J Epidemiol. 2014;180:359–66.
4. Amatullah H, North ML, Akhtar US, Rastogi N, Urch B, Silverman FS, Chow CW, Evans GJ, Scott JA. Comparative cardiopulmonary effects of size-fractionated airborne particulate matter. Inhal Toxicol. 2012;24:161–71.
5. Bell ML, Ebisu K, Leaderer BP, Gent JF, Lee HJ, Koutrakis P, Wang Y, Dominici F, Peng RD. Associations of PM(2).(5) constituents and sources with hospital admissions: analysis of four counties in Connecticut and Massachusetts (USA) for persons >/= 65 years of age. Environ Health Perspect. 2014;122:138–44.
6. Bouchon A, Facchetti F, Weigand MA, Colonna M. TREM-1 amplifies inflammation and is a crucial mediator of septic shock. Nature. 2001; 410:1103–7.
7. Bouthillier L, Vincent R, Goegan P, Adamson IY, Bjarnason S, Stewart M, Guenette J, Potvin M, Kumarathasan P. Acute effects of inhaled urban particles and ozone: lung morphology, macrophage activity, and plasma Endothelin-1. Am J Pathol. 1998;153:1873–84.
8. Breznan D, Karthikeyan S, Phaneuf M, Kumarathasan P, Cakmak S, Denison MS, Brook JR, Vincent R. Development of an integrated approach for comparison of in vitro and in vivo responses to particulate matter. Part Fibre Toxicol. 2016;13:41.
9. Brook RD, Cakmak S, Turner M C, Brook J R, Crouse D L, Peters P A, van D A, Villeneuve P J, Brion O, Jerrett M, Martin R V, Rajagopalan S, Goldberg M S, Pope C A, III Burnett RT. Long-term fine particulate matter exposure and mortality from diabetes mellitus in Canada. Diabetes Care. 2013;36(10):3313–20.
10. Burnett RT, Brook J, Dann T, Delocla C, Philips O, Cakmak S, Vincent R, Goldberg MS, Krewski D. Association between particulate- and gas-phase components of urban air pollution and daily mortality in eight Canadian cities. Inhal Toxicol. 2000;12(Suppl 4):15–39.
11. Canova C, Dunster C, Kelly FJ, Minelli C, Shah PL, Caneja C, Tumilty MK, Burney P. PM10-induced hospital admissions for asthma and chronic obstructive pulmonary disease: the modifying effect of individual characteristics. Epidemiology. 2012;23:607–15.
12. Chauhan V, Breznan D, Thomson E, Karthikeyan S, Vincent R. Effects of ambient air particles on the Endothelin system in human pulmonary epithelial cells (A549). Cell Biol Toxicol. 2005;21:191–205.
13. Chu B, Wang J, Wang Y, Yang G. Knockdown of PKM2 induces apoptosis and Autophagy in human A549 alveolar Adenocarcinoma cells. Mol Med Rep. 2015;12:4358–63.
14. Fujii T, Hayashi S, Hogg JC, Vincent R, van Eeden SF. Particulate matter induces cytokine expression in human bronchial epithelial cells. Am J Respir Cell Mol Biol. 2001;25:265–71.
15. Gan WQ, FitzGerald JM, Carlsten C, Sadatsafavi M, Brauer M. Associations of ambient air pollution with chronic obstructive pulmonary disease hospitalization and mortality. Am J Respir Crit Care Med. 2013;187:721–7.
16. Gonzalez RJ, Tarloff JB. Evaluation of hepatic subcellular fractions for Alamar blue and MTT Reductase activity. Toxicol in Vitro. 2001;15:257–9.
17. Goodnight JH and Harvey WR. Least-Squares Means in the Fixed-Effects General Linear Models. SAS Technical Report R-103. 1978. SAS Institute Inc., SAS Technical Report. SAS Technical Report R-103. Ref Type: Report.
18. Guan L, Rui W, Bai R, Zhang W, Zhang F and Ding W. Effects of Size-Fractionated Particulate Matter on Cellular Oxidant Radical Generation in Human Bronchial Epithelial BEAS-2B Cells. Int J Environ Res Public Health. 2016;13(483):1–14.
19. Huang Q, Zhang J, Peng S, Tian M, Chen J, Shen H. Effects of water soluble PM2.5 extracts exposure on human lung epithelial cells (A549): a proteomic study. J Appl Toxicol. 2014;34:675–87.
20. Huang W, Zhu T, Pan X, Hu M, Lu SE, Lin Y, Wang T, Zhang Y, Tang X. Air pollution and autonomic and vascular dysfunction in patients with cardiovascular disease: interactions of systemic inflammation, overweight, and gender. Am J Epidemiol. 2012;176:117–26.
21. Jedrychowski WA, Perera F P, Camann D, Spengler J, Butscher M, Mroz E, Majewska R, Flak E, Jacek R Sowa A. Prenatal Exposure to Polycyclic Aromatic Hydrocarbons and Cognitive Dysfunction in Children. Environ Sci Pollut Res Int. 2015;22(5):3631–9.
22. Jiang Y, Li X, Yang W, Hawke DH, Zheng Y, Xia Y, Aldape K, Wei C, Guo F, Chen Y, Lu Z. PKM2 regulates chromosome segregation and mitosis progression of tumor cells. Mol Cell. 2014;53:75–87.
23. Julvez J, Ribas-Fito N, Torrent M, Forns M, Garcia-Esteban R, Sunyer J. Maternal smoking habits and cognitive development of children at age 4 years in a population-based birth cohort. Int J Epidemiol. 2007;36:825–32.
24. Kumarathasan P, Blais E, Saravanamuthu A, Bielecki A, Mukherjee B, Bjarnason S, Guenette J, Goegan P, Vincent R. Nitrative stress, oxidative stress and plasma Endothelin levels after inhalation of particulate matter and ozone. Part Fibre Toxicol. 2015;12:28.
25. Kumarathasan P, Breznan D, Das D, Salam M A, Siddiqui Y, Mackinnon-Roy C, Guan J, de S N, Simard B and Vincent R. Cytotoxicity of Carbon Nanotube Variants: A Comparative in Vitro Exposure Study With A549 Epithelial and J774 Macrophage Cells. Nanotoxicology. 2015;9(2):148–61.
26. Liu L, Yu LY, Mu HJ, Xing LY, Li YX, Pan GW. Shape of concentration-response curves between long-term particulate matter exposure and morbidities of chronic bronchitis: a review of epidemiological evidence. J Thorac Dis. 2014;6:S720–7.
27. MacIntyre EA, Brauer M, Melen E, Bauer CP, Bauer M, Berdel D, Bergstrom A, Brunekreef B, Chan-Yeung M, Klumper C, Fuertes E, Gehring U, Gref A, Heinrich J, Herbarth O, Kerkhof M, Koppelman GH, Kozyrskyj AL, Pershagen G, Postma DS, Thiering E, Tiesler CM, Carlsten C. GSTP1 and TNF gene variants and associations between air pollution and incident childhood asthma: the traffic, asthma and genetics (TAG) study. Environ Health Perspect. 2014;122:418–24.
28. Merlo F, Costantini M, Reggiardo G, Ceppi M, Puntoni R. Lung cancer risk among refractory brick workers exposed to crystalline silica: a retrospective cohort study. Epidemiology. 1991;2:299–305.
29. Mutze K, Vierkotten S, Milosevic J, Eickelberg O, Konigshoff M. Enolase 1 (ENO1) and protein disulfide-Isomerase associated 3 (PDIA3) regulate Wnt/Beta-catenin-driven trans-differentiation of Murine alveolar epithelial cells. Dis Model Mech. 2015;8:877–90.
30. Peng RD, Dominici F, Pastor-Barriuso R, Zeger SL, Samet JM. Seasonal analyses of air pollution and mortality in 100 US cities. Am J Epidemiol. 2005;161:585–94.
31. Pisani C, Gaillard JC, Nouvel V, Odorico M, Armengaud J, Prat O. High-throughput, quantitative assessment of the effects of low-dose silica Nanoparticles on lung cells: grasping complex toxicity with a great depth of field. BMC Genomics. 2015;16:315.
32. Pope CA III, Burnett RT, Krewski D, Jerrett M, Shi Y, Calle EE, Thun MJ. Cardiovascular mortality and exposure to airborne fine particulate matter and cigarette smoke: shape of the exposure-response relationship. Circulation. 2009;120:941–8.
33. Pope CA III, Burnett RT, Turner MC, Cohen A, Krewski D, Jerrett M, Gapstur SM, Thun MJ. Lung cancer and cardiovascular disease mortality associated with ambient air pollution and cigarette smoke: shape of the exposure-response relationships. Environ Health Perspect. 2011;119:1616–21.
34. Prieditis H, Adamson IY. Comparative pulmonary toxicity of various soluble metals found in urban particulate dusts. Exp Lung Res. 2002;28:563–76.
35. R Core Team. R: A language and environment for statistical computing. 2013. http://www.R-project.org/. Ref Type: Online Source.

36. Rao X, Patel P, Puett R, Rajagopalan S. Air pollution as a risk factor for type 2 diabetes. Toxicol Sci. 2015;143:231–41.
37. Reich M, Liefeld T, Gould J, Lerner J, Tamayo P, Mesirov JP. GenePattern 2.0. Nat Genet. 2006;38:500–1.
38. Roskoski R Jr. ERK1/2 MAP Kinases: structure, function, and regulation. Pharmacol Res. 2012;66:105–43.
39. Sakamoto N, Hayashi S, Gosselink J, Ishii H, Ishimatsu Y, Mukae H, Hogg JC, van Eeden SF. Calcium dependent and independent cytokine synthesis by air pollution particle-exposed human bronchial epithelial cells. Toxicol Appl Pharmacol. 2007;225:134–41.
40. Schenk M, Bouchon A, Seibold F, Mueller C. TREM-1–expressing intestinal macrophages crucially amplify chronic inflammation in experimental colitis and inflammatory bowel diseases. J Clin Invest. 2007;117:3097–106.
41. Schneider A, Hampel R, Ibald-Mulli A, Zareba W, Schmidt G, Schneider R, Ruckerl R, Couderc JP, Mykins B, Oberdorster G, Wolke G, Pitz M, Wichmann HE, Peters A. Changes in deceleration capacity of heart rate and heart rate variability induced by ambient air pollution in individuals with coronary artery disease. Part Fibre Toxicol. 2010;7:29.
42. Scott JA. Fog and deaths in London, December 1952. Public Health Rep. 1953;68:474–9.
43. Searle SR, Speed FM, Miliken GA. The population marginal means in the linear model: an alternative to least squares means. Am Stat. 1980;34:216–21.
44. Siemiatycki J, Dewar R, Lakhani R, Nadon L, Richardson L, Gerin M. Cancer risks associated with 10 inorganic dusts: results from a case-control study in Montreal. Am J Ind Med. 1989;16:547–67.
45. Snow SJ, De Vizcaya-Ruiz A, Osornio-Vargas A, Thomas RF, Schladweiler MC, McGee J, Kodavanti UP. The effect of composition, size, and solubility on acute pulmonary injury in rats following exposure to Mexico City ambient particulate matter samples. J Toxicol Environ Health A. 2014;77:1164–82.
46. Stocks P. Cancer and bronchitis mortality in relation to atmospheric deposit and smoke. Br Med J. 1959;1:74–9.
47. Su MW, Tsai CH, Tung KY, Hwang BF, Liang PH, Chiang BL, Yang YH, Lee YL. GSTP1 is a hub gene for gene-air pollution interactions on childhood asthma. Allergy. 2013;68:1614–7.
48. Sun B, Pokhrel S, Dunphy DR, Zhang H, Ji Z, Wang X, Wang M, Liao YP, Chang CH, Dong J, Li R, Madler L, Brinker CJ, Nel AE, Xia T. Reduction of acute inflammatory effects of Fumed silica Nanoparticles in the lung by adjusting Silanol display through Calcination and metal doping. ACS Nano. 2015a;9:9357–72.
49. Sun H, Zhu A, Zhang L, Zhang J, Zhong Z, Wang F. Knockdown of PKM2 suppresses tumor growth and invasion in lung Adenocarcinoma. Int J Mol Sci. 2015b;16:24574–87.
50. Suzuki Y, Imai Y, Nakayama H, Takahashi K, Takio K, Takahashi R. A serine protease, HtrA2, is released from the mitochondria and interacts with XIAP, inducing cell death. Mol Cell. 2001;8:613–21.
51. Thomson E, Kumarathasan P, Goegan P, Aubin RA, Vincent R. Differential regulation of the lung Endothelin system by urban particulate matter and ozone. Toxicol Sci. 2005;88:103–13.
52. Thomson EM, Breznan D, Karthikeyan S, Mackinnon-Roy C, Charland JP, Dabek-Zlotorzynska E, Celo V, Kumarathasan P, Brook JR, Vincent R. Cytotoxic and inflammatory potential of size-fractionated particulate matter collected repeatedly within a small urban area. Part Fibre Toxicol. 2015;12:24.
53. Thomson EM, Vladisavljevic D, Mohottalage S, Kumarathasan P, Vincent R. Mapping acute systemic effects of inhaled particulate matter and ozone: multiorgan gene expression and Glucocorticoid activity. Toxicol Sci. 2013; 135:169–81.
54. Tonne C, Elbaz A, Beevers S, Singh-Manoux A. Traffic-related air pollution in relation to cognitive function in older adults. Epidemiology. 2014;25:674–81.
55. Verma V, Rico-Martinez R, Kotra N, King L, Liu J, Snell TW, Weber RJ. Contribution of water-soluble and insoluble components and their hydrophobic/hydrophilic subfractions to the reactive oxygen species-generating potential of fine ambient aerosols. Environ Sci Technol. 2012;46:11384–92.
56. Vincent R, Bjarnason SG, Adamson IY, Hedgecock C, Kumarathasan P, Guenette J, Potvin M, Goegan P, Bouthillier L. Acute pulmonary toxicity of urban particulate matter and ozone. Am J Pathol. 1997a;151:1563–70.
57. Vincent R, Goegan P, Johnson G, Brook JR, Kumarathasan P, Bouthillier L, Burnett RT. Regulation of promoter-CAT stress genes in HepG2 cells by suspensions of particles from ambient air. Fundam Appl Toxicol. 1997b; 39:18–32.
58. Vincent R, Kumarathasan P, Goegan P, Bjarnason S G, Guenette J, Berube D, Adamson I Y, Desjardins S, Burnett R T, Miller F J and Battistini B. Inhalation toxicology of urban ambient particulate matter: acute cardiovascular effects in rats. Res Rep Health Eff Inst. 2001;(104):5–54. discussion 55–62.
59. Voet D, Voet JG. Biochemistry. 4th ed. New Jersey: Wiley; 2010.
60. Vora R, Zareba W, Utell MJ, Pietropaoli AP, Chalupa D, Little EL, Oakes D, Bausch J, Wiltshire J, Frampton MW. Inhalation of ultrafine carbon particles alters heart rate and heart rate variability in people with type 2 diabetes. Part Fibre Toxicol. 2014;11:31.
61. Vuong NQ, Goegan P, De R F, Breznan D, Thomson E M, O'Brien J S, Karthikeyan S, Williams A, Vincent R and Kumarathasan P. Responses of A549 Human Lung Epithelial Cells to Cristobalite and Alpha-Quartz Exposures Assessed by Toxicoproteomics and Gene Expression Analysis. J Appl Toxicol. 2017;37(6):721–31.
62. Vuong NQ, Goegan P, Mohottalage S, Breznan D, Ariganello M, Williams A, Elisma F, Karthikeyan S, Vincent R, Kumarathasan P. Human lung epithelial cell A549 proteome data after treatment with titanium dioxide and carbon black. Data Brief. 2016b;8:687–91.
63. Vuong NQ, Goegan P, Mohottalage S, Breznan D, Ariganello M, Williams A, Elisma F, Karthikeyan S, Vincent R, Kumarathasan P. Proteomic changes in human lung epithelial cells (A549) in response to carbon black and titanium dioxide exposures. J Proteome. 2016c;149:53–63.
64. Yang W, Zheng Y, Xia Y, Ji H, Chen X, Guo F, Lyssiotis CA, Aldape K, Cantley LC, Lu Z. ERK1/2-dependent Phosphorylation and nuclear translocation of PKM2 promotes the Warburg effect. Nat Cell Biol. 2012;14:1295–304.
65. Yi S, Zhang F, Qu F, Ding W. Water-insoluble fraction of airborne particulate matter (PM10) induces oxidative stress in human lung epithelial A549 cells. Environ Toxicol. 2014;29:226–33.
66. Zanobetti A, Franklin M, Koutrakis P, Schwartz J. Fine particulate air pollution and its components in association with cause-specific emergency admissions. Environ Health. 2009;8:58.
67. Zhao G, Lu H, Li C. Proapoptotic activities of protein disulfide Isomerase (PDI) and PDIA3 protein, a role of the Bcl-2 protein Bak. J Biol Chem. 2015; 290:8949–63.
68. Zhou X, Zhang Y, Han N, Guo S, Xiao T, Cheng S, Gao Y, Zhang K. Alpha-Enolase (ENO1) inhibits epithelial-Mesenchymal transition in the A549 cell Lineby suppressing ERK1/2 Phosphorylation. Zhongguo Fei Ai Za Zhi. 2013; 16:221–6.

7

Predicting the in vivo pulmonary toxicity induced by acute exposure to poorly soluble nanomaterials by using advanced in vitro methods

Thomas Loret[1,2], Françoise Rogerieux[1], Bénédicte Trouiller[1], Anne Braun[1], Christophe Egles[2,3] and Ghislaine Lacroix[1*]

Abstract

Background: Animal models remain at that time a reference tool to predict potential pulmonary adverse effects of nanomaterials in humans. However, in a context of reduction of the number of animals used in experimentation, there is a need for reliable alternatives. In vitro models using lung cells represent relevant alternatives to assess potential nanomaterial acute toxicity by inhalation, particularly since advanced in vitro methods and models have been developed. Nevertheless, the ability of in vitro experiments to replace animal experimentation for predicting potential acute pulmonary toxicity in human still needs to be carefully assessed.
The aim of the study was to evaluate the differences existing between the in vivo and the in vitro approaches for the prediction of nanomaterial toxicity and to find advanced methods to enhance in vitro predictivity. For this purpose, rats or pneumocytes in co-culture with macrophages were exposed to the same poorly soluble and poorly toxic TiO_2 and CeO_2 nanomaterials, by the respiratory route in vivo or using more or less advanced methodologies in vitro. After 24 h of exposure, biological responses were assessed focusing on pro-inflammatory effects and quantitative comparisons were performed between the in vivo and in vitro methods, using compatible dose metrics.

Results: For each dose metric used (mass/alveolar surface or mass/macrophage), we observed that the most realistic in vitro exposure method, the air-liquid interface method, was the most predictive of in vivo effects regarding biological activation levels. We also noted less differences between in vivo and in vitro results when doses were normalized by the number of macrophages rather than by the alveolar surface. Lastly, although we observed similarities in the nanomaterial ranking using in vivo and in vitro approaches, the quality of the data-set was insufficient to provide clear ranking comparisons.

Conclusions: We showed that advanced methods could be used to enhance in vitro experiments ability to predict potential acute pulmonary toxicity in vivo. Moreover, we showed that the timing of the dose delivery could be controlled to enhance the predictivity. Further studies should be necessary to assess if air-liquid interface provide more reliable ranking of nanomaterials than submerged methods.

Keywords: Poorly soluble nanomaterials, Acute exposure, Pulmonary toxicity, Alternative toxicity testing, Air-liquid interface, In vivo - in vitro comparison

* Correspondence: ghislaine.lacroix@ineris.fr
[1]Institut National de l'Environnement Industriel et des Risques (INERIS), (DRC/VIVA/TOXI), Parc Technologique ALATA - BP 2, F-60550 Verneuil-en-Halatte, France
Full list of author information is available at the end of the article

Background

Inhalation is an important exposure route for many metallic and poorly soluble nanomaterials (NMs) [1], including TiO_2 or CeO_2, which are among the most commonly used in nanotechnologies [2]. To assess the pulmonary toxicity of these NMs after acute exposure, in vivo assays using animal models remain the most reliable approach to predict potential adverse effects in humans [3], because of similar levels of complexity. Nevertheless, considering the high number of NMs used and their physico-chemical diversity, it seems difficult, for ethical and financial reasons, to rely on animal experimentation only. It is therefore necessary to find reliable methods that can be used as alternatives to in vivo models in this context.

In vitro studies using lung cells represent an inexpensive and easy-to-use alternative to assess pulmonary acute toxicity after exposure to NMs [4]. Usually in vitro, the cells are exposed in submerged conditions to suspensions of NMs for 24 h. However, these simplistic experimental conditions do not accurately mimic the interactions between particles and lungs in the human body [5]. This may lead to different biological responses between in vivo and in vitro approaches. Recently, many progresses have been made to simulate in vitro the cell–particle interactions occurring in the lungs in vivo. Importantly, advanced cellular models including co-cultures or 3D-cultures [6] and physiological exposure methods, including systems allowing exposure of cells at the air-liquid interface (ALI) to aerosols of NMs [7], have been developed. These new methodologies could help to predict more reliably the pulmonary effects observed in vivo.

Comparisons of NMs toxicity between in vivo and in vitro approaches were performed in several studies to assess if similar toxicity patterns could be found. Qualitative *vivo-vitro* comparisons were performed. In their study, Sayes et al. [8] compared cytotoxic and inflammatory responses, between rats exposed in vivo by intratracheal instillation and alveolar epithelial cells and macrophages exposed in vitro in submerged conditions to silicium and ZnO NMs. The authors didn't observe correlations between the in vitro and in vivo results. Nevertheless, Rushton et al. [9] highlighted that better *vivo-vitro* correlations could be obtained when the toxicological responses were normalized by the NM surface areas. In this work, the authors normalized the data published by Sayes et al. by the surface area of the NMs and showed that the NMs used could be ranked similarly in vivo and in vitro in function of their toxicity. Recently, it has also been shown that advanced comparisons could be performed by using similar dose metrics between in vivo and in vitro approaches. For example, Kim et al. [10] performed quantitative comparisons between mice exposed in vivo by oropharyngeal aspiration and lung slices or alveolar macrophages exposed in vitro to suspensions of TiO_2 and CeO_2 NMs. For some NMs, they showed pro-inflammatory effects at similar doses in vivo and in vitro when the doses were expressed in mass of NM per surface unit, both in vivo and in vitro. Teeguarden et al. [11] compared the pulmonary toxicity between mice exposed in vivo by inhalation and alveolar epithelial cells or macrophages exposed in vitro in submerged conditions to iron oxide NMs. They showed inflammatory effects at lower doses in vivo compared to in vitro when the doses were expressed in $\mu g/cm^2$ and better similarity when the doses were expressed in mass of NM per number of macrophages. Donaldson et al. [12] showed good correlations between pro-inflamatory responses in vivo in rats (neutrophil influx) and in vitro (IL-8 expression) in A549 cells when the doses expressed in $\mu g/cm^2$ where normalized by NM surface areas. Nevertheless, only few in vitro experiments performed in submerged conditions were compared to in vivo experiments and it remains unclear whether better prediction could be obtained by using more advanced in vitro methods, like ALI exposures.

In this context, the aim of our study was to assess the ability of several in vitro methods, more or less advanced, to predict the adverse effects observed in vivo after exposure to poorly toxic and poorly soluble metallic NMs. The perspective is to promote reliable alternative methodologies to predict the potential inhalation toxicity of NMs in humans. For this purpose, in vivo and in vitro experiments were performed using the same TiO_2 and CeO_2 NMs. In vivo, rats were exposed to the NMs by intratracheal instillation and then sacrificed after 24 h of exposure. In vitro, alveolar epithelial cells in co-culture with macrophages were exposed for 24 h at the ALI to aerosols or in submerged conditions to suspensions of NMs. Moreover, different deposition kinetics were tested. The results of the in vitro study were published previously by our team [13]. In this paper we showed toxic effects at lower doses when cells were exposed at the ALI to aerosols of NMs compared to exposure to suspensions. We also showed the relevance of timing consideration for the dose delivery when assessing poorly soluble NM toxicity in vitro. Both in vivo and in vitro, cytotoxic, inflammatory and oxidative stress responses were assessed after 24 h of exposure and qualitative and quantitative comparisons were performed. To perform in vivo - in vitro comparisons, common dose metrics were selected between in vivo and in vitro methods and normalizations were performed.

Results

The ability of several in vitro methods (ALI and submerged) to predict potential adverse effects in vivo in lungs, after exposure to poorly toxic and poorly soluble metallic NMs, was assessed in this study.

For this purpose, we performed in vivo and in vitro experiments using the same TiO_2 (NMs 105, 101 and 100) and CeO_2 (NM212) NMs. The physico-chemical characteristics of the four NMs were characterized in exposure media (Table 1). Furthermore, the number size distributions and densities of NMs in suspensions (for exposure of cells in submerged conditions in vitro or rats by intratracheal instillation in vivo) and in aerosols (for exposure of cells at the ALI) were assessed. Surprisingly, similar results were observed between NM suspended in water and in culture medium [13]. Number size distributions and densities determined in exposure media were then used to calculate the mean surface area of NM agglomerates in suspensions and in aerosols (for ALI exposures only). Based on our previous electron microscopy observations [13], agglomerates were considered spherical for the calculation. The mean surface area calculated in exposure media was then used for *vivo-vitro* comparisons.

The major innovation of this study was to compare NM toxicities between in vivo and in vitro approaches, using several more or less advanced in vitro methods and testing different timings of the dose delivery in vitro. The Fig. 1, which was adapted from our previous published paper [13] to take into account our new in vivo experiments, is presented here and proposes an overview of the study design. For the study, we focused on the doses deposited into the lungs (in vivo) or on cells (in vitro) because we postulated that metallic and poorly soluble NMs exert their toxicity by direct contact with the cells.

In vivo, rats were exposed to NMs by intratracheal instillation and sacrificed after 24 h of exposure. In vitro, alveolar epithelial cells in co-culture with macrophages were exposed for 24 h at the ALI to aerosols or in submerged conditions to the NMs. At the ALI, the cells were exposed to aerosols of NMs for 3 h, meaning that the final deposited dose was reached within 3 h. The cells were then kept in the incubator for the remaining 21 h at the ALI with the NMs deposited on their surface. In submerged conditions, we used two different timings of the dose delivery. Nevertheless, as shown in our previous paper [13], NMs concentration in suspensions were adjusted to obtain similar deposited doses (Additional file 1: Table S1). First, cells were exposed to suspensions in inserts and the NM deposition was maintained for 3 h. After 3 h of exposure, the deposition was stopped and the cells were kept during the remaining 21 h in submerged condition in the incubator. Secondly, cells were exposed in plates to suspensions of NMs for 24 h. In that situation, the NM deposition was maintained for the whole exposure time, meaning that the final deposited dose was reached within 24 h. After 24 h of exposure, inflammation, cytotoxicity and oxidative stress were assessed. Lowest Observed Adverse Effects Levels (LOAELs) and critical effect dose intervals were then determined, using first significant effects measured or benchmark dose response modeling, respectively. Focusing on these LOAELs and critical effect dose intervals, quantitative and qualitative comparisons were performed between in vivo and in vitro results. With dose intervals, contrary to with LOAELs, dose-response curves were taken into account and uncertainty was included in the data. Comparisons were performed with LOAELs and dose intervals to assess if similar conclusions could be made using the two criteria of effect dose. For these comparisons, normalizations were performed to have common dose metrics between in vivo and in vitro approaches. NM surface areas were also considered for ranking comparisons.

Pro-inflammatory responses in vivo and in vitro

In vivo and in vitro, the biological responses were assessed after 24 h of exposure to three TiO_2 (NMs 105, 101, 100) and one CeO_2 (NM212) NMs.

In vivo, pro-inflammatory effects (neutrophil influx and levels of the pro-inflammatory mediators IL-1β, IL-6, KC-GRO and TNF-α) were assessed in bronchoalveolar lavage fluids (BALF) of rats exposed by intratracheal instillation (IT) to the NMs (around 4.5 mL recovered for each sample). We observed significant effects with TiO_2 NMs 105 and 101 and CeO_2 NM212, but not with TiO_2 NM100. Significant pro-inflammatory

Table 1 Physico-chemical properties of TiO_2 (NMs 105, 101, 100) and CeO_2 (NM212) nanomaterials in exposure media

	Critallinity	Coating	Primary particle size (nm)	Primary density (g/cm^3)	Primarysurface area, BET (m^2/g)	Mean size in exposure media (nm)		Mean density in exposure media (g/cm^3)		Mean surface area in exposure media (m^2/g)	
						Susp	Aero	Susp	Aero	Susp	Aero
NM105	80% anatase / 20% rutile	No	21	4.2	46.1	318	240	1.4	0.7	13.5	37.7
NM101	Anatase	Hydrophobic	8	3.9	316	567	80	1.6	0.9	6.7	83.3
NM100	Anatase	No	100	3.9	10	286	320	1.8	0.6	11.7	31.3
NM212	Cubic cerionite	No	29	7.2	27	233	200	2.1	1.1	12.5	27.3

Susp Suspension, *Aero* Aerosol

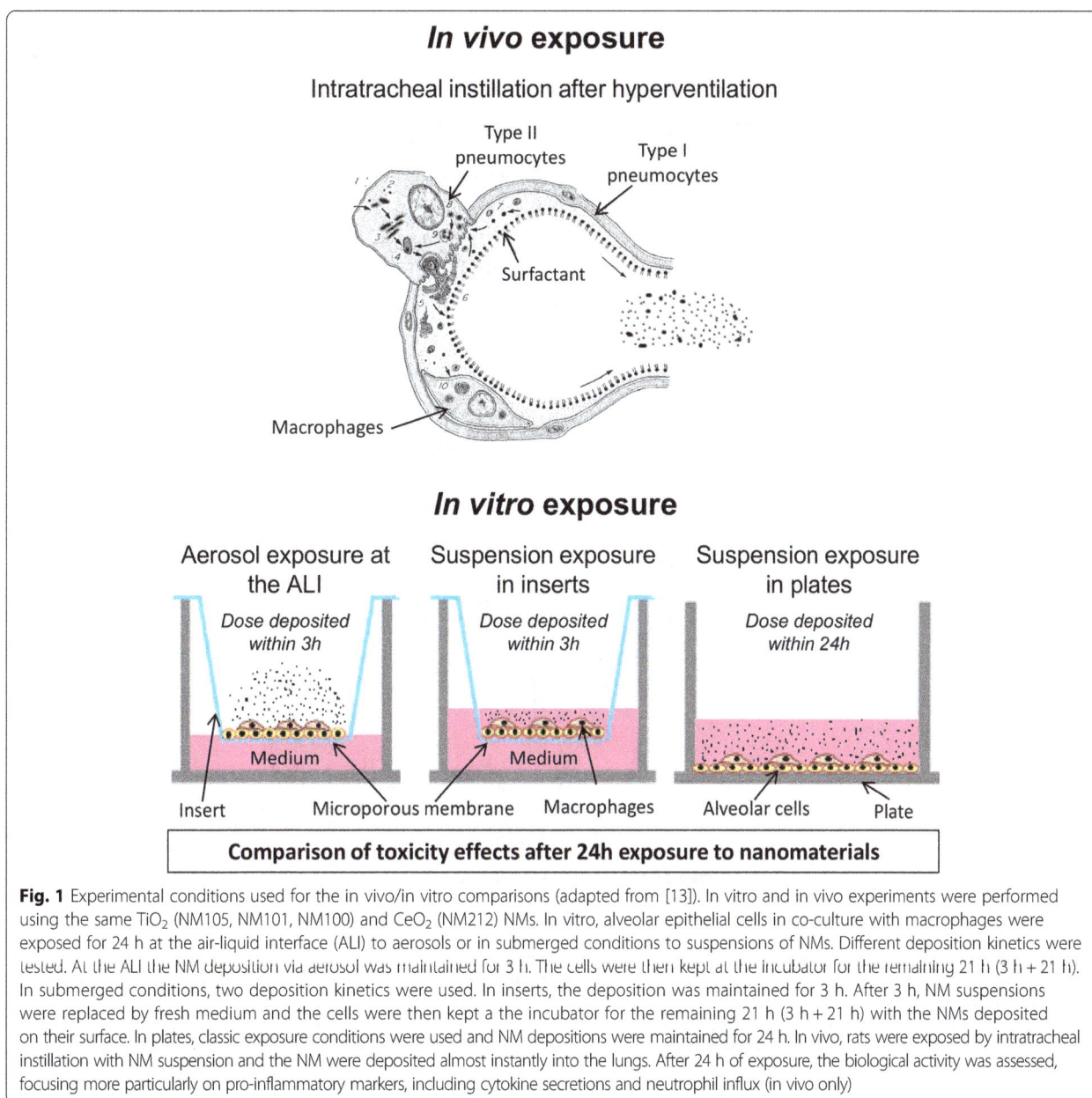

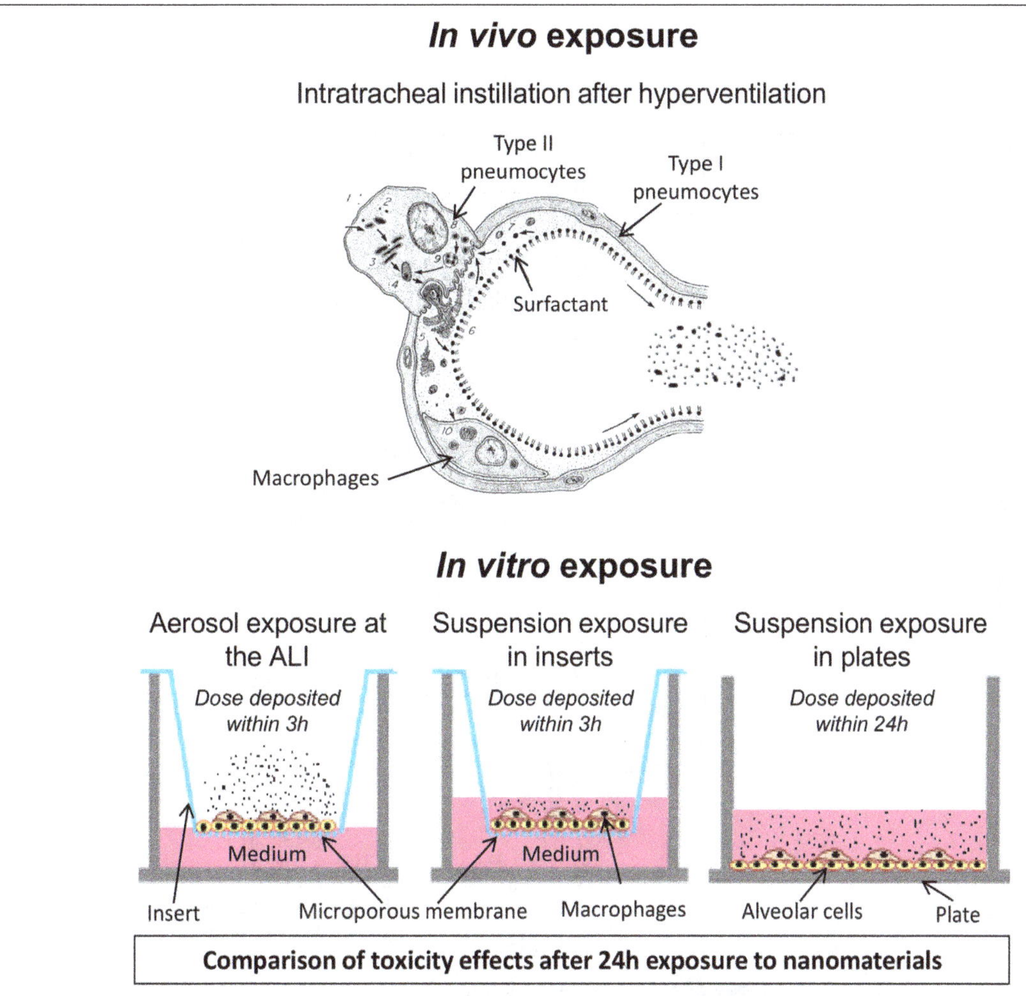

Fig. 1 Experimental conditions used for the in vivo/in vitro comparisons (adapted from [13]). In vitro and in vivo experiments were performed using the same TiO_2 (NM105, NM101, NM100) and CeO_2 (NM212) NMs. In vitro, alveolar epithelial cells in co-culture with macrophages were exposed for 24 h at the air-liquid interface (ALI) to aerosols or in submerged conditions to suspensions of NMs. Different deposition kinetics were tested. At the ALI the NM deposition via aerosol was maintained for 3 h. The cells were then kept at the incubator for the remaining 21 h (3 h + 21 h). In submerged conditions, two deposition kinetics were used. In inserts, the deposition was maintained for 3 h. After 3 h, NM suspensions were replaced by fresh medium and the cells were then kept a the incubator for the remaining 21 h (3 h + 21 h) with the NMs deposited on their surface. In plates, classic exposure conditions were used and NM depositions were maintained for 24 h. In vivo, rats were exposed by intratracheal instillation with NM suspension and the NM were deposited almost instantly into the lungs. After 24 h of exposure, the biological activity was assessed, focusing more particularly on pro-inflammatory markers, including cytokine secretions and neutrophil influx (in vivo only)

effects were noted at the maximum dose tested: 400 µg/lungs, corresponding to around 0.1 µg/cm^2 or 20 µg/10^6 macrophages after normalization by the alveolar surface (4000 cm^2) or the number of alveolar macrophages (25 million), respectively (Fig. 2). After exposure to TiO_2NMs 105 and 101, this was characterized by a significant neutrophil influx in BALF supernatants, associated with increased concentrations of TNF-α for the NMs 105 and 101 and KC-GRO for NM105 only. We also noted significant increases in IL-1β, IL-6 and TNF-α secretion with NM212, although no significant neutrophil influx was detected. The absence of significant neutrophil influx with NM212 may have been due to a high variability in the control sample. No significant increases in neutrophils or cytokines were noted for TiO_2 NM100. Moreover, for all the NMs tested, we did not observe any significant changes in macrophages or total cell numbers.

Based on the significant responses detected in vivo, lowest observed adverse effects levels (LOAELs) were determined for pro-inflammatory effects with NMs 105, 101 and 212, but not with NM100. These LOAELs were used in the present study to compare in vivo and in vitro results. We also used benchmark dose-response modeling to determine critical effect doses for a 20% increase of cytokine/chemokine response with an interval of doses corresponding to a 90% confidence, to compare in vivo and in vitro results.

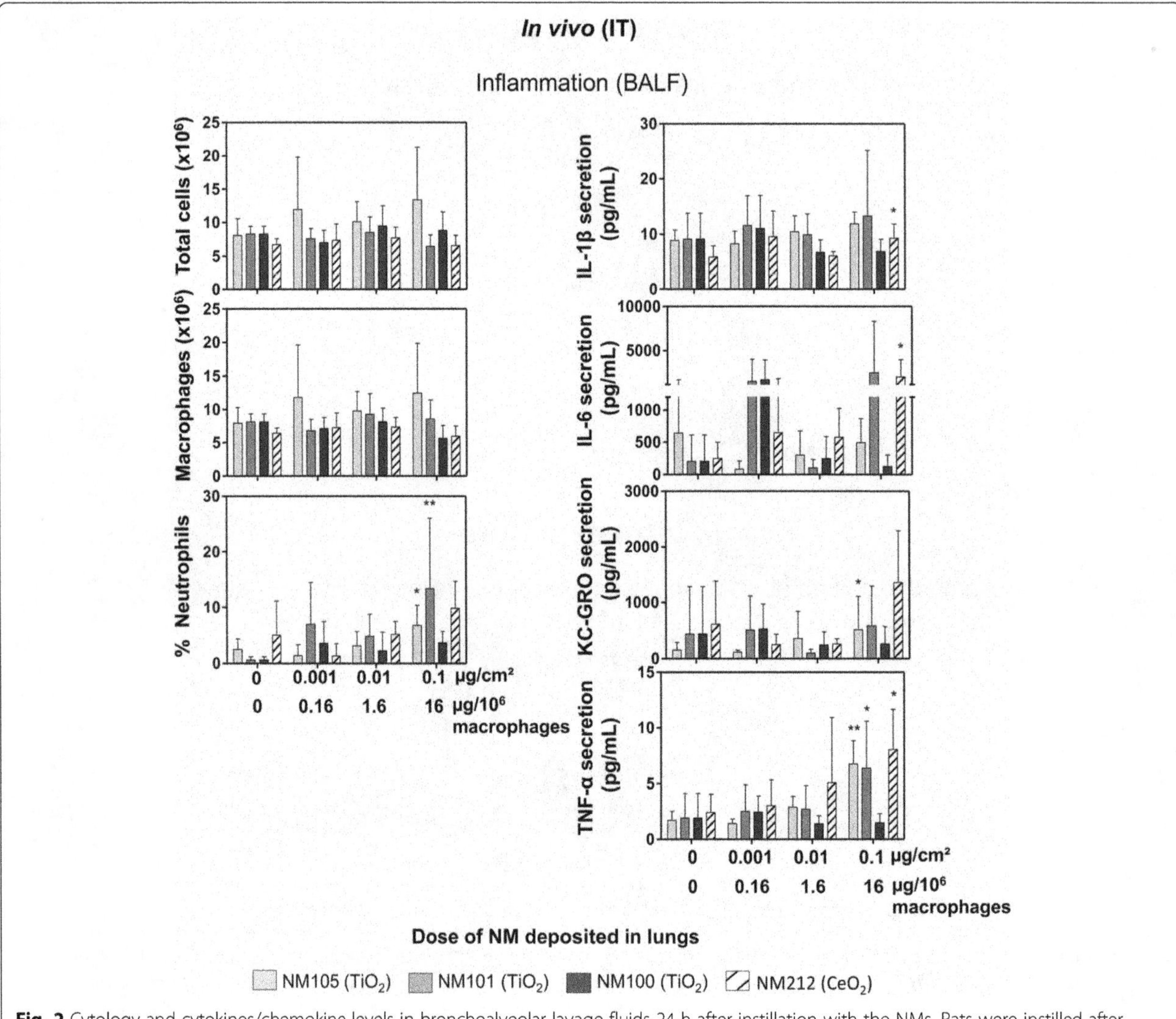

Fig. 2 Cytology and cytokines/chemokine levels in bronchoalveolar lavage fluids 24 h after instillation with the NMs. Rats were instilled after hyperventilation with suspensions of TiO_2 (NM105, NM101, NM100) and CeO_2 (NM212). After sacrifice, bronchoalveolar lavages were performed using PBS. The bronchoalveolar lavage fluids were recovered and centrifuged to separate cells from supernatant. For cytology analysis, the cells were resuspended in RMPI medium and then seeded on slides at 300000 cells/spots using a cytospin and then fixated and coloured in May-Grunwald Giemsa. The percentage of different cell types in BALF was determined using optical microscopy. For cytokine/chemokine analysis, supernatants were dosed using ELISA multiplex to determine IL-1β, IL-6, KC-GRO and TNF-α levels. Data represent the mean ± SD of six animals. Kruskal-Wallis test followed by Dunn's post-hoc test were performed to compare treated groups to controls (*$p < 0.05$; **$p < 0.01$; ***$p < 0.001$)

In vitro, pro-inflammatory responses were assessed after 24 h of exposure by evaluating the levels of pro-inflammatory mediators IL-1β, IL-6, IL-8 and TNF-α in cell supernatants. After ALI exposure to aerosols of NM in inserts, cytokine levels were only measured in the basolateral compartment (containing 2 mL of culture medium) as the cells were maintained at the ALI for the 3 h of exposure to the aerosols and for the remaining 21 h into the incubator with the NMs deposited on their surface. After exposure in submerged conditions to suspensions in inserts, using the similar dose rate timing of the dose delivery than at the ALI (3 h), cytokine levels were assessed both in the apical and basolateral compartments of the inserts (containing 1 and 2 mL of culture medium, respectively). In submerged conditions in plates, which represents the classic exposure conditions usually used in vitro, the NM deposition was maintained for the 24 h of exposure and cytokine levels were exclusively measured on the apical side of the cells (containing 0.5 mL of culture medium) due to the absence of a basolateral compartment.

Briefly, as demonstrated in our previous in vitro study [13], we observed significant pro-inflammatory responses at the ALI with all tested NMs. We also observed effects in submerged conditions in inserts and in plates, but mainly with NMs 105 and 101. A compilation of the pro-inflammatory results published in our previous study [13] is available in the Additional files of the present paper (Additional file 1: Figure S1). According to the first significant pro-inflammatory responses detected, LOAELs were determined for each assay performed (Additional file 1: Table S2). For all NMs, the LOAELs were determined at lower doses at the ALI compared to submerged conditions in inserts and also at lower doses when the final dose was deposited within 3 h rather than within 24 h. In the present study, benchmark dose-response modeling was also used with the in vitro data to determine an interval of dose for a 20% increase of cytokine/chemokine response with a 90% confidence, to compare in vivo and in vitro results.

Cytotoxicity and oxidative stress effects in vivo and in vitro

Cytotoxicity and oxidative stress responses were also assessed, both in vivo and in vitro. In vivo, LDH levels were evaluated in BALF supernatants and Reactive Oxygen Species (ROS) levels were measured in BALF cells. Although significant pro-inflammatory responses were noted, we did not observe any significant cytotoxic or oxidative stress effects after 24 h of exposure to the NMs (Table 2 and Additional file 1: Figure S2). In vitro, cytotoxicity was assessed by using the alamar blue test and by measuring LDH levels in cell supernatants. ROS levels were measured in cells as marker of oxidative stress. We observed few significant cytotoxicity and oxidative responses at the ALI (and only with the NMs 105 and 101). LOAELs were also determined for cytotoxicity and oxidative stress in submerged conditions and more particularly in inserts (Table 2). As described in our previous article [13], it was not possible to perform clear quantitative comparisons between the different in vitro exposure method using these two parameters because too little significant cytotoxicity and oxidative stress effects were detected in vitro. However, it could not be excluded that less cytotoxicity and oxidative stress effects were observed compared to pro-inflammatory effects, both in vivo and in vitro, because of a lack of sensitivity of the assays performed.

Vivo-vitro comparisons using the inflammation results

As described previously, inflammation was the most sensitive marker of biological responses at 24 h in our study, both in vivo and in vitro. For this reason, we focused on the pro-inflammatory responses to perform *vivo-vitro* comparisons. To perform quantitative comparisons, the LOAELs determined in vivo and in vitro for the first significant pro-inflammatory responses observed were first used. Dose-response comparisons were then performed using dose intervals determined by benchmark modeling. For dose intervals calculation, we determined a critical effect dose corresponding to a 20% increase of pro-inflammatory mediator levels compared to non-exposed controls and the Benchmark Dose Lower confidence limit (BMDL) and the Benchmark Dose Upper confidence limit (BMDU) of the interval for a 90% confidence. This was performed for each pro-inflammatory mediator, each exposure method and each NM used. Examples of benchmark dose-response modeling for the calculation of critical effect doses and dose intervals are shown in the Additional file 1: Figure S3. For each NM and each exposure method, we then calculated the median value of the BMDL and the median value of the BMDU for the four pro-inflammatory mediators (IL-1β, IL-6, IL-8/KC-GRO, TNF-α), to determine a median dose interval for general pro-inflammatory response, as shown in the Table 3. We

Table 2 LOAELs (μg/cm^2) for cytotoxicity and oxidative stress effects determined after 24 h of exposure

LOAELs (μg/cm^2)		Cytotoxicity[a]				Oxidative stress			
		In vitro			In vivo	In vitro			In vivo
		ALI[b] (3 h + 21 h)	Subm[c] (3 h + 21 h)	Subm[d] (24 h)	IT[e]	ALI[b] (3 h + 21 h)	Subm[c] (3 h + 21 h)	Subm[d] (24 h)	IT[e]
	NM105	1	10	10	≥>0.1	≥>3	10	10	≥>0.1
TiO_2	NM101	≥>3	10	10	≥>0.1	1	≥>10	≥>20	≥>0.1
	NM100	≥>3	10	≥>20	≥>0.1	≥>3	10	≥>20	≥>0.1
CeO_2	NM212	≥>3	10	≥>20	≥>0.1	≥>3	≥>10	≥>20	ND

[a]LOAELs indicated represent significant cytotoxicity > 5%

(red) Significant effects allowing the determination of a LOAEL

(green) No significant adverse effects observed

[b]Doses tested at the ALI: 0.1, 1, 3 μg/cm^2

[c]Doses tested in submerged conditions in inserts: 1, 3, 10 μg/cm^2

[d]Doses tested in submerged conditions in plates: 1, 3, 10, 20 μg/cm^2

[e]Doses tested in vivo: 0.001, 0.01, 0.1 μg/cm^2

calculated the median dose interval of the four cytokines because similar results could be observed in our study when pooling the results of the four cytokines and when comparing dose intervals of each cytokine one by one. We believe that comparisons performed in our study were easier to follow when a general pro-inflammatory response was used instead of comparing the dose intervals of each cytokine one by one. With dose intervals, contrary to with LOAELs, dose-response curves were taken into account and uncertainty was included in the data. Comparisons were performed with LOAELs and dose intervals to assess if similar conclusions could be made using the two criteria of dose. For the comparisons, LOAELs and dose intervals were expressed using different dose metrics which were compatible between in vivo and in vitro methods.

Selection of relevant dose metrics

Common dose metrics that could be used with all exposure methods (submerged, ALI, instillation or inhalation) were selected, as shown in Fig. 3, to compare NM toxicity between in vivo and in vitro approaches. To generate common dose metrics, we normalized the deposited masses by the alveolar surface or by the macrophage number [14]. These two normalizations were performed as they take into account the direct contact between the NMs and the tissues, that was shown to be the main cause of toxicity for poorly soluble NMs [15–17]. To express the metric in mass per alveolar surface unit, masses deposited into the lungs or on the cells were divided by the total alveolar surface in vivo (4000 cm^2) [18, 19] or by the surface of the cell layer in vitro (4,67 cm^2 in inserts and 2 cm^2 in plates), respectively. To express the metric in mass per macrophage number, the mass of NM in lungs (in vivo) or the deposited mass per cm^2 (in vitro) were divided by the total number of alveolar macrophages in vivo (around 25 million) [18, 20] or in vitro (60,000 or 25,000/cm^2 in inserts or in plates, respectively) [13]. The doses expressed in mass/macrophages were also normalized by the surface area for each NM. This normalization was performed because it was shown that the surface area was the most effective dose metric to explain acute NM toxicity in the lung [15–17]. For that, doses expressed in mass/macrophages were multiplied by NM surface areas, calculated using NM primary characteristics in powders (BET method) or mean sizes and densities in exposure media. Based on our previous observations, NMs were assumed to be spherical for surface area calculations in exposure media [13]. Nevertheless, it was not possible to ensure that NM agglomerates were strictly spherical and relative uncertainties remain regarding the mean surface area calculated in exposure media.

Doses could also be expressed in number of NMs per surface area or per cell. Nevertheless, these metrics were not chosen due to the difficulty to characterize NM size

Table 3 Dose intervals (in μg/cm^2) determined for each NM and each methodology

	Cytokines	NM105			NM101			NM100			NM212		
		Dose interval			Dose interval			Dose interval			Dose interval		
		BMDL	BMDU	Median	BMDL	BMDU	Median	BMDL	BMDU	Median	BMDL	BMDU	Median
In vitro, suspension (24 h)	IL-1β	0.10	11.90	4.63–11.20	0.53	2.85	2.82–6.36	10.68	32.59	10.96–26.19	0.06	10.26	0.430–14.168
	IL-6	4.50	11.11		4.86	10.47		ND	ND		ND	ND	
	IL-8	ND	ND		ND	ND		ND	ND		ND	ND	
	TNF-α	4.76	11.20		2.82	6.36		11.25	19.80		0.80	18.08	
In vitro, suspension (3 h + 21 h)	IL-1β	0.43	2.25	0.26–1.51	0.60	6.61	0.80–6.19	3.47	53.23	3.47–55.64	3.47	54.81	3.37–52.50
	IL-6	0.20	1.36		1.28	8.17		ND	ND		2.30	50.25	
	IL-8	0.11	1.11		0.84	3.73		3.35	58.05		3.42	9.64	
	TNF-α	0.31	1.66		0.76	5.78		3.83	52.87		3.31	54.75	
ALI (3 h + 21 h)	IL-1β	0.051	0.80	0.061–0.82	0.061	0.74	0.099–0.80	0.006	0.91	0.045–0.90	0.63	2.61	0.88–2.71
	IL-6	0.037	0.81		0.089	0.77		0.012	0.88		0.88	2.71	
	IL-8	0.078	0.83		1.13	11.87		0.078	0.90		ND	ND	
	TNF-α	0.070	0.82		0.11	0.84		0.24	0.97		ND	ND	
In vivo	IL-1β	0.0011	0.067	0.0007–0.075	ND	ND	0.0022–0.084	ND	ND	ND	ND	ND	0.0000–0.074
	IL-6	0.00069	0.13		0.0044	0.086		ND	ND		0.000	0.019	
	IL-8	0.00019	0.084		ND	ND		ND	ND		0.0033	0.082	
	TNF-α	0.00075	0.0091		0.000	0.082		ND	ND		0.000	0.074	

BMDL Benchmark Dose Lower confidence limit, *BMDU* Benchmark Dose Upper confidence limit. Median: Median BMDL and BMDU values calculated by pooling the four cytokines, to have a dose-interval for a general pro-inflammatory response

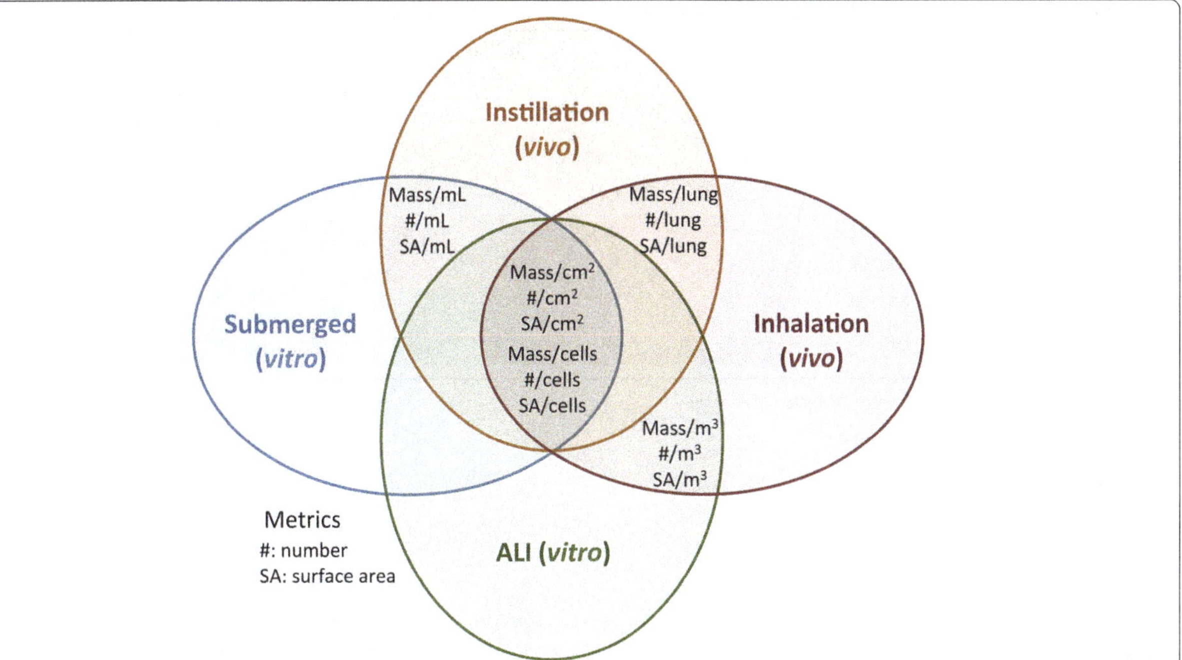

Fig. 3 Compatibility of the different dose metrics between in vivo and in vitro approaches. In order to compare in vitro and in vivo conditions it is important to use common dose metrics. The doses are often expressed as concentrations, including mass/volume of liquid in vitro in submerged conditions and mass/volume of air in vivo in inhalation studies. However, these metrics cannot be used within the different in vivo (inhalation or instillation) and in vitro (ALI or submerged) methodologies. Moreover, using concentrations in mass/volume does not take into account the real contact between the NMs and the cells or tissues. Thus it does not seem appropriate to use such dose metrics for in vivo-in vitro comparisons; more particularly for poorly soluble NMs as their toxicity is attributable to their surface reactivity. In vivo, the total mass of NMs administered per lungs, animal or mass is often used as dose metric. This dose metric takes into account the deposition in the overall organ, but cannot be used in vitro. Nevertheless, common dose metrics can be used by normalizing the mass deposited on cells in vitro or into the lungs in vivo by the surface of the tissues or by the number of cells. Doses expressed in mass can also be normalized NM surface areas, that has been shown to be the most effective dose metric for acute NM toxicity in the lung

distributions in the lungs. Moreover, the number metric was not shown to be more relevant than the mass metric when assessing NM toxicity [16].

Comparisons in mass/alveolar surface

Doses of NMs were first expressed in μg/cm^2, after normalization of the deposited doses by the total alveolar surface in vivo (4000 cm^2) or by the surface of the cell layer in vitro. All the LOAELs and the dose intervals determined for pro-inflammatory effects were expressed using this dose metric (Tables 3 and 4, Fig. 4a) and *vivo-vitro* comparisons were performed. Generally, for each NM, we noted pro-inflammatory effects at lower doses in vivo compared to in vitro. We also observed that the LOAELs and the dose intervals determined in vitro after exposure at the ALI were closer to those in vivo than those determined in vitro in submerged conditions. Moreover, we noted that the LOAELs determined in vitro were closer to those in vivo when the final dose was achieved in vitro within 3 h rather than within 24 h. When comparing the LOAELs for each NM, differences of a factor of 10, 30 and 100 were noted for exposure at the ALI to aerosols (3 h + 21 h), exposure in submerged conditions in inserts (3 h + 21 h) and in submerged conditions in plates (24 h), compared to in vivo, respectively.

Comparisons in mass/macrophages

Doses were also normalized by the total number of macrophages and expressed in μg/10^6 macrophages to compare in vivo and in vitro LOAELs and dose intervals (Table 5, Fig. 4b and Additional file 1: Table S3). For that purpose, in vivo doses expressed in μg were normalized by the number of alveolar macrophages. In vitro, deposited doses expressed in μg/cm^2 were normalized by the total number of alveolar macrophages-like cells per cm^2. We noticed that the LOAELs and the dose intervals determined in vitro were closer to those observed in vivo when the doses were normalized by the number of macrophages rather than by the alveolar surface (Table 5 and Fig. 4). When looking at the LOAELs, the pro-inflammatory responses were observed at similar doses in vivo and in vitro at the ALI, whereas a difference of at least a factor of 10 was observed when the LOAELs were expressed in μg/cm^2. Differences of around a factor of 3 and 20 were observed between the

Table 4 LOAELs (in μg/cm² for 24 h of exposure) determined for pro-inflammatory effects

LOAELs (μg/cm²)		Inflammation				
		In vitro *(cytokines)*			In vivo *(cytokines)*	In vivo *(Neutrophils)*
		ALI[a] (3 h + 21 h)	Subm[b] (3 h + 21 h)	Subm[c] (24 h)	IT[d]	IT[d]
	NM105	1	3	10 20	0.1	0.1
TiO_2	NM101	1	3	10	0.1	0.1
	NM100	1 3	10	> 20	> 0.1	> 0.1
CeO_2	NM212	1 3	10	> 20	0.1	> 0.1

Significant effects allowing the determination of a LOAEL

No significant adverse effects observed

[a]Doses tested at the ALI: 0.1, 1, 3 μg/cm²

[b]Doses tested in submerged conditions in inserts: 1, 3, 10 μg/cm²

[c]Doses tested in submerged conditions in plates: 1, 3, 10, 20 μg/cm²

[d]Doses tested in vivo: 0.001, 0.01, 0.1 μg/cm²

in vivo experiments and the in vitro experiments performed in submerged conditions in inserts (3 h + 21 h) and in plates (24 h), respectively.

Ranking of the NMs according to the methodology used

For each methodology used, a ranking of the four NMs used was provided according to the inflammation results and the dose intervals that had been determined. Ranking comparisons were performed using dose intervals only, because better screening could be performed between NMs by using this criterion of effect compared to the use of LOAELs. Comparisons were performed to assess whether the four poorly toxic and poorly soluble NMs could be ranked similarly, based on the different methodologies tested. The dose intervals were also normalized by NM primary surface areas and agglomerate surface areas to understand the differences in toxicity existing between the NMs. A toxicity ranking of the NMs according to the different methodologies and dose metrics used is presented in the Fig. 5.

Ranking using mass as dose metric

In mass (μg/cm² or μg/10^6 macrophages) some differences were observed between in vivo and in vitro conditions (Fig. 5). In vivo, NMs 105, 101 and 212 were observed to be clearly more toxic than NM100, as we did not observe any significant effects with the NM100. In vitro, we noticed pro-inflammatory responses for NMs 105 and 101, at lower doses than for NM212, at the ALI and in submerged conditions. NM100, similarly as NM105 and NM101, seemed to elicit more pro-inflammatory responses at the ALI than NM212, but this was not observed in submerged conditions.

Ranking using the surface area as dose metric

Doses in mass/macrophages were normalized by the surface area of each NM, to assess how the surface reactivity influenced the biological responses in vivo and in vitro. The dose intervals were expressed in $cm^2/10^6$ macrophages (Additional file 1: Tables S4 and S5) and a ranking was provided for the four poorly toxic and poorly soluble NMs used in our study. Doses in mass/alveolar surface could also be normalized by the surface area, generating the same ranking of the NMs as using the mass/macrophages dose metric (Fig. 5).

First, the dose intervals were normalized by the calculated surface area using the NM primary sizes and densities (BET method) (Additional file 1: Table S4). This normalization had an influence on the ranking of the NMs. The NM101 was ranked with a lower toxicity than expected, both in vivo and in vitro (Fig. 5). In vivo, we observed dose intervals at lower doses for NM105 and NM212 than for NM101, however, it was not possible to include NM100 in this ranking, as no significant effects were observed, probably because significantly lower doses (in $cm^2/10^6$ macrophages) were tested compared to the three other NMs, due to a lower surface area. In vitro, when dose intervals were expressed in $cm^2/10^6$ macrophages, using surface area calculated according to primary sizes, we also observed effects at lower doses for the NM100, the NM105 and the NM212 than for the NM101.

Secondly, the dose intervals were normalized by the surface area calculated according to NM agglomerate mean sizes and densities in exposure media (suspensions or aerosols) (Additional file 1: Table S5). Interestingly, less changes in the ranking of the NMs were observed when performing this normalization, for all the methodologies used (in vitro ALI, in vitro in submerged and in vivo) (Fig. 5). In vivo, no clear discrepancy could be

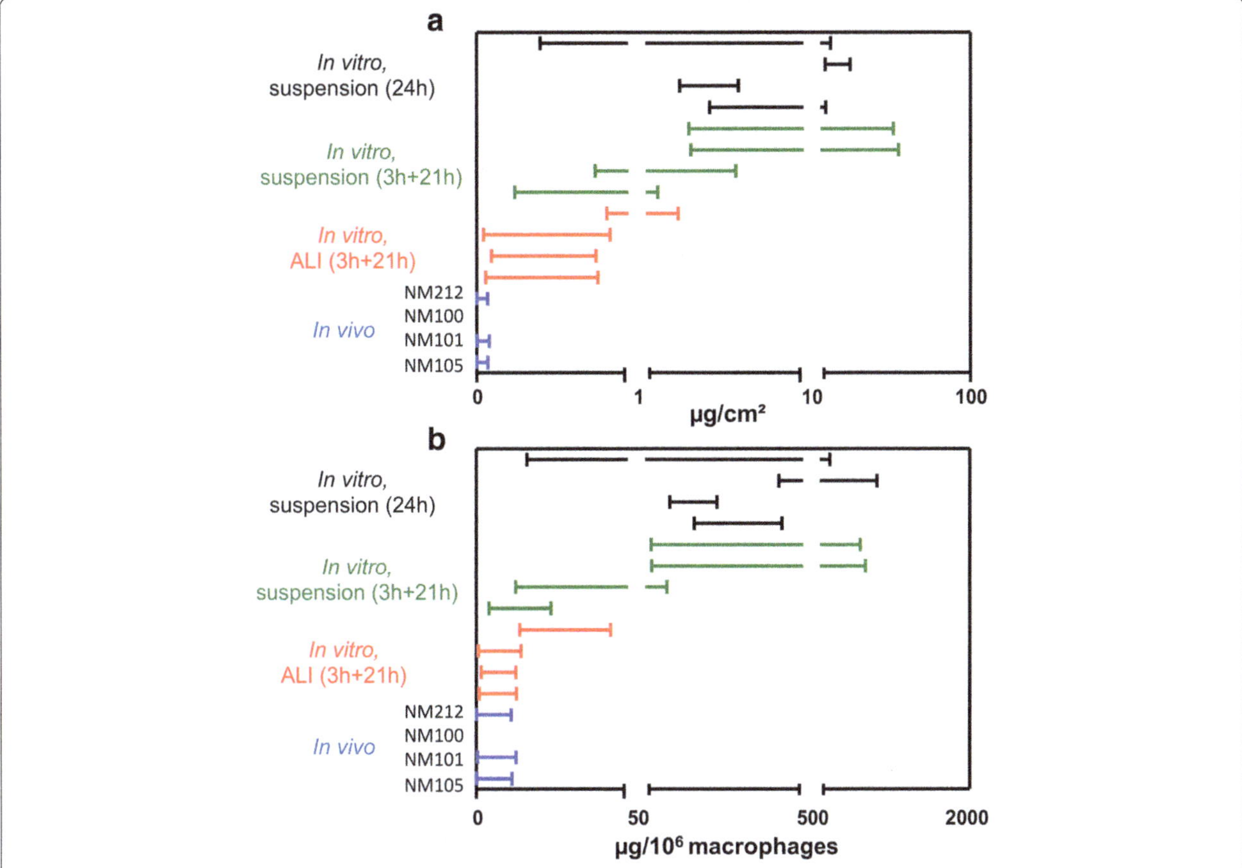

Fig. 4 Dose intervals calculated for a 20% increase in inflammation markers in function of methodologies used. Comparisons of dose intervals were performed between the in vivo and in vitro methods used. The comparisons were performed using two dose metrics: the mass/alveolar surface (**a**) or the mass/macrophages (**b**). In vitro and in vivo experiments were performed using the same TiO_2 (NM105, NM101, NM100) and CeO_2 (NM212) NMs. In vitro, alveolar epithelial cells in co-culture with macrophages were exposed for 24 h at the air-liquid interface (ALI) to aerosols or in submerged conditions to suspensions of NMs. Different deposition kinetics were tested. At the ALI the NM deposition via aerosol was maintained for 3 h. The cells were then kept at the incubator for the remaining 21 h (3 h + 21 h). In submerged conditions, two deposition kinetics were used. In inserts, the deposition was maintained for 3 h. After 3 h, NM suspensions were replaced by fresh medium and the cells were then kept a the incubator for the remaining 21 h (3 h + 21 h) with the NMs deposited on their surface. In plates, classic exposure conditions were used and NM depositions were maintained for 24 h. In vivo, rats were exposed by intratracheal instillation with NM suspensions and the NMs were deposited almost instantly into the lungs. After 24 h of exposure, the biological activity was assessed, focusing more particularly on pro-inflammatory mediators. For each exposure method and for each NM, benchmark dose-response modeling was used to estimate the critical dose related to a 20% increase of pro-inflammatory mediator level and the lowest (BMDL) and the highest (BMDU) dose of the interval corresponding to confidence interval of 90%. A median dose intervals was then calculated by pooling the dose intervals of the four cytokine to have a general pro-inflammatory response

made between NMs 105, 101 and 212; all three were observed to be more toxic than NM100. In vitro at the ALI, NMs 105, 101 and 100 were observed toxic at lower dose than NM 212, although this was clearly more pronounced for NM105 and NM100. In submerged conditions, similarly as when the dose intervals were expressed in mass/macrophages, NMs 105 and 101 were observed to be more toxic than NMs 100 and 212. This better correlation in the ranking between doses expressed in mass and doses expressed in surface area, when normalizing the dose intervals by mean agglomerates surface area rather than by primary surface areas, indicates that toxicity may be due to NM agglomerates rather than isolated NMs.

Discussion

The aim of this study was to assess the ability of several more or less advanced in vitro methods, to predict the pulmonary adverse effects observed in vivo after acute exposure to poorly toxic and poorly soluble metallic NMs. The perspective is to promote reliable alternative methodologies to animal testing for the prediction of pulmonary toxicity of NMs in humans.

Table 5 LOAELs (µg/10^6 macrophages for 24 h exposure) determined for pro-inflammatory-effects

LOAELs (µg/10^6 macrophages)		Inflammation				
		In vitro *(cytokines)*			In vivo *(cytokines)*	In vivo *(Neutrophils)*
		ALI[a] (3 h + 21 h)	Subm[b] (3 h + 21 h)	Subm[c] (24 h)	IT[d]	IT[d]
TiO_2	NM105	16.7	50	400–800	16	16
	NM101	16.7	50	400	16	16
	NM100	16.7–50	167	≥>800	≥>16	≥>16
CeO_2	NM212	16.7–50	167	≥>800	16	≥>16

Significant effects allowing the determination of a LOAEL

No significant adverse effects observed

[a]Doses tested at the ALI: 1.67, 16.7, 50 µg/10^6 macrophages
[b]Doses tested in submerged conditions in inserts: 16.7, 50, 167 µg/10^6 macrophages
[c]Doses tested in submerged conditions in plates: 40, 120, 400, 800 µg/10^6 macrophages
[d]Doses tested in vivo: 0.16, 1.6, 16 µg/10^6 macrophages

The selection of relevant in vivo and in vitro models to predict potential biological responses in humans was thus very important. In vivo, the rat was selected because it is the recommended species to assess inhalation toxicity in humans [21]. In vitro, human rather than rat cells were chosen because they were more likely to model responses of cells in the human body. Moreover, because the principal pulmonary target for inhaled NMs remains the alveoli [22], we focused on this part of the lungs. At the alveolar surface in vivo, macrophages are in close contact with epithelial cells (i.e type and I and II pneumocytes), at a ratio of approximately one macrophage to ten pneumocytes [18, 20]. The main role of the macrophage is to engulf particles to eliminate them from the alveolar space [23]. Type I pneumocytes serve as a thin gas-permeable epithelial barrier [24]. Type II pneumocytes have a role in defense of the alveoli thanks to their physiological abilities [25]. In the alveoli, macrophages and epithelial cells are at the ALI and are covered by a thin layer of surfactant secreted at the apical side by the type II pneumocytes.

To mimic the cell organization at the alveolar surface and the potential interactions between the cells and the NMs, a co-culture using two cell types was selected in vitro. The A549 alveolar epithelial cell line was selected for its ability to form a cell layer and to secrete surfactant [23, 26]. The THP-1 monocyte cell line was chosen for its capacity to differentiate into macrophage-like cells with Phorbol Myristate Acetate (PMA) [27]. This model was selected for its increased sensitivity compared to mono-cultures of alveolar epithelial cells at the ALI [13] and in submerged conditions [28–30]. We also postulated that with this co-culture model, the deposited NMs could become covered with surfactant before they interact with the cells, as observed in the alveoli in vivo [22]. Nevertheless, because the presence of surfactant was not evaluated in our study, it remains unclear whether the cells and the NMs were covered by surfactant.

Different exposure methods were assessed. In vivo, rats were exposed for 24 h by intratracheal instillation of NM suspensions, after hyperventilation. In vitro, cells were exposed using more or less advanced methods. Co-cultures were exposed at the ALI in inserts to simulate more closely the interactions between NMs and alveolar cells occurring in vivo, and to avoid contamination with culture medium. The ALI exposure system used in our study [13] was selected for its ability to deposit sufficient amounts of NMs on cells to observe biological adverse effects [31, 32]. In parallel we also used a more classical exposure method and cells were exposed to NM suspensions in submerged conditions to assess the general impact of the culture medium surrounding poorly soluble NMs on the cell biological response.

Both in vivo and in vitro, the toxicity was assessed after 24 h of exposure to the same TiO_2 and CeO_2 NMs. For that, we focused on the deposited doses on cells or into the lungs, because metallic and poorly soluble NMs exert their toxicity mainly by direct contact with the cells [17]. Moreover, we tested different timings of the dose delivery in vitro, to assess if that factor could influence the cell response. In vivo, the final doses of NMs were deposited by instillation almost instantly into the lungs. At the ALI in vitro, NMs were deposited on the cells using a very low aerosol flow rate of 5 mL/min to prevent cell damages due to the air flux. To deposit a dose sufficient to observe biological effects, cells were exposed for 3 h to aerosols. After exposure, the cells were then kept in the incubator for the remaining 24 h with NMs deposited on their surface. In submerged conditions, it was not possible to deposit the NMs instantly on the cells either, as the deposition kinetics depended mostly on their sedimentation rate. In

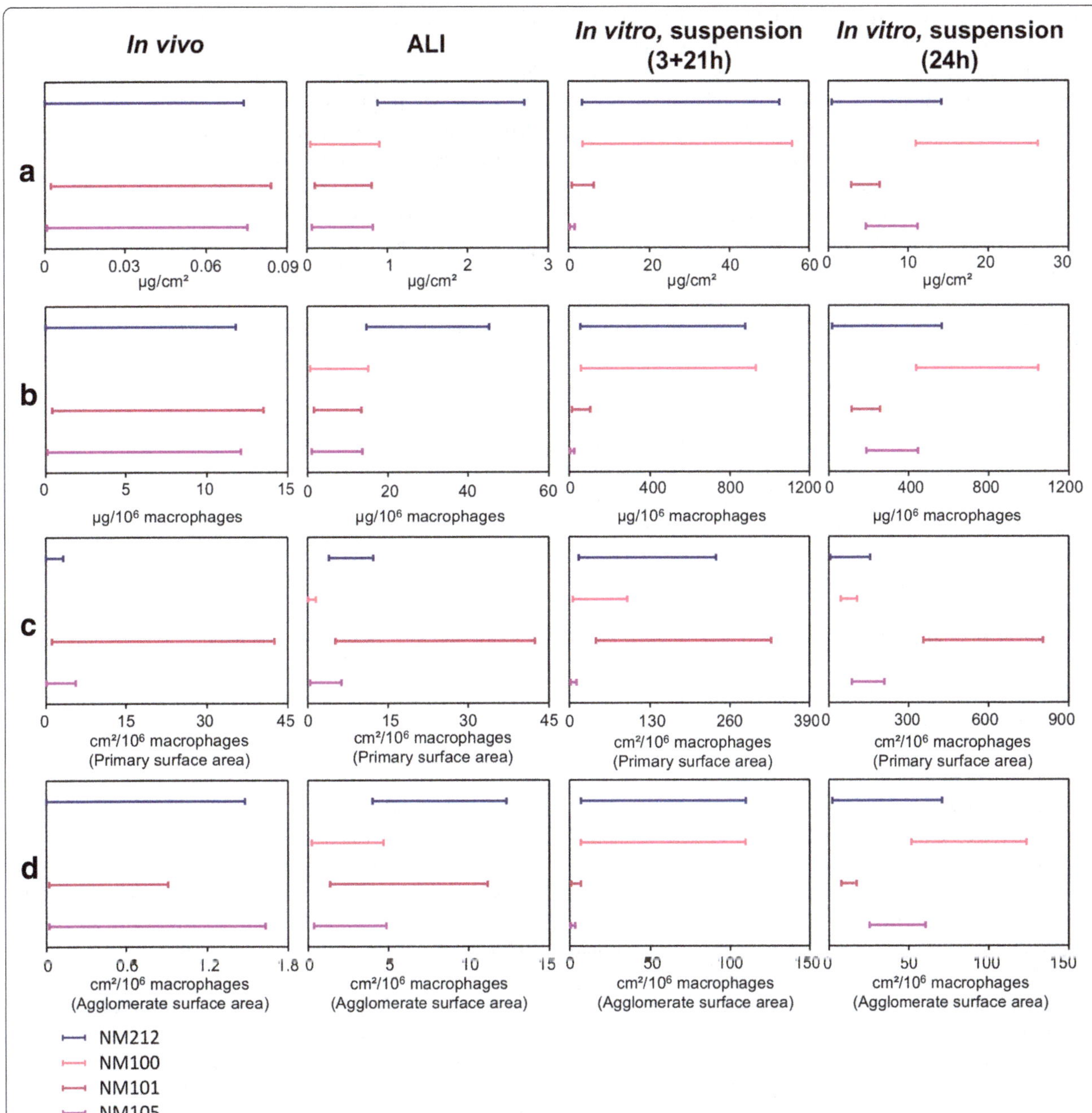

Fig. 5 Dose intervals of NMs for inflammation according to methodologies and dose metrics used. Dose intervals calculated for general acute pro-inflammatory response were used to compare the ranking of each NM in function of each exposure method used. Comparisons were also performed according to the four dose metrics used in our study (**a**: mass/alveolar surface), (**b**: mass/macrophages), (**c**: dose in mass/macrophages normalized by primary surface area), (**d**: dose in mass/macrophages normalized by agglomerate surface area). In vitro, alveolar epithelial cells in co-culture with macrophages were exposed for 24 h at the air-liquid interface (ALI) or in submerged conditions to suspensions of NMs. In vivo, rats were exposed by intratracheal instillation of NM suspensions. After 24 h of exposure, the biological activity was assessed, focusing on pro-inflammatory mediators. For each exposure method, each NM and each cytokine, benchmark dose-response modeling was used to estimate the critical dose related to a 20% increase of pro-inflammatory mediator level and the lowest (BMDL) and the highest (BMDU) dose of the interval corresponding to a confidence interval of 90%. A median dose intervals was then calculated by pooling the dose intervals of the four cytokine to have a general pro-inflammatory response

inserts, we used the duration of 3 h for the dose delivery, in order to provide comparisons as accurate as possible between ALI and submerged exposure. As for the ALI, the cells were kept for the remaining 21 h with NMs deposited on their surface. In submerged conditions in plates, we used classical exposure conditions and the NM deposition on the cells was maintained for 24 h.

Similar endpoints were selected to compare in vivo and in vitro toxicity. The biological responses were assessed after 24 h of exposure to the NMs, by performing cytotoxicity, oxidative stress and inflammation assays, to determine the absolute toxicity of each NM. Both in vivo and in vitro, we observed that inflammation was the most sensitive parameter for detection of biological responses at 24 h. After NM exposure, we detected significantly more pro-inflammatory effects than cytotoxicity and oxidative stress responses, and generally at lower doses. We were not surprised about the absence of clear pulmonary cytotoxic effects in our study as poorly soluble TiO_2 and CeO_2 NMs were shown to be not very cytotoxic at 24 h both in vivo and in vitro [33]. Regarding oxidative stress production, as ROS are known to interact quickly with molecules present in the cells, better detection could have been achieved by performing several measurements during the 24 h of exposure. Moreover, in our protocol, cells were incubated with DCFDA probe after exposure and not before exposure which may have reduced assay sensitivity [34]. Nevertheless, in absence of cytotoxicity at 24 h, which is the case in our study, the authors did not show a clear increase of ROS measurement sensitivity when the probe was added before NM exposure [34].

For these reasons, comparisons were performed mostly with inflammation markers as readout for NM toxicity. Nevertheless, it has to be noted that the inflammatory effects were observed at high doses (at least 10-fold higher) compared to realistic human exposure scenarios [7]. The markers of inflammation used in our study were selected according to their relevance in representing the pro-inflammatory acute response in the lungs after exposure to particles [35, 36]. Similar pro-inflammatory mediators were chosen in vitro and in vivo, however those significantly secreted in vitro were not necessarily predominant in vivo. On the basis of this finding we assumed that better comparisons could be provided in our study by considering the global inflammatory response, more particularly the secretion of pro-inflammatory mediators that can be measured both in vivo and in vitro.

To perform quantitative comparisons, LOAELs were first determined according to the significant pro-inflammatory responses observed. Secondly, we used benchmark dose-response modeling to determine dose intervals related to increase in pro-inflammatory mediator levels. There are multiple advantages of using benchmark dose modeling instead of a No Observed Adverse Level (NOAEL) or LOAEL approach in hazard assessment. Using NOAEL/LOAEL approach, toxic effects are reduced to a yes/no question and are typically determined based on the presence or absence of statistical significance. Moreover, the uncertainty in the NOAELs or LOAELs cannot be quantified and can be considerable as it sticks only to the dose tested. Thus NOAELs and LOAELS determined depend strongly on the study design [37–39]. On the contrary, dose intervals determined by benchmark modeling take the potency of NMs to induce an effect into account and take uncertainty in the data into account. The question is not whether an effect is induced or not, but at what dose an effect of interest is induced. These dose intervals provide more accurate comparisons between in vivo and in vitro data. [37–39].

Although there were clear advantages in using dose intervals, some uncertainties remain in our study regarding their determination due to limited log dose data intervals and because the pro-inflammatory effects were observed mostly at the highest doses tested. This highlights the importance of providing experimental data that should allow to model a reasonable response slope by either providing a clear dose-response pattern of toxicity (that implies the use of toxic compounds) or more refined tested doses in case of low toxicity. The more experimental doses are tested, the more accurate is the analysis and this is true also for NOAEL/LOAEL assessment.

Comparisons were performed with LOAELs and dose intervals to assess if similar conclusions could be made using the two criteria of effect dose. As the LOAELs and dose intervals were associated with dose metrics, the key point for the comparisons was to select similar metrics for both in vivo and in vitro methodologies. For that, we focused on the deposited masses because it take into account the direct contact between the NMs and the tissues, that was shown to be the main cause of toxicity for poorly soluble NMs [15–17]. Doses in mass were first normalized to the total alveolar surface in vivo or to the surface of the cell layer in vitro. This normalization was based on the assumption that the alveolar epithelium may be the main target after acute exposure to NMs [14, 22].

Expressing results in mass/alveolar surface, we observed responses at doses around ten times lower in vivo (LOAELs at 0.1 $\mu g/cm^2$ and BMDU around 0.08 $\mu g/cm^2$) than in vitro at the ALI (LOAELs at 1 $\mu g/cm^2$, BMDU from 0.8 to 2.7 $\mu g/cm^2$). The differences were slightly more pronounced in submerged conditions when the dose was delivered in 3 h (at least 20-fold compared to in vivo) (LOAELs at 3 $\mu g/cm^2$, BMDU from 1.5 to 55 $\mu g/cm^2$), and much more important, with a factor of around 100, when the deposition of the NMs was continuous during the 24 h of in vitro exposure (LOAELs at 10 $\mu g/cm^2$, BMDU from 6.4 to 26 $\mu g/cm^2$). Interestingly, when comparing in vivo and in vitro biological activation levels using the mass/alveolar surface metric, similar differences were observed with LOAELs and dose intervals determined using benchmark dose-response modeling. This indicates that similar conclusions could be made using these two criteria of effect, when comparing biological activation levels in vivo and in vitro.

In vivo and in vitro results expressed in mass/alveolar surface were also compared in three noteworthy studies [10, 11, 40]. In their study, Kim et al. [10] observed similar pro-inflammatory profiles when expressing the doses in μg/cm^2, after exposing mice by oropharyngeal aspiration and macrophages or lung slices to suspensions of TiO_2, CeO_2 and SiO_2 NMs. Nevertheless, the real masses of NMs deposited in vitro and ex vivo were not assessed and no clear quantitative comparisons were performed between the in vivo and the in vitro approaches, which renders the interpretation of the results from their study difficult. Jing et al. [40] compared the responses after acute exposure to Cu NPs, in mice lungs and in alveolar epithelial cells at the ALI. They observed similar responses (chemokine and LDH release) but apparently at lower doses in vitro compared to in vivo, when expressing the dose in ng/cm^2. Nevertheless, the responses were assessed at 2 h or 4 h in vitro and at 24 h or 40 h in vivo, which brings uncertainties towards their comparative results. Teeguarden et al. [11] exposed mice in vivo by inhalation or lung epithelial cells in vitro with suspensions of FeO NMs for 4 h with similar timings of the dose delivery and assessed the mass and regional deposition of the NMs. When focusing on the tracheobronchal part of the lung, they observed pro-inflammatory responses with doses about 10 to 100-time lower in vivo than in vitro. However, they did not study the response of the alveolar part of the lung with this metric. Instead, they normalized the doses in mass by the number of alveolar macrophages in vivo and in vitro. Indeed, monocultures of murine macrophages were also exposed to suspensions in their study [11]. When focusing on the alveolar macrophages, they showed that pro-inflammatory responses were triggered at similar doses in vitro and in vivo.

Interestingly, we also observed significant effects at much closer doses in vivo (LOAELs at 16 μg/10^6 macrophages, BMDU around 12 μg/10^6 macrophages) and in vitro using this dose metric, and more particularly at the ALI (LOAELs at 16.7 μg/10^6 macrophages, BMDU from 13 to 45 μg/10^6 macrophages) and when the dose was deposited in submerged conditions on the cells within 3 h (LOAELs at 50 μg/10^6 macrophages, BMDU from 25 to 900 μg/10^6 macrophage), rather than in 24 h (LOAELs at 400 μg/10^6 macrophages, BMDU from 250 to 1000 μg/10^6 macrophage). As shown by using the mass/alveolar surface metric, similar differences were observed using LOAELs and dose intervals, when comparing in vivo and in vitro biological activation levels using the mass/macrophage metric. Nevertheless, for the NMs 100 and 212 the differences of toxicity observed between submerged exposure in inserts for 3 h and submerged exposure in plates for 24 h were less obvious when looking at the interval of doses instead of the LOAELs. Finally, pro-inflammatory effects were still observed at higher doses in vitro in submerged conditions compared to at the ALI or in vivo. Although serum was added in our in vitro experiments in submerged conditions to keep the cells in their best physiological conditions, we hypothesized that the presence of serum may have reduced potential NM toxicity. Indeed, it has been shown that NMs were less toxic in vitro in presence of serum in suspensions compared to in absence of serum [41, 42]. Taking that into account, better correlations at 24 h may be provided in absence of serum, however this point still has to be demonstrated.

Although differences exist regarding the cellular and animal models and the duration of exposure between the Teeguarden study and ours, this seems to indicate that focusing on the cell number might better explain the general acute pro-inflammatory response elicited by NMs in the alveoli, both in vivo and in vitro. However, in our study we did not discriminate between the responses from the alveolar epithelial cells and the macrophages. Moreover, it should be noted that although a ratio of one macrophage for ten pneumocytes was used to mimic in vitro the ratio present in vivo in rat or human lungs [18], the number of macrophages/cm^2 (60,000/cm^2 in inserts or 25,000/cm^2 in plates) was higher in vitro compared to in vivo (around 6000 macrophages/cm^2) because the A549 cell surface in vitro was much lower than the alveolar epithelial cell surface in vivo. This could explain why in vivo and in vitro results were matching better when the doses were expressed in mass/macrophages rather by in mass/alveolar surface.

Ranking comparisons were also performed between the four NMs tested. For ranking comparisons, we focused on dose intervals only. Indeed, LOAELs are depending a lot on the experimental design as they are strictly determined according to the doses tested. In the case of few doses are tested and when NMs are observed to be toxic only at the highest doses tested, like in our study, LOAELs do not allow to make clear differences between the NMs. However, with dose intervals determined using benchmark dose-response modeling, more accurate effect doses were determined for each NM and each exposure method. Thanks to this criterion of dose, a better screening of the four NMs has been performed. The comparisons were performed using the mass metric but also with the surface area metric, since it was shown that the surface area was the most effective dose metric to explain acute NM toxicity in the lung [16, 17, 43].

Expressing the doses in mass (mass/alveolar surface or mass/macrophages), similarity in the rankings were observed between in vivo and in vitro conditions for the three TiO_2 NMs. Both in vivo and in vitro, NMs 105 and 101 appeared more toxic than NM100, except at the

ALI were similar toxicity was observed for the three TiO_2 NMs. However, it was not the case for the CeO_2 NM212. NM212 was observed as toxic as NMs 105 and 101 and more toxic than NM100 in vivo, whereas it was observed to be less toxic than the TiO_2 NMs 105 and 101 in vitro. Moreover, we noticed that the ranking of the NMs could change according to the dose metric used. Generally, when using the NM mass as dose metric, the NM101 appeared as toxic as the NM105 and more toxic than the NMs 212 and 100. Nevertheless, although we observed similarities in nanomaterial rankings between in vivo and in vitro approaches, benchmark dose intervals were too large to make clear ranking comparisons, due to the insufficient quality of the data-set. This underlines the importance of providing good quality data to perform reliable comparisons. Because of the insufficient quality of the data-set, it remains thus undetermined if ALI exposure methods could provide better predictivity than submerged methods regarding the ranking of the NMs.

When doses in mass were normalized by NM primary surface areas, the NM101, that has the highest surface activity, was observed to be less toxic than expected and clearly appeared less toxic than the other NMs. Indeed, based on the surface reactivity theory which implies that higher NM surface areas induce higher potential toxicities [44], similar responses were to be expected from these three NMs when normalizing the dose by surface area. This has been shown in vivo [45] and in vitro [16]. Because this was not the case, we hypothesized that the hydrophobic surface coating that surrounds the NM101 but not NM105, NM100 and NM212 may have contributed to reduce the toxic potential of NM101. This was not surprising as it was shown in several studies that NM acute toxicity was more dependent on coating than on core properties [46, 47].

However, when the doses in mass/macrophages were normalized by surface areas calculated using mean agglomerate sizes and densities, we did not observe this clear change in the NM101 ranking. Indeed, similarities in the rankings were observed between doses expressed in mass/macrophages and in cm^2/macrophages when surface areas were calculated using mean agglomerate sizes and densities. This indicates that focusing on mean surface areas in exposure media rather than on primary surface areas may better explain the biological responses observed with poorly soluble NMs. Nevertheless, further investigations are necessary to confirm this allegation.

Comparing several in vitro methods to the in vivo approach, that was considered as the reference method in our study to estimate the potential toxicity of NMs in humans, allowed us to evaluate the predictive ability of different in vitro system in absolute terms. Finally, according to our results, it seems that the use of advanced and realistic in vitro methodologies allows to predict more closely the biological responses observed in vivo and thus might give a better estimation of the potential absolute toxicity in humans.

Nevertheless, further improvements still need to be made to draw clear conclusions. In our study, the animals were exposed by suspension instillation and not by inhalation of aerosols containing NMs. The instillation method remains less physiologic than the inhalation route, especially because the dose is instantly deposited into the lungs using a bolus. This could induce a greater biological response compared to inhalation, where the final dose is generally deposited within 4 h [48]. Moreover, although the instillation method allows to deposit NMs more deeply into the lungs [49], there was a lack of accurate dosimetry in our study as the Multiple-Path Particle Dosimetry Model (MPPD) [50] could not be used. Thus, the regional deposition and more particularly the real dose distributed to the alveoli was not accurately evaluated.

Furthermore, some limitations remain regarding the assessment of dose delivery in vitro, more particularly in submerged conditions as the deposited dose on cells was estimated using the ISDD model and not directly measured. Nevertheless, the relative uncertainty was probably low as good similarities were observed between the estimated and measured deposited doses of poorly soluble NMs at 24 h [51]. At 3 h, the uncertainty may have been higher and could have led to an underestimation of the deposited dose [51]. This may have contributed to increased differences between the ALI and the submerged exposures in terms of biological activation levels.

Another reason why it is difficult to conclude clearly that the use of advanced and realistic in vitro methodologies might give a better estimation of the potential absolute toxicity in humans is that some uncertainties exist regarding the dose metrics selected. To compare the in vivo to the in vitro approach, we normalized the dose in vivo in mass by the total alveolar surface. We decided to use the value of 4000 cm^2 [18, 19], which seemed suitable for 7 weeks old male rats. Nevertheless, this may represent an overestimation as alveolar surfaces of around 2000 [52], and 3400 cm^2 [53] have also been calculated for 6 weeks and 60 days old rats, respectively. To normalize the dose by the number of macrophages, we assumed that around 25 million of macrophages were in the alveoli in vivo and we used the number of counted macrophages in vitro. Although we based ourselves on two publications [18, 54] to determine the number of alveolar macrophages in vivo, it remains unclear whether all of them were in contact and contributed to the biological response elicited by the NMs, more particularly considering that only around 8 million of macrophages were retrieved in the BALF in vivo.

Nevertheless, we decided to use the value of 25 million of macrophages instead of the measured value of 8 million because we observed that the number of macrophages retrieved from the BALF was depending a lot on the experimenter and because the protocol used in our study was not implemented to retrieve all the alveolar macrophages.

Some uncertainties also remain because our experimental data-set did not allow to provide a clear dose-response pattern of toxicity. That may had an impact on the accuracy of our comparisons. For example in vivo, there was a difference of a factor of ten between each dose tested; this might prevent us to determine accurate LOAELs and dose intervals. This is particularly true because the pro-inflammatory effects were observed at the highest dose tested. Although using intermediary doses might have enabled to determine more precisely LOAELs and critical dose intervals, this has no impact on our general conclusions regarding comparison of biological activation levels between the different exposure methods used in our study: regardless the criterion of comparison used, the in vivo methodology remains the most sensitive one in our study, to predict potential adverse effects after acute exposure to poorly soluble NMs. Regarding NM rankings, we observed that it was difficult to use LOAELs to rank NMs in function of each exposure methodology used and that determining dose intervals using benchmark dose-response modeling was very important for this purpose. However, because the data-set quality used in our study was not optimal, the dose intervals determined were too large to provide clear and reliable comparisons of NM rankings between each methodology used. To perform in vivo - in vitro comparisons we thus recommend to test more doses and to reduce the interval between each doses, in order to determine more accurate dose intervals.

Conclusion

Quantitative comparisons were performed between in vivo and in vitro acute pro-inflammatory responses using compatible dose metrics. Biological activation levels were compared and we showed better in vivo- in vitro correlations when doses were expressed in mass/macrophages rather than in mass/alveolar surface. Using the determined LOAELs and critical effect dose intervals, we assessed the ability of each in vitro method used in our study to predict the biological responses in vivo. We showed that the most realistic in vitro exposure method: the ALI method, was the most predictive in terms of absolute toxicity, whatever the dose metric used. In vitro, we also showed better *vivo-vitro* correlations while using timings of dose delivery of 3 h rather than 24 h. For each exposure method, we ranked NMs in function of their toxicity and we highlighted that critical effect dose intervals could be used instead of LOAELs to provide more accurate comparisons between the NMs. Regarding toxicity rankings of NMs, relative similarities were shown between in vivo and in vitro methodologies. Nevertheless, we could not conclude clearly about each in vitro methodology ability to predict the NM rankings observed in vivo because the quality of the data-set was insufficient to determine accurate dose intervals. Interestingly, we also observed when normalizing the doses by NM surface areas, that the toxic effects were probably more attributable to agglomerates, rather than to isolate NMs.

In conclusion, we showed that advanced methods could be used to enhance the in vitro experiments ability to predict potential acute pulmonary toxicity in vivo. Moreover, we highlighted that careful consideration of some key methodological points in vitro could contribute to improve in vitro methods predictivity, including control of the timing of the dose delivery. Although these conclusions are inferred from our experimental data-set and should be further confirmed with other nanomaterials, including more toxic NMs, this study brings new perspectives regarding the usage and development of advanced in vitro methods.

Methods

Nanomaterials

Four poorly toxic and poorly soluble NMs were used in the study. The TiO_2 NM100 and NM101 and the CeO_2 NM212 were obtained from the Joint research center (JRC). The TiO_2 NM105 was obtained from Evonik Industries (AEROXIDE® TiO_2 P25). Data indicated in our study regarding primary sizes and specific surface areas (BET) were provided by the manufacturer (Table 1). TiO_2 and CeO_2 primary physico-chemical properties were also well characterized by the JRC. [55, 56]. The endotoxin levels of the NMs were tested by partners of the European project NANoREG. They were below the limit of detection (data not shown).

In vivo study

Animals

Pathogens free 7 weeks old male rats (WISTAR RjHan:WI, JANVIER LABS, France; 250 g), were housed in polycarbonate cages, in a temperature and humidity controlled room, and had free access to food and water ad libitum. All the in vivo experiments were approved by the "Comité Régional d'Ethique en Matière d'Expérimentation Animale de Picardie" (CREMEAP) (C2EA – 96).

Preparation of NM suspensions

Similarly as for the in vitro study, suspensions of TiO_2 (NM105, NM101, NM100) and CeO_2 (NM212) at 10 mg/mL in Mili-Q water were prepared and then sonicated at amplitude 100 during 2 min (1 min on, 1 min off, 1 min on) using a cuphorn sonicator (QSONICA, Q700). Suspensions in Milli-Q water at 5; 0.5 and 0.05 mg/mL were prepared to expose rats to 500; 50 and 5 μg/animal, respectively.

Characterization of NM suspensions

For each NM, DLS measurements were performed (Malvern, Zetasizer Nano S) on NM suspensions to measure the hydrodynamic diameter and to assess the size distribution of the particles in suspensions. DLS results on water suspensions used to instill animals are presented in the Additional files section (Additional file 1: Figure S4). Regarding in vitro experiments, DLS measurements were performed after sonication in stock suspensions (2.56 mg/mL in milli-Q water) and just after dilution in 0.4 mg/mL suspensions in culture medium. These in vitro results were presented in our previous article [13]. Surprisingly, similar results were observed between NM suspended in water and in culture medium.

Intratracheal instillation

Rats were anesthetized (0.5 mg/kg ketamine hydrochloride, 0.1 mg/kg atropine and 1 mg/kg xylazine), endotracheal intubation was performed using a canula and animals were connected to a respirator (Harvard Apparatus, ventilator model 683) for 30 s to create a hyperventilation. Rats were disconnected from the apparatus, 100 μL of NMs suspension in water or vehicle (Mili-Q water) was added in the cannula and suspensions were directly aerosolized into rat lungs by physiological aspiration. It was chosen to disperse NMs in Milli-Q water and not in physiological saline buffer to enhance NM stability in suspension. This choice was made since it was shown that intratracheal instillation of distilled water in rats, like physiological saline, did not induce significant inflammatory responses at 24 h [9].

Dosing and biodistribution analysis

After instillation, rats were sacrificed 3 h after instillation to evaluate the lung burden ($n = 2$). Mass of NM was measured in collected lungs by inductively coupled plasma mass spectrometry (ICP-MS) analysis. Briefly, a procedure consisting of incubation with a mixture of nitric acid (HNO3) and hydrofluoric acid (HF), and heating was applied to digest lungs and TiO_2 nanomaterials in order to determine the total Ti content by ICP-MS [57].

Assessment of biological activity

Animals ($n = 6$) were sacrificed 24 h after instillation and bronchoalveolar lavages were performed with PBS. A first bronchoalveolar lavage was performed using 5 mL of PBS for biochemical analysis. Two other lavages were then performed with 10 mL of PBS to collect more cells. Collected BALFs were centrifuged at 350 g for 10 min and 4 °C, to separate the cells from the supernatant. The supernatants recovered from the first lavage (around 4.5 mL for each sample) were aliquoted in eppendorf tubes and stored at − 80 °C until analysis.

Cell counting After centrifugation, the cell pellets were resuspended in 5 mL of RPMI medium (Gibco, 61870), 20 μL of cell suspension were mixed with 20 μL of propidium iodide containing accridine solution (Nexcelom, CS2-0106) and the cells were counted using a cell counter equipped with a fluorometer (Nexcelom, Cellometer® Auto 2000), to differentiate the dead cells and the erythrocytes from the pulmonary cells.

BALF cytology After counting, the cells were diluted in RPMI, seeded on slides at 300000 cells/spots using a cytospin (300 g, 5 min) (Shandon, cytospin2) and then fixated and coloured in May-Grunwald Giemsa (MGG). Briefly, the slides were fixated in MG pure for 3 min followed by 2 min in MG diluted at 50% in Mili-Q water, rinsed 2 times with Mili-Q water for 20 min and then coloured in Giemsa. The percentage of the different cell types (macrophages, neutrophils, eosinophil) in BALF was then determined using optical microscopy.

Intracellular ROS levels (DCF assay) After counting, the BALF cells were seeded at 1×10^6 cells/mL in 24 well plates (Falcon, 353047) (in RPMI medium supplemented with 10% of FCS: 0,5 mL/well), and were then incubated for 18 h at 37 °C and with 5% of CO_2 to let the cells (mostly macrophages) to adhere on the plate. The cells were then rinsed with PBS and incubated for 35 min with 10 μM of 5-(and-6)-chloromethyl-2′,7′-dichlorodihydrofluorescein diacetate (CM-H_2DCFDA) probe (Life technologies, C6827) in PBS (0.5 mL/well). After 30 min of incubation, the probe was removed in some control wells, 1 mM of H_2O_2 in PBS was added and the cells were incubated for 5 min, to serve as positive control. After incubation, the cells were washed with PBS and incubated for 5 min in 90% of Dimethyl Sulfoxide (DMSO) (Sigma-Aldrich, D2438) in PBS (0.5 mL/well). The cells were then scraped using scrapers (TPP, 99002), the well contents were retrieved in tubes (Eppendorf, 3810X) and the tubes were centrifuged at 10000 g and 4 °C for 5 min, to eliminate the dead cells and to remove the remnants particles. The tube contents were transferred in 96 well black plate (150 μL/well) (Greiner Bio-one, 655076) and the fluorescence of the samples was read (excitation: 488 nm, emission: 530 nm) using a spectrophotometer (TECAN, infinite 2000). The value of each sample was expressed in percentage of intracellular ROS compared to the control.

Pro-inflammatory release in BALF supernatants Il-1β, IL-6, IL-8 and TNF-α releases were measured in collected supernatants using a commercial available ELISA multiplex kit (Mesoscale discovery, Proinflammatory Panel 2, N05059A-1) and a multiplex reader (Mesoscale discovery, Sector Imager 24000) according to supplier recommendations.

LDH release and protein levels in BALF supernatants LDH release were quantified in BALF using a commercially available kit (Promega, CytoTox-ONE Homogeneous Membrane Integrity assay). Proteins levels were measured in BALF using a Bradford assay (Biorad, protein assay kit).

Statistical analysis All data were expressed as mean ± standard deviation (SD) ($n = 6$). Statistical analyses were performed using Graphpad Prism 5.0 (GraphPad Software Inc., San Diego, CA). Results were analyzed by a non-parametric Kruskal-Wallis test followed by Dunn's post-hoc test to compare the different treated groups to the non-exposed control.

In vitro study

All materials and methods used in the in vitro study are fully detailed in the following article [13]. Briefly, alveolar epithelial cells (A549) in co-culture with macrophages (THP-1) were exposed either at the ALI to aerosols or in submerged condition to suspensions of TiO_2 and CeO_2 NMs. A ratio of ten A549 for one THP-1 was used to mimic the ratio existing in vivo in the lungs.

Different timings of the dose delivery were used in vitro. At the ALI, cells were exposed to aerosol of NMs using a Vitrocell® system. In this system, the NM deposition was maintained for 3 h, meaning that the final dose was reached within 3 h. The cells were then kept in the incubator for the remaining 21 h at the ALI with the NMs deposited on their surface. In submerged conditions, two different dose rates were used. Cells were exposed to suspensions of NMs in inserts using similar timing of the dose delivery as at the ALI. The NM deposition was maintained for 3 h. After 3 h of exposure, the deposition was stopped by replacing NM suspensions by fresh medium and cells were then kept during the remaining 21 h in submerged condition in the incubator. Cells were also exposed in plates to suspensions of NMs for 24 h, to represent the exposure conditions usually used in vitro. In that situation, the NM deposition was maintained for the whole exposure time, meaning that the final dose was reached within 24 h. After 24 h of exposure, the biological activity of the cells was assessed for all methodologies using cytotoxicity (Alamar blue, LDH), inflammation (IL-1b, IL-6, IL-8, TNF-α levels in culture medium (ELISA)), and oxidative stress assays (DCF assay).

Deposited dose assessment

In vivo, the mass of each NM instilled into the lungs was measured by ICP-MS. The nominal doses (5; 50; 500 μg/animal) were corrected to 4; 40 and 400 μg/animal according to dosage results (Additional file 1: Figure S5). According to the lung alveolar surface (4000 cm^2) or the number of alveolar macrophages (25 million), this corresponds to theoretical deposited doses in lungs of around 0.1; 0.01; 0.001 μg/cm^2 or 16; 1.6; 0.16 μg/10^6 macrophages, respectively.

In vitro, the real mass deposited on the cells was either assessed by ICP-MS dosage (for ALI exposures) or estimated (in submerged conditions) using the in vitro sedimentation diffusion and dosimetry model (ISDD) [58], after measuring the hydrodynamic diameter by dynamic light scattering and the effective density of the agglomerates following the Volumetric Centrifugation Method (VCM) [59]. The detailed material and methods used in vitro and all the deposition data are available in the following paper [13]. Deposited masses on cells in vitro are also presented in the Additional files section of the present manuscript (Additional file 1: Tables S1 and S6). The final measured or calculated doses tested were around 0,1; 1; 3 μg/cm^2 at the ALI (for 3 h of maintained deposition + 21 h without deposition in the incubator), 1; 3; 10 μg/cm^2 in submerged in inserts (for 3 h of maintained deposition + 21 h without deposition in the incubator) and 1, 3, 10, 20 μg/cm^2 in submerged in plates (24 h of maintained deposition).

Determination of critical dose intervals using benchmark dose-response modeling

All the in vivo and in vitro data were analyzed using the benchmark dose-response modeling software PROAST (RIVM, Bilthoven, The Netherlands). The PROAST software selects the optimal data fitting model from an exponential family of models. Briefly, for each cytokine and each exposure method used (in vivo, ALI (3 h + 21 h), submerged in inserts (3 h + 21 h), submerged in plates (24 h)), we determined the critical effect dose corresponding to a 20% increase of pro-inflammatory mediator levels compared to non-exposed controls and the benchmark dose lower confidence limit (BMDL) and the benchmark dose upper confidence limit (BMDU) of the interval for a 90% confidence. For each exposure method used and each NM, we then calculated the median value of the BMDL and the median value of the BMDU of the four pro-inflammatory mediators (IL-1β, IL-6, IL-8/KC-GRO, TNF-α), to determine a median dose interval for general pro-inflammatory response. We decided to calculate the median dose interval of the four cytokines because similar results could be observed when pooling the results of the four cytokines and when comparing dose intervals of each cytokine one by one. We believe that our comparisons were easier to interpret in our study when using a general pro-inflammatory response. We choose a critical effect of 20% based on the magnitude of effect in several notable studies [16, 60, 61].

Additional files

Additional file 1: Figure S1. Levels of pro-inflammatory mediators in cell supernatants in vitro (adapted from [13]). **Figure S2.** Levels of proteins, LDH (cytotoxicity) and intracellular ROS (oxidative stress) in BALF. **Figure S3.** Examples of critical effect doses (CED) and dose intervals (CEDL/BMDL and CEDU/BMDU) determined using benchmark dose response modeling. **Figure S4.** Size distribution of the NMs in the suspensions used to expose rats. **Figure S5.** Initial lung burden in vivo assessed by ICP-MS 3 h after instillation ($n = 2$). **Table S1.** Doses deposited in vitro in submerged conditions in function of nominal concentrations in suspensions (First published in [13]). **Table S2.** LOAELs (in $\mu g/cm^2$) determined in vitro with the pro-inflammatory effects for each exposure method used (First published in [13]). **Table S3.** Dose intervals (in $\mu g/10^6$ macrophages) determined for each NM and each methodology. **Table S4.** Dose intervals normalized by primary surface areas (in $cm^2/10^6$-macrophages) for each NM and methodology. **Table S5.** Dose intervals normalized by agglomerate surface areas (in $cm^2/10^6$ macrophages) for each NM and methodology. **Table S6.** Characterization of mass deposited in vitro on cells after 3 h exposure at the ALI to aerosols of NMs (Adapted from [13]). (DOCX 831 kb)

Abbreviations

ALI: Air-Liquid Interface; BALF: BronchoAlveolar Lavage Fluids; BET: Brunauer–Emmett–Teller; BMDL: Benchmark Dose Lower confidence limit; BMDU: Benchmark Dose Upper confidence limit; DLS: Dynamic Light Scattering; DMSO: Dimethyl Sulfoxide; ICP-MS: Inductively Coupled Plasma - Mass Spectrometry; ISDD: In vitro Sedimentation Diffusion and Dosimetry; JRC: Joint Research center; LDH: Lactate DeHydrogenase; LOAEL: Lowest Observed Adverse Effect Level; MGG: May-Grunwald Giemsa; NM(s): NanoMaterial(s); NOAEL: No Observed Adverse Effect Level; PMA: Phorbol Myristate Acetate; ROS: Reactive Oxygen Species; SD: Standard Deviation; VCM: Volumetric Centrifugation Method

Acknowledgements

We thank Christelle Gamez, Kelly Blazy, Franck Robidel, Anthony Lecomte and Emanuel Peyret for their technical assistance regarding animal experimentations. We thank Camille Rey for the critical revision and the language corrections.

Funding

This work was supported by the French ministry of environment ("Programme 190") and by the EU-FP7 (NANoREG project).

Authors' contributions

The manuscript was written through contributions of all authors. All authors gave approval to the final version of the manuscript. TL designed and performed the experiments, analyzed and interpreted the data, wrote and revised the manuscript. FR was involved in the design, the performance of in vivo experiments. BT, AB, CE were involved in the writing and the revisions. GL designed the study and was involved in the performance of the in vivo experiments, the writing and the revisions.

Competing interests

The authors declare that they have no competing interests.

Author details

Institut National de l'Environnement Industriel et des Risques (INERIS), (DRC/VIVA/TOXI), Parc Technologique ALATA - BP 2, F-60550 Verneuil-en-Halatte, France. [2]Université de Technologie de Compiègne (UTC), Laboratoire BioMécanique et BioIngénierie (BMBI), UMR CNRS 7338, 60205 Compiègne, France. [3]Department of Biomedical Engineering, Tufts University, Medford, MA, USA.

References

1. Bakand S, Hayes A, Dechsakulthorn F. Nanoparticles: a review of particle toxicology following inhalation exposure. Inhal Toxicol. 2012;24(2):125–35.
2. Piccinno F, Gottschalk F, Seeger S, Nowack B. Industrial production quantities and uses of ten engineered nanomaterials in Europe and the world. J Nanopart Res. 2012;14(9):1109.
3. Oomen AG, Bos PM, Fernandes TF, Hund-Rinke K, Boraschi D, Byrne HJ, et al. Concern-driven integrated approaches to nanomaterial testing and assessment–report of the NanoSafety Cluster Working Group 10. Nanotoxicology. 2014;8(3):334–48.
4. Nel A, Xia T, Meng H, Wang X, Lin S, Ji Z, et al. Nanomaterial toxicity testing in the 21st century: use of a predictive toxicological approach and high-throughput screening. Acc Chem Res. 2013;46(3):607–21.
5. Joris F, Manshian BB, Peynshaert K, De Smedt SC, Braeckmans K, Soenen SJ. Assessing nanoparticle toxicity in cell-based assays: influence of cell culture parameters and optimized models for bridging the in vitro-in vivo gap. Chem Soc Rev. 2013;42(21):8339–59.
6. BeruBe K, Aufderheide M, Breheny D, Clothier R, Combes R, Duffin R, et al. In vitro models of inhalation toxicity and disease. The report of a FRAME workshop. ATLA. 2009;37(1):89–141.
7. Paur HR, Cassee FR, Teeguarden J, Fissan H, Diabate S, Aufderheide M, et al. In-vitro cell exposure studies for the assessment of nanoparticle toxicity in the lung—a dialog between aerosol science and biology. J Aerosol Sci. 2011;42(10):668–92.
8. Sayes CM, Reed KL, Warheit DB. Assessing toxicity of fine and nanoparticles: comparing in vitro measurements to in vivo pulmonary toxicity profiles. Toxicol Sci. 2007;97(1):163–80.
9. Rushton EK, Jiang J, Leonard SS, Eberly S, Castranova V, Biswas P, et al. Concept of assessing nanoparticle hazards considering nanoparticle dosemetric and chemical/biological response metrics. J Toxicol Environ Health A. 2010;73(5):445–61.
10. Kim YH, Boykin E, Stevens T, Lavrich K, Gilmour MI. Comparative lung toxicity of engineered nanomaterials utilizing in vitro, ex vivo and in vivo approaches. J Nanobiotechnol. 2014;12:47.
11. Teeguarden JG, Mikheev VB, Minard KR, Forsythe WC, Wang W, Sharma G, et al. Comparative iron oxide nanoparticle cellular dosimetry and response in mice by the inhalation and liquid cell culture exposure routes. Part Fibre Toxicol. 2014;11:46.
12. Donaldson K, Schinwald A, Murphy F, Cho WS, Duffin R, Tran L, et al. The biologically effective dose in inhalation nanotoxicology. Acc Chem Res. 2013;46(3):723–32.
13. Loret T, Peyret E, Dubreuil M, Aguerre-Chariol O, Bressot C, le Bihan O, et al. Air-liquid interface exposure to aerosols of poorly soluble nanomaterials induces different biological activation levels compared to exposure to suspensions. Part Fibre Toxicol. 2016;13(1):58.
14. U.S. EPA. Air quality criteria for particulate matter (Final Report, 2004). U.S. Environmental Protection Agency, Washington, DC, EPA 600/P-99/002aF-bF. 2004. https://cfpub.epa.gov/si/si_public_record_report.cfm?dirEntryId=87903.
15. Schmid O, Stoeger T. Surface area is the biologically most effective dose metric for acute nanoparticle toxicity in the lung. J Aerosol Sci. 2016;99:133–43.
16. Braakhuis HM, Cassee FR, Fokkens PHB, de la Fonteyne LJJ, Oomen AG, Krystek P, et al. Identification of the appropriate dose metric for pulmonary

inflammation of silver nanoparticles in an inhalation toxicity study. Nanotoxicology. 2016;10(1):63–73.
17. Duffin R, Tran L, Brown D, Stone V, Donaldson K. Proinflammogenic effects of low-toxicity and metal nanoparticles in vivo and in vitro: highlighting the role of particle surface area and surface reactivity. Inhal Toxicol. 2007;19(10): 849–56.
18. Stone KC, Mercer RR, Gehr P, Stockstill B, Crapo JD. Allometric relationships of cell numbers and size in the mammalian lung. Am J Respir Cell Mol Biol. 1992;6(2):235–43.
19. Ohashi T, Pinkerton K, Ikegami M, Jobe AH. Changes in alveolar surface-area, surfactant protein-A, and saturated phosphatidylcholine with postnatal rat lung growth. Pediatr Res. 1994;35(6):685–9.
20. Crapo JD, Barry BE, Gehr P, Bachofen M, Weibel ER. Cell number and cell characteristics of the normal human lung. Am Rev Respir Dis. 1982;126(2):332–7.
21. OECD. Guidance document on acute inhalation toxicity testing. ENV/JM/MONO(2009)28. Series on testing and assesment: number 39. 2009.
22. Geiser M, Kreyling WG. Deposition and biokinetics of inhaled nanoparticles. Part Fibre Toxicol. 2010;7:2.
23. Lehnert BE. Pulmonary and thoracic macrophage subpopulations and clearance of particles from the lung. Environ Health Perspect. 1992;97: 17–46.
24. Mann-Jong M, Shih L, Wu R. Pulmonary epithelium: cell types and functions. In: Proud M, editor. The pulmonary epithelium in health and disease. West Sussex: Wiley; 2008.
25. Fehrenbach H. Alveolar epithelial type II cell: defender of the alveolus revisited. Respir Res. 2001;2(1):33–52.
26. Blank F, Rothen-Rutishauser BM, Schurch S, Gehr P. An optimized in vitro model of the respiratory tract wall to study particle cell interactions. J Aerosol Med. 2006;19(3):392–405.
27. Park EK, Jung HS, Yang HI, Yoo MC, Kim C, Kim KS. Optimized THP-1 differentiation is required for the detection of responses to weak stimuli. Inflamm Res. 2007;56(1):45–50.
28. Wottrich R, Diabate S, Krug HF. Biological effects of ultrafine model particles in human macrophages and epithelial cells in mono- and co-culture. Int J Hyg Environ Health. 2004;207(4):353–61.
29. Napierska D, Thomassen LC, Vanaudenaerde B, Luyts K, Lison D, Martens JA, et al. Cytokine production by co-cultures exposed to monodisperse amorphous silica nanoparticles: the role of size and surface area. Toxicol Lett. 2012;211(2):98–104.
30. Rothen-Rutishauser B, Blank F, Muhlfeld C, Gehr P. In vitro models of the human epithelial airway barrier to study the toxic potential of particulate matter. Expert Opin Drug Metab Toxicol. 2008;4(8):1075–89.
31. Kim JS, Peters TM, O'Shaughnessy PT, Adamcakova-Dodd A, Thorne PS. Validation of an in vitro exposure system for toxicity assessment of air-delivered nanomaterials. Toxicol in Vitro. 2013;27(1):164 73.
32. Xie YM, Williams NG, Tolic A, Chrisler WB, Teeguarden JG, Maddux BLS, et al. Aerosolized ZnO nanoparticles induce toxicity in alveolar type II epithelial cells at the air-liquid interface. Toxicol Sci. 2012;125(2):450–61.
33. Landsiedel R, Sauer UG, Ma-Hock L, Schnekenburger J, Wiemann M. Pulmonary toxicity of nanomaterials: a critical comparison of published in vitro assays and in vivo inhalation or instillation studies. Nanomedicine (Lond). 2014;9(16):2557–85.
34. Hoet PH, Nemery B, Napierska D. Intracellular oxidative stress caused by nanoparticles: what do we measure with the dichlorofluorescein assay? Nano Today. 2013;8(3):223–7.
35. Driscoll KE, Carter JM, Hassenbein DG, Howard B. Cytokines and particle-induced inflammatory cell recruitment. Environ Health Perspect. 1997;105:1159–64.
36. Oberdorster G, Finkelstein JN, Johnston C, Gelein R, Cox C, Baggs R, et al. Acute pulmonary effects of ultrafine particles in rats and mice. Res Rep Health Eff Inst. 2000;96:5–74; disc 5–86
37. Organization WH. Guidance document on evaluating and expressing uncertainty in hazard characterization. 2018.
38. Hardy A, Benford D, Halldorsson T, Jeger MJ, Knutsen KH, More S, et al. Update: use of the benchmark dose approach in risk assessment. EFSA J. 2017;15(1):4658.
39. Slob W. Dose-response modeling of continuous endpoints. Toxicol Sci. 2002;66(2):298–312.
40. Jing X, Park JH, Peters TM, Thorne PS. Toxicity of copper oxide nanoparticles in lung epithelial cells exposed at the air-liquid interface compared with in vivo assessment. Toxicol in Vitro. 2015;29(3):502–11.
41. Panas A, Marquardt C, Nalcaci O, Bockhorn H, Baumann W, Paur HR, et al. Screening of different metal oxide nanoparticles reveals selective toxicity and inflammatory potential of silica nanoparticles in lung epithelial cells and macrophages. Nanotoxicology. 2013;7(3):259–73.
42. Wiemann M, Vennemann A, Sauer UG, Wiench K, Ma-Hock L, Landsiedel R. An in vitro alveolar macrophage assay for predicting the short-term inhalation toxicity of nanomaterials. J Nanobiotechnol. 2016;14:16.
43. Stoeger T, Schmid O, Takenaka S, Schulz H. Inflammatory response to TiO2 and carbonaceous particles scales best with BET surface area. Environ Health Perspect. 2007;115(6):A290-A1.
44. Oberdorster G, Oberdorster E, Oberdorster J. Nanotoxicology: an emerging discipline evolving from studies of ultrafine particles. Environ Health Perspect. 2005;113(7):823–39.
45. Braakhuis HM, Giannakou C, Peijnenburg WJ, Vermeulen J, van Loveren H, Park MV. Simple in vitro models can predict pulmonary toxicity of silver nanoparticles. Nanotoxicology. 2016;10(6):770–9.
46. Fubini B, Ghiazza M, Fenoglio I. Physico-chemical features of engineered nanoparticles relevant to their toxicity. Nanotoxicology. 2010;4(4):347–63.
47. Demokritou P, Gass S, Pyrgiotakis G, Cohen JM, Goldsmith W, McKinney W, et al. An in vivo and in vitro toxicological characterisation of realistic nanoscale CeO2 inhalation exposures. Nanotoxicology. 2013;7(8):1338–50.
48. Baisch BL, Corson NM, Wade-Mercer P, Gelein R, Kennell AJ, Oberdorster G, et al. Equivalent titanium dioxide nanoparticle deposition by intratracheal instillation and whole body inhalation: the effect of dose rate on acute respiratory tract inflammation. Part Fibre Toxicol. 2014;11:5.
49. Wong BA. Inhalation exposure systems: design, methods and operation. Toxicol Pathol. 2007;35(1):3–14.
50. Anjilvel S, Asgharian B. A multiple-path model of particle deposition in the rat lung. Fundam Appl Toxicol. 1995;28(1):41–50.
51. Cohen JM, Teeguarden JG, Demokritou P. An integrated approach for the in vitro dosimetry of engineered nanomaterials. Part Fibre Toxicol. 2014;11:20.
52. Pinkerton KE, Barry BE, Oneil JJ, Raub JA, Pratt PC, Crapo JD. Morphologic changes in the lung during the lifespan of Fischer 344 rats. Am J Anat. 1982;164(2):155–74.
53. Massaro GD, Mortola JP, Massaro D. Sexual dimorphism in the architecture of the lungs gas-exchange region. Proc Natl Acad Sci U S A. 1995;92(4):1105–7.
54. Miller FJ. Dosimetry of particles in laboratory animals and humans in relationship to issues surrounding lung overload and human health risk assessment: a critical review. Inhal Toxicol. 2000;12(1):19–57.
55. Singh C, Friedrichs S, Ceccone G, Gibson N, Jensen K, Levin M, et al. Cerium dioxide, NM-211, NM-212, NM-213. Characterisation and test item preparation, JRC repository: NM-series of representative manufactured nanomaterials Ispra, Italy: European Commission Joint Research Centre Institute for health and consumer protection. 2014.
56. Rasmussen K, Mast J, De Temmerman P-J, Verleysen E, Waegeneers N, Van Steen F, et al. Titanium dioxide, NM-100, NM-101, NM-102, NM-103, NM-104, NM-105: characterisation and physico-chemical properties. JRC science and policy reports. 2014.
57. Krystek P, Tentschert J, Nia Y, Trouiller B, Noel L, Goetz ME, et al. Method development and inter-laboratory comparison about the determination of titanium from titanium dioxide nanoparticles in tissues by inductively coupled plasma mass spectrometry. Anal Bioanal Chem. 2014;406(16):3853–61.
58. Hinderliter PM, Minard KR, Orr G, Chrisler WB, Thrall BD, Pounds JG, et al. ISDD: a computational model of particle sedimentation, diffusion and target cell dosimetry for in vitro toxicity studies. Part Fibre Toxicol. 2010;7(1):36.
59. DeLoid G, Cohen JM, Darrah T, Derk R, Rojanasakul L, Pyrgiotakis G, et al. Estimating the effective density of engineered nanomaterials for in vitro dosimetry. Nat Commun. 2014;5:3514.
60. Gosens I, Mathijssen LE, Bokkers BG, Muijser H, Cassee FR. Comparative hazard identification of nano- and micro-sized cerium oxide particles based on 28-day inhalation studies in rats. Nanotoxicology. 2014;8(6):643–53.
61. Stoeger T, Reinhard C, Takenaka S, Schroeppel A, Karg E, Ritter B, et al. Instillation of six different ultrafine carbon particles indicates a surface area threshold dose for acute lung inflammation in mice. Environ Health Perspect. 2006;114(3):328–33.

8

Concentration-dependent systemic response after inhalation of nano-sized zinc oxide particles in human volunteers

Christian Monsé[1*], Olaf Hagemeyer[1], Monika Raulf[1], Birger Jettkant[1], Vera van Kampen[1], Benjamin Kendzia[1], Vitali Gering[1], Günther Kappert[2], Tobias Weiss[1], Nadin Ulrich[1], Eike-Maximilian Marek[1], Jürgen Bünger[1], Thomas Brüning[1] and Rolf Merget[1]

Abstract

Background: Inhalation of high concentrations of zinc oxide particles (ZnO) may cause metal fume fever. In an earlier human inhalation study, no effects were observed after exposure to ZnO concentrations of 0.5 mg/ m^3. Further data from experimental studies with pure ZnO in the concentration range between 0.5 and 2. 5 mg/m^3 are not available. It was the aim of this experimental study to establish the concentration-response relationship of pure nano-sized ZnO particles.

Methods: Sixteen healthy subjects were exposed to filtered air and ZnO particles (0.5, 1.0 and 2.0 mg/m^3) for 4 h on 4 different days, including 2 h of cycling with a low workload. The effects were assessed before, immediately after, and about 24 h after each exposure. Effect parameters were symptoms, body temperature, inflammatory markers and clotting factors in blood, and lung function.

Results: Concentration-dependent increases in symptoms, body temperature, acute phase proteins and neutrophils in blood were detected after ZnO inhalation. Significant effects were detected with ZnO concentrations of 1.0 mg/m^3 or higher, with the most sensitive parameters being inflammatory markers in blood.

Conclusion: A concentration-response relationship with nano-sized ZnO particles in a low concentration range was demonstrated. Systemic inflammatory effects of inhaled nano-sized ZnO particles were observed at concentrations well below the occpational exposure limit for ZnO in many countries. It is recommended to reassess the exposure limit for ZnO at workplaces.

Keywords: Zinc oxide, Nanoparticles, Concentration-response relationship, Systemic effects, Inhalation study

Background

Zinc oxide fumes produced by activities such as thermal cutting, welding and melting may induce zinc fever after inhalation. Besides fever, typical symptoms include throat irritation, cough, minor respiratory symptoms, metallic taste, as well as flu-like symptoms, such as a general feeling of illness, myalgia, arthralgia or headache [1]. Typically, the symptoms occur after a latency period of 4 - 12 h, and resolve themselves within 48 h. Tolerance, which may develop after repeated exposures, has been shown to be reversible after several exposure-free days [1]. Generally, zinc fever is assumed to have no long-term sequels, but there is no valid epidemiologic information available.

In previous human experimental inhalation studies, nearly all volunteers developed zinc fever after exposure to 5 mg/m^3 ZnO for 2 h [2, 3]. Conversely, lower ZnO concentrations of 2.5 mg/m^3 for 2 h only induced a slight but significant increase in body temperature [3].

Thus far, only one study has analyzed leukocytes in blood after ZnO exposure, with the authors reporting no increase in polymorphonuclear neutrophilic granulocytes (ZnO concentration range 2.76 to 37 mg/m^3; 15 to 120 min. Exposure duration) [4].

* Correspondence: monse@ipa-dguv.de
[1]Institute for Prevention and Occupational Medicine of the German Social Accident Insurance, Institute of the Ruhr-Universität Bochum (IPA), Bürkle-de-la-Camp-Platz 1, 44789 Bochum, Germany
Full list of author information is available at the end of the article

Exposure to 0.5 mg/m^3 ultrafine and fine ZnO particles produced no effects (symptoms, body temperature, blood and sputum parameters) in 12 subjects after inhalation for 2 h at rest [5].

Earlier studies showed an increase of blood leukocytes about 20 h after exposure to welding fumes of galvanized steel [6, 7]. An asymptomatic increase in high-sensitive C-reactive protein (hsCRP) in the blood of 12 subjects after inhalation of metal inert gas (MIG) welding fumes of zinc-coated steel for 6 h at a zinc concentration of 1.5 mg/m^3 was reported [8]. In a further study by the same working group, an increase in blood CRP (measured with a high sensitive (hs) ELISA) was detected after exposure to different concentrations of MIG brazing fumes of zinc-coated materials for 6 h. The authors defined a No Observed Effect Level (NOEL) for systemic inflammation for welding fume concentrations (PM_{10}) between 1.4 and 2.0 mg/m^3 (containing 1.1 to 1.5 mg/m^3 ZnO), but did not rule out that the effects may be different for other processes, even with the same zinc content [9]. Three different welding fumes containing Zn, traces of aluminum with/without copper showed a maximal increase in interleukin-6 (IL-6) 10 h after exposure, but no qualitative differences were observed in inflammatory parameters like CRP and serum amyloid A (SAA), even 29 h after exposure [10].

In summary, experimental inhalation studies investigating zinc containing welding fumes report that zinc-related inflammatory effects occur below 2.0 mg/m^3 ZnO. However, one study with low concentrations of pure ZnO (0.5 mg/m^3) reported no effects [5]. Thus, a precise NOEL cannot be defined with the available data, and as a consequence we aimed in the present study to define the concentration-response relationship for pure ZnO in this lower concentration range.

Methods

Generation and characterization of ZnO nanoparticles

The principle of the particle synthesis was based on the pyrolysis of atomized aqueous zinc formate solutions with a hydrogen-oxygen flame [11]. The mobility diameter of the generated primary particles was about 10 nm. Depending on the ZnO concentration the primary particles formed aggregates and agglomerates in a range from 48 nm (0.5 mg/m^3 ZnO) to 86 nm (2.0 mg/m^3 ZnO). The particle diameters are comparable to those observed in an emission study of galvanized materials with different welding techniques [12]. A ceiling fan was used to homogenize the freshly generated ZnO nanoparticle atmospheres in the exposure unit [13]. Briefly, constant target concentrations with 0.5, 1.0 and 2.0 mg/m^3 ZnO were planned. Sham exposures (0 mg/m^3 ZnO) were also performed with the flame generator operated with purified water without zinc salt.

There were negligible differences between target and measured concentrations (Table 1). The particle size distributions were monomodal with relatively small geometric standard deviations of 1.66 to 1.69.

The purity of the airborne ZnO was 99.71%. Three precursor solutions were prepared by dissolving 11.0, 22.5 and 46.0 g zinc formate dihydrate ($Zn(CH_2O)_2 * 2 H_2O$, purity 98%, Alfa Aesar GmbH, Karlsruhe, Germany) in 3.0 mL acetic acid (HAc), which acted as a stabilizer (purity 99%, Merck GmbH, Darmstadt, Germany), and brought to a total volume of 1000 mL with purified water to yield Zn concentrations of 0.057, 0.118 and 0.240 mol/L, respectively. The hydrogen volumetric flow rate was set to 10.0 L/min and the oxygen flow to 5.0 L/min. Argon flow rate was 4.0 L/min. The atomizing gas was nitrogen (nitrogen generator, model NGM 22, cmc instruments GmbH, Eschborn, Germany), and the atomizing pressure was set to 0.30 bar. Typical flow rates of the aqueous zinc formate solutions were in the range of 0.90-1.00 mL/min.

The air exchange rate was set at 12 per hour (360 m^3/h) with a room temperature of 23.5 °C (+/− 0.3 °C) and a relative humidity of 47.0% (+/− 1.7%).

A Scanning Mobility Particle Sizer (SMPS, model 3080, TSI Inc., Shoreview MN, USA, equipped with a long differential mobility analyzer and a butanol condensation particle counter, TSI model 3776) measured the particle size distributions in the exposure unit. The number concentration and size distributions were determined every 5 min. Mass concentration measurements of airborne ZnO were recorded at 1-min intervals using a tapered elemental oscillating microbalance (TEOM, model 1400a, Rupprecht and Patashnik, Albany NY, USA). Trace gas analyses of nitric oxides (NO, NO_2) were performed via online chemical ionization mass spectroscopy at 1-s intervals (Airsense.net, MS4 GmbH, Rockenberg, Germany) to control the pyrolysis process. All measurement results of airborne ZnO concentrations, mobility particle diameter, geometric standard deviations as well as particle number concentration are listed in Table 1 (averaged over all exposure days for each exposure condition) (Fig. 1).

Participants

Sixteen healthy nonsmoking volunteers (8 women, 8 men) with a median age of 26 (range 19-42) years participated in the study (Table 2). The subjects had no previous exposure to airborne zinc compounds and did not show bronchial hyperresponsiveness to methacholine as assessed with a reservoir method [14]. Standard baseline laboratory parameters were within normal ranges. Seven subjects sensitized to ubiquitous aeroallergens (atopy screen sx1, Phadiatop, ImmunoCAP system, Thermo-Fisher Scientific, Phadia AB, Uppsala, Sweden) without any clinical manifestation were included, but exposures were performed outside of the allergy season.

Table 1 Measured parameters of airborne ZnO nanoparticles

Target concentration [mg/m^3]	Measured concentration [mg/m^3]	Mobility particle diameter [nm]	Geometric standard deviation [GSD]	Particle number concentration [#/cm^3]
0.0	0.016 (+/− 71.8%)	–	–	< 500
0.5	0.514 (+/− 2.4%)	47.8 (+/− 2.4%)	1.66	1.69E + 06 (+/− 3.5%)
1.0	1.013 (+/− 1.1%)	62.8 (+/− 2.7%)	1.68	2.03E + 06 (+/− 4.1%)
2.0	2.014 (+/− 1.2%)	85.8 (+/− 4.0%)	1.69	2.53E + 06 (+/− 9.2%)

Study design

Exposures were performed in an exposure unit at our institute [15]. Subjects were exposed for 4 h, with 2 weeks intervals for each subject. The subjects were generally at rest, except for short periods of moderate physical activity on a cycle ergometer set to 15 L/min/m^2 (corresponding to a work load of 60 watt (range 30-96 watt), which was separated into 4 blocks of 30 min each (total 120 min)). Exposures were randomized and double blinded, with the exception of the exposures to 2.0 mg/m^3 ZnO, which were not blinded according to instructions by the ethics committee. Medical examinations were performed before, directly after, and approximately 24 h after the start of exposure. Additionally, examinations were performed before the first (baseline test) and after the last exposure (final test) (Fig. 2).

At each examination, subjects answered a questionnaire and underwent a physical examination, blood sampling, lung function testing, and measurements of fractional exhaled nitric monoxide (FeNO) and body temperature. In addition, vital functions (electrocardiogram, blood pressure) were monitored during the exposures.

Questionnaire

All subjects answered a questionnaire addressing flu-like symptoms (at least 1 of 3 symptoms: feeling of fever, feeling sick and muscle pain), and additionally all symptoms were graded according to severity (not at all (1 score point), barely (2 points), little (3 points), moderate (4 points), strong (5 points), very strong (6 points)). To avoid any information bias we added questions about itching nose, abdominal pain, metallic taste in mouth, dry nose, throat irritation, headache, cough, burning eyes, feeling warm, itching skin, nausea, shortness of breath, dry eyes, sweating, irritation of the eyes, general irritability, feeling cold, chills, runny nose, feeling unwell, bleeding eyes and muscle cramps.

Body temperature

Subjects measured their own body temperatures using an infrared method that recorded the temperature in both ears. This was performed at each examination, and at intervals of 2 h from the beginning of the exposure to 24 h afterwards, but not during sleep (Braun Thermoscan Pro 4000, WelchAllyn, Hechingen, Germany).

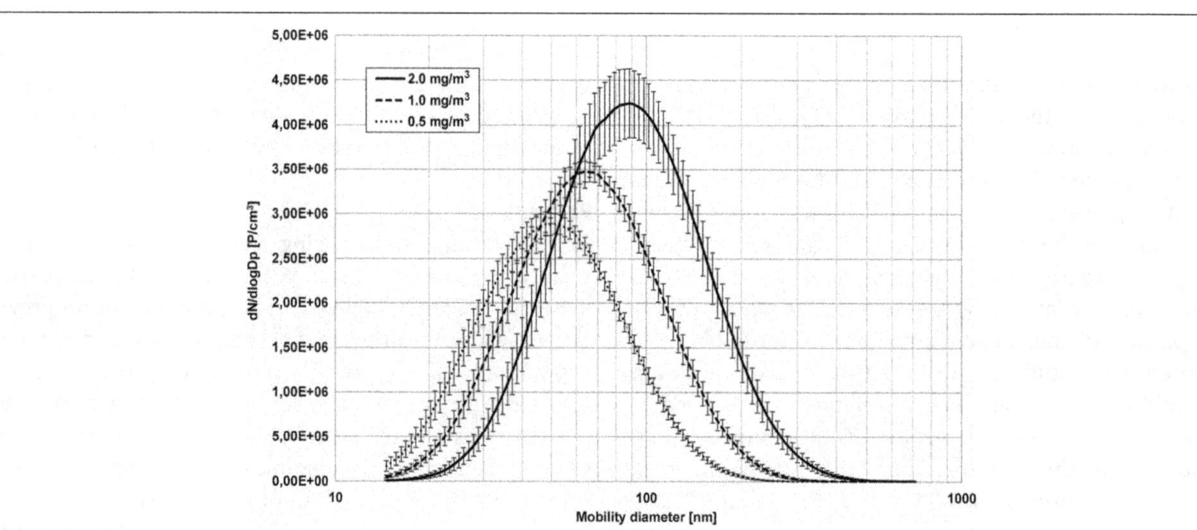

Fig. 1 Particle size distributions of airborne ZnO concentrations at 0.5, 1.0 and 2.0 mg/m^3. In addition, the error bars of each individual size channel are shown

Table 2 Characteristics of the study subjects

	Total $n = 16$	Male $n = 8$	Female $n = 8$
Age [years]	26 (19-42)	28 (19-42)	24 (23-32)
Height [cm]	178 (155-191)	182 (176-191)	164 (155-182)
Weight [kg]	72 (51-104)	83 (61-104)	59 (51-91)
BMI [kg/m^2]	24 (19-29)	25 (20-29)	23 (19-27)
Total IgE [kU/L]	31 (2-329)	79 (2-208)	28 (20-329)
sx1 [$n \geq 0.35$ kUA/L]	7	4	3

Medians, minimum and maximum values are listed. BMI = body mass index. Sx1 is an indicator of sensitization to environmental allergens

Blood parameters

Markers of inflammation (blood cell counts, CRP, SAA, Club cell protein (CC16), IL-6) and coagulation (prothrombin F 1.2, endothelial microparticles, fibrinogen, D-dimers) were analyzed. The total and differential blood cell counts were determined using standard procedures with UniCell DxH800 (Beckman Coulter Inc., Brea CA, USA). Sandwich ELISA were used to measure CC16 (BioVendor, Brno, Czech Republic, range 1.57-50 ng/mL), IL-6 (R & D Systems, Wiesbaden, Germany, range 4.7-600 pg/mL), SAA (Invitrogen™ Novex ™ SAA Human ELISA Kit which detect serum amyloid A1 cluster, Carlsbad CA, USA, range 9.4-600 ng/mL), and CRP (high sensitive ELISA from Siemens Healthcare Diagnostics Products GmbH, Marburg, Germany, precision levels down to or below 0.3 mg/L) in serum.

The clotting factors were measured in plasma according to the manufacturer's instructions: Prothrombin cleavage fragment F1.2 with Enzygnost F1.2 (Siemens, range 69-229 pmol/L), endothelial microparticles with ZYMUPHEN MP (Hyphen Biomed, Neuville-sur-Oise, France, precision levels down to or below 5 nM), fibrinogen with a modified method from Clauss with Multifibren U (Siemens, range 180-350 mg/dL), and D-dimers with Behring Coagulation System XP (BCS XP) and INNOVANCE D-Dimer (Siemens, precision levels down to or below 0.5 mg/L).

Biomonitoring

Biomonitoring was performed by determination of zinc levels in blood and urine. Plastic materials were used for sample preparation to prevent contamination. Prior to usage, the vessels were cleaned with 1% nitric acid for 2 h, rinsed with ultrapure water and dried at room temperature. After thawing the frozen aliquots, 50 µL of the blood samples were diluted 1:100, and 500 µL of the urine samples were diluted 1:10 with 0.1 M HCl solution and 100 µL of a 0.2% solution of Triton-X. Rhodium was used as internal standard. Analysis was carried out using a 7700 ICP-MS system from Agilent Technologies in He-mode (flow rate 5 mL/min) with a collision cell to avoid interferences. Skimmer and sampler cones were made of nickel. Calibration and calculation of the Zn concentrations were carried out using standards at eight different concentrations. LOQ was 4.0 µg/L. Materials from RECIPE (ClinChek Whole Blood Level, lyophil. For Trace Elements I and II, REF 8840, LOT 227; ClinChek Urine Control lyophil. For Trace Elements I and II, REF 8847-8849, LOT 122) and SERONORM (Trace Elements Whole Blood Level I and II, LOT 1103129, Trace Elements Urine Level I and II, LOT 1011644) served as internal control.

FeNO

Fractional exhaled nitric oxide was measured using a portable electrochemical analyzer (NIOX Mino, Aerocrine, Solna, Sweden) taking into account the guidelines of the American Thoracic Society and European Respiratory Society [16].

Lung function testing

Lung function was recorded using both body plethysmography [17] and spirometry [18] in a linked maneuver with a MasterLab (Jaeger, Würzburg, Germany). A battery of different parameters was evaluated (e.g. airway resistance, lung volumes, and flows).

Data analysis

Descriptive analysis was performed for each variable stratified by exposure (sham, 0.5, 1.0 and 2.0 mg/m^3 ZnO) and time of measurement (before, during, immediately

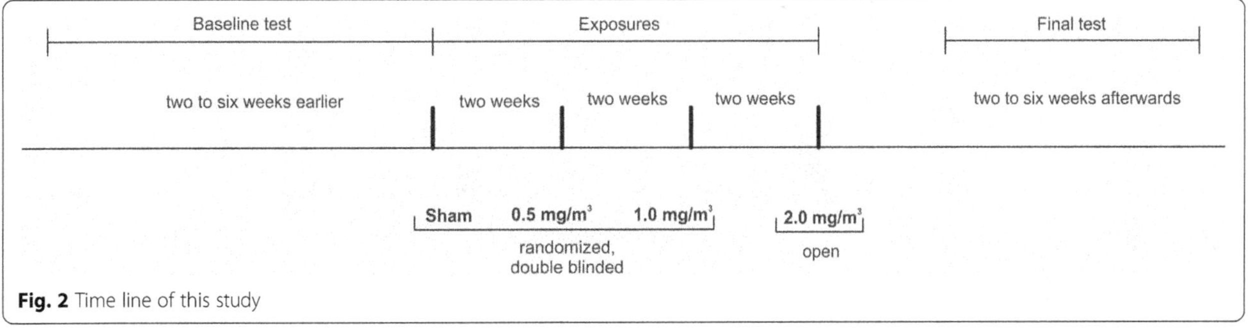

Fig. 2 Time line of this study

after, and 24 h post exposure). Characteristics of subjects were expressed as medians, 25%- and 75%-quantiles, as well as minimum and maximum. Graphical representations were illustrated with boxplots. Effects were compared between the before, immediately after, and 24 h after exposure. In addition, the effects after sham were compared to exposure after ZnO. Exposure groups were compared using paired Student's t-test for normal or log-normal distributed variables. The problem of multiple comparisons was counteracted using the Bonferroni correction, by dividing the overall desired statistical significance level $\alpha = 0.05$ by the number of hypotheses tested. Individual descriptive analyses were performed for body temperature with a cut-off of ≥37.5 °C. Spearman correlation coefficients (r_S) were calculated to predict the monotone association between parameters.

Rank order tables were developed to give another estimate of increased effects which follow a concentration-response relationship. Increased effects were defined as values bigger than the largest value of baseline test, examinations before each exposure and final test ($n = 6$) plus the double median absolute deviation (MAD) of these 6 values (> max (baseline test, final test, initial investigation before start of exposure) + 2 MAD). Each of the ZnO related effects was assigned to ranks 1 to 4, the lowest value represented by rank 1 and the highest by rank 4, respectively. All parameters were evaluated with both group comparisons and rank order tables.

Results

The results obtained from baseline tests, examinations done before each exposure, and from final tests ($n = 6$) were not significantly different from one another. In addition, when the final tests were conducted at the end of the study (minimum 14 days after the last exposure), all parameters had returned to levels that were within the range of the initial values. Consequently, only those parameters with significant changes are presented below. ZnO exposure had no effect on CC16, IL-6, clotting factors (prothrombin F 1.2, endothelial microparticles, fibrinogen, D-dimers) in blood, FeNO, and all lung function parameters.

Questionnaire

There was a small increase in the number of subjects with flu-like symptoms 24 h after exposure to 2.0 mg/m^3 ZnO when compared to the number of complaints directly after exposure (Fig. 3). The same results were also obtained if the grading of severity of symptoms was considered (data not shown). Also there were no concentration-related effects with any other questions (data not shown).

Body temperature

With the exception of one male subject who suffered from an abdominal infection during the sham exposure, there was no significant increase in body temperature (≥ 37.5 °C) in subjects exposed to either sham or 0.5 mg/m^3 ZnO. Only two subjects exposed to 1.0 mg/m^3 ZnO reported increased temperatures of ≥37.5 °C; whereas, six subjects had elevated temperatures upon exposure to 2.0 mg/m^3 ZnO. Furthermore, only one subject reported increased body temperature after exposure to both 1.0 and 2.0 mg/m^3 ZnO. All temperature increases occurred between 8 to 10 h post exposure, with the maximum reported temperature of 39.5 °C in females and 38.6 °C in males. Importantly, the increase in temperature in all subjects was not significantly different within group comparisons.

Blood parameters

The concentration of the acute phase proteins CRP and SAA were highly correlated ($r_S = 0.78$) as illustrated in Fig. 4. The Spearman correlation coefficient of $r_S = 0.78$ was calculated including all values at all exposure conditions. Coefficients for each concentration yielded similar results (0 mg/m^3 ZnO: $r_S = 0.68$, 0.5 mg/m^3

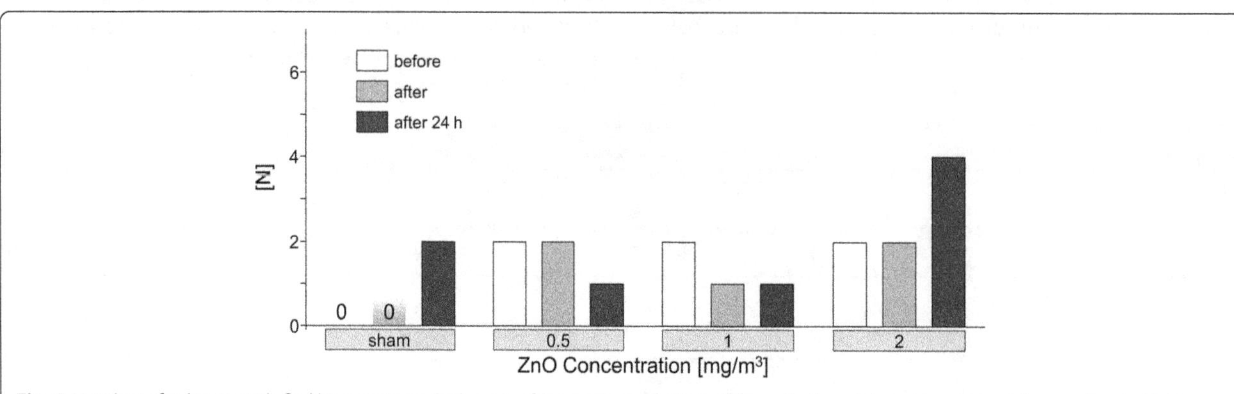

Fig. 3 Number of subjects with flu-like symptoms (at least 1 of 3 symptoms: feeling of fever, feeling sick and muscle pain) according to ZnO concentrations and time points

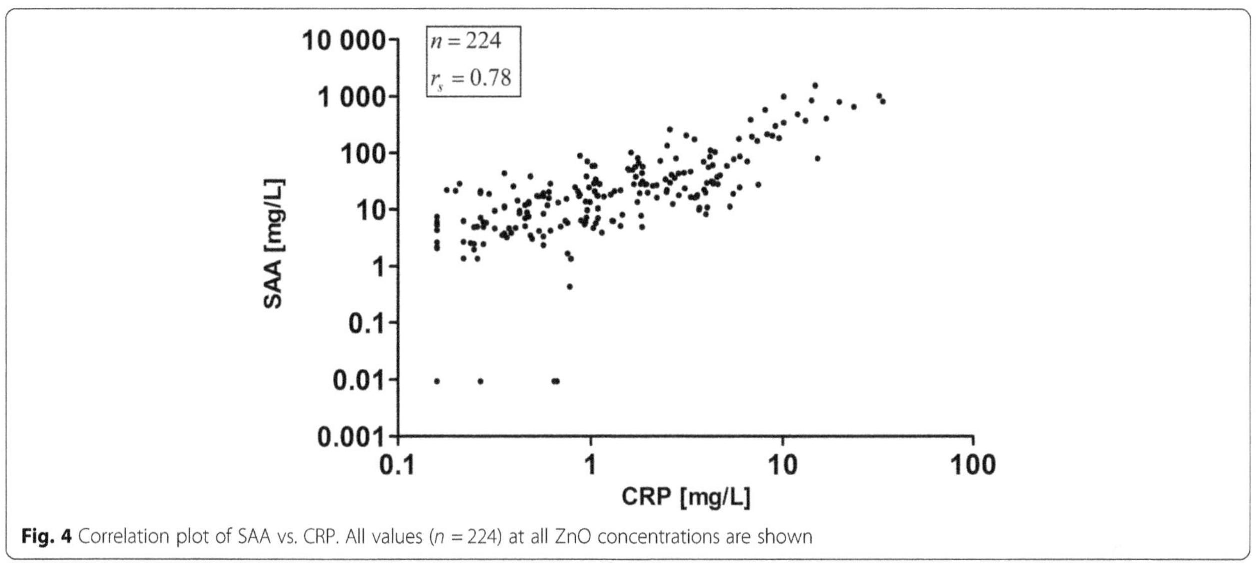

Fig. 4 Correlation plot of SAA vs. CRP. All values (n = 224) at all ZnO concentrations are shown

ZnO: r_S = 0.86, 1.0 mg/m^3 ZnO: r_S = 0.74 and 2.0 mg/m^3 ZnO: r_S = 0.89).

Exposure to ZnO led to a concentration-dependent increase in both CRP and SAA levels in the blood 24 h after exposure. When compared to the levels before exposure, blood CRP levels significantly increased with all ZnO concentrations 24 h after exposure. Conversely, SAA levels increased 24 h after exposure to 1.0 and 2.0 mg/m^3 ZnO (Fig. 5). Compared to the sham exposure, ZnO exposures yielded significantly higher CRP values 24 h after exposure to 2.0 mg/m^3 ZnO, and higher SAA values after 1.0 and 2.0 mg/m^3 ZnO (Fig. 5).

Absolute and relative numbers of neutrophil granulocytes were similar to each other and as a result only the relative numbers were shown as a percentage (Fig. 5c) (absolute numbers not shown). In contrast to the acute phase proteins, neutrophil levels increased significantly immediately after all exposure scenarios (including sham), but not in a concentration-dependent relationship, suggesting an effect of the physical exercise [19]. A concentration-response was observed only after 24 h after exposure. Neutrophil levels increased 24 h after exposure to 1.0 and 2.0 mg/m^3 ZnO compared to levels before the exposure (Fig. 5). Furthermore, compared to the sham exposure, all concentrations of ZnO elicited significant increases in neutrophils 24 h later (Fig. 5).

Four subjects showed increased CRP levels upon exposure to sham exposures as illustrated in the rank order tables, including the one subject (ID 3) with an acute abdominal infection (Table 3). The effect increased with increasing ZnO concentrations with 6 subjects (CRP) after 0.5 mg/m^3 ZnO, 12 subjects (CRP and SAA) after 1.0 mg/m^3 ZnO, and up to 15 subjects (CRP) after 2.0 mg/m^3 ZnO. The acute phase proteins (CRP and SAA) increased in a concentration dependent manner after exposures to 1.0 and 2.0 mg/m^3 ZnO. In contrast, neutrophils and body temperature significantly increased only after 2.0 mg/m^3 ZnO. No susceptible subjects were identified, because increased effects occurred in all subjects, without increased frequency in single subjects (Table 3).

There were no differences between males and females, as well as between subjects with and without sensitizations to environmental allergens (data not shown). Levels of Zn in blood and urine were unaffected by ZnO inhalation at any concentration (data not shown). This is due to the naturally occurring high zinc concentrations in the blood, which are in the range between 4 to 7.5 mg/L whole blood [20]. In addition, the concentration shows large fluctuations, influenced by food intake, but the diet of our subjects was not standardized in this study.

Calculation of deposition rates of inhaled ZnO particles

We used the ICRP model [21] to identify possible differences of deposition rates of ZnO particles with different median diameters in the tracheobronchial and alveolar region. Due to the way of particle generation, the median diameter of the ZnO particles at 0.5 mg/m^3 with 47.8 nm increases at 1.0 mg/m^3 ZnO to 62.8 nm and at 2.0 mg/m^3 ZnO to 85.8 nm. The estimations of the deposition rates were performed under the following conditions: The ZnO particles are ideal spheres, the measured mobility diameter corresponds to the activity median aerodynamic diameter in the ICRP model and the density of the particles is 1 g/cm^3. We used the data of the "Reference Worker" in this model. Table 4 shows the estimation of deposition rates in dependence of different particle size and lung compartments.

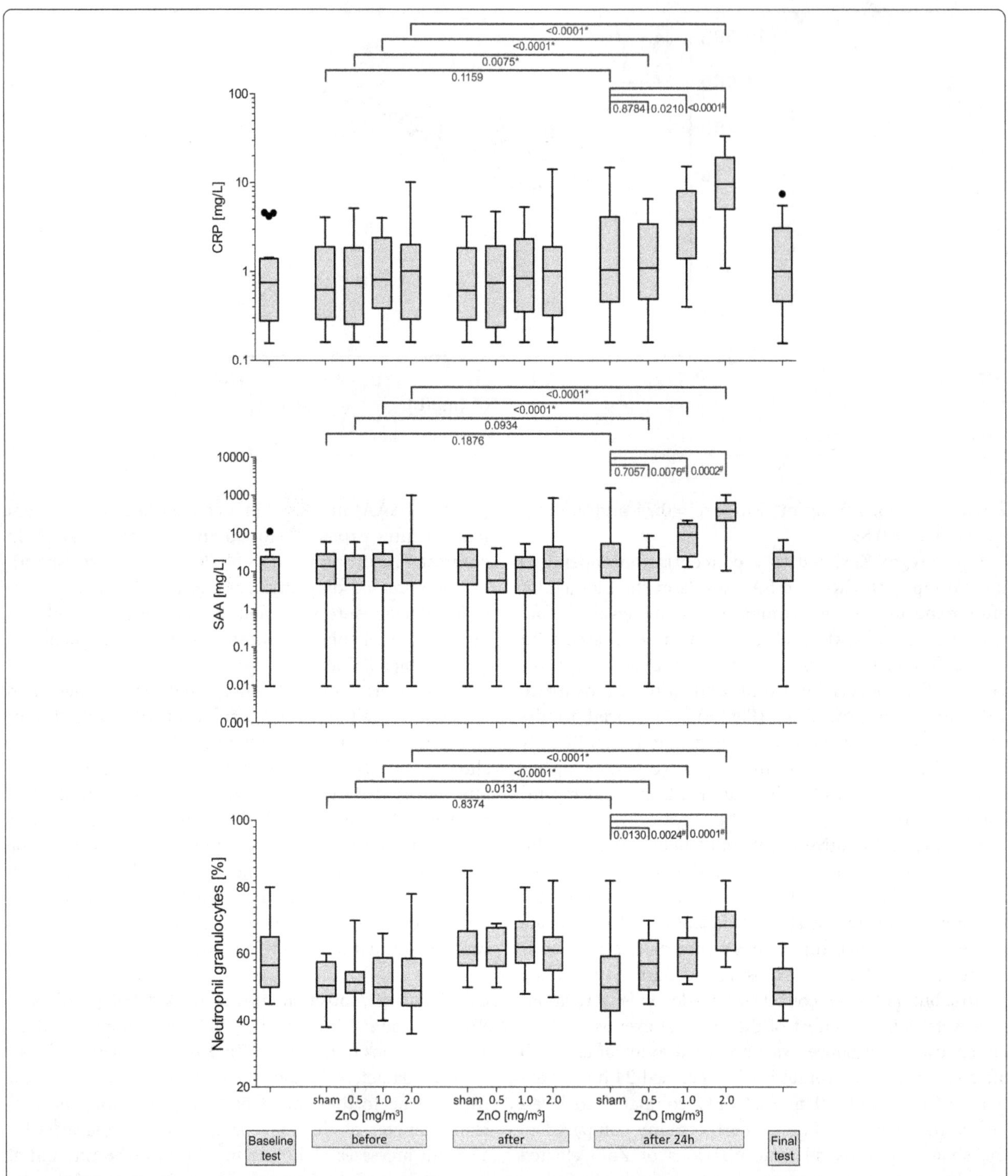

Fig. 5 Selected blood parameters according to ZnO concentrations and time points. *significant values with significance level $\alpha = 0.0125$ (after Bonferroni correction). #significant values with significance level $\alpha = 0.0167$ (after Bonferroni correction). Outliers are defined as values above median + 1.5 x interquartile range or values below median – 1.5 x interquartile range

Discussion

Experimental inhalation studies in humans with nanoparticles, which use multiple concentration steps in order to describe a concentration-response relationship are extremely sparse. The present study is, to our knowledge, the first human inhalation study with pure nano-sized ZnO in the concentration range of 0.5 to 2.0 mg/m^3. A key result of this study is the demonstration of

Table 3 Rank order tables

ID	Temperature				CRP				SAA				Neutrophils [%]			
	ZnO-Conc. [mg/m³]				ZnO-Conc. [mg/m³]				ZnO-Conc. [mg/m³]				ZnO-Conc. [mg/m³]			
	0	0.5	1.0	2.0	0	0.5	1.0	2.0	0	0.5	1.0	2.0	0	0.5	1.0	2.0
1	3	1	2	4	1	2	3	4	1	2	3	4	1	2	3	4
2	1	2	3	4	1	2	3	4	1	2	3	4	2	1	3	4
3	4	1	2	3	4	1	2	3	4	1	2	3	4	3	1	2
4	1	4	3	2	2	1	3	4	2	1	3	4	4	1	2	3
5	1	2	4	3	1	2	3	4	2	1	3	4	1	2	3	4
6	1	3	2	4	1	1	3	4	2	1	3	4	1	3	2	4
7	1	2	3	4	1	2	3	4	2	1	3	4	1	2	3	4
8	3	4	1	1	1	2	3	4	4	1	2	3	1	2	3	4
9	3	1	4	2	1	2	3	4	1	2	3	4	1	4	2	3
10	1	1	3	4	2	1	3	4	2	1	3	4	1	1	3	4
11	2	1	3	4	1	2	3	4	1	2	3	4	1	2	3	4
12	4	1	2	3	1	2	3	4	2	1	3	4	1	2	2	4
13	4	1	4	4	1	3	2	4	3	1	2	4	1	3	2	3
14	1	3	1	4	1	2	3	4	1	2	3	4	1	2	3	4
15	2	1	4	3	2	1	3	4	1	2	3	4	1	2	3	4
16	2	1	3	4	2	1	3	4	1	2	3	4	1	4	3	2

Grey colored cells represent increased effects defined as > max value of baseline test, final test and initial investigation before start of exposure plus double median absolute deviation (MAD) of these 6 values. Numbers indicate ranks of effects

such a concentration-response relationship. The most sensitive outcomes were the increase in acute phase proteins (CRP and SAA) and neutrophils in blood, followed by an increase in body temperature and the occurrence of flu-like symptoms at and above 1 mg/m³ ZnO.

No relevant effects were detectable after sham exposures, but initial increases of acute phase proteins were observed with a concentration of 0.5 mg/m³ ZnO after 24 h. Pronounced effects on acute phase proteins and neutrophils occurred after 1.0 mg/m³ ZnO, together with increases in body temperature in some subjects. All the effects were strongest after 2.0 mg/m³ ZnO, with flu-like symptoms and elevated body temperature measured in several subjects.

The results of this study are in accordance with previous studies that reported effects (flu-like symptoms, increase in temperature and inflammatory markers) after exposure to ≥2.5 mg/m³ ZnO [2–4]. The only previous study that investigated lower concentrations, i.e. 0.5 mg/m³ ZnO [5] showed no effects, but importantly, the duration of exposure was only 2 h without physical exercise, resulting in an approximately 4 fold lower inhaled dose (with linear extrapolation) of ZnO in comparison with our lowest ZnO dose. The findings of the present study are also compatible with a previous study investigating ZnO-containing welding fumes [8], which showed an increase in CRP levels after 6 h exposure to 1.5 mg/m³ zinc with short periods of physical exercise.

Our investigations were conducted with ZnO as a single component in the nanoscale range at maximal concentrations considered to represent high workplace exposures [12]. The observed effects in this study were caused only by the different airborne ZnO concentrations. Any influences from secondary components of welding fume and trace gases are negligible. Possible effect differences due to different deposition rates of ZnO particles with concentration-dependent median diameters (see Table 1) can be nearly excluded. Our estimation with the help of the ICRP model revealed similar deposition rates of the different particle sizes in this study in terms of both total deposition (sum of alveolar, inhalable and tracheobronchial) and alveolar deposition alone (see Table 4).

The effects measured in this study are indicative of systemic inflammation which may be explained by either primary local inflammation of the respiratory tract/lung and secondary resorption of inflammatory markers, or by primary systemic inflammation due to resorbed zinc ions. The latter mechanism is supported by the 4.8 to 19.2 h half-life

Table 4 Estimated depostion rates of ZnO in the current study

Particle concentration [mg/m³]	Median particle diameter [nm]	ZnO deposition rate (sum of tracheobronchial, inhalable and alveolar)	ZnO deposition rate (alveolar)
0.5	47.8	78%	48%
1.0	62.8	74%	47%
2.0	85.8	66%	44%

of ZnO particles in rat lungs [22, 23]. In addition, Cho et al. [24] hypothesized that the rapid pH-dependent dissolution of ZnO particles inside phagosomes is the main cause of ZnO-induced diverse progressive lung injuries. It has been shown in an ex-vivo study that the release of Zn ions from ZnO nanoparticles, due to their instability in the acidic compartment of lysosomes, increases reactive oxygen species generation and damage of lysosomal membranes and activation of executioner caspase-3 and caspase-7 [25]. The ZnO-induced effects strongly argue for a zinc-specific mechanism, since the distinct clinical presentations of metal fume fever by ZnO as well as other metal compounds, have not been observed after exposure to poorly soluble particles (PSP) [26].

While the acute phase proteins in blood clearly increased after ZnO inhalation, effects on further inflammatory parameter in the blood, such as IL-6 and the secreted CC16 as of a marker of increased lung permeability could not be detected and thus a complete inflammatory response could not be observed in the blood samples obtained at the selected time points. Very recently, it was shown that IL-6 increased 10 h after the start of a 6 h exposure to zinc-containing welding fumes, but this increase was not seen 29 h after the start of exposure [10]. Thus, it is probable that an increase in IL-6 concentration in the blood was overlooked due to the time intervals of the blood sampling in the present study. The increase in body temperature in a subset of subjects suggests susceptibility. Interestingly, increases in inflammatory markers were observed in all subjects - a finding that does not support the concept that only susceptible individuals are affected.

Generally, chronic effects cannot be derived from acute human inhalation experiments. The observation that zinc fever occurs predominantly on the first day after periods without exposure to zinc-containing fumes suggests poorly understood adaptation processes. Zinc fever is proposed to be an acute disease, but epidemiologic information on the long-term consequences of exposure is limited. Our data clearly demonstrate that all observed effects were reversible at the time of the final tests.

Inflammatory systemic biomarkers have been proposed as biomarkers of cancer [27, 28], heart diseases [29–31] and chronic obstructive pulmonary disease and comorbidities [32] in epidemiological studies. However, it is unknown whether the association between inflammatory markers and disease is causal. A number of controlled studies in humans report increased levels of CRP or SAA after particle inhalation, and it is believed that this acute phase pulmonary and systemic response following particle inhalation may indeed constitute a causal link between particle inhalation and for example cardiovascular disease [33]. Very recently, it was shown for the first time that anti-inflammatory therapy led to a significantly lower rate of recurrent cardiovascular events than placebo [34]. This finding strengthens the view that inflammation is indeed causal, thus prevention of cardiovascular disease should comprise, among other measures, minimization of particle inhalation.

It has been reported earlier that pulmonary inflammatory responses following zinc oxide particle inhalation were much stronger than after inhalation of PSP like magnesium oxide. Thus particle composition is a major contributor to inflammation [26]. Epidemiological studies with cancer and cardiovascular disease as endpoints do not exist in predominantly ZnO exposed occupational cohorts. A dose-dependent association between welding fumes and lung cancer has been described for welders [35], and there are weak indications that welding fumes are a risk factor for cardiovascular diseases [36, 37]. The inflammatory acute response after ZnO inhalation in our study was reversible within a few weeks. It remains to be assessed whether repeated or chronic exposure to ZnO increase the risk for diseases which have been shown to be associated with environmental particle inhalation.

One weakness of the present study is that the effect parameters were recorded at limited time points, suggesting that some effects were overlooked due to their shorter or longer kinetics. However, the time points of the increases in the most sensitive parameters - CRP and SAA - in this study correspond well with other evaluations [10]. A further weakness is the lack of blinding of the highest ZnO concentration. In general, inhalation studies should be blinded, but for security reasons due the high ZnO concentrations, this was not performed. However, confounding of objective inflammatory markers in blood should be negligible.

For most of the effect parameters in this study, reference values do not exist or show large inter-individual variability. Thus, with the exception of body temperature (with well-known reference values), descriptive analyses with respect to reference values and interpretations of the magnitudes of the effects were not considered. In this study, two different group comparisons (before / after exposure; sham / ZnO) and additional intra-individual analyses by rank order tables were used. The latter were developed in order to overcome the problem of multiple testing and associated definition of significant effects. Here six control scenarios were available, thus accidental variabilities were minimized. A strength of this study is the lack of effects after sham exposures, with the exception of one subject with an abdominal infection, as well as rare and minor unexplained increases of CRP (but not SAA) in three females. The lack of increased effects in sham exposures, and the consistent concentration-related effects in almost all subjects add to the credibility of the study results.

Conclusions

In summary, this study was able to demonstrate a concentration-response relationship of ZnO nanoparticles with clear systemic effects at and above 1 mg/m^3 ZnO. The results are in accordance with previous experimental studies that showed no effects at 0.5 mg/m^3 ZnO [5] and clear effects concerning CRP with concentrations between 1.1 and 1.5 mg/m^3 ZnO-containing welding fumes [9]. Similarly an increase of SAA was observed after inhalation of zinc or copper containing welding fumes [38], but the different exposure scenarios within these studies have to be considered. A No Effect Exposure Level (NOEL) derived from our study would be defined between 0.5 and 1 mg/m^3, although, in contrast to a previous study with 2 h exposures at rest [5], initial effects were seen with ZnO exposures of 0.5 mg/m^3 concerning CRP and SAA, which were the most sensitive parameters. Exposure limits of ZnO in many countries (e.g. USA, United Kingdom, Australia, Canada) were set to 5.0 mg/m^3 [39]. As this and more recent experimental studies showed effects far below this concentration, it is highly recommended to reassess the exposure limit for ZnO at workplaces.

Abbreviations

BMI: Body mass index; CC16: Club cell protein; CRP: C-reactive protein; FeNO: fractional exhaled nitric monoxide; GSD: geometric standard deviation; IL-6: interleukin-6; MAD: median absolute deviation; MIG: metal inert gas welding; NO: nitrogen monoxide; NO_2: nitrogen dioxide; NOEL: No observed effect level; PM_{10}: Particulate matter with an aerodynamic diameter smaller than 10 µm; PSP: Poorly soluble particles; r_S: Spearman correlation coefficients; SAA: Serum amyloid A; SMPS: Scanning mobility particle sizer; TEOM: Tapered elemental oscillating microbalance; ZnO: Zinc oxide

Acknowledgments

We are grateful to our volunteers for their participation. The authors thank Sabine Bernard, Gerda Borowitzki, Anja Deckert, Jennifer Gili, Evelyn Heinze, Claudia Litzenberger, Ursula Meurer, Melanie Ulbrich and Susann Widmer for their excellent technical assistance. We acknowledge the valuable contribution to the discussion of the results of this study of Martin Wieske (German Association of non-ferrous Metals), Heiko Udo Käfferlein, Dirk Pallapies, Dirk Taeger and Gerhard Schlüter (IPA).

Funding

This work was supported by the German Association of non-ferrous Metals.

Authors' contributions

Conception and design: CM, OH, MR, JB, TB, RM. Analysis and interpretation: BJ, VK, BK, VG, GK, EM, CM, OH, RM. Biomonitoring: TW, NU. Drafting the manuscript for important intellectual content: CM, OH, RM. All authors read and approved the final manuscript.

Competing interests

The authors declare that they have no competing interests.

Author details

[1] Institute for Prevention and Occupational Medicine of the German Social Accident Insurance, Institute of the Ruhr-Universität Bochum (IPA), Bürkle-de-la-Camp-Platz 1, 44789 Bochum, Germany. [2]Gerinnungszentrum Rhein-Ruhr, Königstraße 13, 47051 Duisburg, Germany.

References

1. Nemery B. Metal toxicity and the respiratory tract. Eur Respir J. 1990;3:202–19.
2. Gordon T, Chen LC, Fine JM, Schlesinger RB, Su WY, Kimmel TA, Amdur M. Pulmonary effects of inhaled zinc oxide in human subjects, guinea pigs, rats, and rabbits. Am Ind Hyg Assoc J. 1992;53:503–9.
3. Fine J, Gordon T, Chen LC, Kinney P, Falcone G, Beckett W. Metal fume fever: Caracterization of clinical and plasma IL-6 responses in controlled human exposures to zinc oxide fume at and below the threshold limit value. J Occup Environ Med. 1997;39:722–6.
4. Kuschner WG, D'Alessandro A, Wintermeyer SF, Wong H, Boushey HA, Blanc PD. Pulmonary responses to purified zinc oxide fume. J Investig Med. 1995;43:371–8.
5. Beckett WS, Chalupa DF, Puly-Brown A, Speers DM, Stewart JC, Frampton MW, Utell MJ, Huang LS, Cox C, Zareba W, Oberdörster G. Comparing inhaled ultrafine versus fine zinc oxide particles in healthy humans. Am J Respir Crit Care Med. 2005;171:1129–35.
6. Blanc P, Wong H, Bernstein MS, Boushey HA. An experimental human model of metal fume fever. Ann Int Med. 1991;114:930–6.
7. Blanc PD, Boushey HA, Wong H, Wintermeyer SF, Bernstein MS. Cytokines in metal fume fever. Am Rev Respir Dis. 1993;147:134–8.
8. Hartmann L, Bauer M, Bertram J, Gube M, Lenz K, Reisgen U, Schettgen T, Kraus T, Brand P. Assessment of the biological effects of welding fumes emitted from metal inert gas welding processes of aluminium and zinc-plated materials in humans. Int J Hyg Environ Health. 2014;217:160–8.
9. Brand P, Bauer M, Gube M, Lenz K, Reisgen U, Spiegel-Ciobanu VE, Kraus T. Relationship between welding fume concentration and systemic inflammation after controlled exposure of human subjects with welding fumes from metal inert gas brazing of zinc-coated materials. J Occup Environ Med. 2014;56:1–5.
10. Baumann R, Joraslafsky S, Markert A, Rack I, Davatgarbenam S, Kossack V, Gerhards B, Kraus T, Brand P, Gube M. IL-6, a central acute-phase mediator, as an early biomarker for exposure to zinc-based metal fumes. Toxicology. 2016;373:63–73.
11. Monsé C, Monz C, Dahmann D, Asbach C, Stahlmecke B, Lichtenstein N, Buchwald K-E, Merget R, Bünger J, Brüning T. Development and evaluation of a nanoparticle generator for human inhalation studies with airborne zinc oxide. Aerosol Sci Technol. 2014;48:418–26.
12. Reisgen U, Olschok S, Lenz K, Spiegel-Ciobanu VE. Ermittlung von Schweißrauchdaten und Partikelkenngrößen bei verzinkten Werkstoffen. Schweissen und Schneiden. 2012;64:788–96.
13. Pillar F, Kahl A, Brüning T, Monsé C. Validierungsuntersuchungen eines Berechnungsmodells zur Ausbreitung von Gefahrstoffen. Gefahrst Reinhalt L. 2016;76:19–25.
14. Merget R, Heinze E, Neumann L, Taeger D, Bruening T. Comparison of the Pari Provotest II reservoir- and the ATS dosimeter method for the assessment of bronchial hyperresponsiveness. In: Bruening T, Harth V, Zaghow M, editors. Proceedings of the 45th annual meeting of the German Society for Occupational and Environmental Medicine. Stuttgart: Gentner Publishing Company; 2005. p. 624–5.
15. Monsé C, Sucker K, van Thriel C, Broding HC, Jettkant B, Berresheim H, Wiethege T, Käfferlein H, Merget R, Bünger J, Brüning T. Considerations for the design and technical setup of a human whole-body exposure chamber. Inhal Toxicol. 2012;24:99–108.
16. American Thoracic Society and European Respiratory Society (ATS/ERS). Recommendations for standardized procedures for the online and offline measurement of exhaled lower respiratory nitric oxide and nasal nitric oxide, 2005. Am J Respir Crit Care Med. 2005;171:912–30.
17. Criée CP, Sorichter S, Smith HJ, Kardos P, Merget R, Heise D, Berdel D, Köhler D, Magnussen H, Marek W, Mitfessel H, Rasche K, Rolke M, Worth H, Jörres RA. Bodyplethysmography - its principles and clinical use. Respir Med. 2011;105:959–73.
18. American Thoracic Society. Standardization of spirometry, 1994 update. Am J Respir Crit Care Med. 1995;152:1107–36.

19. Szlezak AM, Szlezak SL, Keane J, Tajouri L, Minahan C. Establishing a dose-response relationship between acute resistance-exercise and the immune system: protocol for a systematic review. Immunol Lett. 2016;180:54–65.
20. Thomas L. Labor und Diagnose: Indikation und Bewertung von Laborbefunden für die medizinische Diagnostik. 2007. ISBN-10: 3980521567, ISBN-13: 978-3980521567.
21. International Commission for Radiological Protection (ICRP). Human respiratory tract model for radiological protection. ICRP publication 66 Ann ICRP. 1994;24:1–3.
22. Hollinger MA, Raabe OG, Giri SN, Freywald M, Teague SV, Tarkington B. Effect of the inhalation of zinc and dietary zinc on paraquat toxicity in the rat. Toxicol Appl Pharmacol. 1979;49:53–61.
23. Pauluhn J. Derivation of occupational exposure levels (OELs) of low-toxicity isometric biopersistent particles: how can the kinetic lung overload paradigm be used for improved inhalation toxicity study design and OEL-derivation? Part Fibre Toxicol. 2014;11:72.
24. Cho WS, Duffin R, Howie SE, Scotton CJ, Wallace WA, Macnee W, Bradley M, Megson IL, Donaldson K. Progressive severe lung injury by zinc oxide nanoparticles; the role of Zn2+ dissolution inside lysosomes. Part Fibre Toxicol. 2011;8:27.
25. Syama S, Sreekanth PJ, Varma HK, Mohanan PV. Zinc oxide nanoparticles induced oxidative stress in mouse bone marrow mesenchymal stem cells. Toxicol Mech Methods. 2014;24:644–53.
26. Kuschner WG, Wong H, Dalessandro A, Quinlan P, Blanc PD. Human pulmonary responses to experimental inhalation of high concentration fine and ultrafine magnesium oxide particles. Environ Health Perspect. 1997;105:1234–7.
27. Allin KH, Bojesen SE, Nordestgaard BG. Baseline C-reactive protein is associated with incident cancer and survival in patients with cancer. J Clin Oncol. 2009;27:2217–24.
28. Allin KH, Nordestgaard BG. Elevated C-reactive protein in the diagnosis, prognosis, and cause of cancer. Crit Rev Clin Lab Sci. 2011; 48:155–70.
29. Rietzschel E, De Buyzere M. High-sensitive C-reactive protein: universal prognostic and causative biomarker in heart disease? Biomark Med. 2012;6:19–34.
30. Kounis NG, Soufras GD, Tsigkas G, Hahalis G. White blood cell counts, leukocyte ratios, and eosinophils as inflammatory markers in patients with coronary artery disease. Clin Appl Thromb Hemost. 2015;21:139–43.
31. Getz GS, Krishack PA, Reardon CA. Serum amyloid a and atherosclerosis. Curr Opin Lipidol. 2016;27:531–5.
32. Thomsen M, Dahl M, Lange P, Vestbo J, Nordestgaard BG. Inflammatory biomarkers and comorbidities in chronic obstructive pulmonary disease. Am J Respir Crit Care Med. 2012;186:982–8.
33. Saber AT, Jacobsen NR, Jackson P, Poulsen SS, Kyjovska ZO, Halappanavar S, Yauk CL, Wallin H, Vogel U. Particle-induced pulmonary acute phase response may be the causal link between particle inhalation and cardiovascular disease. Wiley Interdiscip Rev Nanomed Nanobiotechnol. 2014;6:517–31.
34. Ridker PM, Everett BM, Thuren T, MacFadyen JG, Chang WH, Ballantyne C, Fonseca F, Nicolau J, Koenig W, Anker SD, JJP K, Cornel JH, Pais P, Pella D, Genest J, Cifkova R, Lorenzatti A, Forster T, Kobalava Z, Vida-Simiti L, Flather M, Shimokawa H, Ogawa H, Dellborg M, PRF R, RPT T, Libby P, Glynn RJ, CANTOS Trial Group. Antiinflammatory therapy with Canakinumab for atherosclerotic disease. N Engl J Med. 2017;377:1119–31.
35. : Kendzia B, Behrens T, Jöckel KH, Siemiatycki J, Kromhout H, Vermeulen R, Peters S, Van Gelder R, Olsson A, Brüske I, Wichmann HE, Stücker I, Guida F, Tardón A, Merletti F, Mirabelli D, Richiardi L, Pohlabeln H, Ahrens W, Landi MT, Caporaso N, Consonni D, Zaridze D, Szeszenia-Dabrowska N, Lissowska J, Gustavsson P, Marcus M, Fabianova E, 't Mannetje A, Pearce N, Tse LA, Yu IT, Rudnai P, Bencko V, Janout V, Mates D, Foretova L, Forastiere F, McLaughlin J, Demers P, Bueno-de-Mesquita B, Boffetta P, Schüz J, Straif K, Pesch B, Brüning T. Welding and lung cancer in a pooled analysis of case-control studies. Am J Epidemiol 2013;178:1513-1525.
36. Li H, Hedmer M, Kåredal M, Björk J, Stockfelt L, Tinnerberg H, Albin M, Broberg K. A cross-sectional study of the cardiovascular effects of welding fumes. PLoS One. 2015;10:e0131648.
37. Ibfelt E, Bonde JP, Hansen J. Exposure to metal welding fume particles and risk for cardiovascular disease in Denmark: a prospective cohort study. Occup Environ Med. 2010;67:772–7.
38. Baumann R, Gube M, Markert A, Davatgarbenam S, Kossack V, Gerhards B, Kraus T, Brand P. Systemic serum amyloid A as a biomarker for exposure to zinc and/or copper-containing metal fumes. J Expo Sci Environ Epidemiol 2017 [Epub ahead of print].
39. GESTIS Substance Database. Information system on hazardous substances of the German Social Accident Insurance. 2017; http://limitvalue.ifa.dguv.de

9

Short-term effects of fine particulate matter and ozone on the cardiac conduction system in patients undergoing cardiac catheterization

Siqi Zhang[1*], Susanne Breitner[1], Wayne E Cascio[2], Robert B Devlin[2], Lucas M Neas[2], David Diaz-Sanchez[2], William E Kraus[3], Joel Schwartz[4], Elizabeth R Hauser[3], Annette Peters[1] and Alexandra Schneider[1]

Abstract

Background: Air pollution-induced changes in cardiac electrophysiological properties could be a pathway linking air pollution and cardiovascular events. The evidence of air pollution effects on the cardiac conduction system is incomplete yet. We investigated short-term effects of particulate matter ≤ 2.5 μm in aerodynamic diameter ($PM_{2.5}$) and ozone (O_3) on cardiac electrical impulse propagation and repolarization as recorded in surface electrocardiograms (ECG).

Methods: We analyzed repeated 12-lead ECG measurements performed on 5,332 patients between 2001 and 2012. The participants came from the Duke CATHGEN Study who underwent cardiac catheterization and resided in North Carolina, United States (NC, U.S.). Daily concentrations of $PM_{2.5}$ and O_3 at each participant's home address were predicted with a hybrid air quality exposure model. We used generalized additive mixed models to investigate the associations of $PM_{2.5}$ and O_3 with the PR interval, QRS interval, heart rate-corrected QT interval (QTc), and heart rate (HR). The temporal lag structures of the associations were examined using distributed-lag models.

Results: Elevated $PM_{2.5}$ and O_3 were associated with four-day lagged lengthening of the PR and QRS intervals, and with one-day lagged increases in HR. We observed immediate effects on the lengthening of the QTc interval for both $PM_{2.5}$ and O_3, as well as delayed effects for $PM_{2.5}$ (lagged by 3 – 4 days). The associations of $PM_{2.5}$ and O_3 with the PR interval and the association of O_3 with the QRS interval persisted until up to seven days after exposure.

Conclusions: In patients undergoing cardiac catheterization, short-term exposure to air pollution was associated with increased HR and delays in atrioventricular conduction, ventricular depolarization and repolarization.

Keywords: Air pollution, Electrocardiogram, PR interval, QT interval, QRS interval

Background

The associations between ambient air pollution and cardiovascular morbidity and mortality are well established [1–3]. One potential pathway of the linkage might be through the air pollution-induced changes in cardiac electrophysiological properties. The cardiac conduction system initiates and conducts electrical impulses as recorded in the electrocardiogram (ECG). Cardiac conduction abnormalities, such as first-degree atrioventricular block (first-degree AVB) or prolonged ventricular repolarization, are associated with increased incidence and prevalence of atrial fibrillation (AF), total mortality, and sudden cardiac death [4, 5].

The acute effects of air pollution on the cardiac conduction system could be mediated by physiological mechanisms including autonomic imbalance and systemic inflammation, which trigger both immediate and delayed responses over a period ranging from hours to days [6, 7]. Epidemiological studies have reported associations of a lengthening of the heart rate-corrected

* Correspondence: siqi.zhang@helmholtz-muenchen.de
[1]Institute of Epidemiology, Helmholtz Zentrum München, Ingolstädter Landstr. 1, P.O. Box 11 29, D-85764 Neuherberg, Germany
Full list of author information is available at the end of the article

QT interval (QTc), a measure of ventricular repolarization, with particulate matter in the elderly and patients having diabetes or preexisting ischemic heart disease [6, 8–11]. However, such associations were not observed in a panel study of cardiac rehabilitation patients [7]. In addition to the inconsistent results of particulate matter, evidence of ambient ozone (O_3) effects on the QTc interval is still limited [12, 13], and the impacts of air pollution on atrioventricular conduction and ventricular depolarization have not been fully investigated [9, 14].

Hypothesizing that air pollution exposure would be associated with cardiac conduction delay, we performed this study to investigate the short-term effects of $PM_{2.5}$ and O_3 on the electrocardiographic intervals reflecting impulse propagation and repolarization in high-risk patients from a cardiovascular cohort.

Methods

Study population

The data used in this study were obtained from the Catheterization Genetics (CATHGEN) Study, a cohort of 9,334 patients who underwent cardiac catheterization at Duke University Medical Center from 2001 through 2010. More details of the CATHGEN Study can be found elsewhere [15].

Our analyses were restricted to 6,209 individuals who had ECG measurements and resided in North Carolina, United States (NC, U.S.) at catheterization. From the CATHGEN database, we collected information on participant demographic characteristics (age, sex, and race), body mass index (BMI), smoking status, and the history of myocardial infarction (MI). The Coronary Artery Disease Prognostic index (CAD index) was assessed during the catheterization procedure. The CAD index is an indicator of the severity of coronary artery disease (CAD) based upon cardiovascular outcomes. A CAD index > 23 represents at least one ≥ 75% occlusion in one major epicardial coronary artery [16]. Data on area-level educational attainment and urban/rural status were obtained from the 2000 U.S. Census based on each patient's home address at catheterization. Area-level educational attainment refers to the percentage of adults (≥ 25 years old) in the block group with less than a high school education; it was categorized into low (≥ 25%) and high (< 25%) levels.

ECG measurement

During the study period (2001–2012), 71,194 12-lead ECGs were performed at the time of catheterization and in follow-up examinations, and analyzed automatically using the Philips TraceMaster ECG system (Andover, MA). ECG parameters of interest were the PR interval (ms), QRS interval (ms), QT interval (ms), and heart rate (HR, beats/min). The PR interval is measured from the beginning of the P wave to the beginning of the QRS complex, reflecting the electrical impulse conduction from the sinus node through the atrioventricular node and His-Purkinje system. The QRS interval is the time from the onset of the Q wave to the end of the S wave, which represents ventricular depolarization. The QT interval is defined as the duration from the beginning of the Q wave to the end of the T wave. The QT interval is dependent on HR; after HR-correction, the QTc interval is a measure of ventricular repolarization. The QT correction for HR was performed using the Bazett formula in our main analyses [17].

We first excluded 13,632 ECGs with the diagnosis of atrial fibrillation, atrial flutter, multifocal atrial tachycardia, or paced rhythms. For participants with multiple ECGs on the same day or ECGs on consecutive days, we only included the first of the day and the first on consecutive days to reduce the potential impact of intervening medical treatment. To reduce bias caused by artifacts, we excluded ECGs with non-physiological parameter values in the following ranges: (1) PR interval < 100 ms or > 400 ms, (2) QRS interval < 50 ms or > 170 ms, (3) QTc < 350 ms or > 600 ms, (4) HR < 20 beats per minute (bpm) or > 180 bpm. We further excluded participants with bundle branch block (BBB, QRS interval > 120 ms), leaving 28,741 eligible ECGs on 5,376 participants.

Exposure assessment

Daily concentrations of $PM_{2.5}$ (daily average in $\mu g/m^3$) and O_3 (daily 8-h maximum in ppb) for NC were predicted at a 1 km × 1 km spatial grid resolution from 2000 to 2012. Predictions were made using a neural network-based hybrid model, incorporating input variables such as chemical transport model outputs, satellite-based aerosol optical depth data, absorbing aerosol index, land-use terms, and meteorological variables. The ten-fold cross-validation indicated good model performances with coefficients of determination of 0.86 and 0.68 for $PM_{2.5}$ and O_3, respectively. Detailed descriptions and predictive performance of the model were reported elsewhere [18, 19].

Daily air temperature in NC was also predicted at a 1 km × 1 km grid resolution for the study period. The modeling process involved satellite-derived daily surface temperature, daily air temperature from NC weather stations, normalized difference vegetation index, and predictors of air temperature (percent of urban areas, elevation, and distance to water body). A three-stage modeling approach was used, allowing the prediction in grid cells without weather monitors or grid cells/days without data on satellite surface temperature [20].

The latitude and longitude of each participant's residential address were geocoded by the Children's

Environmental Health Initiative in the Duke Nicholas School of the Environment (https://cehi.rice.edu/). For individuals who moved during the study period, we used the address most closely linked with the date on which the ECG was performed. The geocoded addresses were matched with air pollution and temperature data based on the spatial location and date. Daily air pollutant concentrations and air temperature on the same day and 1–14 days prior to the ECG measurement were assigned to each ECG.

Statistical analysis

Short-term effects of $PM_{2.5}$ and O_3 on ECG parameters were investigated using generalized additive mixed models with random intercepts for patients. The ECG parameters were log-transformed in our regression models to increase the conformity to a normal distribution of residuals. To control for systematic variation over time, we included a penalized spline for long-term time trend with four degrees of freedom per year, and two categorical variables for season (spring: March–May; summer: June–August; autumn: September–November; winter: December–February) and day of the week. Air temperature was adjusted for by modeling low and high temperatures separately [21]. For days with average temperature on the previous four days (lag1–4) lower than the median annual temperature, we introduced a natural spline with two degrees of freedom for lag1–4 temperature. Similarly, for days with average temperature on the current and previous day (lag0–1) higher than the median annual temperature, we introduced a natural spline for lag0–1 temperature with three degrees of freedom. Besides, we controlled for individual characteristics at each measurement time point, including age (continuous), sex (male or female), race (European-Americans, African-Americans, or others), area-level educational attainment (low or high), BMI (continuous), smoking status (never smoker, or current/former smoker), and living area (rural or urban). The adjusted confounders were identical across models for the various air pollutants and ECG parameters. We investigated the effects of air pollution on the concurrent day (lag0), for single-day lags from one to four days (lag0–lag4), and for a multi-day lag of five days (lag04).

For pollutant-outcome pairs showing significant delayed associations four days after exposure, we examined lagged effects up to 14 days using distributed-lag models [22]. We therefore built a cross-basis matrix with a third degree polynomial function of lags, which was then incorporated into the generalized additive mixed model adjusted for the same confounders as in the main model.

To explore effect modification and identify the subgroups that might be more susceptible to the effects of $PM_{2.5}$ and O_3, we incorporated interaction terms between air pollution and individual characteristics in the model. The examined potential modifiers included sex, age (< 60 years vs. ≥ 60 years), area-level educational attainment, obesity (BMI < 30 kg/m^2 vs. ≥ 30 kg/m^2), smoking status, urban/rural status, CAD index (CAD index ≤ 23 vs. > 23), and history of MI.

In sensitivity analyses, we excluded ECGs with single-day (lag0–lag4) exposure levels of $PM_{2.5}$ above 35 $\mu g/m^3$ or O_3 above 70 ppb to examine the effects of air pollution below the current U.S. National Ambient Air Quality Standards (NAAQS) [23]. As the electrophysiological parameters are potentially dependent on the HR, we further adjusted for the HR in models for the PR interval, QRS interval, and the raw QT interval without HR-correction. In addition, we used Fridericia formula in QT correction [24], and investigated air pollution effects on corrected JT interval (JTc), which was defined by subtracting the QRS from QTc. The JTc interval is also an indicator to measure the duration of ventricular repolarization and is reported to reduce the impact of wide QRS complex on the QTc interval [25]. To examine the influence of BBB on associations between air pollution and ECG parameters, we performed analyses using 33,117 eligible ECG measurements on 5,819 participants regardless of the presence of BBB. We tested the robustness of the results by building two-pollutant models with $PM_{2.5}$ and O_3 of the same lag, restricting the analyses to participants with two or more ECG measurements, changing the degree of freedom for the trend spline, excluding season as a categorical variable, and applying generalized additive mixed models with linear spatial correlation structure given that the dependency between repeated ECG measurements might decrease with increasing time interval. Furthermore, we added long-term air pollution exposure (365-day moving average of air pollution of 0–364 days prior to each ECG measurement) to our models and replaced the daily mean concentration with the deviation between daily mean and long-term average. In this way, we sought to investigate the acute effect of temporal variation of pollutants with the control for spatial variation. The linearity of the exposure-response relationships was examined by including a spline for air pollution variables in models.

The effect estimates are reported as percent changes of the geometric mean (GM) of outcomes and 95% confidence intervals (95% CI) corresponding to an interquartile range (IQR) increase in $PM_{2.5}$ and O_3. We performed the analyses with the software R (version 3.5.1), using the 'gamm4', 'mgcv', and 'dlnm' packages. The significance level was set at 0.05.

Results

Participant characteristics and exposure concentrations

After further exclusion of 44 patients without complete data on ECG parameters of interest, air pollution concentrations, or main covariates, we analyzed a final sample of 28,578 ECGs on 5,332 participants (See Additional file 1: Figure S1). Among them, 4,009 participants had two or more eligible ECG recordings during the study period. The mean age and BMI at enrollment were 59.8 years and 30.1 kg/m^2, respectively (Table 1). 60.7% of the participants were male, over half were never smokers, and the majority were European-American (72.3%). More individuals lived in rural areas and areas with a high level of educational attainment. Compared to excluded individuals, the participants included in our main analyses tended to be younger and more likely to live in urban areas, have a higher proportion of African-Americans and a higher level of educational attainment (See Additional file 1: Table S1).

Table 2 shows the descriptive statistics of ECG parameters in all ECG recordings. The correlations between ECG parameters were weak or negligible. During the study period, the average concentrations of $PM_{2.5}$ and O_3 in geocoded areas with participants were 11.2 μg/m^3 and 40.5 ppb, respectively (Table 3). Most daily $PM_{2.5}$ and O_3 levels (99.9% for $PM_{2.5}$ and 98.7% for O_3) were below the current NAAQS (daily average concentration of 35 μg/m^3 for $PM_{2.5}$ and daily maximum 8-hour concentration of 70 ppb for O_3). $PM_{2.5}$ and O_3 were moderately correlated with a Spearman correlation coefficient of 0.49.

Table 1 Descriptive statistics of the study population at baseline (n=5332)

	Mean ± SD / N (%)
Age (years)	59.8 ± 11.7
BMI (kg/m^2)	30.1 ± 7.2
Sex (male)	3237 (60.7)
Race	
European-Americans	3854 (72.3)
African-Americans	1188 (22.3)
Others	290 (5.4)
Smoking (never smoker)	2753 (51.6)
Education (high)	3231 (60.6)
Area (rural)	2953 (55.4)
CAD-index > 23 (yes)[a]	2418 (50.4)
History of MI (yes)	1449 (27.2)

SD standard deviation, *BMI* body mass index, *CAD* coronary artery disease, *MI* myocardial infarction
[a]Data on CAD-index were available for 4801 participants

Air pollution and ECG parameters

Increments in $PM_{2.5}$ and O_3 were significantly associated with the lengthening of the PR interval lagged three or four days, and with the concurrent as well as lagged lengthening of the QTc interval (Table 4). Positive associations with the QRS interval were significant for O_3 at lag4 and marginally significant for $PM_{2.5}$ at lag1 and lag4. We also observed significant increases in the HR associated with elevated $PM_{2.5}$ and a marginally significant increase for O_3, with the strongest single-day effects at lag1.

We used polynomial distributed-lag models for PR, QRS, and QTc intervals as they showed delayed responses to air pollution. Estimates of the distributed-lag models indicated that the effects of $PM_{2.5}$ and O_3 on the PR interval and the effect of O_3 on the QRS interval persisted until seven days after exposure. For the QTc interval, we did not find lagged effects of $PM_{2.5}$ beyond four days (Fig. 1).

Effect modification

We observed stronger effects of O_3 on the QRS and QTc intervals in patients living in rural areas, and stronger air pollution effects on the QTc interval in patients with low educational attainment or obesity. We did not find significant or consistent effect modification by other examined potential modifiers (See Additional file 1: Figure S2).

Sensitivity analyses

Analyses of exposure below the NAAQS showed slightly attenuated associations between air pollution and ECG parameters; the effects of air pollution on the PR interval, QTc interval, and HR remained significant (See Additional file 1: Table S2). Associations of air pollution with the PR, QRS, and QT intervals were not sensitive to the adjustment for HR (See Additional file 1: Figure S3). We observed reduced effects of air pollution on the QTc interval calculated using the Fridericia formula compared to using the Bazett formula at lag0–lag2 (See Additional file 1: Figure S4). However, the associations between air pollution and ventricular repolarization were generally consistent across different indicators. Including participants with BBB reduced the air pollution effects on the QRS and QTc intervals and did not significantly affect the effects on the PR interval and HR (See Additional file 1: Figure S5).

We did not observe substantial changes in effect estimates in two-pollutant models, except for the attenuated effect of $PM_{2.5}$ on the PR interval at lag4 when adjusted for O_3 and vice versa (See Additional file 1: Figure S6). The associations of $PM_{2.5}$ and O_3 with ECG parameters were robust to excluding participants with only one ECG measurements, changing the degree of freedom of trend spline, excluding season, controlling for long-term

Table 2 Descriptive statistics and Spearman correlation coefficients of ECG parameters (n=28578)

	Mean ± SD		Min	25%	Median	75%	Max	Correlation coefficients		
	Geometric	Arithmetic						PR	QRS	QTc
PR (ms)	170 ± 1	173 ± 31	100[a]	152	168	188	400[a]	--		
QRS (ms)	91 ± 1	91 ± 12	53	83	90	99	120[a]	0.18	--	
QTc (ms)	434 ± 1	435 ± 33	350[a]	412	433	456	587	-0.02	0.24	--
HR (bpm)	73 ± 1	74 ± 17	31	62	72	85	160	-0.28	-0.09	0.32

SD standard deviation, *Min* minimum, *25%* the 25th percentile, *75%* the 75th percentile, *Max* maximum, *QTc* heart rate-corrected QT interval, *HR* heart rate, *bpm* beats per minute

[a]The minimum and maximum values were set by the exclusion criteria

exposure to air pollution, or applying spatial correlation structure in mixed-effects models. The linear exposure-response relationships between air pollution and ECG parameters held true when air pollution variables were included in models as splines (results not shown).

Discussion

In high-risk patients undergoing cardiac catheterization, we observed associations of increments in $PM_{2.5}$ and O_3 with the lengthening of the PR, QRS, and QTc intervals and increased HR. The effects of $PM_{2.5}$ and O_3 on the PR interval and the effect of O_3 on the QRS interval persisted until up to one week in distributed lag models. These findings supported our hypothesis that short-term exposure to air pollution was associated with atrioventricular and intraventricular conduction delay.

An increased PR interval could relate to parasympathetic activation, sympathetic withdrawal, or the block of inward calcium current through membrane channels. A lengthening of the PR interval, even below the diagnostic threshold for first-degree AVB (PR interval > 200 ms), is associated with increased incidence of AF, pacemaker implantation, and all-cause mortality [5]. Few prior studies investigated the effect of air pollution on the PR interval. The Air Pollution and Cardiac Risk and its Time Course (APACR) Study found a 0.09% increase in the PR interval for each 10 μg/m^3 increment in $PM_{2.5}$ [14]. Since individuals with cardiovascular disease are potentially more sensitive to air pollution effects, the smaller effect estimate compared to our study (0.25%) could be due to the healthier participants in the APACR Study. The distinct lag times of associations (1.5–2 hours in the APACR Study and 3–4 days in our study) might also partly explain the difference. In addition to $PM_{2.5}$, our study provided evidence for an association between O_3 and the PR interval, which to our knowledge has not been reported previously.

The associations between air pollution and the QRS interval in our study indicated the effects of air pollution

Table 3 Descriptive statistics of air pollution and temperature in geocoded areas with participants during the study period

	Mean ± SD	Min	25%	Median	75%	Max	IQR
$PM_{2.5}$ (μg/m^3)	11.2 ± 5.5	0.9	7.3	10.1	14.2	54.5	7.0
O_3 (ppb)	40.5 ± 12.8	8.6	30.4	39.5	49.8	97.6	19.4
Air temperature (°C)	16.8 ± 8.1	-4.7	10.2	17.8	24.0	31.0	13.8

SD standard deviation, *Min* minimum, *25%* the 25th percentile, *75%* the 75th percentile, *Max* maximum, *IQR* interquartile range, *$PM_{2.5}$* particulate matter ≤ 2.5 μm in aerodynamic diameter, *O_3* ozone, *ppb* parts per billion

Table 4 Percent change (95% CI) of the geometric mean of ECG parameters per interquartile range increase in pollutants

ECG parameter	Lag (day)	$PM_{2.5}$	O_3
		% Change (95% CI)	% Change (95% CI)
PR	0	-0.07 (-0.23, 0.08)	-0.01 (-0.24, 0.23)
	1	-0.07 (-0.23, 0.09)	0.03 (-0.21, 0.27)
	2	-0.07 (-0.23, 0.09)	-0.12 (-0.36, 0.12)
	3	0.17 (0.01, 0.33)*	0.02 (-0.22, 0.26)
	4	0.18 (0.03, 0.34)*	0.29 (0.05, 0.53)*
	04	0.07 (-0.18, 0.32)	0.09 (-0.26, 0.43)
QRS	0	0.11 (0.00, 0.22)	-0.04 (-0.21, 0.12)
	1	0.03 (-0.08, 0.14)	0.00 (-0.17, 0.16)
	2	0.01 (-0.10, 0.12)	-0.05 (-0.22, 0.11)
	3	0.04 (-0.07, 0.15)	0.04 (-0.13, 0.21)
	4	0.11 (0.00, 0.21)	0.21 (0.04, 0.37)*
	04	0.15 (-0.03, 0.32)	0.06 (-0.18, 0.30)
QTc	0	0.11 (0.02, 0.19)*	0.17 (0.04, 0.30)**
	1	0.05 (-0.04, 0.14)	0.18 (0.04, 0.31)**
	2	0.05 (-0.04, 0.14)	0.07 (-0.06, 0.21)
	3	0.11 (0.03, 0.20)*	0.02 (-0.11, 0.15)
	4	0.13 (0.05, 0.22)**	0.04 (-0.09, 0.17)
	04	0.23 (0.09, 0.36)**	0.20 (0.01, 0.39)*
HR	0	0.22 (-0.05, 0.49)	0.23 (-0.17, 0.63)
	1	0.47 (0.20, 0.75)**	0.40 (0.00, 0.81)
	2	0.28 (0.01, 0.56)*	0.28 (-0.13, 0.69)
	3	-0.11 (-0.38, 0.16)	-0.21 (-0.62, 0.20)
	4	0.04 (-0.23, 0.30)	-0.12 (-0.53, 0.29)
	04	0.44 (0.01, 0.86)*	0.24 (-0.34, 0.83)

CI confidence interval, *ECG* electrocardiogram, *$PM_{2.5}$* particulate matter ≤ 2.5 μm in aerodynamic diameter, *O_3* ozone; *QTc* heart rate-corrected QT interval, *HR* heart rate

*p-Value <0.05; **p-Value <0.01

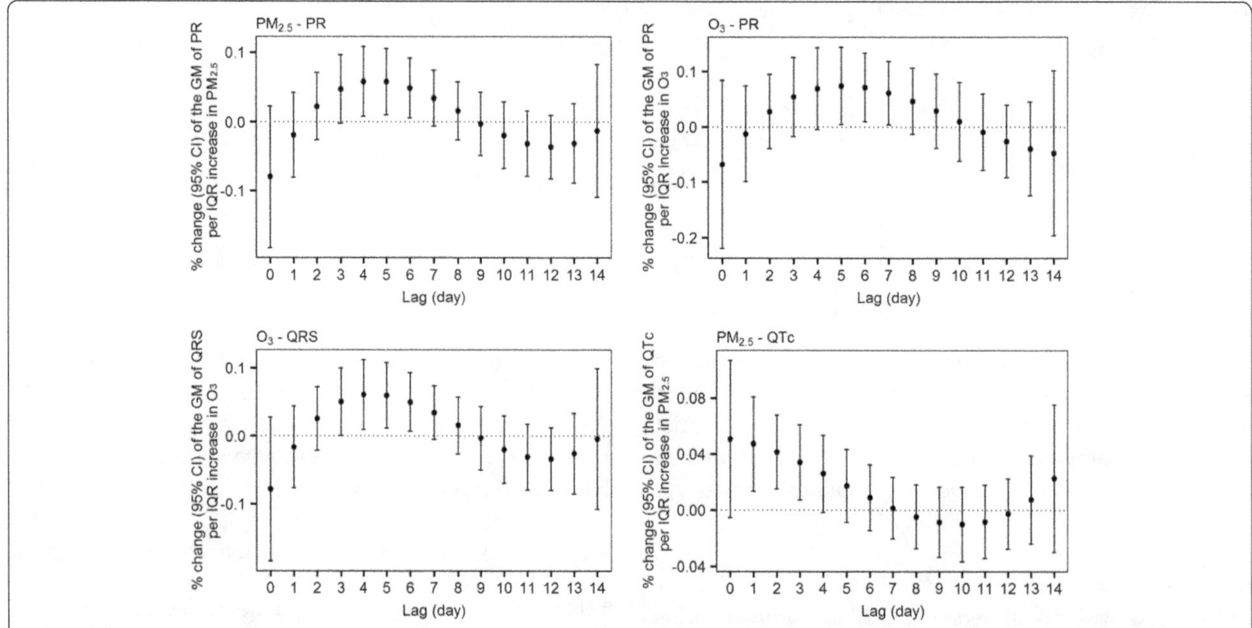

Fig. 1 Percent change (95% CI) of the geometric mean of ECG parameters per interquartile range increase in $PM_{2.5}$ and O_3 in distributed-lag models. *CI* confidence interval, *ECG* electrocardiogram, *$PM_{2.5}$* particulate matter ≤ 2.5 μm in aerodynamic diameter, *O_3* ozone *QTc* heart rate-corrected QT interval, *GM* geometric mean, *IQR* interquartile range

on ventricular depolarization among individuals without bundle branch block. An increase in the QRS interval is an independent predictor of cardiovascular mortality [26]. Yet, the evidence of air pollution effects on the QRS interval is still limited. Consistent with our results, a higher prevalence of prolonged QRS interval was associated with long-term residential $PM_{2.5}$ exposure in the U.S. Multi-Ethnic Study of Atherosclerosis (MESA) Cohort. Besides, in a controlled exposure study among individuals with metabolic syndrome, the GSTM1 null participants showed an increased QRS interval after acute exposure to concentrated ambient ultrafine particles [27]. However, the QRS interval was not associated with $PM_{2.5}$ in the APACR Study [9], and an immediate decrease of 5.8% (95%CI: -10.5, -1.0) in the QRS interval after exposure to O_3 was observed in a crossover study among healthy volunteers [13]. The mechanism by which air pollution might lead to a change in QRS complex remains unclear and needs to be clarified by further epidemiological and experimental studies. Some theoretical explanations could be the impact of air pollution on the inward sodium current and the extracellular resistance.

Our findings of both concurrent and delayed effects of air pollution on the lengthening of the QTc interval are supported by previous studies [6, 8, 13]. The potential pathway of the immediate associations could be the direct impact of air pollution on the autonomic nervous system, and the delayed effects are possibly mediated by air pollution-induced inflammatory responses [6]. Ambient air pollutants trigger reactive oxygen species production, which in turn induces pulmonary and systemic inflammation. The concentrations of circulating inflammatory biomarkers, such as C-reactive protein (CRP), interleukin 6, and fibrinogen, are increased after acute air pollution exposure [6, 28]. Further, inflammation is a modulator of cardiomyocyte ion currents in the cardiac conduction system, through a pathway involving cytokine- and sympathetic-induced modulation [29]. Elevated levels of circulating inflammatory biomarkers have been proven to be associated with QTc prolongation [30–32].

The QTc interval calculated using the Bazett formula has been reported to be inferior to using the Fridericia formula in the prediction of mortality [33]. In our study, the associations between air pollution and the QTc interval calculated using the Fridericia formula were generally comparable to using the Bazett formula. Similar results were also found in the APACR Study [9]. In addition, since the QT interval encompasses the duration of ventricular depolarization as reflected by the QRS interval, the air pollution-induced lengthening of the QTc interval could be partly attributable to the effects on the QRS interval. When subtracting the QRS from the QTc, we still observed significant associations between air pollution and the JTc interval. The robust results provided strong evidence for the air pollution effects on ventricular repolarization.

The 1–2 days lagged associations between air pollution and HR suggested the effects of air pollution on the autonomic nervous system [8, 34–36]. These associations could be potentially affected by the use of medication. For example, stronger effects of air pollution on HR and heart rate variability are observed among individuals not taking beta-blockers or calcium-channel blockers [8, 34]. On the other hand, taking medication indicates the presence of underlying clinical conditions, which might increase individual's susceptibility to air pollution. Therefore, other studies reported non-significant effect modification by medication or even stronger effects in individuals taking angiotensin-converting-enzyme inhibitor (ACE inhibitor) [37, 38]. The interaction between medication usage and clinical conditions potentially limits the interpretability of the non-significant effect modification by CAD in our study.

Although the effects of air pollution on the cardiac conduction system were relatively small in this study, it is still of public health significance because of its implications for the entire population. Using the World Health Organization air quality guideline for 24-hour mean of $PM_{2.5}$ (25 $\mu g/m^3$) as reference [39], exposure to the maximum $PM_{2.5}$ in this study (54.5 $\mu g/m^3$) would account for an increase of 2.4 ms in the QTc interval in exposed individuals. Moreover, cardiac conduction is affected by many other factors. For instance, preexisting medical conditions (left ventricular hypertrophy, ischemia, etc.) and certain medications can prolong cardiac repolarization [40]. Among patients with these conditions, further exposure to air pollution may add to the effects of other factors, and drive the QT interval across a critical threshold.

Strengths and limitations

A major strength of this study is the large sample size of the study population and the vast number of ECG recordings for analyses, which to the best of our knowledge is the largest cohort for analyzing air pollution effects on ECG parameters. The repeated measures study design provided substantial statistical power and enabled control for unmeasured individual-level confounders. Besides, we investigated the associations of $PM_{2.5}$ and O_3 with ECG parameters that have rarely been examined previously, such as the PR and QRS intervals.

One limitation of the study is the heterogeneity of time intervals caused by unscheduled follow-up visits. In the analyses, we applied mixed-effects models, which can reduce the impact of the unbalanced data structure. Second, we used daily residential exposure assessment instead of personal exposure. This may have resulted in non-differential exposure misclassification and bias the results towards the null [41]. Third, due to the unavailability of data, we were not able to control for medication intake, and the smoking status was roughly divided into current/former smoker or never smoker, which may have led to inaccuracy in assessing effect modification by pre-existing morbidities and residual confounding. Finally, our study was performed in high-risk patients receiving cardiac catheterization; thus, the results may not be generalizable to the general population. However, it enabled us to assess the association in a population subgroup at greater risk of cardiovascular events and potentially more susceptible to the adverse effects of air pollution.

Conclusions

In summary, short-term exposure to $PM_{2.5}$ and O_3 was associated with lengthening of the PR, QRS, and QTc intervals, and increasd heart rate in patients with cardiovascular disease. These findings provide evidence for the acute effects of air pollution on atrioventricular conduction and ventricular deporlarization and repolarization, which could potentially mediate the associations of air pollution with cardiac arrhythmias and cardiovascular mortality.

Additional file

Additional file 1: Table S1. Comparison of individual characteristics between participants included and excludes in main analyses. **Table S2.** Percent change (95% CI) of the geometric mean of ECG parameters per interquartile range increase in $PM_{2.5}$ and O_3 below the NAAQS. **Figure S1.** Flow chart of the exclusion procedure. **Figure S2.** Effect modification (percent change with 95% CI) by participant characteristics on the associations of air pollution with ECG parameters. **Figure S3.** Percent change (95% CI) of the geometric mean of the PR, QRS, and raw QT intervals per interquartile range increase in $PM_{2.5}$ and O_3 in models with adjustment for HR. **Figure S4**. Comparison of the air pollution effects (percent change with 95% CI) on different ventricular repolarization indicators. **Figure S5.** Percent change (95% CI) of the geometric mean of ECG parameters per interquartile range increase in $PM_{2.5}$ and O_3 among participants with QRS ≤ 120 ms and participants with QRS in the full range (50 ms ≤ QRS ≤ 170 ms). **Figure S6.** Percent change (95% CI) of the geometric mean of ECG parameters per interquartile range increase in $PM_{2.5}$ and O_3 in sensitivity analyses. (DOC 884 kb)

Abbreviations

AF: Atrial fibrillation; AVB: Atrioventricular block; BBB: Bundle branch block; BMI: Body mass index; BPM: Beats per minute; CAD: Coronary artery disease; CI: Confidence interval; CRP: C-reactive protein; ECG: Electrocardiogram; GM: Geometric mean; HR: Heart rate; IQR: Interquartile range; MI: Myocardial infarction; NAAQS: National Ambient Air Quality Standards; O_3: Ozone; $PM_{2.5}$: Particulate matter ≤ 2.5 μm in aerodynamic diameter; QTc: Heart rate-corrected QT interval; SD: Standard deviation

Funding

This work was partially supported by Health Effects Institute 4946-RFPA10-3/14-7 to WEK (PI) with subagreement 3838618 to Helmholtz Zentrum München, AS (subrecepient PI), and a scholarship under the State Scholarship Fund by the China Scholarship Council (File No. 201606010330).

Disclaimer

Authors' contributions

SZ performed the statistical analyses and drafted the manuscript. AS, SB, AP, WC were substantially involved in the design of the study and interpretation of the data, and revised the manuscript critically. RD, LN, DDS, WK, and EH were involved in the acquisition of the CATHGEN data and reviewed the manuscript critically. JS was involved in the acquisition of the air pollution and temperature data and reviewed the manuscript critically. All authors read and approved the final manuscript.

Competing interests

The authors declare that they have no competing interests

Author details

[1]Institute of Epidemiology, Helmholtz Zentrum München, Ingolstädter Landstr. 1, P.O. Box 11 29, D-85764 Neuherberg, Germany. [2]National Health and Environmental Effects Research Laboratory, US Environmental Protection Agency, Research Triangle Park, Durham, NC, USA. [3]Duke Molecular Physiology Institute, School of Medicine, Duke University, Durham, NC, USA. [4]Department of Environmental Health, Harvard T.H. Chan School of Public Health, Boston, MA, USA.

References

1. Pope CA, Burnett RT, Thurston GD, Thun MJ, Calle EE, Krewski D, Godleski JJ. Cardiovascular mortality and long-term exposure to particulate air pollution. Circulation. 2004;109(1):71–7.
2. Rückerl R, Schneider A, Breitner S, Cyrys J, Peters A. Health effects of particulate air pollution: a review of epidemiological evidence. Inhal Toxicol. 2011;23(10):555–92.
3. Brook RD, Rajagopalan S, Pope CA 3rd, Brook JR, Bhatnagar A, Diez-Roux AV, Holguin F, Hong Y, Luepker RV, Mittleman MA, et al. Particulate matter air pollution and cardiovascular disease: An update to the scientific statement from the American Heart Association. Circulation. 2010;121(21):2331–78.
4. Straus SM, Kors JA, De Bruin ML, van der Hooft CS, Hofman A, Heeringa J, Deckers JW, Kingma JH, Sturkenboom MC, Stricker BH et al: Prolonged QTc interval and risk of sudden cardiac death in a population of older adults. J Am Coll Cardiol 2006, 47(2):362-367.
5. Cheng S, Keyes MJ, Larson MG, McCabe EL, Newton-Cheh C, Levy D, Benjamin EJ, Vasan RS, Wang TJ. Long-term outcomes in individuals with prolonged PR interval or first-degree atrioventricular block. Jama. 2009; 301(24):2571–7.
6. Schneider A, Neas LM, Graff DW, Herbst MC, Cascio WE, Schmitt MT, Buse JB, Peters A, Devlin RB. Association of cardiac and vascular changes with ambient PM 2.5 in diabetic individuals. Part Fibre Toxicol. 2010; **7**(1):14.
7. Rich DQ, Zareba W, Beckett W, Hopke PK, Oakes D, Frampton MW, Bisognano J, Chalupa D, Bausch J, O'Shea K, et al. Are ambient ultrafine, accumulation mode, and fine particles associated with adverse cardiac responses in patients undergoing cardiac rehabilitation? Environ Health Perspect. 2012;120(8):1162–9.
8. Hampel R, Schneider A, Bruske I, Zareba W, Cyrys J, Ruckerl R, Breitner S, Korb H, Sunyer J, Wichmann HE, et al. Altered cardiac repolarization in association with air pollution and air temperature among myocardial infarction survivors. Environ Health Perspect. 2010;118(12):1755–61.
9. Liao D, Shaffer ML, Rodriguez-Colon S, He F, Li X, Wolbrette DL, Yanosky J, Cascio WE. Acute adverse effects of fine particulate air pollution on ventricular repolarization. Environ Health Perspect. 2010;118(7):1010–5.
10. Baja ES, Schwartz JD, Wellenius GA, Coull BA, Zanobetti A, Vokonas PS, Suh HH. Traffic-related air pollution and QT interval: modification by diabetes, obesity, and oxidative stress gene polymorphisms in the normative aging study. Environ Health Perspect. 2010;118(6):840–6.
11. Henneberger A, Zareba W, Ibald-Mulli A, Rückerl R, Cyrys J, Couderc J-P, Mykins B, Woelke G, Wichmann HE, Peters A. Repolarization Changes Induced by Air Pollution in Ischemic Heart Disease Patients. Environ Health Perspect. 2005;113(4):440–6.
12. Hampel R, Breitner S, Zareba W, Kraus U, Pitz M, Geruschkat U, Belcredi P, Peters A, Schneider A, Cooperative Health Research in the Region of Augsburg Study G. Immediate ozone effects on heart rate and repolarisation parameters in potentially susceptible individuals. Occup Environ Med. 2012;69(6):428–36.
13. Devlin RB, Duncan KE, Jardim M, Schmitt MT, Rappold AG, Diaz-Sanchez D. Controlled exposure of healthy young volunteers to ozone causes cardiovascular effects. Circulation. 2012;126(1):104–11.
14. Liao D, Shaffer ML, He F, Rodriguez-Colon S, Wu R, Whitsel EA, Bixler EO, Cascio WE. Fine particulate air pollution is associated with higher vulnerability to atrial fibrillation--the APACR study. J Toxicol Environ Health A. 2011;74(11):693–705.
15. Kraus WE, Granger CB, Sketch MH Jr, Donahue MP, Ginsburg GS, Hauser ER, Haynes C, Newby LK, Hurdle M, Dowdy ZE, et al. A Guide for a Cardiovascular Genomics Biorepository: the CATHGEN Experience. J Cardiovasc Transl Res. 2015;8(**8**):449–57.
16. Bart BA, Shaw LK, McCants CB, Fortin DF, Lee KL, Califf RM, O'Connor CM. Clinical Determinants of Mortality in Patients With Angiographically Diagnosed Ischemic or Nonischemic Cardiomyopathy. J Am Coll Cardiol. 1997;30(4):1002–8.
17. Bazett HC. An analysis of the time relations of electrocardiograms. Heart. 1920;7:353–70.
18. Di Q, Kloog I, Koutrakis P, Lyapustin A, Wang Y, Schwartz J. Assessing PM2.5 Exposures with High Spatiotemporal Resolution across the Continental United States. Environ Sci Technol. 2016;50(9):4712–21.
19. Di Q, Rowland S, Koutrakis P, Schwartz J. A hybrid model for spatially and temporally resolved ozone exposures in the continental United States. J Air Waste Manag Assoc. 2017;67(1):39–52.
20. Shi L, Liu P, Kloog I, Lee M, Kosheleva A, Schwartz J. Estimating daily air temperature across the Southeastern United States using high-resolution satellite data: A statistical modeling study. Environ Res. 2016;146:51–8.
21. Stafoggia M, Samoli E, Alessandrini E, Cadum E, Ostro B, Berti G, Faustini A, Jacquemin B, Linares C, Pascal M, et al. Short-term associations between fine and coarse particulate matter and hospitalizations in Southern Europe: results from the MED-PARTICLES project. Environ Health Perspect. 2013; 121(9):1026–33.
22. Gasparrini A. Distributed lag linear and non-linear models in R: the package dlnm. J Stat Softw. 2011;43(8):1.
23. National Ambient Air Quality Standards. https://www.epa.gov/criteria-air-pollutants/naaqs-table. Accessed 15 Apr 2018.
24. Fridericia L. The duration of systole in an electrocardiogram in normal humans and in patients with heart disease. Ann Noninvasive Electrocardiol. 2003;**8**(4):343–51.
25. Crow RS, Hannan PJ, Folsom AR. Prognostic significance of corrected QT and corrected JT interval for incident coronary heart disease in a general population sample stratified by presence or absence of wide QRS complex: the ARIC Study with 13 years of follow-up. Circulation. 2003;108(16):1985–9.
26. Desai AD, Yaw TS, Yamazaki T, Kaykha A, Chun S, Froelicher VF. Prognostic Significance of Quantitative QRS Duration. Am J Med. 2006;119(7):600–6.
27. Devlin RB, Smith CB, Schmitt MT, Rappold AG, Hinderliter A, Graff D, Carraway MS. Controlled exposure of humans with metabolic syndrome to concentrated ultrafine ambient particulate matter causes cardiovascular effects. Toxicol Sci. 2014;140(1):61–72.
28. Rückerl R, Greven S, Ljungman P, Aalto P, Antoniades C, Bellander T, Berglind N, Chrysohoou C, Forastiere F, Jacquemin B, et al. Air pollution and inflammation (interleukin-6, C-reactive protein, fibrinogen) in myocardial infarction survivors. Environ Health Perspect. 2007;115(7):1072–80.
29. Lazzerini PE, Capecchi PL, Laghi-Pasini F. Long QT Syndrome: An Emerging Role for Inflammation and Immunity. Front Cardiovasc Med. 2015;2:26.

30. Chang KT, Shu HS, Chu CY, Lee WH, Hsu PC, Su HM, Lin TH, Voon WC, Lai WT, Sheu SH. Association between C-reactive protein, corrected QT interval and presence of QT prolongation in hypertensive patients. Kaohsiung J Med Sci. 2014;30(6):310–5.
31. Kim E, Joo S, Kim J, Ahn J, Kim J, Kimm K, Shin C. Association between C-reactive protein and QTc interval in middle-aged men and women. Eur J Epidemiol. 2006;21(9):653–9.
32. Yue W, Schneider A, Rückerl R, Koenig W, Marder V, Wang S, Wichmann H-E, Peters A, Zareba W. Relationship between electrocardiographic and biochemical variables in coronary artery disease. Int J Cardiol. 2007; 119(2):185–91.
33. Vandenberk B, Vandael E, Robyns T, Vandenberghe J, Garweg C, Foulon V, Ector J, Willems R. Which QT correction formulae to use for QT monitoring? J Am Heart Assoc. 2016;5(6):e003264.
34. Park SK, O'Neill MS, Vokonas PS, Sparrow D, Schwartz J. Effects of Air Pollution on Heart Rate Variability: The VA Normative Aging Study. Environ Health Perspect. 2004;113(3):304–9.
35. Schneider A, Hampel R, Ibald-Mulli A, Zareba W, Schmidt G, Schneider R, Rückerl R, Couderc JP, Mykins B, Oberdörster G. Changes in deceleration capacity of heart rate and heart rate variability induced by ambient air pollution in individuals with coronary artery disease. Part Fibre Toxicol. 2010;**7**(1):29.
36. Zanobetti A, Gold DR, Stone PH, Suh HH, Schwartz J, Coull BA, Speizer FE. Reduction in heart rate variability with traffic and air pollution in patients with coronary artery disease. Environ Health Perspect. 2010;118(3):324.
37. Park SK, Auchincloss AH, O'Neill MS, Prineas R, Correa JC, Keeler J, Barr RG, Kaufman JD, Diez Roux AV. Particulate air pollution, metabolic syndrome, and heart rate variability: the multi-ethnic study of atherosclerosis (MESA). Environ Health Perspect. 2010;118(10):1406–11.
38. Bartell SM, Longhurst J, Tjoa T, Sioutas C, Delfino RJ. Particulate air pollution, ambulatory heart rate variability, and cardiac arrhythmia in retirement community residents with coronary artery disease. Environ Health Perspect. 2013;121(10):1135–41.
39. World Health Organization. WHO Air quality guidelines for particulate matter, ozone, nitrogen dioxide and sulfur dioxide-Global update 2005-Summary of risk assessment, 2006. Geneva: WHO; 2006.
40. Al-Khatib SM, LaPointe NMA, Kramer JM, Califf RM. What clinicians should know about the QT interval. Jama. 2003;289(16):2120–7.
41. Sarnat JA, Brown KW, Schwartz J, Coull BA, Koutrakis P. Ambient gas concentrations and personal particulate matter exposures: implications for studying the health effects of particles. Epidemiology. 2005;16(3):385–95.

10

Maternal engineered nanomaterial inhalation during gestation alters the fetal transcriptome

P. A. Stapleton[1,2†], Q. A. Hathaway[3,4,6†], C. E. Nichols[5], A. B. Abukabda[6,7], M. V. Pinti[3,4], D. L. Shepherd[3,4], C. R. McBride[6,8], J. Yi[6,8], V. C. Castranova[6,7], J. M. Hollander[3,4,6] and T. R. Nurkiewicz[4,6,8*]

Abstract

Background: The integration of engineered nanomaterials (ENM) is well-established and widespread in clinical, commercial, and domestic applications. Cardiovascular dysfunctions have been reported in adult populations after exposure to a variety of ENM. As the diversity of these exposures continues to increase, the fetal ramifications of maternal exposures have yet to be determined. We, and others, have explored the consequences of ENM inhalation during gestation and identified many cardiovascular and metabolic outcomes in the F1 generation. The purpose of these studies was to identify genetic alterations in the F1 generation of Sprague-Dawley rats that result from maternal ENM inhalation during gestation. Pregnant dams were exposed to nano-titanium dioxide (nano-TiO_2) aerosols (10 ± 0.5 mg/m^3) for 7-8 days (calculated, cumulative lung deposition = 217 ± 1 μg) and on GD (gestational day) 20 fetal hearts were isolated. DNA was extracted and immunoprecipitated with modified chromatin marks histone 3 lysine 4 tri-methylation (H3K4me3) and histone 3 lysine 27 tri-methylation (H3K27me3). Following chromatin immunoprecipitation (ChIP), DNA fragments were sequenced. RNA from fetal hearts was purified and prepared for RNA sequencing and transcriptomic analysis. Ingenuity Pathway Analysis (IPA) was then used to identify pathways most modified by gestational ENM exposure.

Results: The results of the sequencing experiments provide initial evidence that significant epigenetic and transcriptomic changes occur in the cardiac tissue of maternal nano-TiO_2 exposed progeny. The most notable alterations in major biologic systems included immune adaptation and organismal growth. Changes in normal physiology were linked with other tissues, including liver and kidneys.

Conclusions: These results are the first evidence that maternal ENM inhalation impacts the fetal epigenome.

Keywords: Nanotechnology, Toxicology, Nanomaterial, Inhalation, Epigenetics, Maternal, Fetal

Background

The Barker Hypothesis [1], Developmental Origins of Health and Disease (DOHaD) [2], and fetal programming [3], all explore the relationship between the health of the gestational environment and fetal development and how this predisposes to future disease or sensitivities. Maternal prenatal health challenges such as nutrient deficiency, undernourishment, gestational diabetes and hypertension have been linked to an elevated risk for postnatal cardiovascular diseases [4]. Recently, maternal environmental toxicant exposures have become of prominent interest in relation to the impact of exposure on the fetal milieu and subsequent progeny health [5]. We have reported that maternal ENM inhalation impairs the ability of uterine arterioles to properly dilate, and this impacts litter health in the form of pup weight, number and gender distribution; as well as impaired microvascular function [21]. While these studies have focused on the maternal development of a hostile gestational environment and subsequent reduction in fetal

* Correspondence: tnurkiewicz@hsc.wvu.edu
†Equal contributors
[4]Mitochondria, Metabolism & Bioenergetics Working Group, West Virginia University School of Medicine, Morgantown, WV, USA
[6]Toxicology Working Group, West Virginia University School of Medicine, Morgantown, WV, USA
Full list of author information is available at the end of the article

nutrients, fetal epigenetic modifications may also occur. Conceptually, this relationship is not novel, but applications of environmental toxicants to the maternal-fetal models are. For example, bisphenol A [6] and air pollution [7] have been shown to negatively impact fetal outcomes. However, the impact of maternal ENM on fetal health and/or epigenetic modification are poorly understood.

Despite the ubiquitous inclusion of engineered nanomaterials in widespread applications, and their projected proliferation in human endeavors, the consequences of maternal ENM inhalation on the developing fetus and their impacts on future health are at best, vague, yet they are increasingly becoming a health concern. The prevalence of ENM covers an immense spectrum: surface coatings and additives in common consumer products (electronics, food, cosmetics), additives in industrial processes (advanced building materials, synthetic fuels), and components of clinical applications (diagnostics, drug delivery, implantable devices). It is widely recognized that throughout the ENM life cycle, the greatest risk for human exposure and subsequent health consequences begins with ENM inhalation, and is typically followed by systemic injuries. We have reported that pulmonary and systemic microvascular inflammation [29, 32] follow ENM inhalation exposure. Consistent with this, other systemic morbidities known to follow pulmonary ENM exposures include: inflammation/apoptosis [8, 9], macrovascular and microvascular dysfunction [10], atherogenesis [11], and organ level ischemia [12]. The developing fetus is equally a systemic target of numerous anthropogenic toxicants [13].

The impact of gestational ENM exposures on maternal and fetal health have been increasingly studied in the past decade. Adverse impact of ENM exposures on maternal health [14] and pregnancy [15, 16] have been reported in animal models. Teratogenic and embryo-lethal effects associated with ENM exposure have been shown [17]. The outcomes from several studies also highlight post-natal behavioral deficits [18, 19], cardiovascular [20, 21], renal [15], immune [22], reproductive [23, 24], pulmonary, and metabolic [20, 25] abnormalities.

Epigenetics, or the transient control of genes through DNA methylation or histone modification, is a recent area of intense focus by governmental agencies recognizing mechanistic links between environmental toxicants and gene expression [26]. These adverse maternal and fetal outcomes strongly reflect the potential risk of ENM exposure during pregnancy that may be linked. However, given the inherent physiological dependencies and complexities of developing and maintaining a healthy pregnancy, linking the mechanisms of pulmonary exposure and gestational effects remains very challenging. Given the magnitude of and the complexity these transgenerational effects, the most effective approach may be to initiate studies from the fetal epigenome and/or transcriptome. This is largely because fetal epigenetic outcomes resulting from maternal ENM exposure consequences may be caused by the creation of a hostile gestational environment [27], and/or the direct impact of ENM interacting with the developing embryo [13]. Because either of these possibilities would compromise health, the purpose of these studies was to identify epigenetic changes in cardiac gene expression within the maternally exposed F1 generations. We hypothesized that because maternal ENM inhalation lead to uterine microvascular dysfunction [21], this contributes to a hostile gestational environment, and altered fetal gene expression results. To test this, pregnant dams were intermittently exposed to nano-TiO_2 aerosols during gestational days 5-19, and their litters were studied on GD 20.

Methods

Animal model

Sprague Dawley rats were purchased from Hilltop Laboratories (250-275 g female; 300-325 g male). All experiments were approved by the West Virginia University Animal Care and Use Committee and experiments adhered to the National Institutes of Health (NIH) Guide for the Care and Use of Laboratory Animals (8th Ed.). Rats were provided food and water ad libitum and housed in an AAALAC approved animal facility at the West Virginia University Health Sciences Center. Before mating, rats were acclimated for a minimum of 72 h, as previously described [20]. Pregnancy was verified by identification of the vaginal plug, after which, rats were randomly placed into one of two nano-TiO_2 exposure groups. These two exposure groups were virtually identical and were created to generate a discrete tissue bank for RNA sequencing, or ChIP sequencing.

Engineered Nanomaterial

Nano-TiO_2 P25 powder was purchased from Evonik (Aeroxide TiO2, Parsippany, NJ), containing anatase (80%) and rutile (20%) TiO_2. Nano-TiO_2 was prepared by drying, sieving, and storing, as previously described [28, 29]. Nano-TiO_2 aerosols were created with our aerosol generator (US Patent No. 8,881,997) [30]. Particle characteristics have been determined including the primary particle size (21 nm), the specific surface area (48.08 m^2/g) [29, 31], and the Zeta potential (–56.6 mV) [32].

Nano-TiO_2 inhalation exposures

The nano-particle aerosol generator (US Patent No. 8,881,997) and whole-body inhalation exposure system used for the current study have been described extensively in previous studies [29, 31]. This collective exposure system consists of a vibrating fluidized bed, a Venturi vacuum pump, cyclone separator, impactor and mixing device, an animal housing chamber, and real-time monitoring devices with feedback control. Nano-TiO_2 was aerosolized via a high velocity air stream passing through the vibrating fluidized bed and into the Venturi vacuum pump. The generated aerosols then entered the cyclone separated, which is designed to remove agglomerates > 400 nm at an input flow rate of 60 l/min of clean dry air before entering the exposure chamber.

Size distribution, mean aerodynamic diameter, and relative mass concentration of the aerosols were monitored in real time (Electrical Low Pressure Impactor (ELPI), Dekati, Tempere, Finland) while the particle size distribution was also measured in real-time with a Scanning Mobility Particle Sizer device (SMPS; TSI Inc., St. Paul, MN). These measurements were verified throughout a given exposure by collecting nanoparticle samples on filters, and making hourly gravimetric measurements with a microbalance. This approach was also used to collect samples for transmission electron microscopy.

Inhalation exposures were initiated on GD 5.78 ± 0.11 and lasted for 7.79 ± 0.26 days of gestation. Exposure days were not consecutive to decrease animal stress. Once the steady state nano-TiO_2 aerosol concentration was achieved, exposure duration was adjusted to produce a daily calculated lung deposition of 31 ± 1.1 µg per day, and the cumulative, calculated dose was therefore 217 ± 1.0 µg. Lung deposition was calculated based on previously described mouse methodology, and normalized to rat weight and to pregnant rat minute ventilation using the equation: $D = F{\cdot}V{\cdot}C{\cdot}T$, where F is the deposition fraction (14%), V is the minute ventilation based on body weight, C equals the mass concentration (mg/m^3), and T equals the exposure duration (minutes) [29, 33]. The target concentration was 10 mg/m^3 and the duration was 4-6 h/exposure (depending on the steady state concentration, as this was used to calculate the lung burden). The last exposure was conducted 24 h prior to sacrifice and experimentation. Control animals were exposed to HEPA filtered air only.

Chromatin Immunoprecipitation (ChIP) sequencing

Isolation

Cardiac tissue was isolated from GD 20 pups in both the nano-TiO_2 exposure and control groups. Each litter was considered an $n = 1$, with cardiac tissue from 5 to 6 pups within each litter being pooled together to collect enough tissue (~25 mg). Chromatin Immunoprecipitation (ChIP) was carried out using the MAGnify™ Chromatin Immunoprecipitation System (Thermo Fisher, Rockford, IL) per manufacturer's instructions. Briefly, hearts were homogenized and treated with 37% formaldehyde, which was prepared fresh. Cross-linking was stopped with 1.25 M glycine. Samples were pelleted through centrifugation and washed in D-PBS before sonication. Using a Sonicator Ultrasonic Processor XL2015 (Misonix Sonicator, Farmingdale, NY) chromatin was sheared to a size of 500-700 base pairs, determined using gel electrophoresis (Fig. 1a). Chromatin was then isolated through ultracentrifugation (20,000 g) and diluted to ~60 uL of chromatin per immunoprecipitation reaction. Samples from both the control and nano-TiO_2 cohorts were incubated with histone 3 lysine 4 tri-methylation (H3K4me3, product number: G.532.8, Thermo Fisher, Rockford, IL) or histone 3 lysine 27 tri-methylation (H3K27me3, product number: G.299.10, Thermo Fisher, Rockford, IL) antibody bound beads. These are two of the most prominently studied and classically applied for activation/repression analysis of gene activity. After incubation, samples were treated to reverse cross-linking solution and Proteinase K to remove bound proteins. DNA was then eluted from beads, using heat, and quantified using a Qubit (Thermo Fisher, Rockford, IL). The TruSeq ChIP Library Preparation Kit (Illumina, Inc., San Diego, CA) was implemented to build the libraries.

ChIP bioinformatics

Samples were processed using the Illumina MiSeq (Illumina, Inc., San Diego, CA) at the West Virginia University Genomics Core, ran as paired-end reads. Fastq files were assessed for quality using FastQC (Babraham Bioinformatics) (Fig. 1b), where it was determined that partial trimming was needed. Trimming of fastq files was accomplished through Trimmomatic [34] (Fig. 1c). Reads were then mapped to the rat genome (rn6) using the default parameters in bowtie2. To perform differential binding analysis on reads while distinguishing peaks, diffReps was used [35]. Bedtools functions were used to delineate upstream promoter regions of genes (bedtools slop) and evaluate the promoter/gene overlay (bedtools intersect). Genes were defined to include 1000 bases upstream from the start of the gene, indicative of our selected "promoter region."

RNA sequencing

Isolation

Cardiac tissue was procured through the same methods as listed above in the ChIP Sequencing section. RNA was then isolated from heart tissue using the Vantage™ Total RNA Purification Kit (Origene, Rockville, MD) per manufacturer's instructions. Briefly, tissue was homogenized and lysis buffer was added to the sample. Sample RNA was spin-column purified and measured for RNA concentration using the Qubit (Thermo Fisher, Rockford, IL). Library preparation was performed using TruSeq RNA Library Prep Kit v2 (Illumina, Inc., San Diego, CA). Quality of RNA was determined using the Agilent 2100 BioAnalyzer (Agilent Technologies, Santa Clara, CA); degradation of cytosolic ribosomal RNAs (28S and

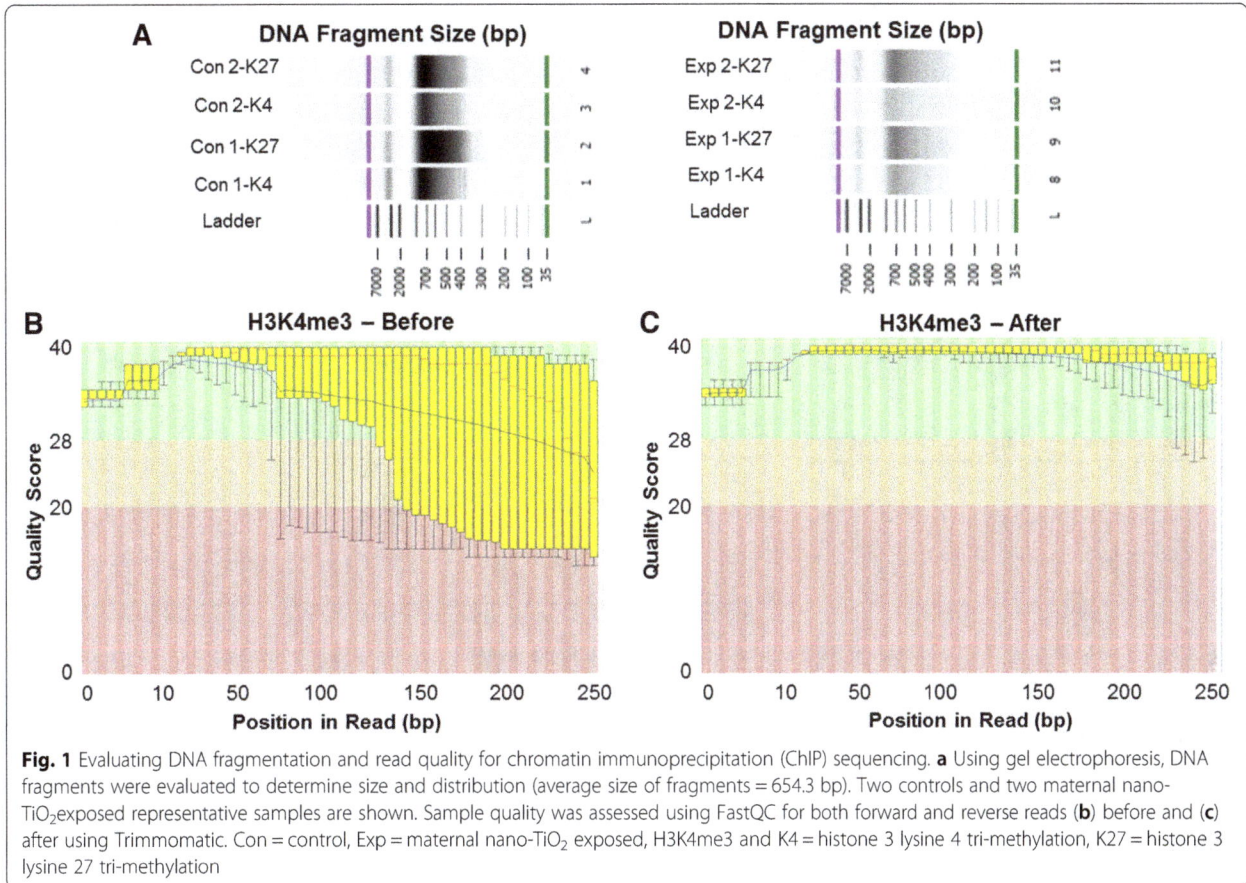

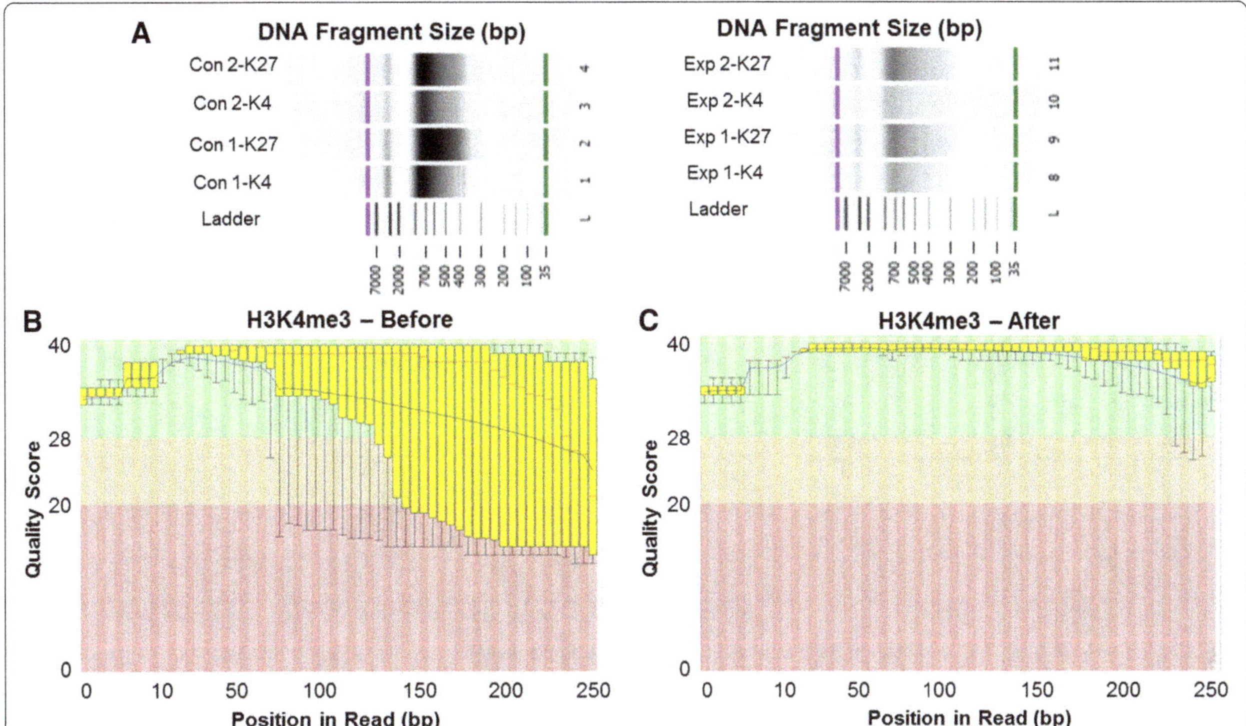

Fig. 1 Evaluating DNA fragmentation and read quality for chromatin immunoprecipitation (ChIP) sequencing. **a** Using gel electrophoresis, DNA fragments were evaluated to determine size and distribution (average size of fragments = 654.3 bp). Two controls and two maternal nano-TiO_2exposed representative samples are shown. Sample quality was assessed using FastQC for both forward and reverse reads (**b**) before and (**c**) after using Trimmomatic. Con = control, Exp = maternal nano-TiO_2 exposed, H3K4me3 and K4 = histone 3 lysine 4 tri-methylation, K27 = histone 3 lysine 27 tri-methylation

18S) are used as a measure of the total RNA Integrity Number (RIN) (Fig. 2a, b).

RNA bioinformatics

Samples were processed using the Illumina HiSeq (illumina, Inc., San Diego, CA) at Marshall University. Samples were run as paired-end reads. Paired-end, fastq files were aligned with HISAT2 [36] to the rat genome (rn6) without trimming. Samtools 1.2 [37] was used for the conversion of SAM to BAM format. Counts data was prepared using Subread 1.5.2 [38], specifically featureCounts [39]. Differential expression analysis was accomplished using DESeq2 [40] in R.

Ingenuity pathway analysis (IPA)

Protein ontology and pathway analysis were completed through QIAGEN's IPA (www.qiagen.com/ingenuity) software. Core analyses and comparative analyses were run on individual and combined ChIP and RNA data sets, respectively. Z-scores are representative of fold change between groups.

RNA IPA Protein Ontology.

The intensity of the color, moving toward blue or red, indicates the degree to which a specific pathway is being decreased or increased, respectively. The change in color, reflective of the z-score, is a quantitative measure of confidence (defined as the cumulative *P*-value of molecules in a specific pathway). This measure of confidence, defined on a color scale, indicates the propensity of all the molecules within that pathway to move in a certain direction, toward either increasing or decreasing the likelihood of developing the listed pathology or condition.

Quantitative PCR

As described above, RNA was isolated from fetal heart tissue. Using the First-strand cDNA Synthesis kit for miRNA (Origene, Rockville, MD, Catalog #: HP100042), per manufacturer's instructions, RNA was converted to cDNA. The cDNA was used for differential quantification of mRNA transcripts Fibroblast Growth Factor Receptor 1 (Fgfr1), Interleukin-18 (Il-18), and Transforming Growth Factor Beta Receptor 2 (Tgfbr2). ChIP-qPCR was used to assess the Tgfbr2 promoter loci. As described above, chromatin was immunoprecipitated with H3K4me3. DNA was then probed at multiple locations along the Tgfbr2 promoter region in order to construct a histone peak profile. Primer design for both the mRNA and ChIP-qPCR are provided (Additional file 1: Table S4). MRNA was normalized to Beta-Actin (β-Actin), while immunoprecipitated DNA was normalized to its respective input control.

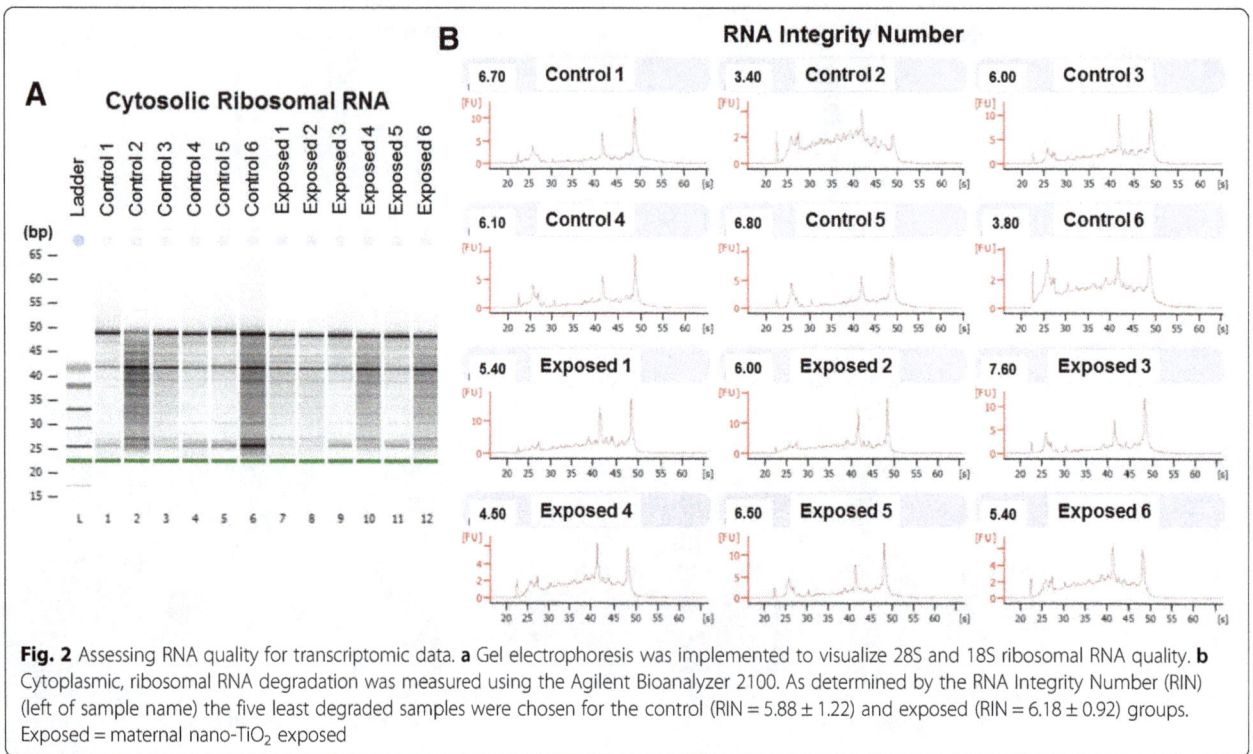

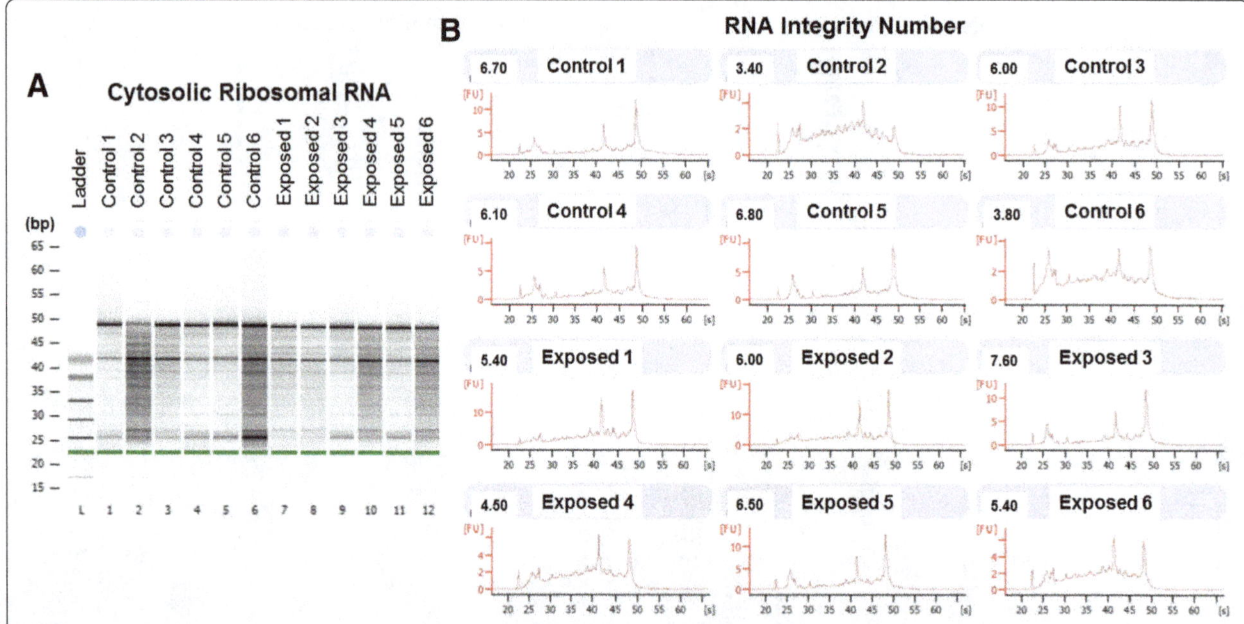

Fig. 2 Assessing RNA quality for transcriptomic data. **a** Gel electrophoresis was implemented to visualize 28S and 18S ribosomal RNA quality. **b** Cytoplasmic, ribosomal RNA degradation was measured using the Agilent Bioanalyzer 2100. As determined by the RNA Integrity Number (RIN) (left of sample name) the five least degraded samples were chosen for the control (RIN = 5.88 ± 1.22) and exposed (RIN = 6.18 ± 0.92) groups. Exposed = maternal nano-TiO_2 exposed

Experiments were performed on the Applied Biosystems 7900HT Fast Real-Time PCR system (Applied Biosystems, Foster City, CA), using 2X SYBR Green Master Mix. Quantification was achieved using the 2-ΔΔCT method.

Statistics

All measures of significance between the control and maternal nano-TiO_2 exposure groups for the sequencing data are presented as adjusted *P*-values. Adjusted P-values are a composition of standard, unadjusted P-values and the stringency of the False Discovery Rate (FDR). Differential expression analysis through DESeq2 implements the Wald Test, using multiple testing against the null hypothesis that P-values are uniformly distributed across a data set, known as the Benjamini-Hochberg procedure. The FDR for this study was set at 0.05. Z-score significance is determined as greater than the absolute value of 2. The z-score is computed as $z = \frac{x}{\sigma_x} = \frac{\sum_i x_i}{\sqrt{n}} = \frac{N_+ - N_-}{\sqrt{N}}$, where N_+ = the number of molecules following a consistent trend, N_- = the number of molecules following an inconsistent trend, and N = the number of interactions within a given pathway. In this way, the z-score, using only values with a significant change ($P \leq 0.05$) can infer direction of a specific pathway while accounting for relationship and data bias and properly weighting the statistical findings (https://www.qiagenbioinformatics.com/products/ingenuity-pathway-analysis/). A consistency score is the non-statistical assignment of confidence to a specific pathway. Where appropriate, a Student's t-test was used with all data presented as ± the standard error mean (SEM). Significance is determined as $P \leq 0.05$.

Results

Animal and Nano-TiO_2 aerosol characteristics

Animal number, age, body weight, and exposure conditions are provided (Table 1). Separate, but similar, inhalation exposures were used for the ChIP and RNA sequencing experiments. No statistical differences were noted between nano-TiO_2 exposure in Experimental Group 1 (ChiP Seq) and Experimental Group 2 (RNA Seq). No statistical differences were noted in either progeny weight or total number of pups between maternal nano-TiO_2 exposed or control groups.

Representative nano-TiO_2 aerosol characterization data are presented in Fig. 3. The target particle concentration was 10 mg/m^3 (Fig. 3a). The real-time nano-TiO_2 mobility diameter was 129 nm (Fig. 3b), and the aerodynamic diameter was 143 nm (Fig. 3c). Nanoparticles were collected on filters, and a representative transmission electron microscopy image is presented in Fig. 3d.

ChIP sequencing

ChIP sample metrics

To better understand the quality and sample dispersion within our cohort for the ChIP sequencing experiment, a series of statistical models were used. To assess the

Table 1 Animal characteristics

Exposure Group	Technique	Number of animals (N)	Age (days)	Body Weight (grams)	Litter Size	Pup Weight (grams)	Aerosol Concentration (mg/m^3)	Electrical Low-Pressure Impactor (nm)	Scanning Particle Mobility Sizer (nm)
Sham Control	RNA Sequencing	7	109 ± 7	402 ± 8.84	13 ± 2	4.06 ± 0.16	0	0	0
Nano-TiO_2	RNA Sequencing	4	113 ± 2	422 ± 13.34	14 ± 1	3.99 ± 0.22	10.35 ± 0.13	136.80 ± 1.44	134.80 ± 1.24
Sham Control	ChIP Sequencing	5	104 ± 2	407 ± 8.09	12 ± 2	5.19 ± 1.02	0	0	0
Nano-TiO_2	ChIP Sequencing	6	98 ± 1	376 ± 19.99	9 ± 5	4.88 ± 1.53	10.5 ± 0.05	143.75 ± 2.32	129.43 ± 3.21

distribution of subpeaks present within the forward and reverse strands of the H3K4me3 and H3K27me3 immunoprecipitations, the average fragment length was determined for each event using the R package csaw [41]. The cross-correlation graph measures the delay distance, or number of base pairs, which separate distinctive subpeaks, also evaluating the consistency of fragment lengths within the data set (Fig. 4a and b). Multidimensional scaling (MDS) plots were used to evaluate individual library homology between both the H3K4me3 and H3K27me3 groups with the R package edgeR [42]. Log fold change (LogFC) determined the differences between libraries (control, red and maternal nano-TiO_2 exposed, blue) within the MDS plots (Fig. 4c and d). To visualize read coverage, the R packages ChIPpeakAnno and Gviz were installed [43]. Complex, differential binding was assessed for both the H3K4me3 (Fig. 4e) and H3K27me3 (Fig. 4f) binding loci. Together, these results suggest that the immunoprecipitation and chromatin fragmentation were successful, and that differential binding is observed between groups.

ChIP IPA Protein Ontology

Differential Binding data for both the H3K4me3 and H3K27me3 marks were uploaded and analyzed in QIAGEN's IPA; all changes are shown as maternal nano-TiO_2 exposed condition relative to the control. Diseases and biological functions (z-score ≥ 2) for H3K4me3 and H3K27me3 are provided in Additional file 1: Table S1 and S2, respectively. Of the diseases and biological functions listed, one of the most prominent pathways for H3K4me3 involved infectious disease (Fig. 5a). The heat

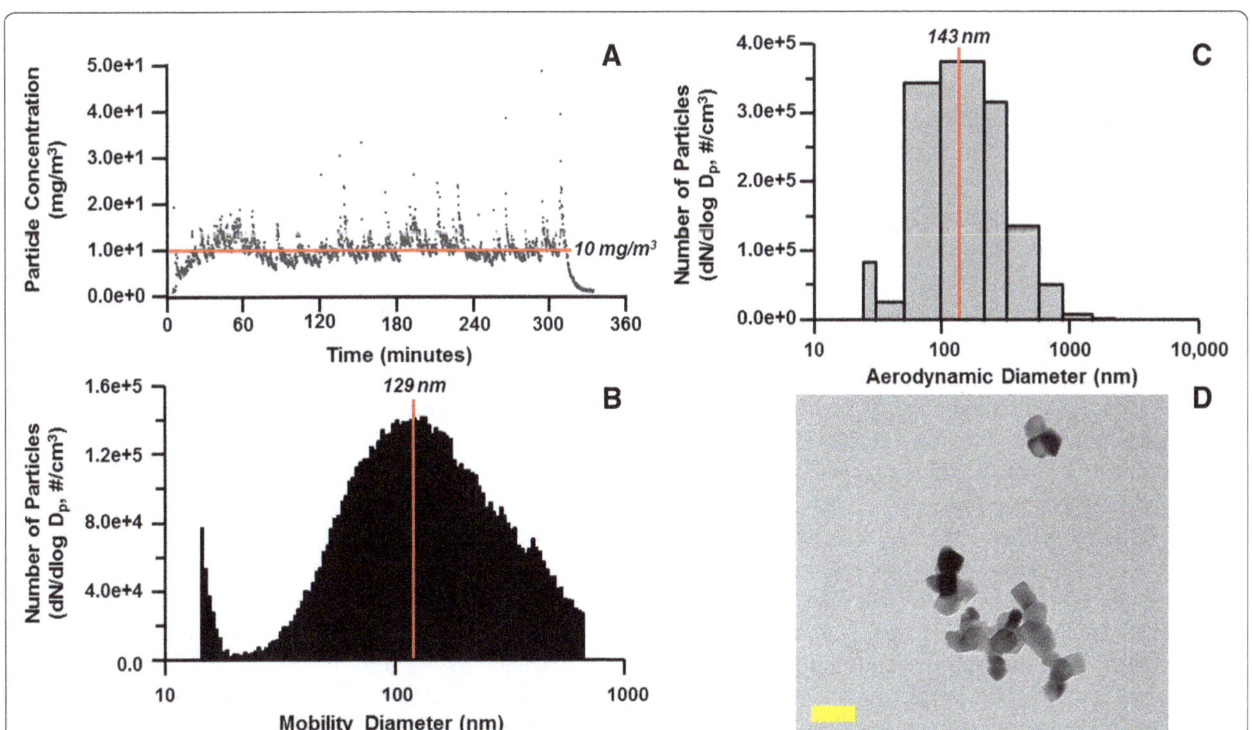

Fig. 3 Maternal nano-TiO_2 exposure particle characterization for RNA sequencing experiments. **a** Total aerosol concentration (10 mg/m^3) of engineered nano-TiO_2 during maternal exposures. **b** Nano-TiO_2 size distribution (mobility diameter, 129.4 nm) using a scanning mobility particle sizer (SMPS). **c** Nano-TiO_2 size distribution (aerodynamic diameter, 143.3 nm) using an electrical low-pressure impactor (ELPI). (D) Transmission electron microscopy image of aerosolized nano-TiO_2 collected via a sampling filter during an exposure

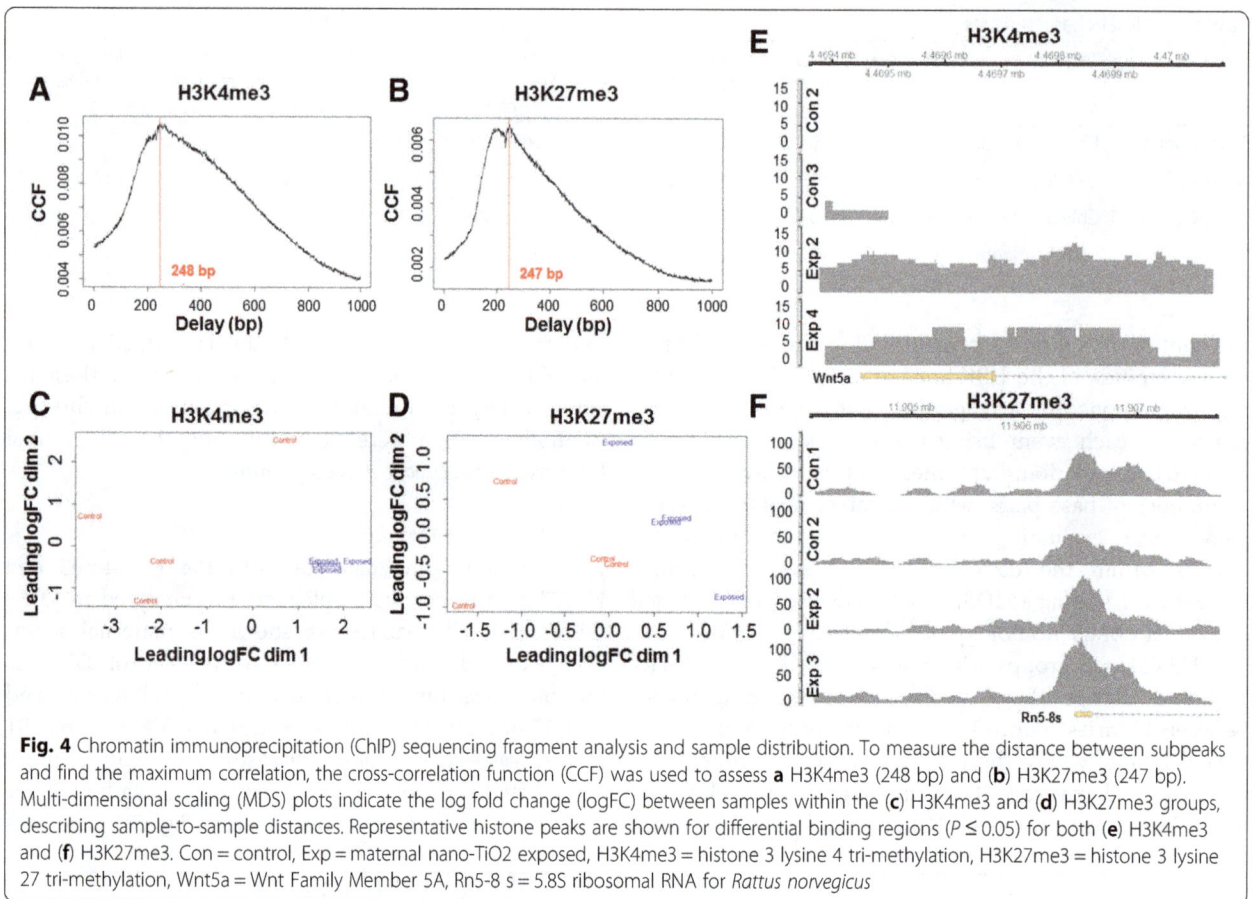

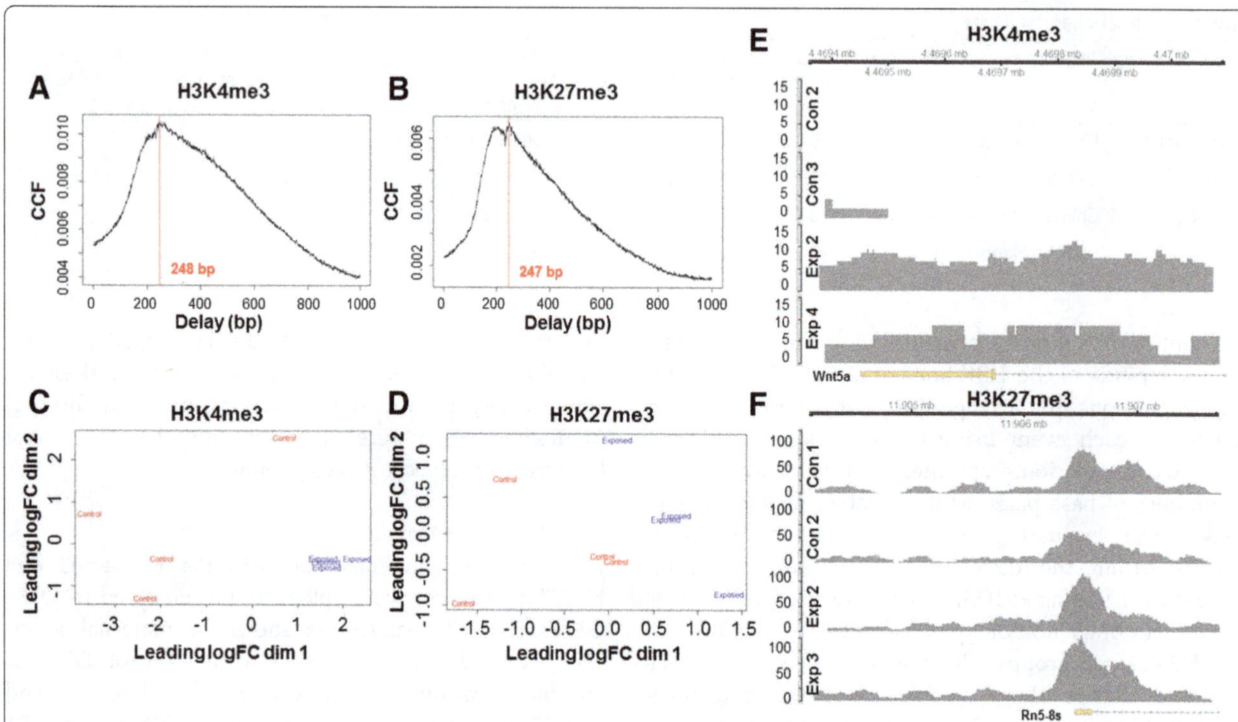

Fig. 4 Chromatin immunoprecipitation (ChIP) sequencing fragment analysis and sample distribution. To measure the distance between subpeaks and find the maximum correlation, the cross-correlation function (CCF) was used to assess **a** H3K4me3 (248 bp) and (**b**) H3K27me3 (247 bp). Multi-dimensional scaling (MDS) plots indicate the log fold change (logFC) between samples within the (**c**) H3K4me3 and (**d**) H3K27me3 groups, describing sample-to-sample distances. Representative histone peaks are shown for differential binding regions ($P \leq 0.05$) for both (**e**) H3K4me3 and (**f**) H3K27me3. Con = control, Exp = maternal nano-TiO2 exposed, H3K4me3 = histone 3 lysine 4 tri-methylation, H3K27me3 = histone 3 lysine 27 tri-methylation, Wnt5a = Wnt Family Member 5A, Rn5-8 s = 5.8S ribosomal RNA for *Rattus norvegicus*

map reveals how changes in molecular signaling could provide an increase susceptibility to infection in maternal nano-TiO_2 exposed offspring. The top canonical pathways (z-score ≥ 2) altered during maternal nano-TiO_2 exposure are presented (Fig. 5b). In general, the canonical pathways altered after exposure involve regulation of growth and cell cycle/apoptosis signaling.

For H3K27me3, the top 10 canonical pathways which are altered are provided (Fig. 5c). For the promoter regions associated with H3K27me3, the majority of signaling changes involve cancer and immunity. A heat map for the toxicological functions of the data representing H3K4me3 is also presented (Fig. 5d). The size and distribution of each major category is proportional to the z-score, which revealed three major organs affected: the heart, kidney and liver. Toxicological pathways associated with the heart, including congenital heart anomaly, heart failure, cardiac hypertrophy (not shown), and cardiac dysfunction (not shown), were found to be significantly decreased in the maternal nano-TiO_2 exposed group. Conversely, toxicological pathways associated with the liver and kidney including, renal necrosis and cell death, liver necrosis and cell death, renal damage, and liver damage (not shown) were found to be increased. Also, an increase in red blood cells, and subsequently the hematocrit, were observed. Increases in H3K4me3 at promoter regions for infection capacity and growth signaling as well as loci involving kidney and liver dysfunction, suggests epigenetic regulation which could significantly alter an organism's susceptibility to disease and potential pre-disposition to future insult. The lack of changes shown for H3K27me3 may suggest an alternative repressive mark implemented as the bivalent companion of H3K4me3.

RNA sequencing

RNA sample metrics

The raw and normalized counts from the RNA sequencing experiment were subjected to a variety of statistical modelling, using the DESeq2 package in R [44], in order to better understand sample parameters. To visualize the variance of the normalized counts data means, the rlog function was used (Fig. 6a). For low-count genes, transformation using rlog, a log2 scale which normalizes data in reference to the library size, helps to better visualize variance-means. Fig. 6a shows limited outliers within the data set for the control vs. control, but increasing variance in the control vs. maternal nano-TiO_2 exposed. Sample-to-sample distance was measured using the PoiClaClu package in R. Sample dissimilarity is depicted as a heat map (Fig. 6b), calculated from the original, not

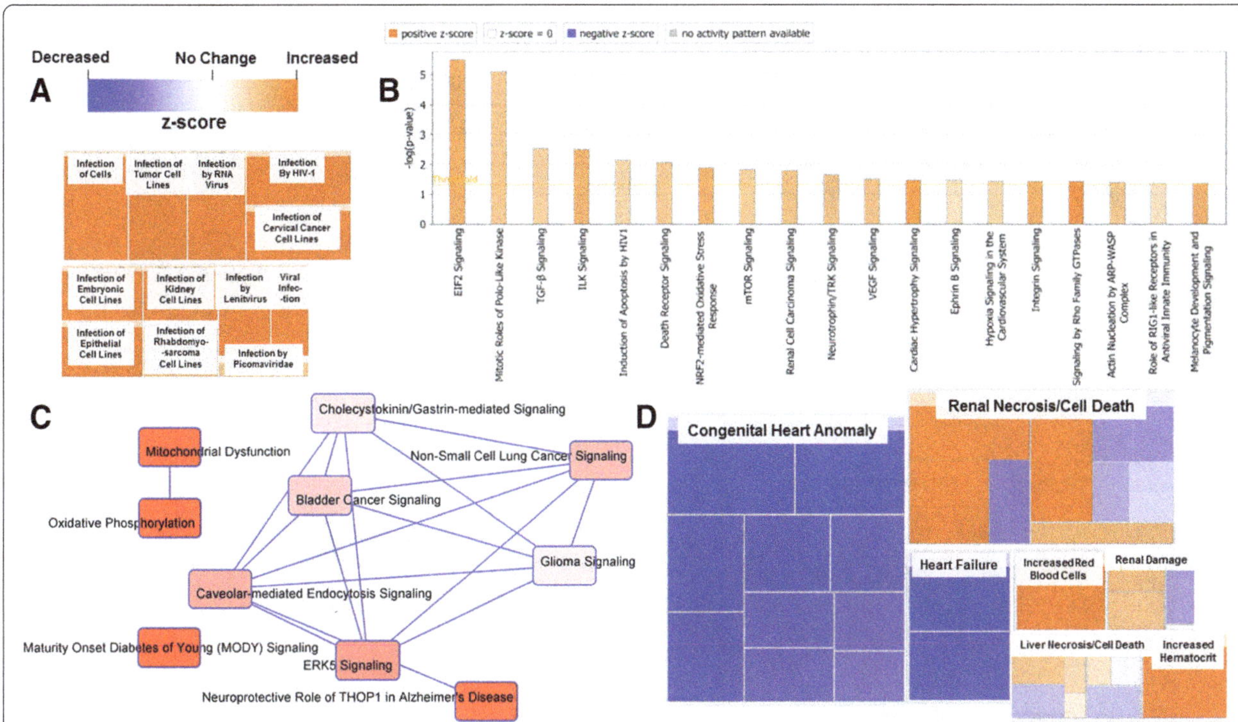

Fig. 5 Assessment of disease and signaling pathways altered epigenetically during maternal nano-TiO_2 exposure. **a** One of the primary disease pathways (z-score = 9.35 ± 1.89) altered epigenetically during exposure was the increased susceptibility to infection in the H3K4me3 group. Disease and toxicological pathways are constructed from specific, individual canonical signaling pathways. **b** Depicts the top canonical pathways for H3K4me3 (z-score ≥ ±2.0) that are significantly ($P \leq 0.05$) impacted, as indicated by the threshold line. **c** The top canonical pathways for H3K27me3 ($P \leq 0.05$) are also shown following exposure (smaller *p*-values are associated with increasing red intensity for pathways). **d** Toxicological functions predicted for genes mapped to H3K4me3 marks

normalized count data. The heat map shows general dissimilarity between the maternal nano-TiO_2 exposed and control groups, with the exception of one of the control samples. Another measure implemented for determining sample distance was a multi-dimensional scaling (MDS) plot based on the rlog-normalized counts (Fig. 6c). Again, the plot shows a general dissimilarity between the maternal nano-TiO_2 exposed and control cohorts. After performing differential expression analysis with DESeq2, we examined the gene with the lowest associated *p*-value (Fig. 6d). The plot illustrates the similar expression of the gene within each group, while showing the disparities across groups. In Fig. 6e, a MA-plot is used to illustrate the number of genes (red) that fall below the *P*-value of 0.05. The statistical models used to assess the RNA sequencing samples indicate that normalized count values between groups are similar and that sample homology is close within groups, but not across groups.

RNA IPA protein ontology

After differential expression analysis processing in R, data was uploaded and analyzed in QIAGEN's IPA; all changes are shown as maternal nano-TiO_2 exposed condition relative to the control. Diseases and biological functions (z-score ≥ 2) for the RNA are provided in Additional file 1: Table S3. Again, a prominent pathway that was found to be increased in the maternal nano-TiO_2 exposed animals involved infectious diseases (Fig. 7a). Both the open promoter conformation (H3K4me3) and the RNA transcript expression reveal an increased propensity for infection. The top canonical pathways (z-score ≥ 3.45) altered during maternal nano-TiO_2 exposure are presented (Fig. 7b). The canonical pathways altered primarily involve inflammatory signaling and organismal development. Examining what factors could be causing differential regulation after maternal nano-TiO_2 exposure, we wanted to evaluate molecular regulator effects. The top molecule (consistency score ≥ 10.453) suggested to play a role in differential regulation of pathways was microRNA-145 (Fig. 7c).

In Fig. 7c, it reveals how decreased expression of microRNA-145 can lead to increased expression of pathways involving cell growth and proliferation. A heat map for the toxicological functions of the data representing the RNA is also shown (Fig. 7d). The size and distribution of each major category is proportional to the z-score and, again consistent with the H3K4me3 mark, three major organs were shown to be affected: the heart, kidney and liver. Toxicological pathways associated with the heart,

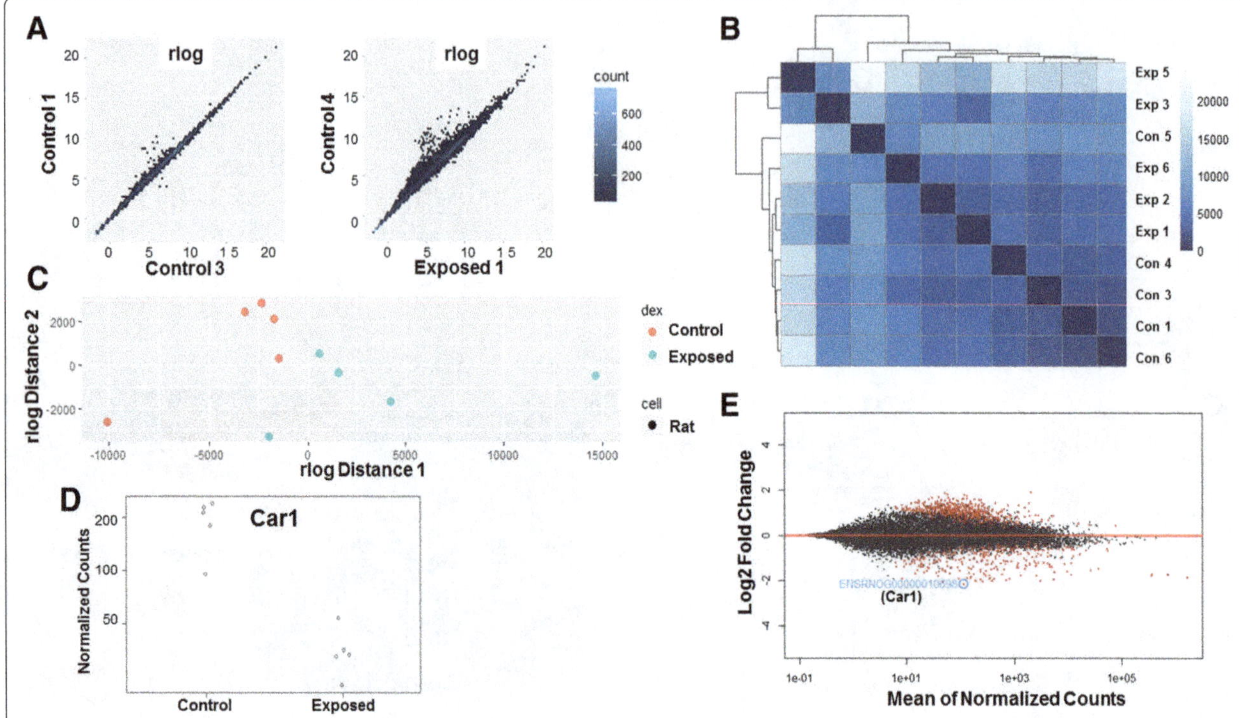

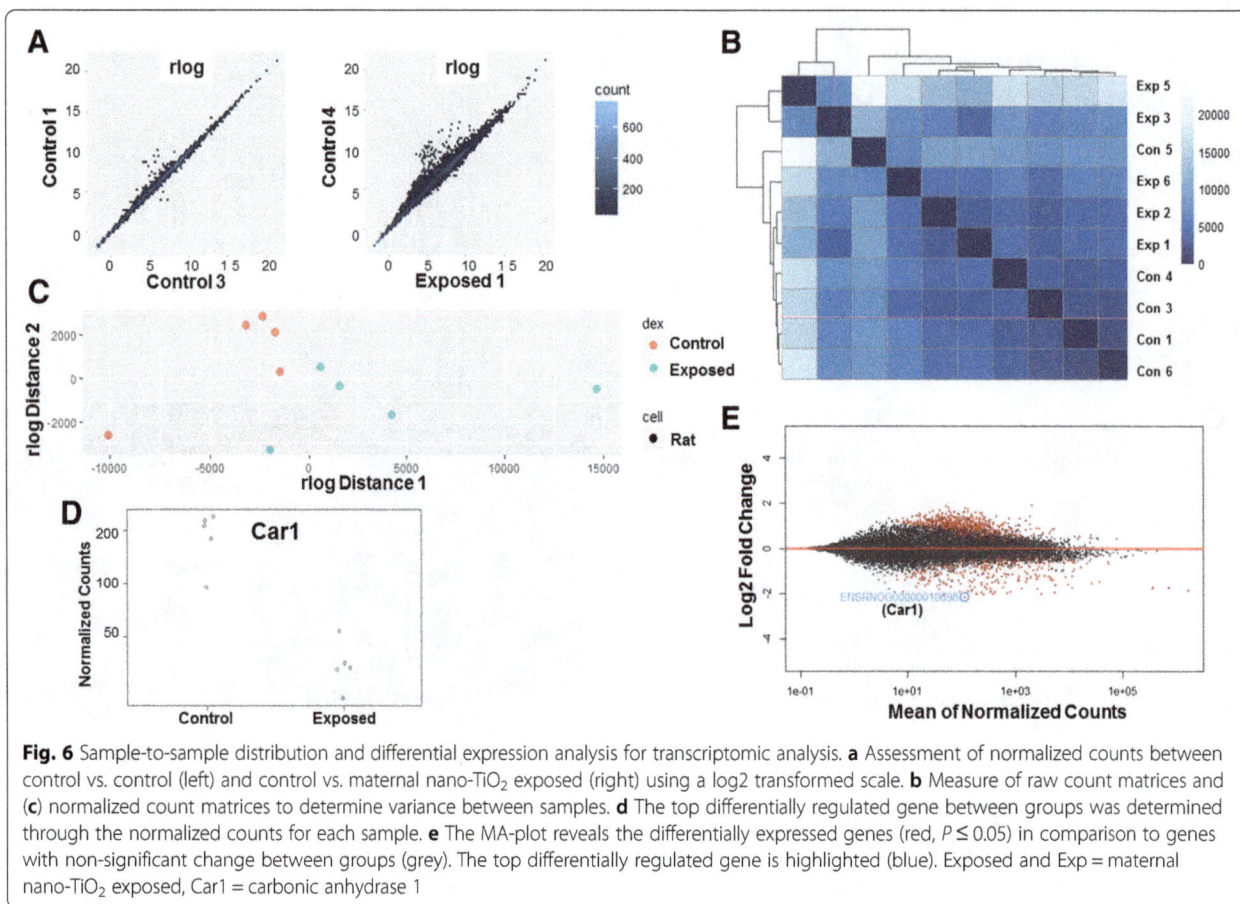

Fig. 6 Sample-to-sample distribution and differential expression analysis for transcriptomic analysis. **a** Assessment of normalized counts between control vs. control (left) and control vs. maternal nano-TiO_2 exposed (right) using a log2 transformed scale. **b** Measure of raw count matrices and (**c**) normalized count matrices to determine variance between samples. **d** The top differentially regulated gene between groups was determined through the normalized counts for each sample. **e** The MA-plot reveals the differentially expressed genes (red, $P \leq 0.05$) in comparison to genes with non-significant change between groups (grey). The top differentially regulated gene is highlighted (blue). Exposed and Exp = maternal nano-TiO_2 exposed, Car1 = carbonic anhydrase 1

including congenital heart anomaly, cardiac hypoplasia, heart failure, cardiac fibrosis, and cardiac damage, were found to be significantly decreased in the maternal nano-TiO_2 exposed group. Alternatively, toxicological pathways associated with the liver and kidney including, renal necrosis and cell death, liver hyperplasia/hyperproliferation, renal proliferation, renal damage, and renal autophagy were found to be increased. As reported for the H3K4me3 promoter regions, increased RNA transcription of genes involving red blood production are shown. Similar to the epigenetic modification H3K4me3, the differential expression of transcripts follows a similar pattern of increased infection and growth of the organism, with increased molecular markers of dysfunction in the liver and kidney.

Epigenetic regulation of transcription

In order to examine how changes between the H3K4me3 mark and RNA transcript data aligned, we performed a comparative analysis through QIAGEN's IPA, all changes are shown as maternal nano-TiO2 exposed condition relative to the control. The top canonical pathways (z-score ≥ 4.5) for both the transcript and ChIP data are shown (Fig. 8a). The combined data sets illustrate the common pathways involving both inflammation and organismal growth signaling. For toxicological functions, the molecular profile for cardiac dysfunction is significantly decreased compared to the controls, while kidney dysfunction is increased (Fig. 8b). A heat map for the cumulative diseases and biological functions is shown (Fig. 8c). The heat map depicts two major molecular changes that could impact the phenotype: increased survival and increased susceptibility to infection. In Fig. 8d, canonical pathways are sorted by *p*-value, depicting pathways with large sets of molecules having significantly altered expression levels. Although, the mitochondrial dysfunction and oxidative phosphorylation pathways do not have significant z-scores and a very small contribution of changes coming from the transcript data, Fig. 8b demonstrates the epigenetic changes occurring at these loci to a large segment of genes. Figure 8e illustrates the NF-κB (Nuclear Factor kappa-light-chain-enhancer of activated B cells) signaling pathway for the RNA (right) and H3K4me3 (left) sequencing experiments. The comparative analysis suggests that maternal nano-TiO_2 exposure can cause significant changes to how the development of the progeny takes place, changing the epigenetic landscape, which can directly affect transcript abundance.

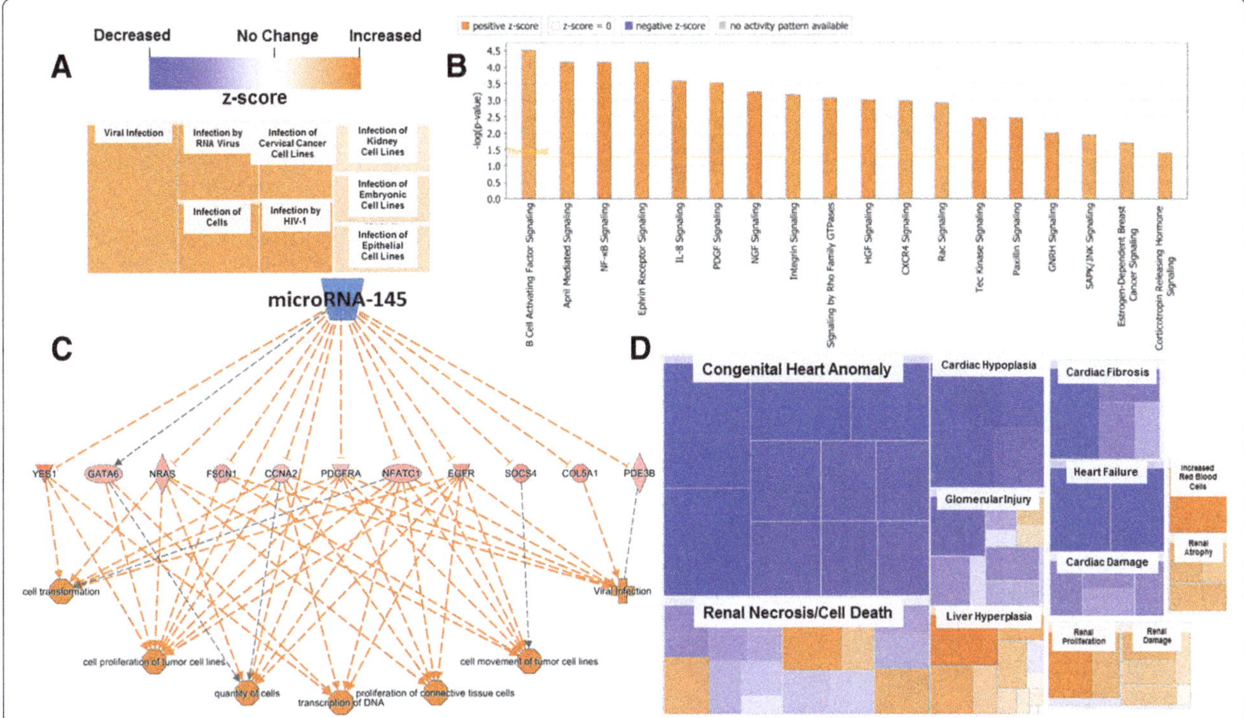

Fig. 7 Assessment of disease and signaling pathways altered transcriptionally during maternal nano-TiO_2 exposure. **a** Similar to the activation by H3K4me3, transcriptional upregulation of genes associated with increased susceptibility to infection (z-score = 2.02 ± 0.96) was found. **b** The top canonical pathways (z-score ≥ ±3.45) that are significantly ($P \leq 0.05$) impacted transcriptionally, as indicated by the threshold line. The canonical pathways for the RNA sequencing reveal a significant increase in inflammatory and growth signaling. **c** The top regulator (consistency score = 10.453) determined through pathway analysis of gene expression (arrows = activation, bars = repression). Increasing gene activation (red) and suppression (blue) reveal targeting of multiple cell functions. **d** Toxicological functions predicted for transcript abundance in the RNA sequencing experiment

Molecular validation of sequencing

To further confirm the reliability of the sequencing data, we implemented qPCR to examine molecules involved in the NF-κB Pathway, which are not shown in the illustrative Fig. 8d, e. The mRNA levels of Fgfr1, Il-18, and Tgfbr2 are reported, and coincide with similar expression profiles seen in the sequencing data (Fig. 9a). In Fig. 9a, the data obtained from RNA sequencing (grey bars) are used as a reference to validate the expression profile of the maternal nano-TiO2 group when running qPCR. Likewise, we also wanted to use ChIP-qPCR to validate that histone modifications were also reliably reported, with the ChIP-Seq revealing epigenetic changes at the Tgfbr2 promoter region. We confirmed the H3K4me3 histone modifications for Tgfbr2, showing higher H3K4me3 association at its promoter region (Fig. 9b). The increased magnitude of the histone peak of the maternal nano-TiO2 group, Fig. 9b, suggests the increased abundance of H3K4me3 and active transcription of the Tgfbr2 gene. Tgfbr2 provides an explicit example of how genes reported to be epigenetically altered (ChIP-Seq, through H3K4me3 localization at the Tgfbr2 promoter region) with subsequent changes in transcription (RNA-Seq, reporting increased expression of Tgfbr2 transcripts) can be further validated using other molecular techniques, such as qPCR. An overview of the experimental design is illustrated in Fig. 9c. Briefly, the figure provides an example of suggested functional outcomes related to maternal nano-TiO2 exposure, with the link between the exposure paradigm and end function being fetal, epigenetic consequences.

Discussion

The gene expression and epigenetic analyses performed in this study provide the first evidence that maternal ENM inhalation may result in significant pathway alterations in the fetus. The two most prominently impacted mechanisms are: inflammatory signaling, and cardiac-renal-hepatic pathology/toxicity.

The nano-TiO_2 exposure paradigm used herein (10 mg/m^3, 4-6 h) resulted in a calculated lung deposition of approximately 217 μg. This lung burden, achieved over 7 days of exposure in the second half of gestation, has been previously shown to impair uterine arteriolar reactivity by almost 50% [40]. To estimate how this lung burden compares to what a human may experience, alveolar surface areas must be known [32]. The rat alveolar surface area is 0.4 m^2/lung. Therefore, the rat

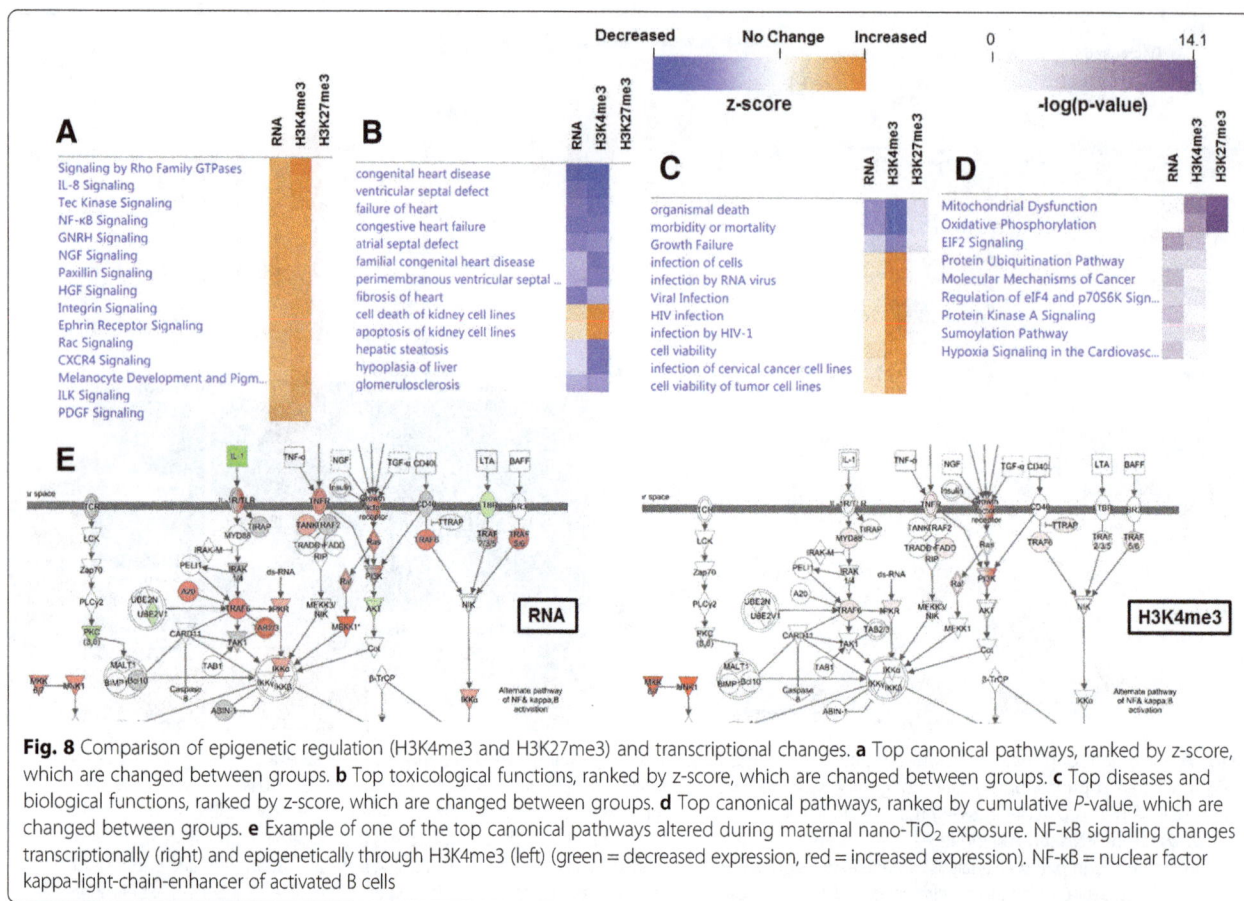

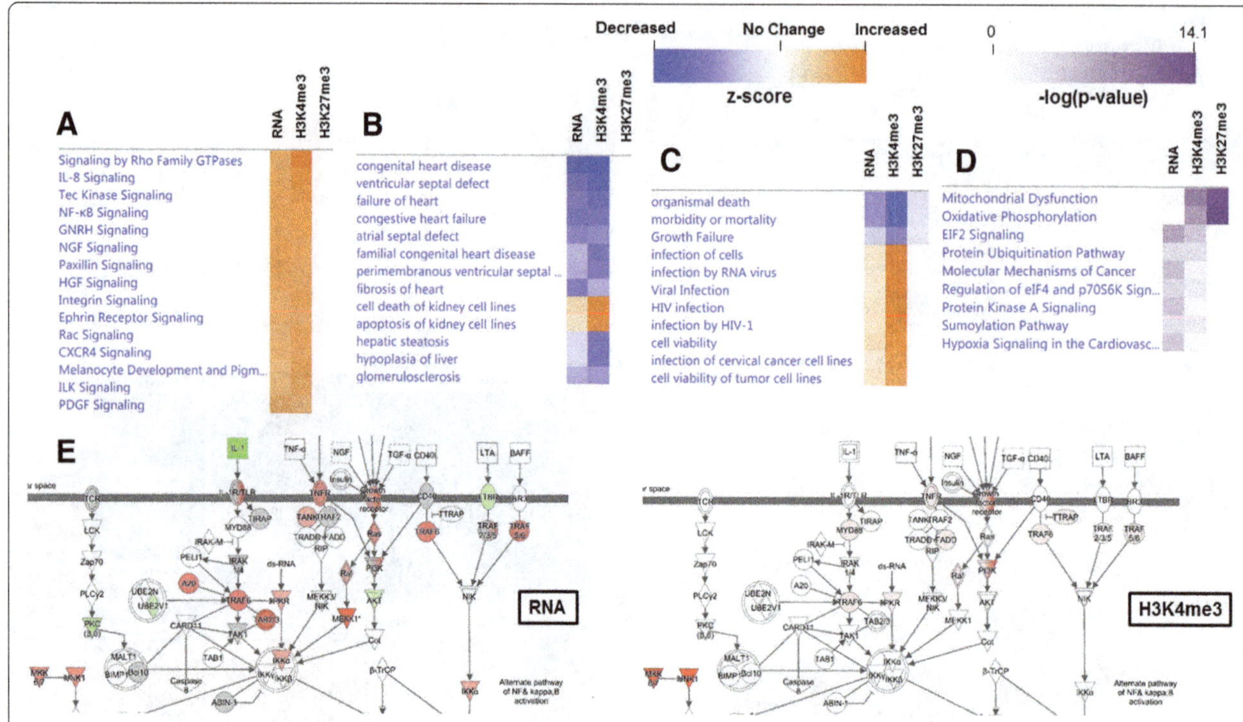

Fig. 8 Comparison of epigenetic regulation (H3K4me3 and H3K27me3) and transcriptional changes. **a** Top canonical pathways, ranked by z-score, which are changed between groups. **b** Top toxicological functions, ranked by z-score, which are changed between groups. **c** Top diseases and biological functions, ranked by z-score, which are changed between groups. **d** Top canonical pathways, ranked by cumulative *P*-value, which are changed between groups. **e** Example of one of the top canonical pathways altered during maternal nano-TiO_2 exposure. NF-κB signaling changes transcriptionally (right) and epigenetically through H3K4me3 (left) (green = decreased expression, red = increased expression). NF-κB = nuclear factor kappa-light-chain-enhancer of activated B cells

burden of 217 μg/lung would result in 542.5 $\mu g/m^2$. Given that the human alveolar surface area is 102 m^2, the equivalent human burden of this exposure paradigm would be 55.3 mg. The next logical question is how long would it take to achieve this burden in humans. In this regard, lung burden may be calculated as:

$$nano\text{-}TiO_2\ aerosol\ concentration \cdot minute\ ventilation \cdot exposure\ duration \cdot deposition\ fraction,$$

with the following values:

$$55.3\ mg = nano\text{-}TiO_2\ aerosol\ concentration \cdot 7600\ ml/\ min \cdot (8\ hr/day \cdot 60\ \ min/hr) \cdot 14\%,$$

and therefore:

$$55.3\ mg = nano\text{-}TiO_2\ aerosol\ concentration \cdot 0.51\ m^3/day.$$

The National Institute for Occupational Safety and Health (NIOSH) Recommended Exposure Limit (REL), or aerosol concentration for nano-TiO_2 is 0.3 mg/m^3 (DHHS, 2011). This would result in a lung burden of 0.15 mg/day. Whereas, the Occupational Safety and Health Administration (OSHA) Permissible Exposure Limit is 5 mg/m^3 (DHHS 2011). This would result in a lung burden of 2.55 mg/day. Considering the NIOSH REL and OSHA PEL together, it would require 1.45 working years or 21.7 working days (respectively) for a human to achieve comparable lung burdens with the exposure paradigm used herein. Because the human gestational period is 9 months, we consider our exposure paradigm highly relevant to the worker population.

Contrary to the functional deficits seen in the young adult [20, 25] we found that both the transcriptomic and epigenetic data support increased cardiac function (Figs. 5d and 7d). Though this seems paradoxical, we suggest that the interplay between the heart, liver, and kidneys is vital in understanding the pathology associated with maternal nano-TiO_2 exposure. It is equally plausible that as hematocrit increases, viscosity of the blood also increases, requiring an elevation in contractile force or a drop in peripheral resistance. Alternatively, it is possible that disruptions in maternal-fetal perfusion balances occur. The pulmonary exposure of the mother is well described, but the secondary effect(s) on the developing progeny is/are likely to come through impacts on the maternal/fetal circulation. Maternal nutrients are delivered to the placenta via the arterial circuit, if blood flow is inadequate, then fetal compensation must occur

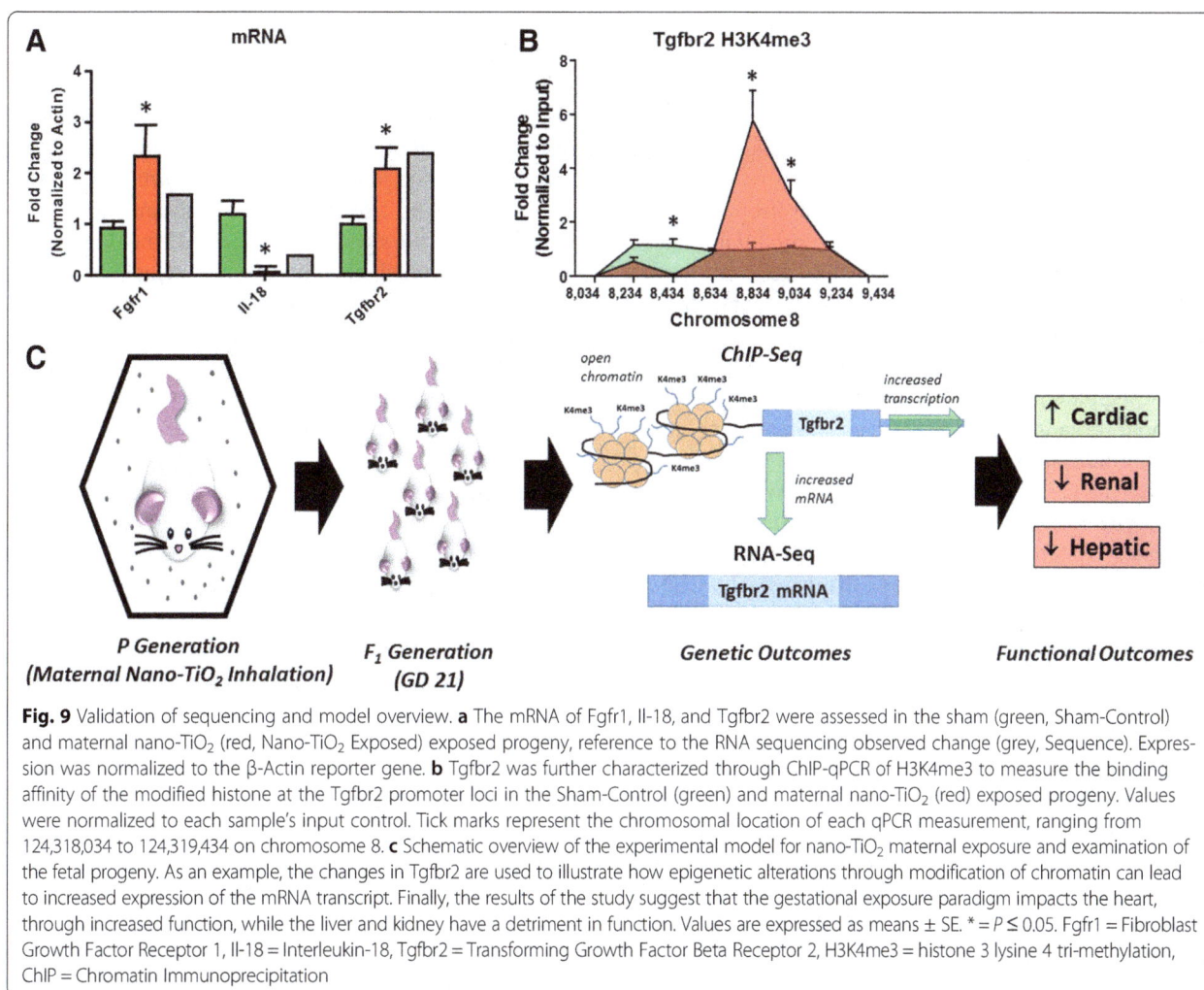

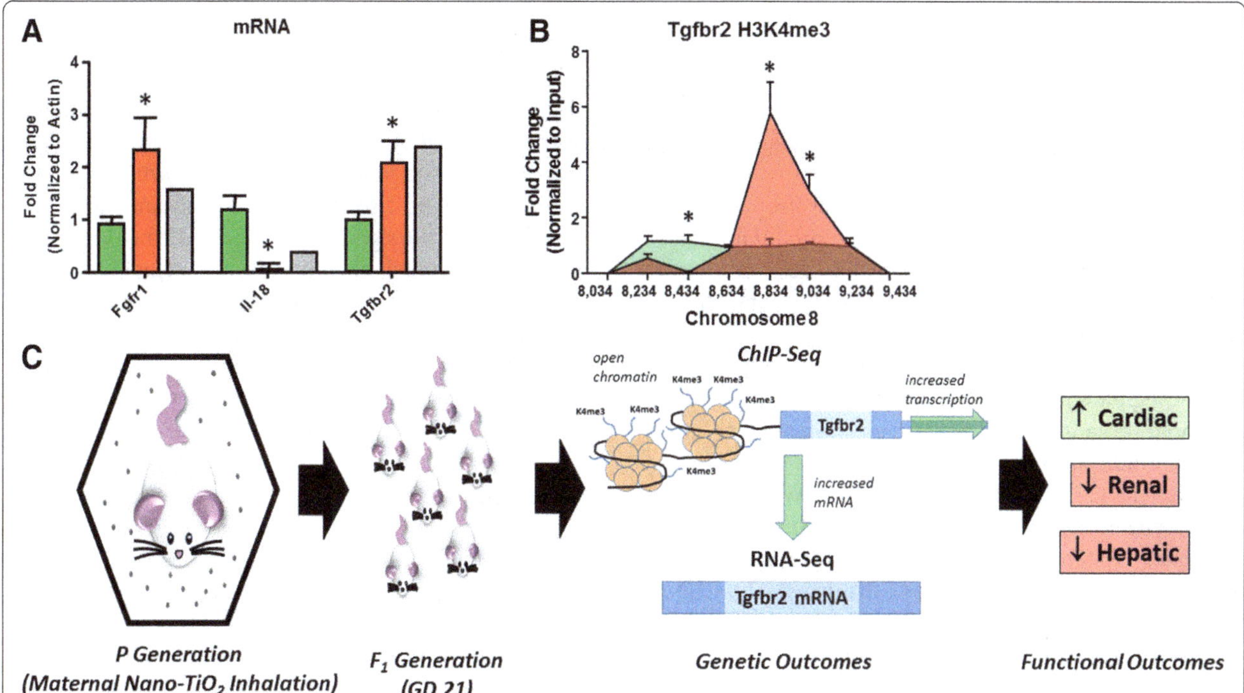

Fig. 9 Validation of sequencing and model overview. **a** The mRNA of Fgfr1, Il-18, and Tgfbr2 were assessed in the sham (green, Sham-Control) and maternal nano-TiO_2 (red, Nano-TiO_2 Exposed) exposed progeny, reference to the RNA sequencing observed change (grey, Sequence). Expression was normalized to the β-Actin reporter gene. **b** Tgfbr2 was further characterized through ChIP-qPCR of H3K4me3 to measure the binding affinity of the modified histone at the Tgfbr2 promoter loci in the Sham-Control (green) and maternal nano-TiO_2 (red) exposed progeny. Values were normalized to each sample's input control. Tick marks represent the chromosomal location of each qPCR measurement, ranging from 124,318,034 to 124,319,434 on chromosome 8. **c** Schematic overview of the experimental model for nano-TiO_2 maternal exposure and examination of the fetal progeny. As an example, the changes in Tgfbr2 are used to illustrate how epigenetic alterations through modification of chromatin can lead to increased expression of the mRNA transcript. Finally, the results of the study suggest that the gestational exposure paradigm impacts the heart, through increased function, while the liver and kidney have a detriment in function. Values are expressed as means ± SE. * = $P \leq 0.05$. Fgfr1 = Fibroblast Growth Factor Receptor 1, Il-18 = Interleukin-18, Tgfbr2 = Transforming Growth Factor Beta Receptor 2, H3K4me3 = histone 3 lysine 4 tri-methylation, ChIP = Chromatin Immunoprecipitation

to support proper nutrient delivery via the umbilical vein to the fetal portal circulation.

At the fetal stage, the heart plays a less significant role in energetics [45]. Whereas, the liver and kidneys play pivotal roles in blood conditioning at this stage of development, and these signaling pathways are altered by maternal ENM inhalation during gestation (Fig. 5). We hypothesize that potential liver and kidney damage from either inflammation, direct ENM translocation or a combination may result in an increased hematocrit, and or maternal-fetal perfusion balance. Together, this may suggest that in maternal nano-TiO_2 exposed progeny, the functional deficits seen later in development may be a result of this initial hepatic and renal insult, with subsequent cardiac overcompensation which may represent a protective mechanism. These findings correspond to reports of hepatic DNA damage in newborn murine offspring after maternal nano-TiO_2 inhalation [46]. Impairments in renal function may have profound effects on tubuloglomerular feedback, the renin angiotensin system, and/or osmotic regulation. These impairments may collectively or individually directly influence cardiovascular health throughout prenatal and postnatal development.

MicroRNA (miRNA) are well known to be altered by transcriptomic and epigenetic regulators. When expressed, miRNA broadly regulate cellular function [47] and have been implicated in numerous epigenetic pathways [48]. In Fig. 7c transcriptomic data is provided that reflects the most consistently altered regulator after maternal nano-TiO_2 inhalation. Decreased expression of miRNA-145 has been suggested to increase protein synthesis of targets directly involved in signaling events that promote organism growth and development. The role of altered miRNAs in progeny after maternal ENM inhalation is poorly understood, and may provide a better understanding of the relationship between ENM toxicities, epigenetics, and gene expression.

Figure 8c presents an overview of the two primary cell signaling pathways that are altered during gestational exposure: immunity and development. Parameters of organismal health and development are presented largely as molecular markers for cardiac signaling and function. The increased gene expression of molecular markers associated with infection and immunity may indicate the likelihood of autoimmune disorders associated with an overactive immune system. This is most evident when considering the inflammatory pathways indicated in Fig. 8a and the target organ (kidney) indicated in Fig. 8b reflected by an increased susceptibility as shown in Fig. 8c. These molecular markers may also represent the consequence presented in Fig. 8a of a proinflammatory environment; such an environment has been associated with chronic conditions including cardiovascular disease and cancer [49]. Pulmonary exposure to carbon black nanoparticles has also been identified to contribute to the development of immunotoxicity, particularly in lymphoid organs [22]. Interestingly, organismal death and morbidity/mortality appears to be decreased in maternal nano-TiO_2 offspring, which may again seem counterintuitive. However, we speculate this may reflect a greater systemic response to compensate for the numerous other mechanisms disturbed by ENM inhalation during gestation.

To better identify the future consequences of ENM exposure, the significance of the pathways was represented as the change in *P*-value (Fig. 8d). Mitochondrial dysfunction and oxidative phosphorylation appeared to have the greatest changes in methylation, indicating that future complications in these pathways may occur. Given their widespread involvement, this epigenetic predisposition may manifest in any tissue. In other words, the epigenetic changes associated with energetics may reflect significant alterations that occur during fetal development. It is important to indicate that these changes may not be manifested in functional transcriptomic or proteomic changes until postnatal development or even later into adulthood. If correct, this would be consistent with the Barker Hypothesis and DOHaD.

Maternal nano-TiO_2 exposure is also associated with a pronounced effect on key inflammatory pathways in the exposed progeny. In Fig. 8e, protein kinase B (AKT) signaling is decreased, potentially resulting in an impairment in calcium-independent nitric oxide signaling which would likely result in dysfunctional endothelium-dependent responses. Indeed, calcium dependent and independent mechanisms, as well as endothelial arteriolar dilation are significantly impaired at 3-4 weeks of age [50]. Furthermore, augmented NF-κB signaling via both alternate and canonical pathways [51] has been reported. Maternal nano-TiO_2 exposure significantly activated the expression of the Lymphotoxin Beta Receptor (LTBR) gene, while suppressing the expression of the regulating enzyme Inhibitor of NF-κB Kinase Subunit Alpha (IKKα) Fig. 8e. This is important in the negative feedback of the NF-κB canonical signaling that limits inflammatory gene activation and suggests that more robust inflammatory responses are possible as evidenced in Fig. 8a. Furthermore, NF-κB plays a central role in the development of inflammation through further regulation of genes encoding not only pro-inflammatory cytokines, but also adhesion molecules such as E-selectin, VCAM-1 (vascular cell adhesion molecule-1) and ICAM-1 (intercellular adhesion molecule-1), chemokines, and inducible nitric oxide synthase (iNOS) [52, 53]. Figure 8e also reflects a significant increase in interleukin-8 (IL-8) signaling, a major chemokine associated with neutrophil chemotaxis and degranulation secreted by macrophages and endothelial cells during acute inflammatory responses [54]. Considered jointly, uncontrolled activation of NF-κB and IL-8 pathways in maternally exposed progeny may predispose towards endothelial-dependent dysfunction and leukocyte adhesion.

Conclusion

The pathway analyses reported herein indicate dysfunction in many physiologic systems. As it is not possible to functionally verify each of these functional implications, the primary goal of the manuscript is to identify those systems as a priority for future study. Systemic impairments associated with acute and chronic nanomaterial exposures is an evolving field as nanotechnology continues to expand. Maternal and fetal outcomes following gestational exposures have recently been considered. While initial functional microvascular assessments have begun, little is known regarding epigenetic alterations within the F1 generation. The findings from this study describe epigenetic changes in the progeny of mothers exposed to nano-TiO_2 aerosols during gestation. The evidence of the study is strengthened by the use of two separate cohorts to separately probe the transcriptomic and epigenetic alterations, suggesting that even in separate discrete experimental populations, changes to the epigenome and RNA transcript levels align and similar exposure paradigms yield consistent results. Changes in the RNA transcripts and histone modifications on DNA suggest that maternal nano-TiO_2 progeny exhibit a propensity toward hepatic and renal disease, increased inflammatory signaling, and growth/survival while showing decreased cardiac dysfunction. What remains to be understood is if and/or how far these epigenetic changes persistent into adulthood, the dose-response relationships, and what stage of development is most sensitive to maternal ENM exposure.

Additional file

Additional file 1: Table S1. Listing of all disease and biological pathways with a positive or negative z-score greater than the absolute value of 2 for H3K4me3. **Table S2.** Listing of all disease and biological pathways with a positive or negative z-score greater than the absolute value of 2 for H3K27me3. **Table S3.** Listing of all disease and biological pathways with a positive or negative z-score greater than the absolute value of 2 for RNA. **Table S4.** Primer design for qPCR experiments.

Primers for the mRNA-qPCR experiments were designed using Primer-BLAST (https://www.ncbi.nlm.nih.gov/tools/primer-blast/). MRNA primers were designed to produced amplicons 100 – 250 bp in length. ChIP-qPCR primers were designed spanning a 1400 bp loci in the promoter region of the Tgfbr2 gene. Primers were designed to measure chromatin H3K4me3 modifications every 200 bp. Primer sequences were constrained to 60-100 bp amplicon lengths, in order to appropriately span sheered chromatin. All primer designs were performed against the *Rattus norvegicus* July 2014 (RGSC 6.0/rn6) genome build. ChIP = Chromatin Immunoprecipitation. (DOCX 41 kb)

Abbreviations

AKT: Protein Kinase B; Car1: Carbonic anhydrase 1; ChIP: Chromatin Immunoprecipitation; DOHad: Developmental Origin of Health and Disease; ENM: Engineered Nanomaterials; FDR: False Discovery Rate; Fgfr1: Fibroblast Growth Factor Receptor 1; GD: Gestational Day; H3K27me3: 3 lysine 27 tri-methylation; H3K4me3: 3 lysine 4 tri-methylation; IACUC: Institutional Animal Care and Use Committee; ICAM-1: Intercellular Adhesion Molecule-1; IKKα: Inhibitor of NF-κB Kinase Subunit Alpha; Il-18: Interleukin-18; IL-8: Interleukin 8; IPA: Ingenuity Pathway Analysis; LogFC: Log Fold Change; LTBR: Lymphotoxin Beta Receptor; NF-κB: Nuclear Factor kappa-light-chain-enhancer of activated B cells; NOS: Nitric Oxide Synthase; PEL: Permissible Exposure Limit; qPCR: Quantitative Polymerase Chain Reaction; REL: Recommended Exposure Limit; RIN: RNA Integrity Number; Rn5-8 s: 5.8S ribosomal RNA for *Rattus norvegicus*; Tgfbr2: Transforming Growth Factor Beta Receptor 2; VCAM-1: Vascular Cell Adhesion Molecule-1; Wnt5a: Wnt Family Member 5A

Acknowledgements

We thank Kevin Engels of the West Virginia University Department of Physiology, Pharmacology and Neuroscience; and Sherri A. Friend of NIOSH for their expert technical assistance.

Funding

This work was supported by: NIH-R00-ES024783 (PAS), R01-ES015022 (TRN), R01 HL-128485 (JMH), AHA-13PRE16850066 (CEN), NSF-1003907 (TRN), DGE-1144676 (QAH, ABA, TRN), and AHA-17PRE33660333 (QAH).

Authors' contributions

PAS-study design, pregnancy model, inhalation exposures, tissue harvesting, manuscript preparation. QAH-transcriptomic analysis, manuscript preparation. CEN- transcriptomic analysis, manuscript preparation. ABA- tissue harvesting, manuscript preparation. MVP-transcriptome preparation. DLS-transcriptome preparation. CRM-pregnancy model, inhalation exposures, tissue harvesting. JY-inhalation exposures. JMH-transcriptome analysis design, manuscript preparation. VCC- lung burden calculations, rodent to human comparisons, manuscript preparation. TRN- study design, pregnancy model, inhalation exposures, tissue harvesting, manuscript preparation. All authors read and approved the final manuscript.

Competing interests

The authors declare that they have no competing interests.

Author details

[1]Department of Pharmacology and Toxicology, Ernest Mario School of Pharmacy, Rutgers University, Piscataway, NJ, USA. [2]Environmental and Occupational Health Sciences Institute, Piscataway, NJ, USA. [3]Division of Exercise Physiology, West Virginia University School of Medicine, Morgantown, WV, USA. [4]Mitochondria, Metabolism & Bioenergetics Working Group, West Virginia University School of Medicine, Morgantown, WV, USA. [5]Immunity, Inflammation, and Disease Laboratory, National Institute of Environmental Health Sciences, Research Triangle Park, NC, USA. [6]Toxicology Working Group, West Virginia University School of Medicine, Morgantown, WV, USA. [7]Department of Pharmaceutical Sciences, West Virginia University School of Pharmacy, Morgantown, USA. [8]Department of Physiology, Pharmacology, and Neuroscience, Robert C. Byrd Health Sciences Center, West Virginia University School of Medicine, 1 Medical Center Drive, Morgantown, WV 26506-9229, USA.

References

1. de Boo HA, Harding JE. The developmental origins of adult disease (barker) hypothesis. Aust N Z J Obstet Gynaecol. 2006;46(1):4–14.
2. Heindel JJ, Vandenberg LN. Developmental origins of health and disease: a paradigm for understanding disease cause and prevention. Curr Opin Pediatr. 2015;27(2):248–53.
3. Lane RH. Fetal programming, epigenetics, and adult onset disease. Clin Perinatol. 2014;41(4):815–31.
4. Alexander BT, Dasinger JH, Intapad S. Fetal programming and cardiovascular pathology. Compr Physiol. 2015;5(2):997–1025.
5. Grason HA, Misra DP. Reducing exposure to environmental toxicants before birth: moving from risk perception to risk reduction. Public Health Rep. 2009;124(5):629–41.
6. He M, et al. Exposure to bisphenol a enhanced lung eosinophilia in adult male mice. Allergy Asthma Clin Immunol. 2016;12:16.
7. Dadvand P, et al. Maternal exposure to particulate air pollution and term birth weight: a multi-country evaluation of effect and heterogeneity. Environ Health Perspect. 2013;121(3):267–373.
8. Perez-Hernandez M, et al. Multiparametric analysis of anti-proliferative and apoptotic effects of gold nanoprisms on mouse and human primary and transformed cells, biodistribution and toxicity in vivo. Part Fibre Toxicol. 2017;14(1):41.
9. Adamcakova-Dodd A, et al. Effects of prenatal inhalation exposure to copper nanoparticles on murine dams and offspring. Part Fibre Toxicol. 2015;12:30.
10. Abukabda AB, Stapleton PA, Nurkiewicz TR. Metal Nanomaterial toxicity variations within the vascular system. Curr Environ Health Rep. 2016; 3(4):379–91.
11. Yan Z, et al. Zinc oxide nanoparticle-induced atherosclerotic alterations in vitro and in vivo. Int J Nanomedicine. 2017;12:4433–42.
12. Holland NA, et al. Impact of pulmonary exposure to gold core silver nanoparticles of different size and capping agents on cardiovascular injury. Part Fibre Toxicol. 2016;13(1):48.
13. Hougaard KS, et al. A perspective on the developmental toxicity of inhaled nanoparticles. Reprod Toxicol. 2015;56:118–40.
14. Jackson P, et al. Exposure of pregnant mice to carbon black by intratracheal instillation: toxicogenomic effects in dams and offspring. Mutat Res. 2012; 745(1-2):73–83.
15. Blum JL, et al. Effects of maternal exposure to cadmium oxide Nanoparticles during pregnancy on maternal and offspring kidney injury markers using a Murine model. J Toxicol Environ Health A. 2015;78(12):711–24.
16. Campagnolo L, et al. Silver nanoparticles inhaled during pregnancy reach and affect the placenta and the foetus. Nanotoxicology. 2017;11(5):687–98.
17. Ema M, et al. Reproductive and developmental toxicity of carbon-based nanomaterials: a literature review. Nanotoxicology. 2016;10(4):391–412.
18. Hougaard KS, et al. Effects of prenatal exposure to surface-coated nanosized titanium dioxide (UV-titan). A study in mice. Part Fibre Toxicol. 2010;7:16.
19. Engler-Chiurazzi EB, et al. Impacts of prenatal nanomaterial exposure on male adult Sprague-Dawley rat behavior and cognition. J Toxicol Environ Health A. 2016;79(11):447–52.
20. Hathaway QA, et al. Maternal-engineered nanomaterial exposure disrupts progeny cardiac function and bioenergetics. Am J Physiol Heart Circ Physiol. 2017;312(3):H446–58.
21. Stapleton PA, et al. Maternal engineered nanomaterial exposure and fetal microvascular function: does the barker hypothesis apply? Am J Obstet Gynecol. 2013;209(3):227. e1-11
22. El-Sayed YS, et al. Carbon black nanoparticle exposure during middle and late fetal development induces immune activation in male offspring mice. Toxicology. 2015;327:53–61.

23. Kyjovska ZO, et al. Daily sperm production: application in studies of prenatal exposure to nanoparticles in mice. Reprod Toxicol. 2013;36:88–97.
24. Hougaard KS, et al. Effects of lung exposure to carbon nanotubes on female fertility and pregnancy. A study in mice. Reprod Toxicol. 2013;41:86–97.
25. Stapleton PA, et al. Microvascular and mitochondrial dysfunction in the female F1 generation after gestational TiO2 nanoparticle exposure. Nanotoxicology. 2015;9(8):941–51.
26. Hu X, et al. Toxicity evaluation of exposure to an atmospheric mixture of polychlorinated biphenyls by nose-only and whole-body inhalation regimens. Environ Sci Technol. 2015;49(19):11875–83.
27. Stapleton PA. Gestational nanomaterial exposures: microvascular implications during pregnancy, fetal development and adulthood. J Physiol. 2016;594(8):2161–73.
28. Knuckles TL, et al. Nanoparticle inhalation alters systemic arteriolar vasoreactivity through sympathetic and cyclooxygenase-mediated pathways. Nanotoxicology. 2012;6(7):724–35.
29. Nurkiewicz TR, et al. Nanoparticle inhalation augments particle-dependent systemic microvascular dysfunction. Part Fibre Toxicol. 2008;5:1.
30. Yi J, et al. Whole-body nanoparticle aerosol inhalation exposures. J Vis Exp. 2013;75:e50263.
31. Sager TM, Kommineni C, Castranova V. Pulmonary response to intratracheal instillation of ultrafine versus fine titanium dioxide: role of particle surface area. Part Fibre Toxicol. 2008;5:17.
32. Nurkiewicz TR, et al. Pulmonary particulate matter and systemic microvascular dysfunction. Res Rep Health Eff Inst. 2011;164:3–48.
33. Stapleton PA, et al. Impairment of coronary arteriolar endothelium-dependent dilation after multi-walled carbon nanotube inhalation: a time-course study. Int J Mol Sci. 2012;13(11):13781–803.
34. Bolger AM, Lohse M, Usadel B. Trimmomatic: a flexible trimmer for Illumina sequence data. Bioinformatics. 2014;30(15):2114–20.
35. Shen L, et al. diffReps: detecting differential chromatin modification sites from ChIP-seq data with biological replicates. PLoS One. 2013;8(6):e65598.
36. Kim D, Langmead B, Salzberg SL. HISAT: a fast spliced aligner with low memory requirements. Nat Methods. 2015;12(4):357–60.
37. Li H, et al. The sequence alignment/map format and SAMtools. Bioinformatics. 2009;25(16):2078–9.
38. Liao Y, Smyth GK, Shi W. The subread aligner: fast, accurate and scalable read mapping by seed-and-vote. Nucleic Acids Res. 2013;41(10):e108.
39. Liao Y, Smyth GK, Shi W. featureCounts: an efficient general purpose program for assigning sequence reads to genomic features. Bioinformatics. 2014;30(7):923–30.
40. Lun AT, Chen Y, Smyth GK. It's DE-licious: a recipe for differential expression analyses of RNA-seq experiments using quasi-likelihood methods in edgeR. Methods Mol Biol. 2016;1418:391–416.
41. Lun AT, Smyth GK. Csaw: a bioconductor package for differential binding analysis of ChIP-seq data using sliding windows. Nucleic Acids Res. 2016;44(5):e45.
42. Robinson MD, McCarthy DJ, Smyth GK. edgeR: a bioconductor package for differential expression analysis of digital gene expression data. Bioinformatics. 2010;26(1):139–40.
43. Hahne F, Ivanek R. Visualizing genomic data using Gviz and bioconductor. Methods Mol Biol. 2016;1418:335–51.
44. Love MI, Huber W, Anders S. Moderated estimation of fold change and dispersion for RNA-seq data with DESeq2. Genome Biol. 2014;15(12):550.
45. Taegtmeyer H, Sen S, Vela D. Return to the fetal gene program: a suggested metabolic link to gene expression in the heart. Ann N Y Acad Sci. 2010;1188:191–8.
46. Jackson P, et al. Pulmonary exposure to carbon black by inhalation or instillation in pregnant mice: effects on liver DNA strand breaks in dams and offspring. Nanotoxicology. 2012;6(5):486–500.
47. Shukla GC, Singh J, Barik S. MicroRNAs: processing, maturation, target recognition and regulatory functions. Mol Cell Pharmacol. 2011;3(3):83–92.
48. Bartel DP. MicroRNAs: target recognition and regulatory functions. Cell. 2009;136(2):215–33.
49. Singh-Manoux A, et al. Association between inflammatory biomarkers and all-cause, cardiovascular and cancer-related mortality. Can Med Assoc J. 2017;189(10):E384–90.
50. Nurkiewicz TR, Boegehold MA. Calcium-independent release of endothelial nitric oxide in the arteriolar network: onset during rapid juvenile growth. Microcirculation. 2004;11(6):453–62.
51. Ze Y, et al. TiO2 nanoparticles induced hippocampal neuroinflammation in mice. PLoS One. 2014;9(3):e92230.
52. Imai Y, et al. Interaction between cytokines and inflammatory cells in islet dysfunction, insulin resistance and vascular disease. Diabetes Obes Metab. 2013;15(Suppl 3):117–29.
53. Sprague AH, Khalil RA. Inflammatory cytokines in vascular dysfunction and vascular disease. Biochem Pharmacol. 2009;78(6):539–52.
54. Harada A, et al. Essential involvement of interleukin-8 (IL-8) in acute inflammation. J Leukoc Biol. 1994;56(5):559–64.

11

Imipramine blocks acute silicosis in a mouse model

Rupa Biswas[1†], Kevin L. Trout[1†], Forrest Jessop[1], Jack R. Harkema[2] and Andrij Holian[1*]

Abstract

Background: Inhalation of crystalline silica is associated with pulmonary inflammation and silicosis. Although silicosis remains a prevalent health problem throughout the world, effective treatment choices are limited. Imipramine (IMP) is a FDA approved tricyclic antidepressant drug with lysosomotropic characteristics. The aim of this study was to evaluate the potential for IMP to reduce silicosis and block phagolysosome membrane permeabilization.

Methods: C57BL/6 alveolar macrophages (AM) exposed to crystalline silica ± IMP in vitro were assessed for IL-1β release, cytotoxicity, particle uptake, lysosomal stability, and acid sphingomyelinase activity. Short term (24 h) in vivo studies in mice instilled with silica (± IMP) evaluated inflammation and cytokine release, in addition to cytokine release from ex vivo cultured AM. Long term (six to ten weeks) in vivo studies in mice instilled with silica (± IMP) evaluated histopathology, lung damage, and hydroxyproline content as an indicator of collagen accumulation.

Results: IMP significantly attenuated silica-induced cytotoxicity and release of mature IL-1β from AM in vitro. IMP treatment in vivo reduced silica-induced inflammation in a short-term model. Furthermore, IMP was effective in blocking silica-induced lung damage and collagen deposition in a long-term model. The mechanism by which IMP reduces inflammation was explored by assessing cellular processes such as particle uptake and acid sphingomyelinase activity.

Conclusions: Taken together, IMP was anti-inflammatory against silica exposure in vitro and in vivo. The results were consistent with IMP blocking silica-induced phagolysosomal lysis, thereby preventing cell death and IL-1β release. Thus, IMP could be therapeutic for silica-induced inflammation and subsequent disease progression as well as other diseases involving phagolysosomal lysis.

Keywords: Silica, Silicosis, Particles, Imipramine, Macrophage, Lysosome, Inflammation, Toxicology

Background

Silicosis is a lung disease caused by inhalation of crystalline silica and is most prevalent as a result of occupational exposures [1, 2]. The seriousness of the disease is reflected by the morbidity and disabling illnesses that continue to occur among workers [3]. Silicosis can be categorized into subtypes based on duration of exposure and associated pathology. In a general sense, chronic silicosis develops after at least 10 years of low concentration exposures, accelerated silicosis develops after 5-10 years of medium concentration exposures, and acute silicosis develops after a few weeks to 5 years of high concentration exposures [4]. Silicoproteinosis is a common distinguishing pathology of acute silicosis, and these terms are often used interchangeably. Most forms of human silicosis are difficult to mimic experimentally due to the long latency period for disease development, but animal models of silica exposure have been shown to produce similar characteristics in a more rapid timeline [5–7]. Currently, treatment choices for silicosis are limited and accompanied by complex adverse outcomes [4]. Therefore, it remains important to understand the mechanism of silica-induced inflammation and disease progression in order to develop effective therapeutics.

When respirable particulates of 2.5 μm or less deposit in the pulmonary alveolus, they are cleared by alveolar

* Correspondence: andrij.holian@umontana.edu
†Equal contributors
[1]Center for Environmental Health Sciences, Department of Biomedical and Pharmaceutical Sciences, University of Montana, Missoula, MT 59812, USA
Full list of author information is available at the end of the article

macrophages (AM) and are predominantly contained in phagosomes [8, 9]. Lysosomes fuse with the phagosomes to form phagolysosomes, in which lysosomal enzymes attempt to degrade phagocytosed particulates. However, a number of particulates including silica cannot be degraded, which may contribute to phagolysosomal membrane permeabilization (LMP) [10, 11]. Nevertheless, the exact cause of particle-induced phagolysosomal instability is not clearly understood.

LMP results in the release of lysosomal proteases to the cytoplasm that have been reported to contribute to cytotoxicity [12–16] and to trigger assembly of the multiprotein complex, NLRP3 inflammasome [17]. The function and regulation of inflammasomes has been reviewed elsewhere [18–22]. NLRP3 inflammasome assembly leads to activation of Caspase-1, which cleaves pro-Interleukin (IL)-1β and pro-IL-18 to their active forms. Another signal is required to activate the NF-κB pathway, such as lipopolysaccharide (LPS), IL-1β, high mobility group box 1 (HMGB1) protein [23], or other damage/pathogen-associated molecular patterns (DAMP/PAMP). NF-κB activation upregulates transcription of inflammasome components, pro-IL-1β, and pro-IL-18. The release of mature IL-1β and IL-18 have been closely associated with acute inflammation and development of lung fibrosis [24, 25]. It should be noted that although inflammasome activation is typically considered to be the primary mechanism for IL-1β processing, it has been suggested that there may also be smaller contributions from inflammasome-independent mechanisms in vivo [20].

Since LMP plays an important regulatory role in NLRP3 inflammasome activation and subsequent inflammation, blocking LMP would be a target for novel therapeutics for inflammatory diseases linked to lysosomal instability. For example, a drug or an agent that can stabilize the lysosome and prevent membrane permeabilization may have the potential to attenuate downstream inflammation. A potential anti-LMP agent is imipramine (IMP), a U.S Food and Drug Administration approved tricyclic antidepressant drug with lysosomotropic properties [26]. Pretreatment with IMP has been reported to attenuate the inflammatory response and improve survival in an LPS-induced acute lung injury model [27]. In another study, the authors reported that IMP and surfactant synergistically suppressed acid sphingomyelinase (aSMase) activity in lung tissue, reduced ceramide generation, and improved pulmonary function in a newborn piglet lavage model [28]. However, IMP has not been examined in models of particulate-induced inflammation. Therefore, the potential of IMP to inhibit inflammation following silica exposure was examined in this study.

We hypothesized that IMP will stabilize lysosomes, thereby decreasing NLRP3 inflammasome activation and downstream inflammation. In vitro studies were conducted using AM from C57Bl/6 mice to evaluate the effect of IMP on IL-1β release and cytotoxicity. In vivo studies with C57Bl/6 mice were conducted to determine if IMP could decrease silica-induced acute inflammation and pathology. Furthermore, we determined the potential of IMP as a protective and a therapeutic agent in a long-term crystalline silica exposure model.

Results

Imipramine inhibited silica-induced IL-1β release and cytotoxicity in vitro

Primary AM were used to evaluate the effects of IMP on IL-1β release and cytotoxicity. Isolated AM were treated ± IMP (25 μM) for 30 min and then exposed to LPS (20 ng/ml) ± silica (100 μg/ml). The results in Fig. 1a show silica leads to a significant increase in IL-1β release compared to cells treated with LPS only. IMP pretreatment significantly inhibited IL-1β release in silica-exposed AM. Similar results were obtained using cell line THP-1 (Additional file 1: Figure S1), which is a human monocytic leukemia line that is commonly used for particle toxicology studies in our laboratory and others [29, 30]. These results demonstrate that IMP can significantly block silica-induced IL-1β release in vitro.

AM cytotoxicity was examined for two purposes: (1) to determine whether the observed decrease in IL-1β was due to any unexpected toxicity of IMP, and (2) to

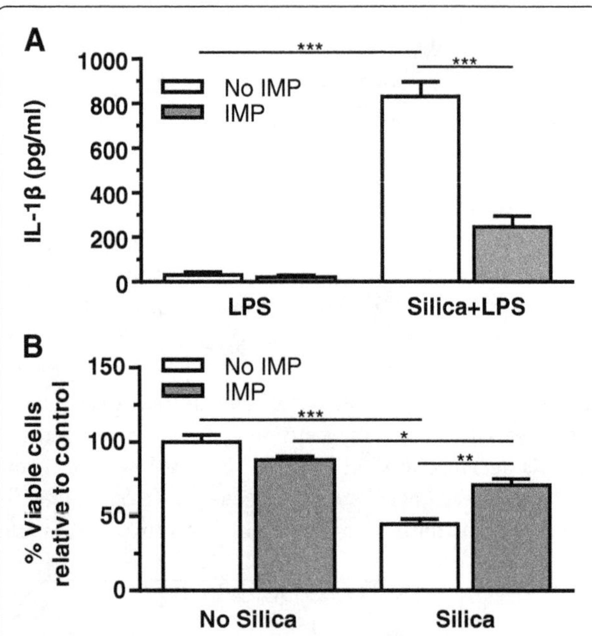

Fig. 1 In vitro IL-1β release and cytotoxicity in AM treated with silica ± imipramine. AM treatment conditions include IMP for 30 min, followed by exposure to LPS and silica for 24 h. **a** IL-1β release was measured by ELISA. **b** MTS assay results are expressed as cell viability relative to no silica, no IMP control. $n \geq 3$ mice per treatment condition

evaluate the effect of IMP on silica-induced cytotoxicity. Isolated AM were pretreated ± IMP for 30 min then exposed to silica overnight. AM exposed to silica showed the expected significant loss in cell viability compared to baseline control (Fig. 1b). Silica-induced cytotoxicity was significantly lowered by IMP pretreatment. Taken together, IMP blocked both the silica-induced IL-1β release and cytotoxicity.

Imipramine pre-treatment reduced short-term silica-induced inflammation in vivo

Since IMP was effective in decreasing silica-induced IL-1β release from macrophages in vitro, it suggested that IMP could be anti-inflammatory in vivo. Therefore, mice were given IMP (25 mg/kg) or vehicle (100 μl) by intraperitoneal (IP) injection 30 min before silica (1 mg/mouse in 25 μl) or vehicle (PBS (sham); 25 μl) exposure. After 24 h, whole lung lavage was analyzed by cell differentials and ELISA for IL-1β. IMP pretreatment did not significantly change the total cell counts (Fig. 2a) and the number of eosinophils and lymphocytes were negligible. In the silica-exposed group there was a significant increase in neutrophils in lavage fluid, and IMP pretreatment significantly inhibited neutrophil infiltration following silica exposure (Fig. 2b). Furthermore, IL-1β levels in lavage fluid were assessed (Fig. 2c). Trends suggest IL-1β is increased by silica, which is reduced by IMP treatment. Though the inhibition of IL-1β release into the lavage fluid did not achieve statistical significance, it followed a similar pattern as observed in vitro.

In order to determine whether IMP had specifically blocked IL-1β production by macrophages in vivo, AM were collected from the lavage fluid in the 24 h experiment above. The lavaged cells were then cultured ex vivo for 24 h ± LPS (20 ng/ml). There was a significant increase in IL-1β release in the silica-exposed group compared to that in the controls, which was significantly reduced by IMP pretreatment (Fig. 2d). Therefore, IMP given IP was sufficient to target AM and block silica-induced release of IL-1β. Overall, the results indicate that the anti-inflammatory effect of IMP following silica exposure followed the same pattern in vitro, in vivo and ex vivo.

Imipramine post-treatment reduced short-term silica-induced inflammation in vivo

In the studies above, IMP was given to mice prior to administration of silica. In order to determine whether IMP would also be effective if given after onset of silica-induced inflammation, mice were first exposed to silica (1 mg/mouse) or vehicle (25 μl). After 30 min, mice were given IMP (25 mg/kg in PBS) or PBS alone by IP injection. After 24 h, whole lung lavage was analyzed by cell differentials and ELISA for IL-1β. IMP post-treatment did not significantly change the total cell counts (Fig. 3a) and the number of eosinophils and lymphocytes were negligible. Silica leads to significant neutrophil influx, which is reduced by IMP treatment (Fig. 3b). IL-1β was significantly higher in the group exposed to silica compared to the vehicle control (Fig. 3c). In order to determine whether IMP was acting on AM specifically in this model, the lavaged cells were cultured ex vivo for 24 h in the presence and absence of LPS (20 ng/ml). There was a significant increase in IL-1β release in the silica-exposed group compared to control (Fig. 3d). IMP pretreatment in vivo significantly decreased IL-1β release from AM following silica exposure.

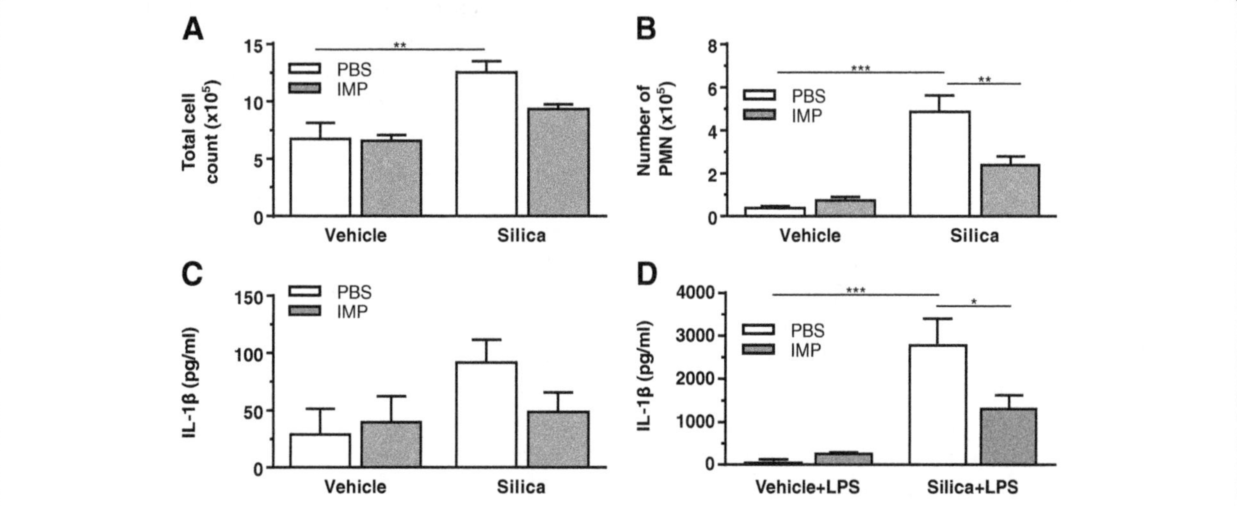

Fig. 2 IMP pre-treatment effect on acute inflammation induced by silica. Mice were treated with IMP or PBS for 30 min, then exposed to silica or vehicle. Whole lung lavage was collected after 24 h. **a** Total number of cells in the lavage fluid. **b** Polymorphonuclear (PMN) leukocytes in lavage were assessed by staining. **c** IL-1β levels in lavage fluid. **d** IL-1β in supernatant of isolated AM exposed to LPS ex vivo for an additional 24 h. $n \geq 3$ mice per treatment condition

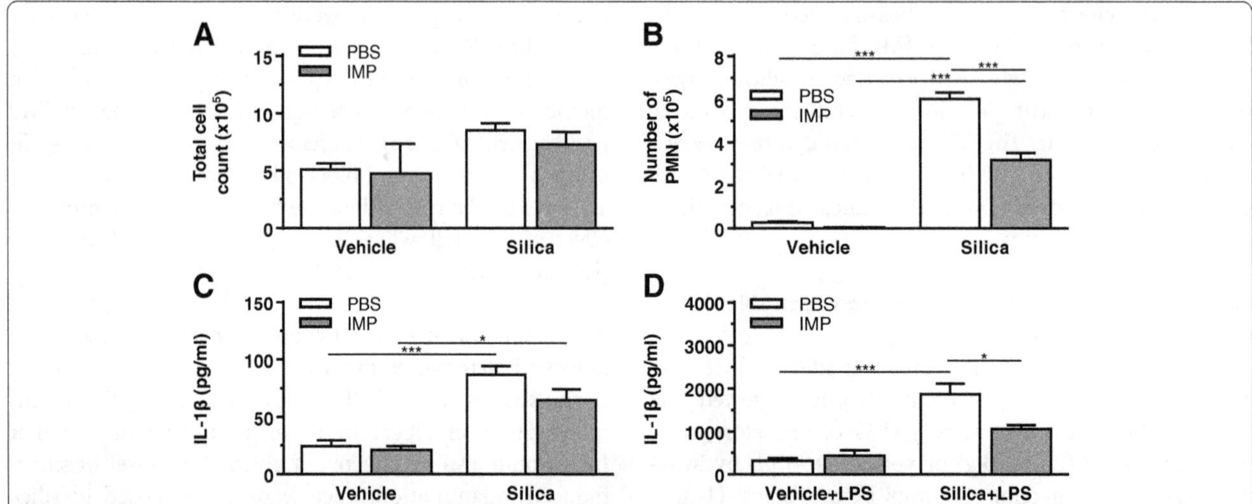

Fig. 3 IMP post-treatment effect on acute inflammation induced by silica. Mice were exposed to silica or vehicle for 30 min, then treated with IMP or PBS. Whole lung lavage was collected after 24 h. **a** Total number of cells in the lavage fluid. **b** Polymorphonuclear (PMN) leukocytes in lavage were assessed by staining. **c** IL-1β levels in lavage fluid. **d** IL-1β in supernatant of isolated AM exposed to LPS ex vivo for an additional 24 h. $n \geq 3$ mice per treatment condition

Similar trends are observed regardless of whether IMP is given before (Fig. 2) or after (Fig. 3) silica.

Imipramine concomitant treatment reduced long-term silica-induced pathology in vivo

The data thus far demonstrated that IMP was effective in blocking acute inflammation caused by silica exposure. Because fibrosis is a result of chronic inflammation, additional studies were completed to determine whether continuous treatment with IMP could block the longer-term effects of silica exposure. Therefore, mice were given IMP in osmotic pump implants to continuously release IMP (or PBS sham) as described in Methods. Simultaneously, the mice were given 1 mg silica and three additional doses of 1 mg silica were given 7, 14 and 21 days later to simulate an extended exposure as previously described [31, 32]. At the end of six weeks, the lungs were examined by histology and quantification of collagen content, a hallmark of lung fibrosis.

A board-certified veterinary pathologist with expertise in respiratory pathobiology of inhaled toxicants in laboratory rodents examined the prepared lung tissue sections by light microscopy. Tissues were examined from at least three mice per treatment group. The pathologist had no knowledge of the exposure history of the individual mice prior to his assessment of pulmonary histopathology. No lung lesions were found in mice that received vehicle alone, regardless of IMP treatment. In contrast, mice instilled with silica without IMP treatment had conspicuous lung lesions consisting of widespread alveolar proteinosis associated with cellular debris and a mixed inflammatory cell influx of neutrophils and mononuclear cells (mainly macrophages/monocytes and lesser numbers of lymphocytes), focal microgranulomas (mainly epithelioid cells and macrophages with lesser numbers of neutrophils), perivascular and peribronchiolar ectopic lymphoid tissue (lymphoplasmacytic), and alveolar type II cell hyperplasia in the affected areas of the lung parenchyma (Figs. 4 and 5).

Immunohistochemically, there were numerous 7/4 antibody-positive inflammatory cells (neutrophils and inflammatory macrophages/monocytes) in mice treated with silica without IMP (Fig. 6). Also, more picrosirius red-positive staining of collagen was found in the lungs of silica-instilled mice as compared to mice that were not instilled with silica (Fig. 7). This greater staining of lung tissue collagen was most associated with the microgranuloma formation in the alveolar parenchyma.

Interestingly, IMP treatment resulted in less severe silica-associated lesions characterized by mild, widely scattered alveolar proteinosis, minimal ectopic lymphoid tissue around blood vessels or conducting airways, and only a few widely scattered microgranulomas with some 7/4 antibody-positive inflammatory cells and modest picrosirius red-positive collagen (Figs. 4d, 5, 6d, and 7d).

Collagen in the lung was measured by hydroxyproline content (Fig. 8). Hydroxyproline content was significantly higher in the silica-exposed group compared to the vehicle-exposed group. IMP treatment significantly attenuated collagen levels in the silica co-administered group. These results demonstrate that the collagen deposition due to extended silica exposure can be attenuated by IMP co-treatment.

Imipramine post-treatment reduced long-term silica-induced lung injury and collagen deposition in vivo

The studies above demonstrated that IMP reduced pathology and collagen deposition when given at the same

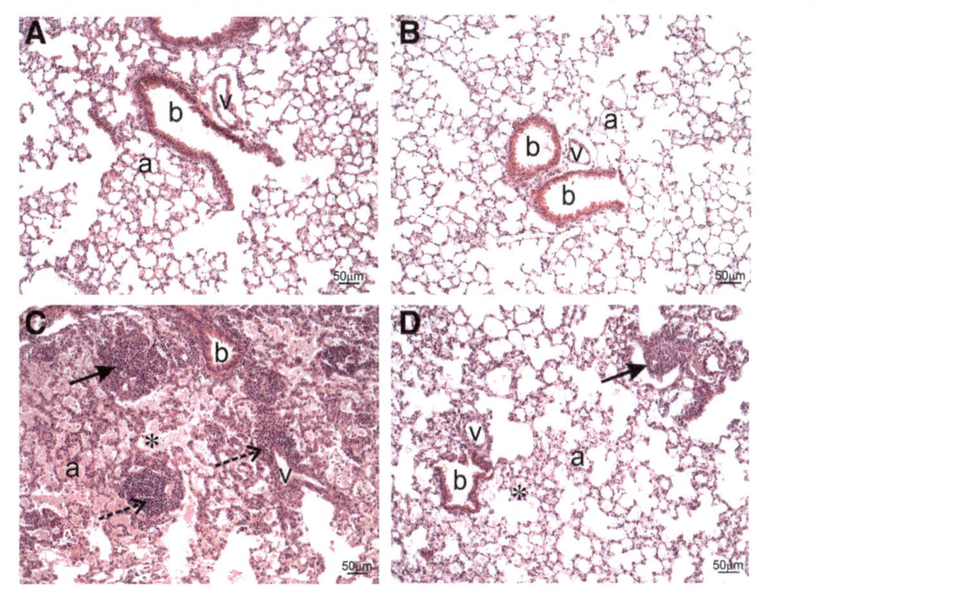

Fig. 4 Histopathology from IMP co-administration study. Mice were exposed to silica or vehicle weekly for the first four weeks, while receiving IMP or PBS by osmotic pump for entire six week duration. Light photomicrographs are H&E-stained lung tissue sections from mice treated with (**a**) vehicle, (**b**) IMP, (**c**) silica, and (**d**) silica + IMP. Silica-induced histopathology included alveolar proteinosis (asterisk), microgranuloma (solid arrow), perivascular and peribronchioloar ectopic lymphoid tissue (dashed arrow; lymphoplasmacytic infiltrate). IMP treatment reduced severity of silica-related lesions, with minimal alveolar proteinosis and a small microgranuloma. Abbreviations: a = alveolar parenchyma; b = bronchiolar airway; v = blood vessel. Tissue was observed from $n \geq 3$ mice per treatment condition

time as silica in a long-term silica exposure mouse model. However, this did not establish the potential of IMP to act as a therapeutic to reverse lung injury and collagen accumulation after disease development. In order to test this potential, disease was first induced by administration of silica for four weeks (as described above), then IMP (or sham) was given to mice for six weeks using osmotic pumps. Protein levels in the lavage fluid, a marker of alveolar-capillary barrier damage, were measured as an indicator of lung injury (Fig. 9a). Lung lavage protein levels were significantly increased in the silica and sham-treated group compared to the controls.

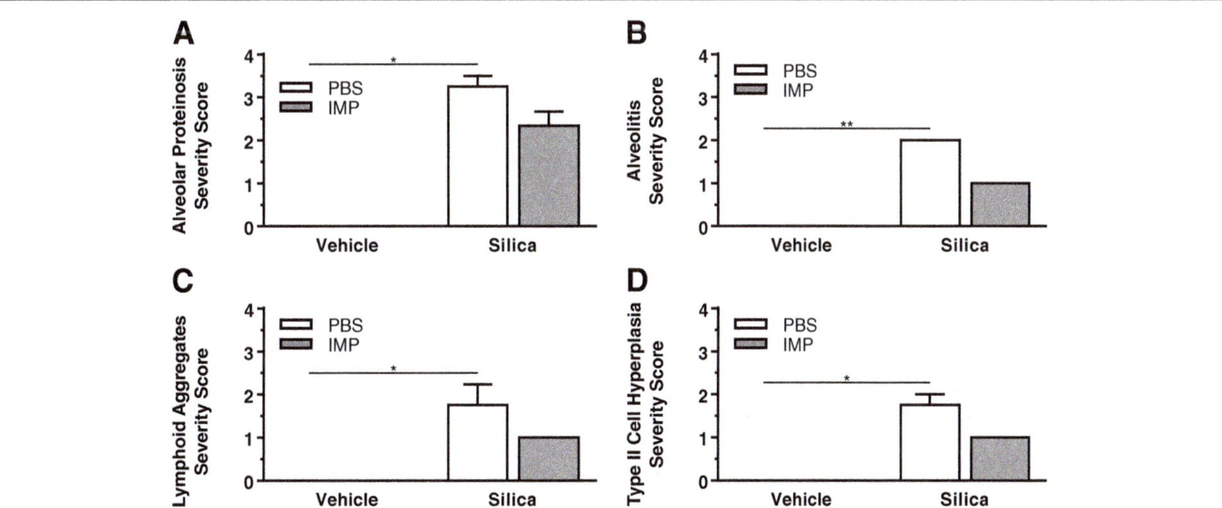

Fig. 5 Semi-quantitative analysis of histopathology. Mice were exposed to silica or vehicle weekly for the first four weeks, while receiving IMP or PBS by osmotic pump for entire six week duration. Multiparametric scoring of H&E-stained lung tissue was completed using an ordinal scale ranging from no significant pathology (score: 0) to severe pathology (score: 5). **a** Alveolar proteinosis. **b** Alveolitis including mixed inflammatory cell infiltrates, microgranulomas, and associated interstitial fibrosis. **c** Perivascular/peribronchiolar lymphoid aggregates. **d** Type II alveolar epithelial cell hyperplasia. Tissue was scored from $n \geq 3$ mice per treatment condition

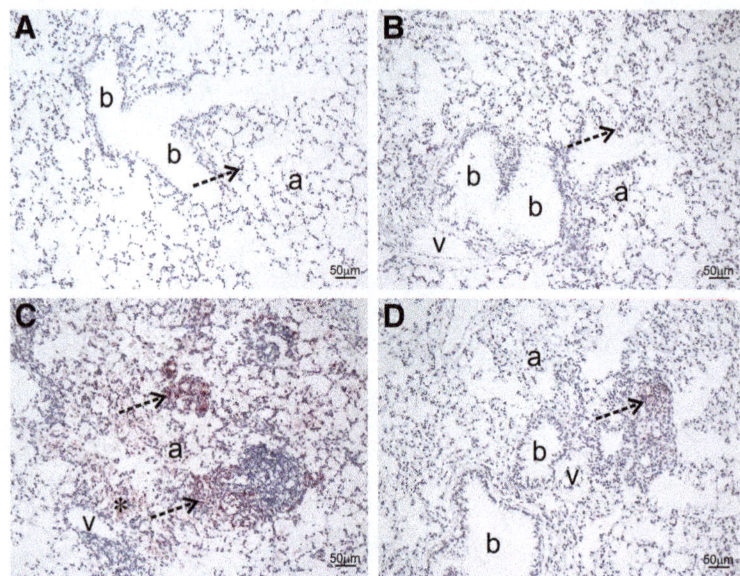

Fig. 6 Immunohistochemistry from IMP co-administration study. Mice were exposed to silica or vehicle weekly for the first four weeks, while receiving IMP or PBS by osmotic pump for entire six week duration. Light photomicrographs are lung sections immunohistochemically stained for neutrophils or inflammatory mononuclear cells (red chromogen; dashed arrows) with hematoxylin counterstain from mice treated with (**a**) vehicle, (**b**) IMP, (**c**) silica, and (**d**) silica + IMP. Mice treated with vehicle- or IMP-only had no areas of pulmonary inflammation, with only a few widely scatter neutrophils in the alveolar septa. Silica treatment resulted in conspicuous aggregates of inflammatory monocytes and neutrophils that are often associated with microgranulomas or adjacent to ectopic lymphoid tissue, as well as alveolar proteinosis (asterisk). IMP reduced this silica-associated pathology to only a small solitary aggregate of inflammatory cells. Abbreviations: a = alveolar parenchyma; b = bronchiolar airway; v = blood vessel. Tissue was observed from n ≥ 3 mice per treatment condition

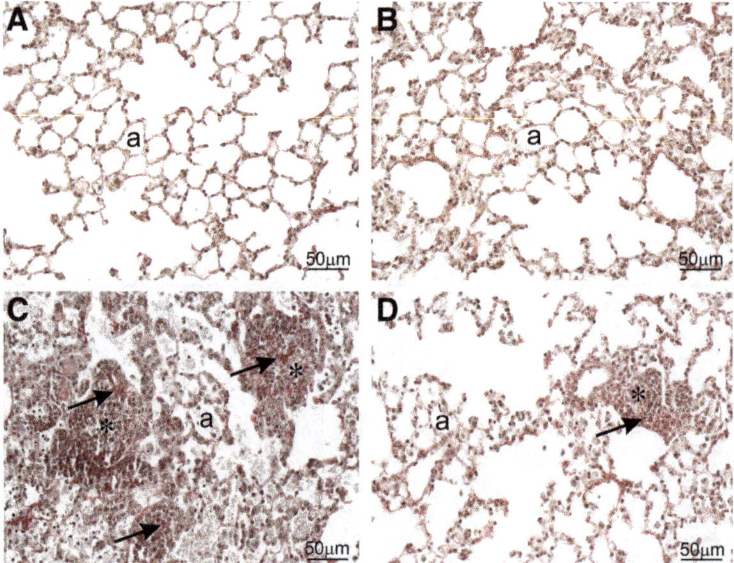

Fig. 7 Collagen staining from IMP co-administration study. Mice were exposed to silica or vehicle weekly for the first four weeks, while receiving IMP or PBS by osmotic pump for entire six week duration. Light photomicrographs are lung sections stained for increased collagen (red chromagen; arrows) with hematoxylin counterstain from mice treated with (**a**) vehicle, (**b**) IMP, (**c**) silica, and (**d**) silica + IMP. Silica treatment resulted in a mild increase in collagen associated with microgranulomas (asterisks), which was reduced by IMP. Abbreviation: a = alveolar parenchyma. Tissue was observed from n ≥ 3 mice per treatment condition

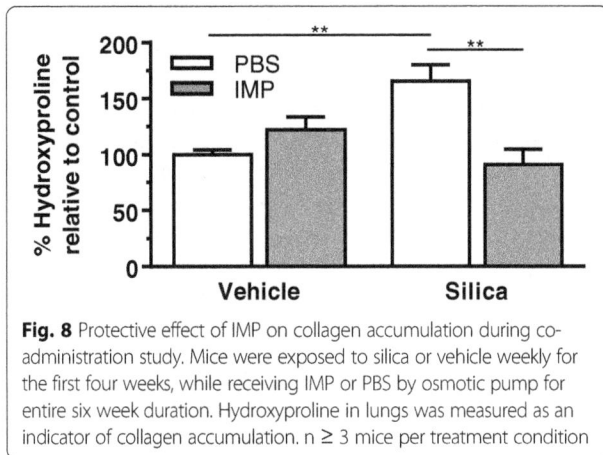

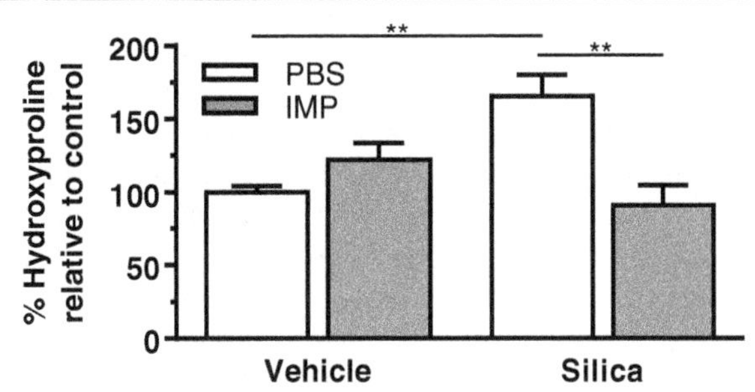

Fig. 8 Protective effect of IMP on collagen accumulation during co-administration study. Mice were exposed to silica or vehicle weekly for the first four weeks, while receiving IMP or PBS by osmotic pump for entire six week duration. Hydroxyproline in lungs was measured as an indicator of collagen accumulation. n ≥ 3 mice per treatment condition

In the silica and IMP-treated group, lung lavage protein levels were significantly lower compared to the silica and sham-treated group. This result demonstrates that IMP treatment reverses silica-induced lung injury.

Hydroxyproline content was higher in the silica and sham-treated group compared to the controls (Fig. 9b). This high hydroxyproline is an indicator of collagen deposition. Mice exposed to silica no longer had significantly increased collagen deposition when they received IMP as a therapy. Taken together, the long-term in vivo results indicated that IMP treatment, after four weeks of silica exposure, did reverse the development of silica-induced lung pathology.

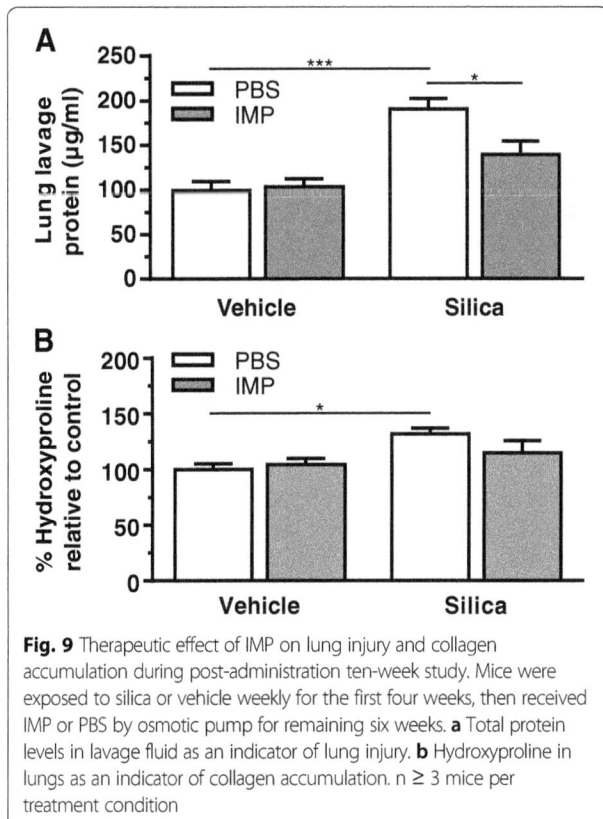

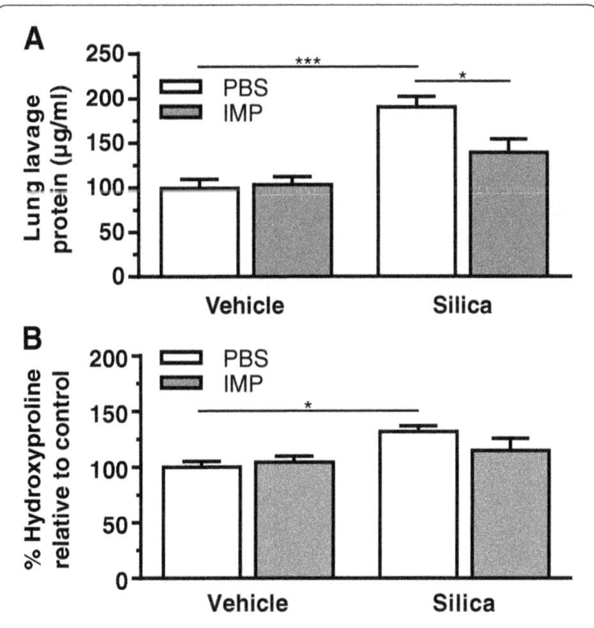

Fig. 9 Therapeutic effect of IMP on lung injury and collagen accumulation during post-administration ten-week study. Mice were exposed to silica or vehicle weekly for the first four weeks, then received IMP or PBS by osmotic pump for remaining six weeks. **a** Total protein levels in lavage fluid as an indicator of lung injury. **b** Hydroxyproline in lungs as an indicator of collagen accumulation. n ≥ 3 mice per treatment condition

Imipramine did not affect silica uptake by macrophages

The above results demonstrate the anti-inflammatory properties of IMP in silica-induced pathology. A potential explanation for this mechanism of action is that IMP inhibits silica uptake, thereby reducing the amount of silica in phagosomes and decreasing LMP. AM silica uptake was investigated by measuring the increase in side scatter using flow cytometry (Fig. 10). AM were pretreated ± IMP for 30 min and then exposed to silica for 90 min before measurement of side scatter. IMP did not affect AM silica uptake. Also, IMP did not affect phagosome maturation into an acidified phagolysosome (Additional file 1: Figure S2). Therefore, the observed IMP inhibition of inflammation and cytotoxicity was not due to an alteration of the silica uptake mechanism.

Imipramine inhibits acid sphingomyelinase (aSMase)

IMP treatment reduces phagolysosome membrane permeabilization caused by silica (Additional file 1: Figure S3). A proposed mechanism by which this occurs is through inhibition of lysosomal acid sphingomyelinase (aSMase) by IMP, leading to a change in lipid balance and stabilization of the phagolysosomal membrane. aSMase catalyzes the hydrolysis of sphingomyelin into ceramide at an acidic pH in lysosomes [33, 34]. aSMase activity was measured in AM as described in Methods. IMP significantly inhibited aSMase activity (Fig. 11), which is consistent with the literature [27, 28, 35, 36].

Discussion

Silica exposure leads to inflammation and fibrosis. Currently, there is no known therapy to reduce this pathology. Following phagocytosis by alveolar macrophages (AM), silica is contained in the phagosome, which subsequently fuses with lysosomes. Crystalline silica leads to phagolysosome membrane permeabilization (LMP) accompanied by

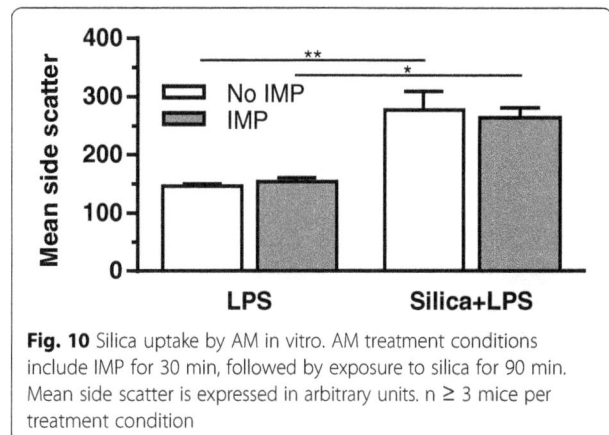

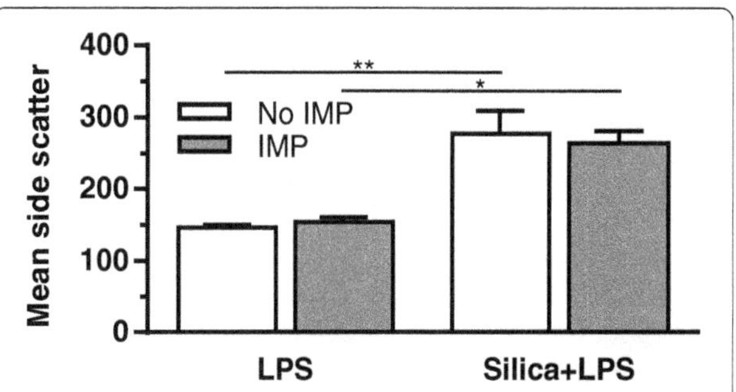

Fig. 10 Silica uptake by AM in vitro. AM treatment conditions include IMP for 30 min, followed by exposure to silica for 90 min. Mean side scatter is expressed in arbitrary units. n ≥ 3 mice per treatment condition

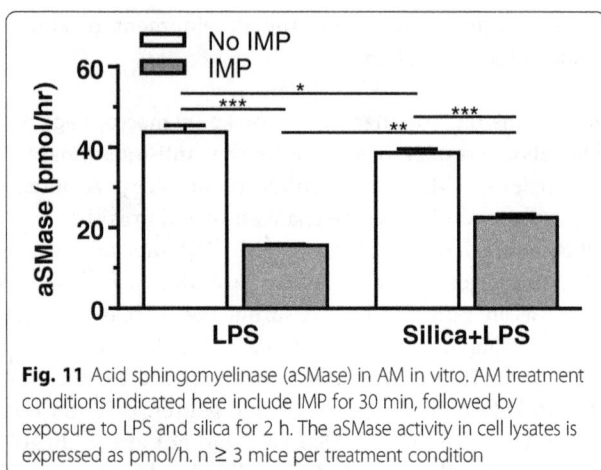

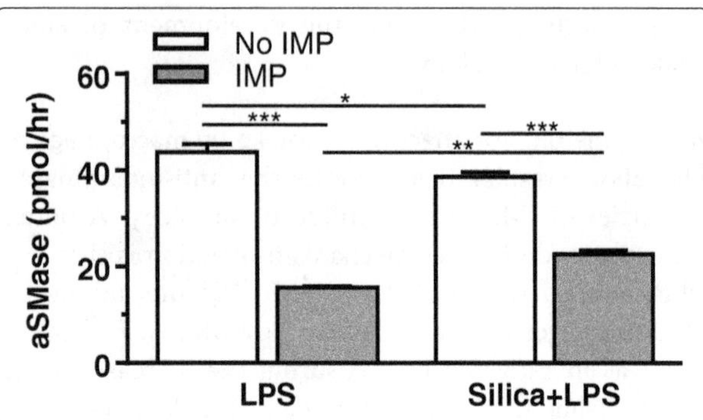

Fig. 11 Acid sphingomyelinase (aSMase) in AM in vitro. AM treatment conditions indicated here include IMP for 30 min, followed by exposure to LPS and silica for 2 h. The aSMase activity in cell lysates is expressed as pmol/h. n ≥ 3 mice per treatment condition

release of a lysosomal cathepsins and other hydrolases into the cytoplasm, which consequently leads to NLRP3 inflammasome assembly and Caspase-1 activation [17, 37]. Furthermore, LMP contributes to silica-induced cell death [12, 16]. Therefore, blocking LMP is a good candidate therapeutic target because its significant role in the onset of inflammation [11].

The focus of this study was to determine the potential of imipramine (IMP) to block LMP and inhibit the pathology following crystalline silica exposure. IMP is a lipophilic weak base that crosses the lysosomal membrane and becomes protonated within the lysosome, resulting in the drug getting trapped inside the acidic environment of the lysosome [26]. We hypothesized that IMP stabilization of the lysosome prevents silica-induced LMP, blocking consequent inflammasome activation and downstream pathology.

IMP was effective in blocking silica-induced IL-1β release and cytotoxicity of AM in vitro. Short-term in vivo studies demonstrated that IMP pretreatment resulted in significantly lower silica-induced neutrophilia and a trend indicating lower IL-1β levels. The target of IMP action was confirmed to be macrophages because AM cultured ex vivo produced significantly lower levels of IL-1β. The results from IMP pre-treatment were similar to post-treatment results, when IMP was administered after silica exposure. It was evident by these short-term studies that the anti-inflammatory effect of IMP occurs rapidly and continues for at least 24 h.

Treatment for silicosis should aim at preventing the progression of the disease, reducing inflammation, decreasing fibrosis, and improving quality of life. Repeated administration of silica over a four-week time period in a murine model has previously been shown to result in pathology similar to silicosis in humans [31, 32]. Therefore, the present study aimed to determine whether IMP has the potential to be both a protective and a therapeutic agent following long-term exposure to silica in a murine model. IMP co-administration with silica attenuated acute silicosis pathology and collagen deposition. Similarly, IMP treatment post-silica exposure attenuated collagen deposition and significantly reduced lung injury. These results suggest that IMP may be a potential therapy for treatment of chronic pulmonary inflammation.

Previous studies in our laboratory demonstrated that macrophage receptor with collagenous structure (MARCO), a class A scavenger receptor, is primarily responsible for silica uptake by AM [38]. However, further studies demonstrated that MARCO-null mice had increased lung inflammation and fibrosis, which was most likely due to decreased clearance of silica from the lung [39, 40]. This is why it was important in the present study to evaluate the influence of IMP on silica uptake. Because IMP did not affect silica uptake in AM, this suggests that the observed decrease in inflammation was not simply a result of altered silica uptake. In addition, it is likely that pathology would not be reversed upon termination of IMP treatment because the clearance is not affected.

Changes in lysosome membrane lipid composition may promote or reduce fusogenicity, and may stabilize or destabilize the membrane [41, 42]. A key regulator of this process is lysosomal acid-sphingomyelinase (aSMase). Inhibition of aSMase has been associated with reducing several pathological conditions such as inflammation, lung injury, and fibrosis [43–46]. It was observed in this study that IMP pretreatment significantly inhibited aSMase activity, which is consistent with existing literature [27, 28, 35, 36]. Inhibition of lysosomal aSMase activity by IMP can be a potential mechanism by which IMP exerts its anti-inflammatory effect.

When the ratio of ceramide to sphingomyelin is decreased due to aSMase deficiency, lysosome fusogenic activity is reduced [34, 42, 47]. Therefore, it was suspected that changes in vesicle membrane composition due to IMP treatment may disrupt cargo trafficking, such as the fusion of lysosomes with particle-containing phagosomes. If this phagosome maturation did not occur, then damaging lysosomal contents would not be present when the particle causes membrane permeabilization. However, experiments tracking the fluorescence of pH-sensitive *E. coli* BioParticles during phagocytosis demonstrated that IMP did not disrupt normal phagosome maturation (Additional file 1: Figure S2). Fluorescence slightly increased during the first 60 min, then decreased. Uptake of BioParticles that were incompletely quenched by trypan blue may be occurring early and BioParticles may begin to be degraded later, while phagosome maturation continues to quench fluorescence throughout. Regardless of the trends over time, it is clear that IMP did not alter BioParticle processing relative to untreated cells.

IMP significantly lowers silica-induced LMP (Additional file 1: Figure S3). This is consistent with literature suggesting sphingomyelin stabilizes membranes [48]. Also, studies show that IMP increases lysosomal cholesterol, likely by inhibiting cholesterol trafficking and sequestering it in the membrane as the lysosome expands in volume [49–52]. The phagolysosome membrane permeabilization assay (Additional file 1) utilized digitonin, which creates membrane pores by replacing cholesterol [53]. Higher cholesterol in lysosomes of IMP-treated cells causes them to be more sensitive to digitonin extraction, which would explain why IMP resulted in slightly higher cathepsin and NAG levels in cells that did not receive silica. Nonetheless, these effects were minor relative to the significant reduction in silica-induced LMP observed in cells treated with IMP.

Conclusions

IMP reduced lung inflammation caused by short- and long-term silica exposure in a C57Bl/6 mouse model. These effects are likely a result of IMP inhibiting lysosomal acid sphingomyelinase and stabilizing the phagolysosomal membrane, while particle uptake and phagosome maturation remain unaffected. Additional studies are needed to more fully determine the mechanism of IMP action in the context of particle-induced inflammation. IMP is a U.S Food and Drug Administration approved tricyclic antidepressant drug that could be repurposed as a protective agent for lung inflammation and subsequent disease progression.

Methods

Mice

C57Bl/6 wild type mice were housed in a specific-pathogen-free laboratory animal facility with controlled environmental conditions and a 12 h light/dark cycle. The mice were provided with ovalbumin-free food and deionized water ad libitum. Age matched (6-8 week) male and female mice were used in all studies. All animal procedures were approved by and in accordance with the Institutional Animal Care and Use Committee at the University of Montana.

Silica preparation

Crystalline silica (Min-U-Sil-5, Pennsylvania Glass Sand Corporation) was washed in 1 M HCl at 100 °C for 1 h followed by three washes with sterile water. Then, the silica was dried in an oven at 200 °C for several hrs to remove all water. Silica was determined endotoxin-free by Limulus Amebocyte Lysate assay (Cambrex, Walkersville, MD), data not shown. Immediately prior to each experiment, stock suspensions of silica (5 mg/ml) in phosphate-buffered saline (PBS) were dispersed by sonicating for 1 min at approximately 50% power in a 500 watt, 20 kHz cup-horn sonicator (Misonix XL-2020, Farmingdale, NY) attached to a Forma Scientific circulating water-bath at 4 °C. Scanning electron microscopy and light scattering techniques were used to determine characteristics of the silica suspensions, which has been previously published by our laboratory [54]. The zeta potential is −16.2 mV and the average particle diameter is approximately 1.5-2.0 μm; however, the particles have a relatively irregular shape and heterogeneous diameters.

Alveolar macrophage (AM) isolation and culture

Mice were euthanized by a lethal injection of sodium pentobarbital (Euthasol, Virbac, Fort Worth, TX) and the lungs were removed with the heart. The lungs were lavaged with 1 ml of cold PBS five times. Pooled cells were centrifuged at RCF (avg) 400 x *g* for 5 min. The lavage fluid was discarded and cells were resuspended in RPMI 1640 culture media supplemented with 10% fetal bovine serum, sodium pyruvate, and an antibiotic-antimycotic solution (Mediatech, Manassas, VA). Lytic reagent (Zap-OGLOBIN II, Beckman Coulter, Brea, CA) was added to a sample of cells prior to counting with a Z2 Coulter particle counter and size analyzer (Beckman Coulter). Cells were resuspended at 1×10^6 cells/ml and 0.1 ml/well was added to flat-bottom, tissue culture-treated 96-well plate (equivalent to approximately 3×10^5 cells/cm^2). Cells were incubated in a 37 °C water-jacketed CO_2 incubator (ThermoForma, Houston, TX). In vitro and ex vivo treatments included IMP (25 μM; Sigma, St. Louis, MO), silica (50 or 100 μg/ml) and/or lipopolysaccharide (LPS, 20 ng/ml, Sigma). This IMP dose was selected because it is used for in vitro studies with various cells [55, 56] and was effective in inhibiting aSMase in alveolar macrophages (Fig. 11). The doses of silica and LPS have been shown previously in our laboratory to stimulate an inflammatory response by alveolar macrophages in vitro [39].

In vivo treatments

Mice were exposed to 25 μl of silica in sterile PBS (1 mg/mouse) or vehicle (sterile PBS only) by oropharyngeal (OP) aspiration. Briefly, the mice were anesthetized by isoflurane inhalation and the volume was delivered into the back of the throat. By holding the tongue to the side, the solution was aspirated into the lungs. This silica concentration was selected because we have shown that it leads to inflammation and fibrosis in mice in our previous studies [31, 32, 57].

Early studies in mice often used intraperitoneal (IP) injections of IMP with doses ranging from approximately 5 to 50 mg/kg. We selected a single dose of 25 mg/kg based on more recent work relevant to our study [27, 58]. For our 24 h short-term study, mice received 100 μl of IMP (25 mg/kg IP) dissolved in sterile PBS or sham (sterile PBS alone). While IP administration is appropriate for mouse models, humans receive IMP tablets for oral administration at adult doses ranging from 50 to 300 mg/day depending on patient condition (refer to FDA label for details on specific products). These dose recommendations are for the treatment of depression; of course, additional studies are required before recommending human dosing of IMP for particle-induced inflammation.

For the six- and ten-week studies, osmotic pumps (Alzet, Cupertino, CA) were used to deliver IMP continuously over an extended period of time. Mice were anesthetized by 100 μl IP injection of a Ketamine (80 mg/kg, Putney Inc., Portland, ME) and Xylazine (12 mg/kg, AnaSed, Lloyd laboratories, Shenandoah, IA) cocktail. Skin over the implantation site was washed and shaved, then betadine was applied. An incision was made adjacent to the mid-scapular region on the back of the animal. Hemostats were then inserted into the incision and a pocket formed by opening and closing the hemostats to spread the subcutaneous tissue. The pocket was large enough to allow some free movement of the pump. The sterile pump, with PBS ± IMP, was inserted into the subcutaneous pocket with the delivery portal inserted first. The incision was then closed using vet bond (3M Animal Care Products, St Paul MN). Mice were given a dose of buprenorphine (0.05-0.10 mg/kg, subcutaneous, Reckett Benckiser Healthcare (UK) Ltd., Hull, England). Mice were monitored until they had recovered from the anesthesia.

All mice were observed daily as part of routine protocol for animal care. No overt abnormalities were reported as a result of IMP treatment.

In vivo treatment timelines

Mice for each study were randomly designated into groups based on treatment combination (PBS ± silica; IMP ± silica). Mice in short-term studies were exposed for 24 h. Some cells isolated from short-term studies were used for additional 24 h ex vivo experiments. Mice in long-term IMP co-treatment studies were exposed to silica or vehicle weekly for the first four weeks and received IMP or sham (PBS) by osmotic pump for the entire duration (six weeks total). Mice in long-term IMP post-treatment studies were exposed to silica or vehicle weekly for the first four weeks, then received IMP or sham (PBS) by osmotic pump for the remaining duration (ten weeks total).

Protein assays

Mouse IL-1β cytokine present in culture supernatants or lavage fluid was quantified using commercially available ELISA kits according to the manufacturer's protocol (R&D Systems, Minneapolis, MN) with a SpectraMax 190 plate reader (Molecular Devices, Sunnyvale, CA). A standard curve was used to calculate the protein concentration as pg/ml. In vitro experiments for assessment of IL-1β involved treatment of AM ± silica (100 μg/ml) for 24 h. Total protein in the whole lung lavage fluid was measured by Pierce bicinchoninic acid (BCA) assay, according to manufacturer protocol (ThermoFisher, Rockford, IL).

Toxicity assay

AM were treated for 24 h with silica (50 μg/ml). Cell viability was determined by MTS assay using the CellTiter[96] assay (Promega, Madison, WI) according to the manufacturer's protocol with one modification described below. This assay used a colorimetric dye read by a colorimetric plate reader (Molecular Devices). In order to avoid artifacts in the optical density values, steps were taken to remove the MTS reaction (transferring it into another plate) from the cell/particle mixture adhered to the plate bottom. The formation of bubbles was avoided and the plate was read at 490 nm. Data was transformed to a percent relative to the no particle, no IMP control cells.

Histology

The lungs from each mouse were inflation-fixed through the trachea with 4% paraformaldehyde-PBS (Electron Microscopy Sciences, Hatfield, PA) and submerged in the same fixative overnight at 4 °C. The lungs were washed with cold PBS, dehydrated with ethanol, embedded in paraffin, and sectioned on a rotary microtome at 4 μm. Hematoxylin and eosin (H&E; RAS Harris Hematoxylin and Shandon Alcohol Eosin) staining was completed using a ThermoShandon automated stainer (ThermoFisher). For immunohistochemistry and picrosirius red staining, sections were placed on charged slides and dried at 56°C overnight then deparaffinized in Xylene and hydrated through descending grades of ethanol to distilled water.

During preparation for immunohistochemistry, deparaffinized slides were placed in Tris buffered saline pH 7.4 (TBS; Scytek Labs, Logan, UT) for 5 min for pH adjustment. Following TBS, slides underwent enzyme induced epitope retrieval utilizing 0.04% pepsin (Sigma) in 0.2 N hydrochloric acid at 37°C for 20 min followed by running tap water rinse as well as several changes of distilled water. Then, standard avidin-biotin complex staining steps were performed at room temperature on a DAKO Autostainer. All staining steps are followed by two rinses in TBS + Tween 20 (Scytek). After blocking for non-specific protein with Normal Rabbit Serum (Vector Labs, Burlingame, CA) for 30 min, sections were incubated with avidin-biotin blocking system for 15 min each (Avidin D, Vector Labs; d-Biotin, Sigma). Primary antibody slides were incubated for 60 min with the monoclonal rat anti-mouse Ly-6B.2 neutrophil marker (clone 7/4; AbD Serotec, Raleigh, NC) diluted 1:2500 in Normal Antibody Diluent (NAD; Scytek). Biotinylated rabbit anti-rat IgG (H + L), mouse absorbed, at 10 μg/ml in NAD was incubated with the slide for 40 min followed by Alkaline Phosphatase Reagent (Kirkegaard & Perry Laboratories, Gaithersburg, MD) for 60 min. Reaction development utilized Vector Substrate Kit 1 (Fast Red) phosphatase chromogen for 8 min. This was followed by counterstain in Gill 2 Hematoxylin (ThermoFisher) for 15 s, differentiation, dehydration, clearing, and mounting with Permount mounting media.

Deparaffinized slides designated for picrosirius red were first stained for nuclei using Weigerts Hematoxylin for 10 min followed by distilled and running tap water rinses. Slides were incubated in 0.2% aqueous Phosphomolybdic acid for 2 min, washed in running tap and distilled water, then stained with 0.1% aqueous Picrosirius Red for 90 min. Stain was followed by several changes of distilled water, dehydration, clearing, and mounting.

Semi-quantitative multiparametric analysis of H&E-stained lung tissue sections was completed using an ordinal scale ranging from no significant pathology (score: 0) to severe pathology (score: 5). Specifically, severity categories were classified according to percentage of affected lung tissue section: less than 10% (minimal: 1), 10-25% (mild: 2), 25-50% (moderate: 3), 50-75% (marked: 4), and greater than 75% (severe: 5). Parameters were alveolar proteinosis, alveolitis (includes mixed inflammatory cell infiltrates, microgranulomas, and associated interstitial fibrosis), perivascular/peribronchiolar lymphoid aggregates, and type II alveolar epithelial cell hyperplasia.

A board-certified veterinary pathologist with expertise in respiratory pathobiology of inhaled toxicants in laboratory rodents examined the prepared lung tissue sections by light microscopy for qualitative and semi-quantitative analysis. Tissues were examined from at least three mice per treatment group, with at least three tissue sections per mouse for scoring. The pathologist had no knowledge of the exposure history of the individual mice prior to his assessment of pulmonary histopathology.

Hydroxyproline assay

Hydroxyproline is an amino acid that is a major component of collagen. The hydroxyproline assay was used to quantify collagen content, as previously described [59]. Lung lobes were excised, weighed, and immediately frozen. The lung tissues were homogenized using a tissue homogenizer (Tissue Tearor model 985,370, Biospec Products, Bartlesville, OK), in 1 ml of sterile PBS. An aliquot of lung homogenate was hydrolyzed in 12 N HCl at 110 °C for 24 h. The mixture was reacted with chloramine T and Ehrlich's reagent to produce a hydroxyproline-chromophore that was quantified by spectrophotometry at 550 nm. Hydroxyproline content was determined by triplicate analysis of the samples to provide an average value.

Particle uptake

Silica particle internalization was determined by flow cytometry using a side-scatter technique previously described [38]. Isolated AM were cultured as described above ± IMP and ± silica (50 μg/ml) for 90 min in suspension cultures using 1.5 mL microfuge tubes and end over end tumbling (Lab Quaker Shaker, ThermoForma). The cells were centrifuged and washed once in PBS. The resulting cell pellet was resuspended in PBS and transferred to filter-top flow cytometry tubes (BD Biosciences, San Jose, CA) for analysis. Data was expressed as mean side scatter for 10^4 cells.

Acid sphingomyelinase assay

Isolated AM were treated ± IMP (25 μM) for 30 min, then exposed to LPS (20 ng/ml) only, or silica (100 μg/ml) and LPS for 2 h. Cell lysates were prepared from the AM using Dounce homogenizer (tight pestle). Cell lysates were assayed for acid sphingomyelinase with commercially available kits according to the manufacturer's protocol (K-3200 Echelon Biosciences Inc., Salt Lake City, UT). Fluorescence analysis was done using a Gemini XS plate reader (Molecular Devices) at 360 nm ex and 460 nm em. Data were expressed as pmol/h of active acid sphingomyelinase.

Statistical analysis

Semi-quantitative analysis of histopathology followed scoring standards that indicate use of an ordinal rating scale, which violates assumptions of normality required by parametric statistical methods [60]. Therefore, unweighted relative effects hypotheses in this two-way factorial design were tested by calculating the ANOVA-type statistic (ATS) [61, 62] followed by nonparametric multiple comparisons by Dunn's test with p-values adjusted in contrasts of interest using the Holm-Bonferroni method. All other statistical analyses involved comparison of means using a two-way ANOVA followed by multiple comparisons using Tukey's honest significant difference (HSD) test to compensate for increased type I error. Statistical significance was defined as a probability of type I error occurring at less than 5%, and significant contrasts of predetermined interest are shown as $^{*}p < 0.05$, $^{**}p < 0.01$, and $^{***}p < 0.001$. Data is represented as the mean ± standard error of at least three independent replications for each experiment. White bars indicate no IMP treatment and gray bars indicate IMP treatment. Graphics and analyses were performed on GraphPad Prism and R statistical software, respectively.

Acknowledgements
The authors acknowledge the technical support of the Center for Environmental Health Sciences facilities: Molecular Histology and Fluorescence Imaging Core, Inhalation and Pulmonary Physiology Core, and Fluorescence Cytometry Core. We would like to thank Lou Herritt and Britten Postma for their technical help and expertise. We also thank Amy Porter for her expertise with picosirius red and 7/4 antibody staining of lung sections.

Funding
The work was supported by a research grant from NIEHS (R01ES015294), Institutional Development Award (IDeA) from NIGMS (P30GM103338), and a grant from NCRR (P20RR017670). The content is solely the responsibility of the authors and does not necessarily represent the official views of the National Institutes of Health.

Authors' contributions
RB and KLT contributed equally to the work. RB and KLT designed and conducted experiments. KLT analyzed data and prepared figs. FJ performed membrane permeability experiments included in supplemental data. JRH was responsible for evaluating the lung pathology. AH contributed to overall project design. All authors contributed to literature review, data interpretation, and manuscript preparation. All authors read and approved the final manuscript.

Competing interests
The authors declare that they have no competing interests.

Author details
[1]Center for Environmental Health Sciences, Department of Biomedical and Pharmaceutical Sciences, University of Montana, Missoula, MT 59812, USA. [2]Department of Pathobiology and Diagnostic Investigation, Michigan State University, East Lansing, MI 48824, USA.

References

1. Bang KM, Mazurek JM, Wood JM, White GE, Hendricks SA, Weston A. Silicosis mortality trends and new exposures to respirable crystalline silica - United States, 2001-2010. MMWR Morb Mortal Wkly Rep. 2015;64:117–20.
2. Crystalline silica, quartz. In: *Concise International Chemical Assessment Documents*. Geneva: World Health Organization; 2000. http://www.who.int/ipcs/publications/cicad/en/cicad24.pdf. Accessed 12 Dec 2016.
3. Health effects of occupational exposure to respirable crystalline silica. Cincinnati, OH: U.S. Department of Health and Human Services, Public Health Service, Centers for Disease Control, National Institute for Occupational Safety and Health; 2002. https://www.cdc.gov/niosh/docs/2002-129/. Accessed 12 Dec 2016.
4. Leung CC, Yu IT, Chen W. Silicosis. Lancet. 2012;379:2008–18.
5. Davis GS, Leslie KO, Hemenway DR. Silicosis in mice: effects of dose, time, and genetic strain. J Environ Pathol Toxicol Oncol. 1998;17:81–97.
6. Lakatos HF, Burgess HA, Thatcher TH, Redonnet MR, Hernady E, Williams JP, et al. Oropharyngeal aspiration of a silica suspension produces a superior model of silicosis in the mouse when compared to intratracheal instillation. Exp Lung Res. 2006;32:181–99.
7. Moore BB, Lawson WE, Oury TD, Sisson TH, Raghavendran K, Hogaboam CM. Animal models of fibrotic lung disease. Am J Respir Cell Mol Biol. 2013; 49:167–79.
8. Hiraiwa K, van Eeden SF. Contribution of lung macrophages to the inflammatory responses induced by exposure to air pollutants. Mediators Inflamm. 2013;2013:619523.
9. Kawasaki H. A mechanistic review of silica-induced inhalation toxicity. Inhal Toxicol. 2015;27:363–77.
10. Hamilton RF Jr, Thakur SA, Holian A. Silica binding and toxicity in alveolar macrophages. Free Radic Biol Med. 2008;44:1246–58.
11. Hornung V, Bauernfeind F, Halle A, Samstad EO, Kono H, Rock KL, et al. Silica crystals and aluminum salts activate the NALP3 inflammasome through phagosomal destabilization. Nat Immunol. 2008;9:847–56.
12. Aits S, Jaattela M. Lysosomal cell death at a glance. J Cell Sci. 2013;126:1905–12.
13. Boya P, Kroemer G. Lysosomal membrane permeabilization in cell death. Oncogene. 2008;27:6434–51.
14. Cesen MH, Pegan K, Spes A, Turk B. Lysosomal pathways to cell death and their therapeutic applications. Exp Cell Res. 2012;318:1245–51.
15. Johansson AC, Appelqvist H, Nilsson C, Kagedal K, Roberg K, Ollinger K. Regulation of apoptosis-associated lysosomal membrane permeabilization. Apoptosis. 2010;15:527–40.
16. Thibodeau MS, Giardina C, Knecht DA, Helble J, Hubbard AK. Silica-induced apoptosis in mouse alveolar macrophages is initiated by lysosomal enzyme activity. Toxicol Sci. 2004;80:34–48.
17. Bunderson-Schelvan M, Hamilton RF, Trout KL, Jessop F, Gulumian M, Holian A. Approaching a unified theory for particle-induced inflammation. In: Otsuki T, Yoshioka Y, Holian A, editors. Biological effects of fibrous and particulate substances. Tokyo: Springer Japan; 2016. p. 51–76.
18. Lamkanfi M, Dixit VM. Inflammasomes and their roles in health and disease. Annu Rev Cell Dev Biol. 2012;28:137–61.
19. Lamkanfi M, Dixit VM. Mechanisms and functions of inflammasomes. Cell. 2014;157:1013–22.
20. Latz E, Xiao TS, Stutz A. Activation and regulation of the inflammasomes. Nat Rev Immunol. 2013;13:397–411.
21. Schroder K, Tschopp J. The inflammasomes. Cell. 2010;140:821–32.
22. Strowig T, Henao-Mejia J, Elinav E, Flavell R. Inflammasomes in health and disease. Nature. 2012;481:278–86.
23. Jessop F, Holian A. Extracellular HMGB1 regulates multi-walled carbon nanotube-induced inflammation in vivo. Nanotoxicology. 2015;9:365–72.
24. Cassel SL, Eisenbarth SC, Iyer SS, Sadler JJ, Colegio OR, Tephly LA, et al. The Nalp3 inflammasome is essential for the development of silicosis. Proc Natl Acad Sci U S A. 2008;105:9035–40.
25. Pedra JH, Cassel SL, Sutterwala FS. Sensing pathogens and danger signals by the inflammasome. Curr Opin Immunol. 2009;21:10–6.
26. MacIntyre AC, Cutler DJ. The potential role of lysosomes in tissue distribution of weak bases. Biopharm Drug Dispos. 1988;9:513–26.
27. Yang J, Qu JM, Summah H, Zhang J, Zhu YG, Jiang HN. Protective effects of imipramine in murine endotoxin-induced acute lung injury. Eur J Pharmacol. 2010;638:128–33.
28. von Bismarck P, Wistadt CF, Klemm K, Winoto-Morbach S, Uhlig U, Schutze S, et al. Improved pulmonary function by acid sphingomyelinase inhibition in a newborn piglet lavage model. Am J Respir Crit Care Med. 2008;177:1233–41.
29. Hamilton RF, Buckingham S, Holian A. The effect of size on Ag nanosphere toxicity in macrophage cell models and lung epithelial cell lines is dependent on particle dissolution. Int J Mol Sci. 2014;15:6815–30.
30. Xia T, Hamilton RF, Bonner JC, Crandall ED, Elder A, Fazlollahi F, et al. Interlaboratory evaluation of in vitro cytotoxicity and inflammatory responses to engineered nanomaterials: the NIEHS Nano GO consortium. Environ Health Perspect. 2013;121:683–90.
31. Beamer CA, Migliaccio CT, Jessop F, Trapkus M, Yuan D, Holian A. Innate immune processes are sufficient for driving silicosis in mice. J Leukoc Biol. 2010;88:547–57.
32. Jessop F, Hamilton RF, Rhoderick JF, Shaw PK, Holian A. Autophagy deficiency in macrophages enhances NLRP3 inflammasome activity and chronic lung disease following silica exposure. Toxicol Appl Pharmacol. 2016;309:101–10.
33. Huang YL, Huang WP, Lee H. Roles of sphingosine 1-phosphate on tumorigenesis. World J Biol Chem. 2011;2:25–34.
34. Kirkegaard T, Roth AG, Petersen NHT, Mahalka AK, Olsen OD, Moilanen I, et al. Hsp70 stabilizes lysosomes and reverts Niemann–Pick disease-associated lysosomal pathology. Nature. 2010;463:549–53.
35. Beckmann N, Sharma D, Gulbins E, Becker KA, Edelmann B. Inhibition of acid sphingomyelinase by tricyclic antidepressants and analogons. Front Physiol. 2014;5:331.
36. Goggel R, Winoto-Morbach S, Vielhaber G, Imai Y, Lindner K, Brade L, et al. PAF-mediated pulmonary edema: a new role for acid sphingomyelinase and ceramide. Nat Med. 2004;10:155–60.

37. Hentze H, Lin XY, Choi MS, Porter AG. Critical role for cathepsin B in mediating caspase-1-dependent interleukin-18 maturation and caspase-1-independent necrosis triggered by the microbial toxin nigericin. Cell Death Differ. 2003;10:956–68.
38. Hamilton RF Jr, Thakur SA, Mayfair JK, Holian A. MARCO mediates silica uptake and toxicity in alveolar macrophages from C57BL/6 mice. J Biol Chem. 2006;281:34218–26.
39. Biswas R, Hamilton RF, Holian A. Role of lysosomes in silica-induced inflammasome activation and inflammation in absence of MARCO. J Immunol Res. 2014;2014:304180.
40. Thakur SA, Beamer CA, Migliaccio CT, Holian A. Critical role of MARCO in crystalline silica-induced pulmonary inflammation. Toxicol Sci. 2009;108:462–71.
41. Appelqvist H, Waster P, Kagedal K, Ollinger K. The lysosome: from waste bag to potential therapeutic target. J Mol Cell Biol. 2013;5:214–26.
42. Utermöhlen O, Herz J, Schramm M, Krönke M. Fusogenicity of membranes: the impact of acid sphingomyelinase on innate immune responses. Immunobiology. 2008;213:307–14.
43. Canals D, Perry DM, Jenkins RW, Hannun YA. Drug targeting of sphingolipid metabolism: sphingomyelinases and ceramidases. Br J Pharmacol. 2011;163:694–712.
44. Dhami R, He X, Schuchman EH. Acid sphingomyelinase deficiency attenuates bleomycin-induced lung inflammation and fibrosis in mice. Cell Physiol Biochem. 2010;26:749–60.
45. Kornhuber J, Tripal P, Reichel M, Muhle C, Rhein C, Muehlbacher M, et al. Functional Inhibitors of Acid Sphingomyelinase (FIASMAs): a novel pharmacological group of drugs with broad clinical applications. Cell Physiol Biochem. 2010;26:9–20.
46. Sakata A, Ochiai T, Shimeno H, Hikishima S, Yokomatsu T, Shibuya S, et al. Acid sphingomyelinase inhibition suppresses lipopolysaccharide-mediated release of inflammatory cytokines from macrophages and protects against disease pathology in dextran sulphate sodium-induced colitis in mice. Immunology. 2007;122:54–64.
47. Schramm M, Herz J, Haas A, Kronke M, Utermohlen O. Acid sphingomyelinase is required for efficient phago-lysosomal fusion. Cell Microbiol. 2008;10:1839–53.
48. Caruso JA, Mathieu PA, Reiners JJ Jr. Sphingomyelins suppress the targeted disruption of lysosomes/endosomes by the photosensitizer NPe6 during photodynamic therapy. Biochem J. 2005;392:325–34.
49. Funk RS, Krise JP. Cationic amphiphilic drugs cause a marked expansion of apparent lysosomal volume: implications for an intracellular distribution-based drug interaction. Mol Pharm. 2012;9:1384–95.
50. Lange Y, Ye J, Steck TL. Circulation of cholesterol between lysosomes and the plasma membrane. J Biol Chem. 1998;273:18915–22.
51. Reiners JJ Jr, Kleinman M, Kessel D, Mathieu PA, Caruso JA. Nonesterified cholesterol content of lysosomes modulates susceptibility to oxidant-induced permeabilization. Free Radic Biol Med. 2011;50:281–94.
52. Roff CF, Goldin E, Comly ME, Cooney A, Brown A, Vanier MT, et al. Type C Niemann-Pick disease: use of hydrophobic amines to study defective cholesterol transport. Dev Neurosci. 1991;13:315–9.
53. Aits S, Jaattela M, Nylandsted J. Methods for the quantification of lysosomal membrane permeabilization: a hallmark of lysosomal cell death. Methods Cell Biol. 2015;126:261–85.
54. Thakur SA, Hamilton R Jr, Pikkarainen T, Holian A. Differential binding of inorganic particles to MARCO. Toxicol Sci. 2009;107:238–46.
55. Miller ME, Adhikary S, Kolokoltsov AA, Davey RA. Ebolavirus requires acid sphingomyelinase activity and plasma membrane sphingomyelin for infection. J Virol. 2012;86:7473–83.
56. Moles A, Tarrats N, Morales A, Dominguez M, Bataller R, Caballeria J, et al. Acidic sphingomyelinase controls hepatic stellate cell activation and in vivo liver fibrogenesis. Am J Pathol. 2010;177:1214–24.
57. Jessop F, Hamilton RF Jr, Rhoderick JF, Fletcher P, Holian A. Phagolysosome acidification is required for silica and engineered nanoparticle-induced lysosome membrane permeabilization and resultant NLRP3 inflammasome activity. Toxicol Appl Pharmacol. 2017;318:58–68.
58. Llacuna L, Mari M, Garcia-Ruiz C, Fernandez-Checa JC, Morales A. Critical role of acidic sphingomyelinase in murine hepatic ischemia-reperfusion injury. Hepatology. 2006;44:561–72.
59. Migliaccio CT, Buford MC, Jessop F, Holian A. The IL-4Ralpha pathway in macrophages and its potential role in silica-induced pulmonary fibrosis. J Leukoc Biol. 2008;83:630–9.
60. Gibson-Corley KN, Olivier AK, Meyerholz DK. Principles for valid histopathologic scoring in research. Vet Pathol. 2013;50:1007–15.
61. Shah DA, Madden LV. Nonparametric analysis of ordinal data in designed factorial experiments. Phytopathology. 2004;94:33–43.
62. Brunner E, Konietschke F, Pauly M, Puri ML. Rank-based procedures in factorial designs: hypotheses about non-parametric treatment effects. J R Stat Soc Series B Stat Methodol. 2016; doi:10.1111/rssb.12222.

Chronic pulmonary exposure to traffic-related fine particulate matter causes brain impairment in adult rats

Chi-Hsiang Shih[1], Jen-Kun Chen[2], Li-Wei Kuo[2], Kuan-Hung Cho[2], Ta-Chih Hsiao[3], Zhe-Wei Lin[1], Yi-Syuan Lin[1], Jiunn-Horng Kang[4,5], Yu-Chun Lo[6], Kai-Jen Chuang[7,8], Tsun-Jen Cheng[9] and Hsiao-Chi Chuang[1,7,10*]

Abstract

Background: Effects of air pollution on neurotoxicity and behavioral alterations have been reported. The objective of this study was to investigate the pathophysiology caused by particulate matter (PM) in the brain. We examined the effects of traffic-related particulate matter with an aerodynamic diameter of < 1 μm (PM_1), high-efficiency particulate air (HEPA)-filtered air, and clean air on the brain structure, behavioral changes, brainwaves, and bioreactivity of the brain (cortex, cerebellum, and hippocampus), olfactory bulb, and serum after 3 and 6 months of whole-body exposure in 6-month-old Sprague Dawley rats.

Results: The rats were exposed to 16.3 ± 8.2 (4.7~ 68.8) μg/m^3 of PM_1 during the study period. An MRI analysis showed that whole-brain and hippocampal volumes increased with 3 and 6 months of PM_1 exposure. A short-term memory deficiency occurred with 3 months of exposure to PM_1 as determined by a novel object recognition (NOR) task, but there were no significant changes in motor functions. There were no changes in frequency bands or multiscale entropy of brainwaves. Exposure to 3 months of PM_1 increased 8-isoporstance in the cortex, cerebellum, and hippocampus as well as hippocampal inflammation (interleukin (IL)-6), but not in the olfactory bulb. Systemic CCL11 (at 3 and 6 months) and IL-4 (at 6 months) increased after PM_1 exposure. Light chain 3 (LC3) expression increased in the hippocampus after 6 months of exposure. Spongiosis and neuronal shrinkage were observed in the cortex, cerebellum, and hippocampus (neuronal shrinkage) after exposure to air pollution. Additionally, microabscesses were observed in the cortex after 6 months of PM_1 exposure.

Conclusions: Our study first observed cerebral edema and brain impairment in adult rats after chronic exposure to traffic-related air pollution.

Keywords: Air pollution, Inflammation, Memonry deficiency, Neurotoxicity, Oxidative stress

Background

Pulmonary exposure to air pollution was reported to cause central nervous system (CNS) toxicity and is associated with a risk of neurological diseases. For example, observations from the U.S. Department of Veterans Affairs Normative Aging Study cohort showed associations of traffic-related pollution and black carbon (BC) with cognition function [1]. They observed an association between traffic-related air pollution and deficiencies in cognitive function in older men. Exposure of high levels of coarse particulate matter ($PM_{2.5-10}$) and fine particulate matter ($PM_{2.5}$) was associated with faster cognitive decline as reported by the Nurses' Health Study Cognitive Cohort in the US [2]. Furthermore, $PM_{2.5}$-exposure was associated with an increase in hospital admission in patients with dementia and Parkinson's disease (PD) in 50 northeastern US cities [3]. Based on these epidemiological reports, pulmonary exposure to air pollution could result in the development of neurological disease. However, the effects of air pollution on neurotoxicity remain unclear.

* Correspondence: r92841005@ntu.edu.tw; chuanghc@tmu.edu.tw
[1]School of Respiratory Therapy, College of Medicine, Taipei Medical University, Taipei, Taiwan
[7]School of Public Health, College of Public Health, Taipei Medical University, Taipei, Taiwan
Full list of author information is available at the end of the article

Toxicological evidence has confirmed the epidemiological associations between neurotoxicity and particulate air pollution. Neuroinflammation is considered to be an important biological response to PM exposure. Pro-inflammatory cytokines such as tumor necrosis factor alpha (TNF-α) and interleukin-1 alpha (IL-1α) were increased in brain after PM exposure [4, 5]. Alteration in IL-6 expression was also observed in the hippocampus after PM exposure [6]. Generally, inflammatory responses in the lungs due to particulate air pollution are known to result in adverse cardiopulmonary health effects [7]; however, brain inflammation occurring due to air pollution is still poorly understood. Inflammation is defined as a non-specific protective response, which is believed to be a critical step in removing injurious stimuli and initiating the healing process. Furthermore, oxidative stress is recognized as a pathogenic mechanism of neurodegenerative diseases. The physicochemistry of PM is an important determinant in regulating PM bioreactivity. Inhaled ultrafine PM (< 100 μm) causes oxidative-inflammatory reactions at sites of deposition [8]. Therefore, exposure to PM may increase oxidative stress and cerebral vascular injury, leading to systemic and local effects in different brain regions [9].

Long-term exposure to air pollutants may cause neurological effects in susceptible groups. Also, the overall risk of neurological disease attributable to air pollution might be considerably higher than previously thought [10]. However, the pathways of PM-induced neurotoxicity remain unclear. A previous study showed that magnetite PM of < 200 nm in diameter was observed in the human brain [11], which demonstrated direct evidence of lung-to-brain effects of PM. Currently, there are three hypothesized pathways of PM's effects on the brain. First, the olfactory bulb is considered to be one route by which inhaled PM can be directly translocated into the brain [11]. Second, smaller PM can directly cross the blood-brain barrier (BBB), which is responsible for keeping harmful particles and chemicals out of the brain [12, 13]. Third, PM directly/indirectly damages barriers, such as the BBB and nasal epithelium [14]. Repeated injury of these barriers is able to impair their integrity, leading to PM and others (e.g. neurotoxic plasma-derived components, cells, and pathogens) crossing the barriers and entering the brain. Additionally, inhaled PM associated with emphysema formation [15] and oxygen desaturation [16, 17], which could lead to hypoxia development. The impairment of oxygen and nutrient supply system may result in brain function alteration. Therefore, exploring the brain pathophysiology that occurs with exposure of PM is urgently needed. The objective of this study was to investigate the effects of particulate air pollution on the brain. Adult Sprague-Dawley (SD) rats were whole-body exposed to traffic-related PM_1 (< 1 μm) for 3 and 6 months, followed by a magnetic resonance imaging (MRI) analysis, behavioral observations, and a brainwave analysis. The particle size distribution, PM_1 mass concentration, particle number concentration, lung deposition surface area (LDSA) concentration, and BC mass concentration were continuously monitored during the study period. Bioreactivity was determined in brain sections (cortex, cerebellum, and hippocampus), the olfactory bulb, and serum.

Results

Exposure to particulate air pollution

The exposure system and experimental design is shown in Fig. 1. Rats were continuously exposed to 24 weeks (6 months) of traffic-related PM_1 during the study period. Daily distributions of the geometric mean diameter (GMD), PM_1 mass concentration, LDSA in the alveolar region, BC, and particle number concentration (PNC) are shown in Fig. 2. The mean value ± SD (min~max) of the GMD over the entire observation period was 55.8 ± 7.3 (40.3~ 74.5) nm. Results showed that most of the particles to which the rats were exposed were in ultrafine size fractions (< 100 nm). We observed that the PM_1 mass concentration was 16.3 ± 8.2 (4.7~ 68.8) $\mu g/m^3$, and the LDSA in the alveolar region was 55.1 ± 21.7 (20.7~ 136.6) $\mu m^2/cm^3$. The BC mass concentration was 1800 ± 784 (219~ 4732) ng/m^3, and the PNC was 11,257 ± 4388 (2218~ 25,733) $\#/m^3$.

Brain volume

To understand the effect of chronic pulmonary exposure to traffic-related PM_1 on the rat brain, we first examined alterations in body weight after 3 and 6 months of exposure. Body weights of rats after exposure to PM_1 are shown in Additional file 1: Figure S1. We observed that the rats in the HEPA and PM_1 groups had significant decreases in body weight after 3 and 6 months of exposure compared to the control group ($p < 0.05$). Next, we analyzed brain images of the control, HEPA, and PM groups by MRI. Brain MRI images were used to calculate the volumes of the whole brain and hippocampus in the control, HEPA, and PM_1 groups as shown in Fig. 3. Although the body weight was significantly lower in rats in the HEPA and PM_1 groups, we observed that the whole brain volume (nm^3) of 3-month PM_1-exposed rats was significantly larger than those of the control and HEPA rats ($p < 0.05$), but there were no significant differences in hippocampal volumes (nm^3) among the control, HEPA, and PM groups. Notably, whole-brain and hippocampal volumes in rats of the HEPA and PM_1 groups were significantly larger than those of control rats at 6 months of exposure ($p < 0.05$). The ratio of the hippocampal volume to whole brain volume (vol%) was next investigated (Fig. 3). We observed that the ratio of the hippocampal to total brain volume (vol%) was slightly lower in the PM_1 group than in the control group after

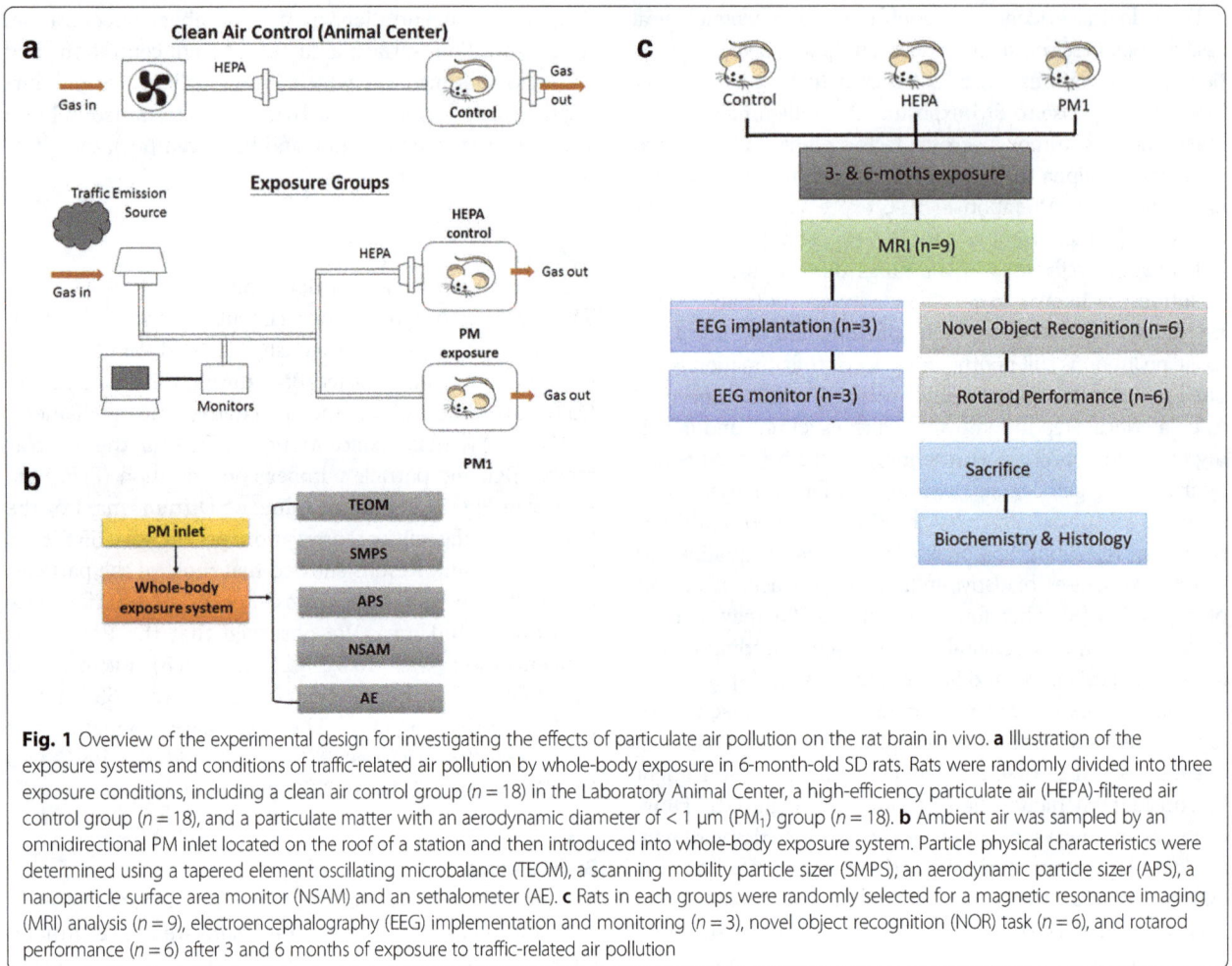

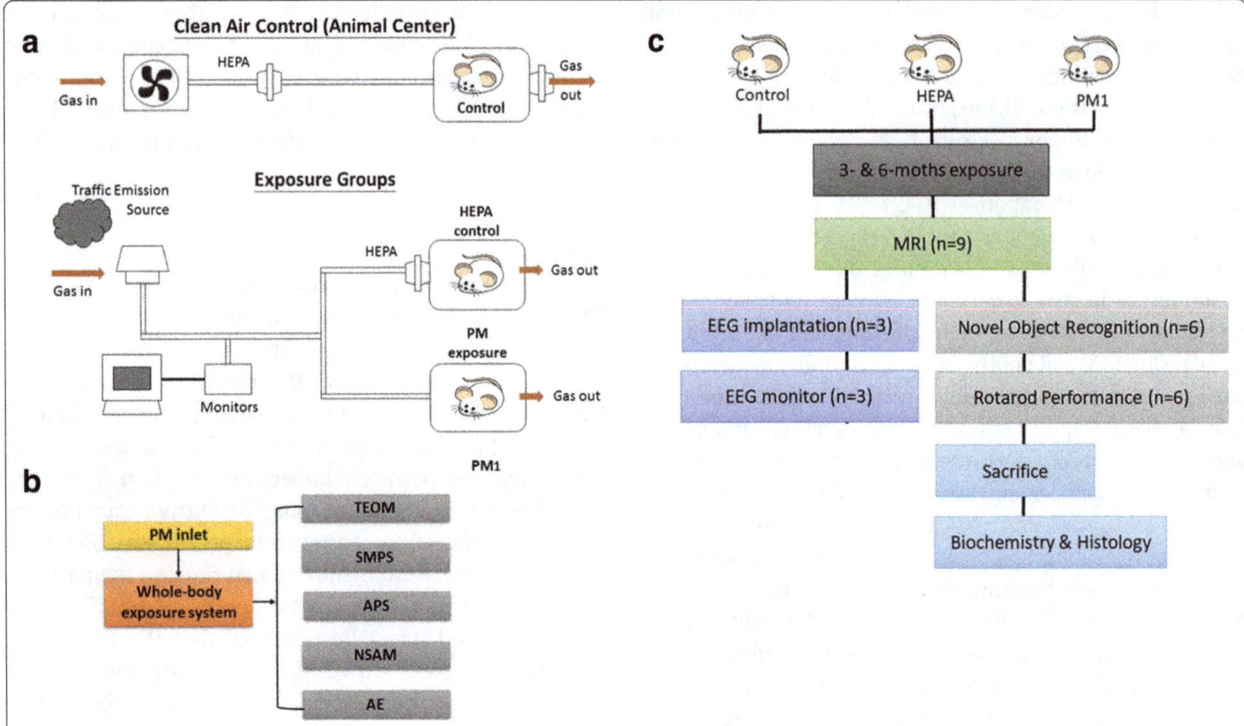

Fig. 1 Overview of the experimental design for investigating the effects of particulate air pollution on the rat brain in vivo. **a** Illustration of the exposure systems and conditions of traffic-related air pollution by whole-body exposure in 6-month-old SD rats. Rats were randomly divided into three exposure conditions, including a clean air control group ($n = 18$) in the Laboratory Animal Center, a high-efficiency particulate air (HEPA)-filtered air control group ($n = 18$), and a particulate matter with an aerodynamic diameter of < 1 μm (PM_1) group ($n = 18$). **b** Ambient air was sampled by an omnidirectional PM inlet located on the roof of a station and then introduced into whole-body exposure system. Particle physical characteristics were determined using a tapered element oscillating microbalance (TEOM), a scanning mobility particle sizer (SMPS), an aerodynamic particle sizer (APS), a nanoparticle surface area monitor (NSAM) and an sethalometer (AE). **c** Rats in each groups were randomly selected for a magnetic resonance imaging (MRI) analysis ($n = 9$), electroencephalography (EEG) implementation and monitoring ($n = 3$), novel object recognition (NOR) task ($n = 6$), and rotarod performance ($n = 6$) after 3 and 6 months of exposure to traffic-related air pollution

3 months of exposure, but lower levels were not observed after 6 months of exposure.

Behavior

Behavioral observations included the NOR test and rotarod performance test, and results are shown in Fig. 4. There were no significant changes in the number of sample objective visits by the control, HEPA, and PM_1 groups after 3 and 6 months of exposure. However, we observed that rats in the PM_1 group had significant fewer novel objective visits after 3 months of exposure compared to the control and HEPA groups ($p < 0.05$). Similarly, after 3 months of exposure to PM_1, rats had a significantly lower recognition index compared to the control ($p < 0.05$). Also, values of the recognition index after 3 and 6 months of exposure to PM_1 were close to the bottom levels (0.50) of recognition memory. We next examined motor function using a rotarod performance test, but there were no significant differences among the control, HEPA, and PM_1 groups after 3 and 6 months of exposure.

Brainwaves

EEG characteristics were analyzed as shown in Fig. 5. The relative power and absolutely power of rats in the control, HEPA, and PM_1 groups after 3 and 6 months of exposure were calculated. There were no significant differences in the four frequency bands (delta, theta, alpha, and beta) of the relative power and absolute power among the control, HEPA, and PM_1 groups after 3 and 6 months of exposure. We further examined the MSE in rats, which showed no significant differences among the control, HEPA, and PM_1 groups after 3 and 6 months of exposure.

Biochemistry

Figure 6 shows biological effects on the brain, olfactory bulb, and serum of rats in the control, HEPA, and PM_1 groups after 3 and 6 months of exposure. First, three sections of the brain were collected, including the cortex, cerebellum, and hippocampus, for 8-isoprostane and IL-6 determinations. We observed that PM_1 exposure significantly increased levels of 8-isoprostane in the cortex ($p < 0.05$; compared to the control and HEPA groups), cerebellum ($p < 0.05$; compared

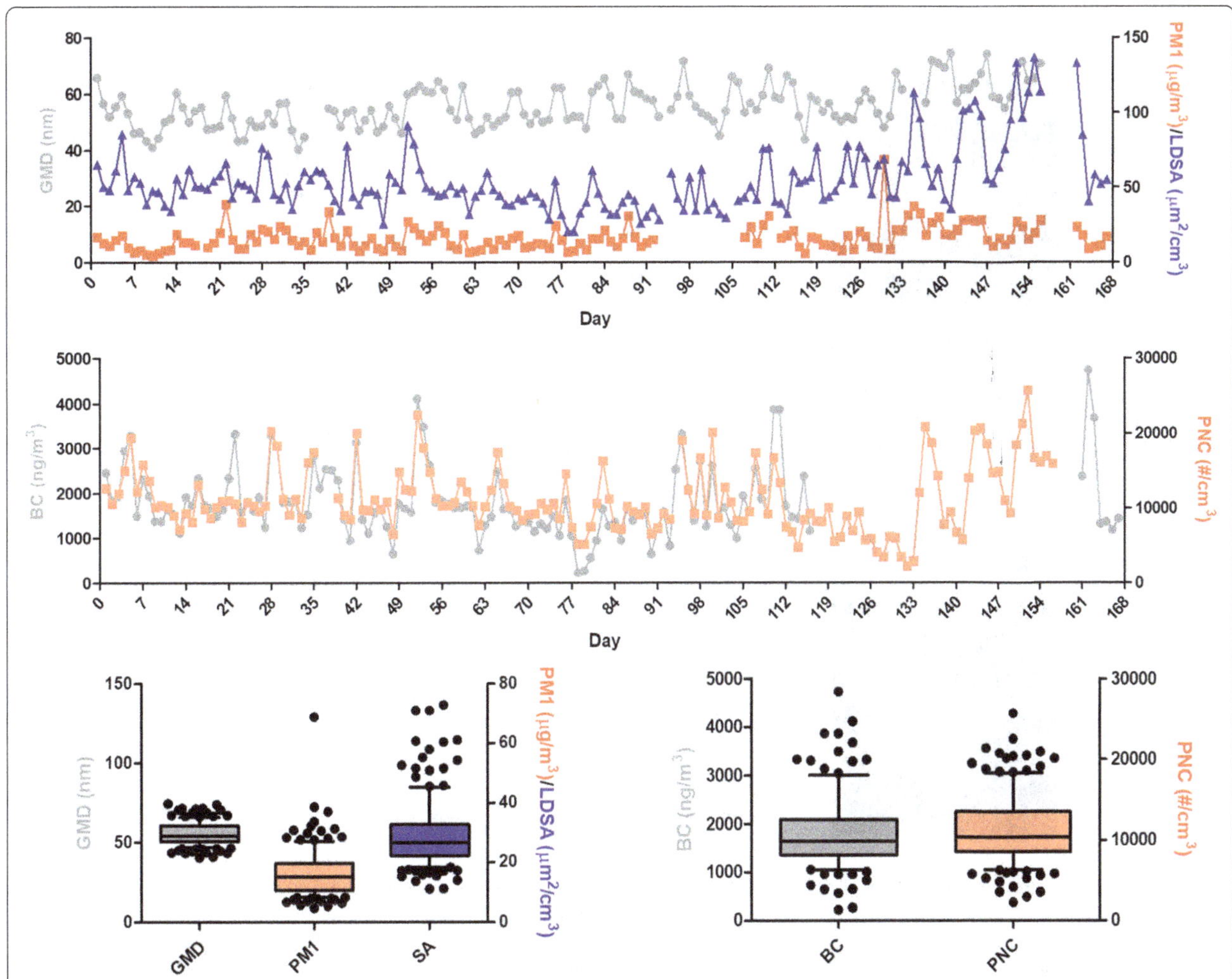

Fig. 2 Measurement of whole-body exposure to particulate air pollution in rats during the study period. Daily distributions of the geometric mean diameter (GMD), particulate matter with an aerodynamic diameter of < 1 μm (PM_1) mass concentration, and lung deposition surface area (LDSA) in the alveolar region concentration, black carbon (BC), and particle number concentration (PNC) during the study period were determined. Characteristics of the traffic-related particles were as follows: the GMD was 55.8 nm; the PM_1 mass concentration was 16.3 μg/m^3; the LDSA was 55.1 μm^2/cm^3; the BC was 1800 ng/m^3; and the PNC was 11257 μg/m^3

to the control group), and hippocampus ($p < 0.05$; compared to the control and HEPA groups) after 3 months of exposure (Fig. 6a). However, differences in the three brain sections were not observed after 6 months of exposure. We observed that IL-6 levels in the hippocampus were significantly increased by 3 months of exposure to PM_1 compared to the control and HEPA groups ($p < 0.05$; Fig. 6a), but a similar situation was not observed in the cortex or cerebellum. Similar to 8-isoprostane, we did not observe significant differences in IL-6 in the cortex, cerebellum, and hippocampus after 6 months of exposure. Next, we observed 8-isoprostane, IL-6 and LDH levels in the olfactory bulb of rats of the control, HEPA, and PM_1 groups after 3 and 6 months of exposure (Fig. 6b). There were no significant alterations in 8-isoprostane, IL-6, or LDH levels in the olfactory bulb in rats among the groups after exposure. We then examined levels of CCL5, CCL11, IL-4, and IL-6 in serum among the three groups after 3 and 6 months of exposure (Fig. 6c). Serum levels of CCL11 were significantly high after 3 and 6 months of exposure to PM_1 compared to control rats ($p < 0.05$), whereas CCL11 was significantly higher after 6 months of exposure to HEPA air compared to control rats ($p < 0.05$). We also observed that serum IL-4 was significantly higher after 6 months of exposure to PM_1 compared to controls rats ($p < 0.05$). There were no significant alterations in serum CCL5 of IL-6 among the three groups after exposure.

LC3II/I and total tau expressions

Expressions of LC3II/I and total tau proteins in the cortex, cerebellum, and hippocampus of rats in the control, HEPA, and PM_1 groups after 3 and 6 months of exposure are shown in Fig. 7. We observed that the LC3II/I ratio was significantly higher after 6 months of exposure

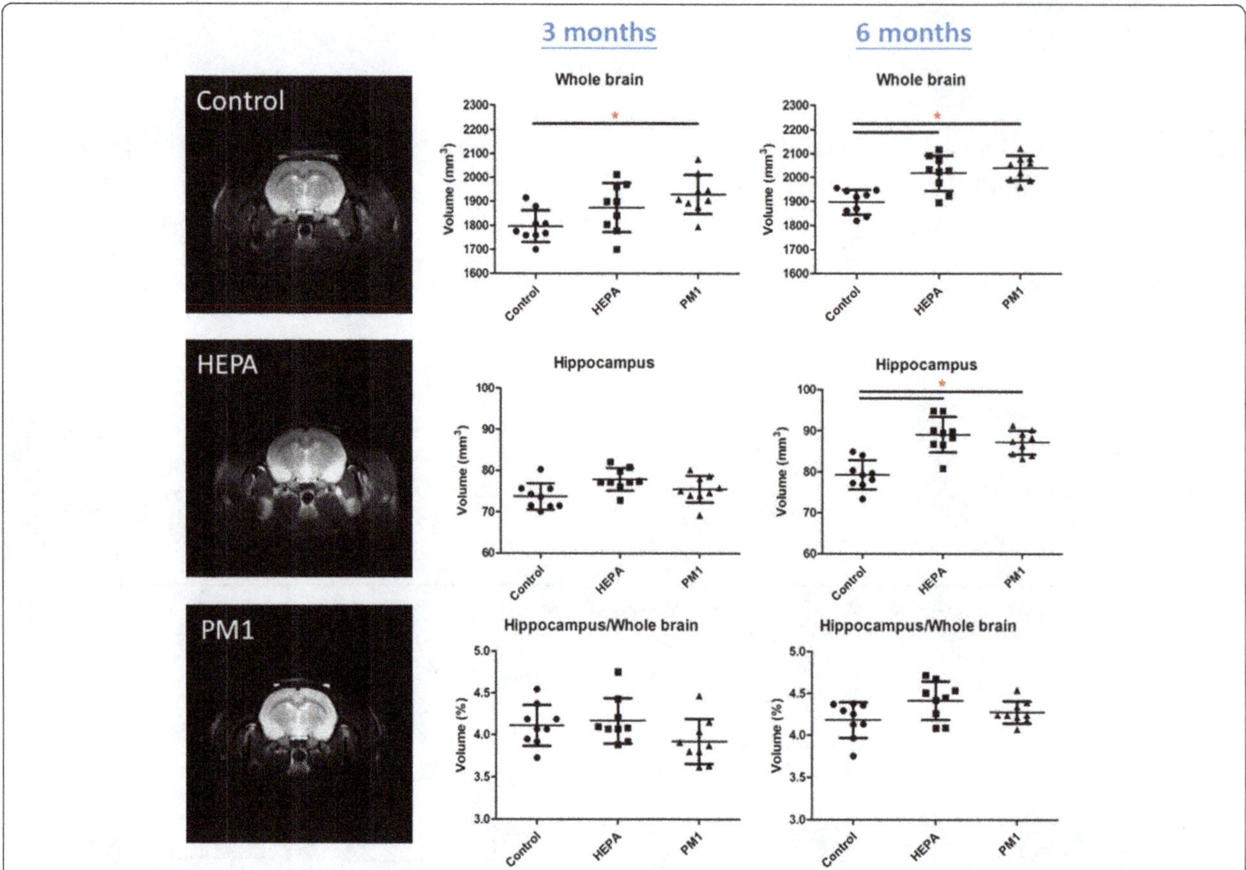

Fig. 3 Magnetic resonance imaging (MRI) analysis of rat brains in the control, high-efficiency particulate air (HEPA), and particulate matter with an aerodynamic diameter of < 1 μm (PM_1) groups ($n = 9$). The whole brain volume, hippocampal volume, and hippocampus to whole brain volume (%) were measured after 3 and 6 months of exposure. Whole brain volumes (nm^3) of rats exposed to PM_1 for 3 months and to HEPA and PM_1 for 6 months were significantly larger than those of the control. Hippocampal brain volumes (nm^3) of rats exposed to HEPA and PM_1 for 6 months were significantly larger than those of the control. * $p < 0.05$

to PM_1 compared to the control ($p < 0.05$). This observation was also confirmed by IHC images. We observed that LC3 expression was significant higher in the hippocampus after PM_1 exposure (6 months; Fig. 8). However, we did not observe a significant difference in the LC3II/I ratio in the cortex or cerebellum among the three groups after exposure, as confirmed by the IHC analysis. There were no significant alterations in tau in the cortex, cerebellum, or hippocampus after 3 and 6 months of exposure. We also did not observe any changes in tau expression by the IHC analysis.

Histology

Figure 9 shows histological changes in the cortex, cerebellum, and hippocampus of rats in the control, HEPA, and PM_1 groups after 3 and 6 months of exposure. We observed that PM_1 caused periventricular spongiosis in the cortex after 3 months of exposure. Neuronal shrinkage in the cortex was also observed after 3 months of HEPA and PM_1 exposure. Increased spongiosis in the superficial molecular layer of the cortex was observed after 6 months of HEPA exposure (as shown in Fig. 9). We also observed neuronal shrinkage in the cortex after 6 months of exposure to PM_1. Notably, microabscesses were identified in the cortex after 6 months of PM_1 exposure (as shown in Fig. 9). Spongiosis in the medulla was observed in the HEPA and PM_1 groups after 6 months of exposure. Hippocampal neuronal shrinkage was observed after 6 months of exposure to HEPA and PM_1 (as shown in Fig. 9).

Discussion

Epidemiological reports indicated that exposure to air pollution is associated with neuropathologies that can instigate neurological disease. However, the pathophysiology of the brain that occurs due to particulate air pollution remains unclear. In the present study, the brain pathophysiology and neurotoxicity were investigated in adult rats after chronic pulmonary exposure to traffic-related PM_1. Six major findings are reported in the present study: (1) the brain volume of rats increased after chronic exposure to PM_1; (2) a deficiency in short-term memory occurred after sub-chronic exposure

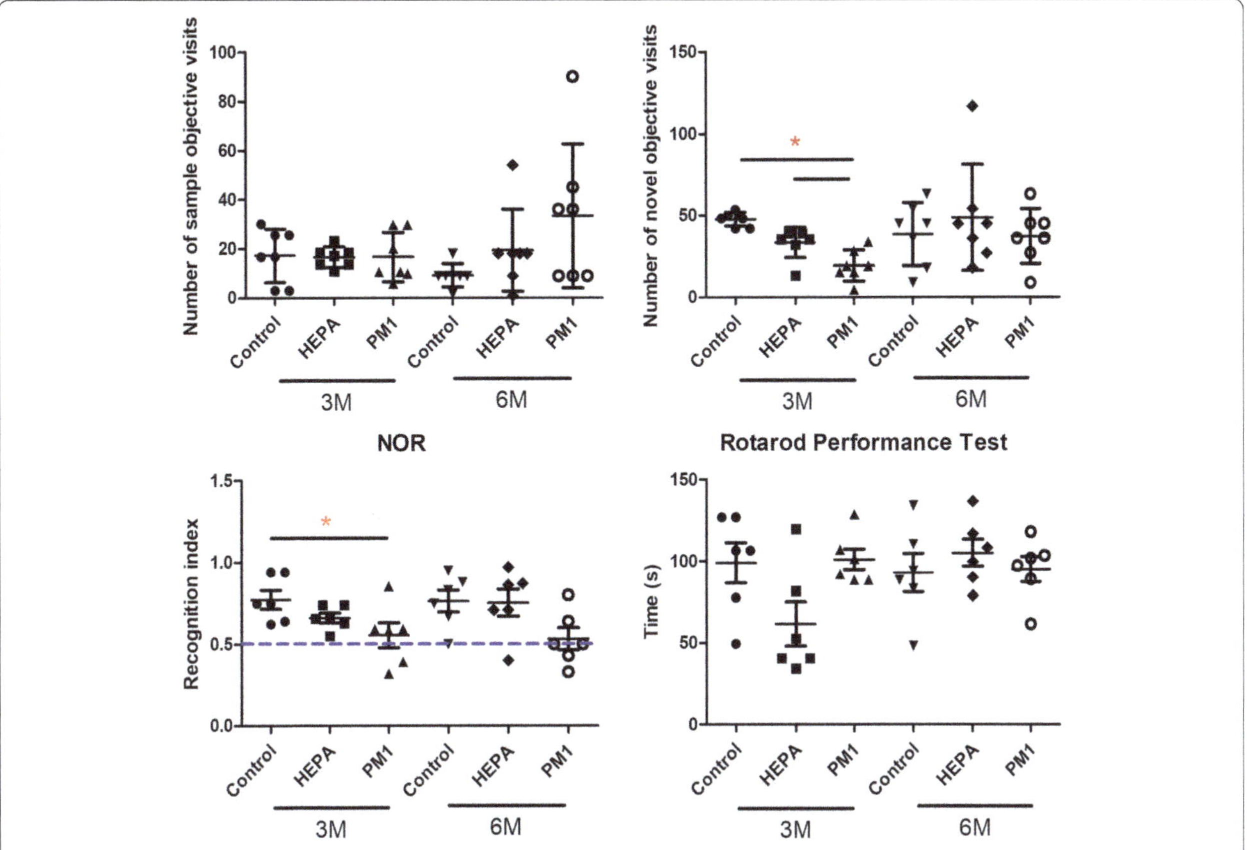

Fig. 4 Behavioral observations in rats after 3 and 6 months of exposure to traffic-related air pollution. The novel object recognition (NOR) task and rotarod performance task ($n = 6$) were conducted in rats of the control, high-efficiency particulate air (HEPA), and particulate matter with an aerodynamic diameter of < 1 μm (PM_1) groups. Three months of exposure to PM_1 caused significant reductions in the number of novel object visits and recognition index compared to the control and HEPA groups. There were no differences in the rotarod performance test among the groups after exposure. * $p < 0.05$

to PM_1; (3) brain oxidative stress and hippocampal inflammation were caused by sub-chronic exposure to PM_1; (4) systemic CCL11 and IL-4 increased after PM_1 exposure; (5) autophagic activation by chronic PM_1 exposure was observed in the hippocampus; and (6) spongiosis, neuronal shrinkage, and microabscesses were observed in the brain after PM_1 exposure.

Traffic-related particulate air pollution has been linked to increased risks of neurological disorders [18]. To study the effects of traffic-related particulate air pollution on the brain, a traffic-dominated urban region in New Taipei City (Taiwan) was selected for the experimental site, where there are lanes with heavy vehicle frequency and a nearby highway and expressway. The temperature, RH, NOx, SO_2, and O_3 during the study periods were referenced from the nearby traffic-related Yonghe air quality monitoring stations (Additional file 2: Table S1), which are operated by the Taiwan Environmental Protection Administration (http://taqm.epa.gov.tw/taqm/tw/) [19]. The temperature was 20 ± 4 (min-max: 12~ 29) °C and RH was 72% ± 9% (min-max: 47%~ 92%). The gaseous pollutants were 32.9 ± 16.4 (min-max: 8.4~ 86.6) ppb for NOx, 2.5 ± 1.0 (min-max: 0.2~ 5.0) ppb for SO_2, and 29.7 ± 11.0 (min-max: 6.7~ 58.2) ppb for O_3 during the study period. All three gaseous pollutants were lower than WHO air quality guidelines [20] during the study. Notably, for particulate air pollution, the mean geometric mean diameter (GMD) was 55.8 nm during the study period (Fig. 2), which suggests that most of the particles the rats were exposed to were dominated by ultrafine-sized fractions. The PM_1 mass concentration was 16.3 μg/m^3, which is similar to our previous observation in Taipei City (Taiwan) [21, 22]. PM_1 levels were relatively lower than the WHO $PM_{2.5}$ guideline of 25 μg/m^3 for the 24-h average [20]. However, there was 18 days of PM_1 mass concentrations higher than the WHO 24-h mean $PM_{2.5}$ guideline, and more than 116 days of PM_1 mass concentrations higher than the WHO annual mean $PM_{2.5}$ guideline. The rats were continually exposed to traffic-related PM_1, the LDSA of which was 55.1 μm^2/cm^3 during the study period. The LDSA level was higher than measured levels (37 μm^2/cm^3) in Barcelona, Spain [23]. This result indicates that the particle size suspended in

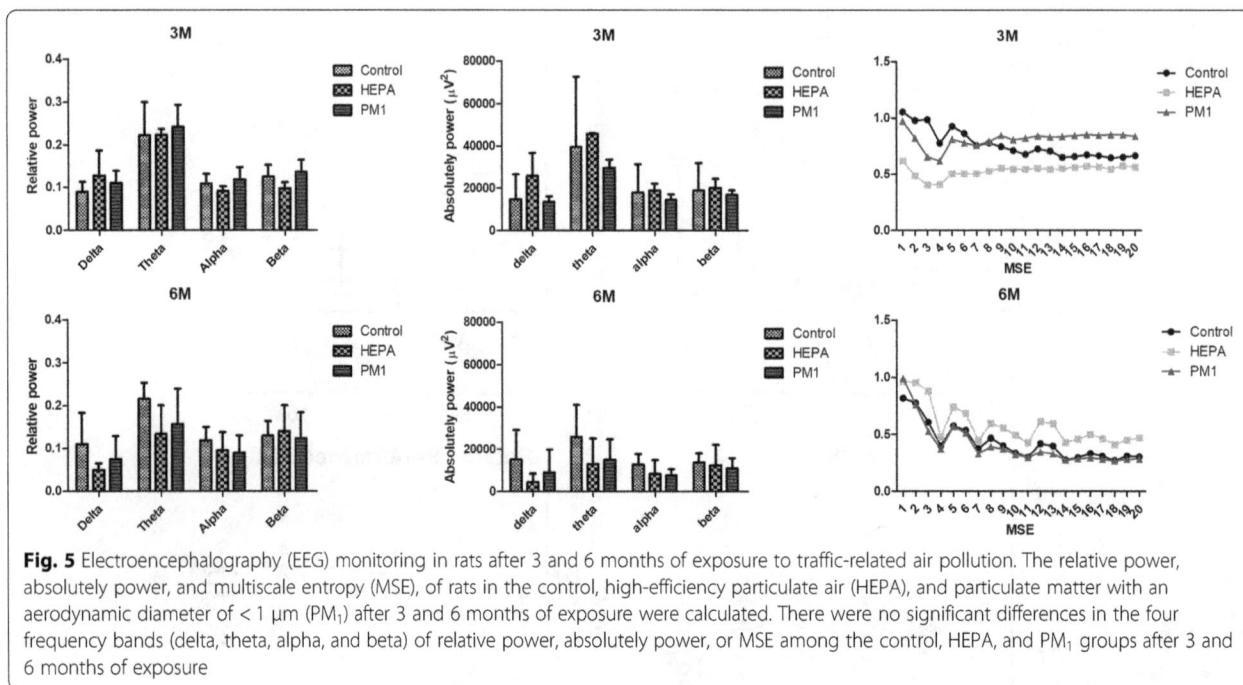

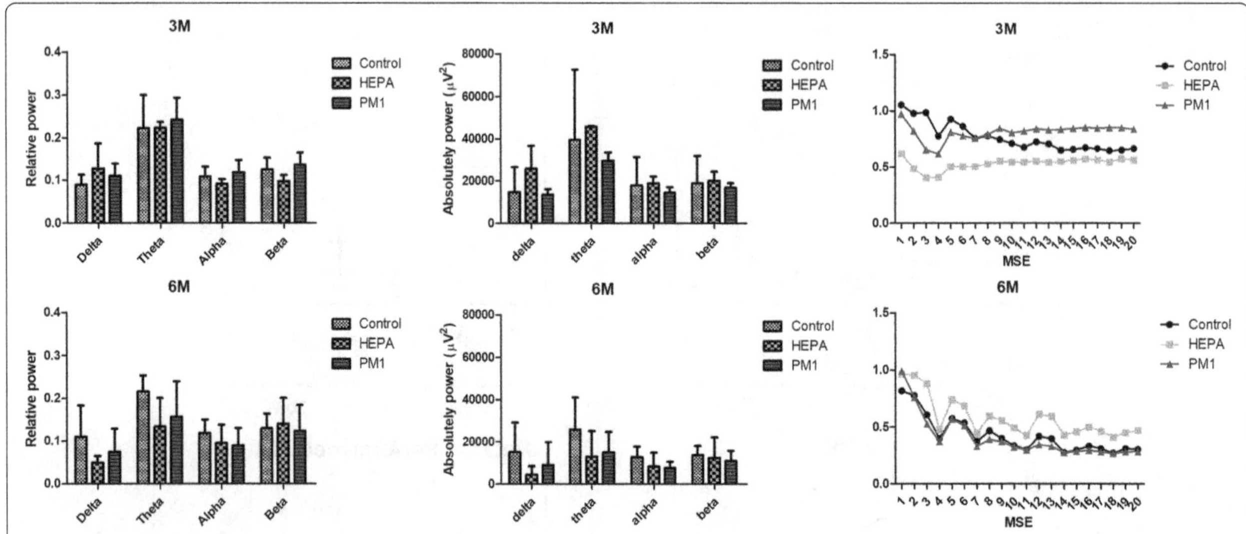

Fig. 5 Electroencephalography (EEG) monitoring in rats after 3 and 6 months of exposure to traffic-related air pollution. The relative power, absolutely power, and multiscale entropy (MSE), of rats in the control, high-efficiency particulate air (HEPA), and particulate matter with an aerodynamic diameter of < 1 μm (PM_1) after 3 and 6 months of exposure were calculated. There were no significant differences in the four frequency bands (delta, theta, alpha, and beta) of relative power, absolutely power, or MSE among the control, HEPA, and PM_1 groups after 3 and 6 months of exposure

the ambient air in New Taipei City was smaller (a higher surface area of particles) than particles measured in Barcelona. The BC concentration (1,899 ng/m^3) and PNC (11,257 #/m^3) determined in the present study were higher than our previous measurements (1,229 ng/m^3 for BC and 6,065 #/m^3 for PNC) [21]. Based on measurements of gaseous and particulate air pollution, the rats were exposed to relatively lower traffic-dominated air pollution during the study period. Therefore, this exposure condition of air pollution provides a good platform to study effects of chronic exposure to air pollution on the brain.

To study the pathophysiology of the brain caused by 3 and 6 months of exposure to particulate air pollution, a clean air control group (control), HEPA group (for gaseous effects), and PM_1 group were evaluated. First, a structural change in the brain by PM_1 in rats was observed by the MRI analysis (Fig. 3). Surprisingly, for the first time, we observed that the whole brain volume in 3-month PM_1-exposed rats was significantly larger than that of control rats. This finding suggests that sub-chronic exposure to PM_1 enlarged the whole brain volume of rats. Furthermore, the whole brain and hippocampal volumes of rats were enlarged by 6 months of exposure to gaseous pollution and PM_1. However, our in vivo observations were inconsistent with previous epidemiological associations. For example, Power and colleagues (2018) observed that long-term exposure to $PM_{2.5}$ was associated with smaller deep-gray volume of the brain in the Atherosclerosis Risk in Communities study. Long-term exposure to $PM_{2.5}$ was associated with increasing loss of both gray matter and white matter of brains of older women [24], but that was not observed for hippocampal volumes [25]. Wilker and colleagues (2015) observed that air pollution was associated with insidious effects on structural brain aging even in dementia- and stroke-free persons. Our observations in rats may have been due to the different statuses of disease progression in the brain due to air pollution. The BBB plays an important role in preventing entry of neurotoxic plasma-derived components, cells, and pathogens into the brain. A breakdown of the BBB may result in alterations in the brain's structures, such as cerebral edema and atrophy. A recent study found that 3-month-old C57BL/6 mice exposed to 100 μg/m^3 of vehicle emissions for 30 days exhibited increased BBB permeability and impaired BBB integrity [26]. Therefore, it is reasonable to hypothesize that chronic exposure to air pollution causes early brain pathologies, such as cerebral edema as observed in our study. Brain edema is defined as an increase in the brain volume as a result of abnormal accumulation of fluid within the cerebral parenchyma, which can be a fatal pathological state of the brain [27]. The abnormal accumulation of fluid due to an increase of the BBB permeability and integrity impairment can cause an increase in the brain volume and elevation of intracranial pressure because of the enclosed rigid skull. Generally, cerebral edema is mainly classified into vasogenic and cytotoxic edema [28, 29]. Vasogenic edema is characterized by extravasation and extracellular accumulation of fluid in the cerebral parenchyma caused by BBB injury, whereas cytotoxic edema is characterized

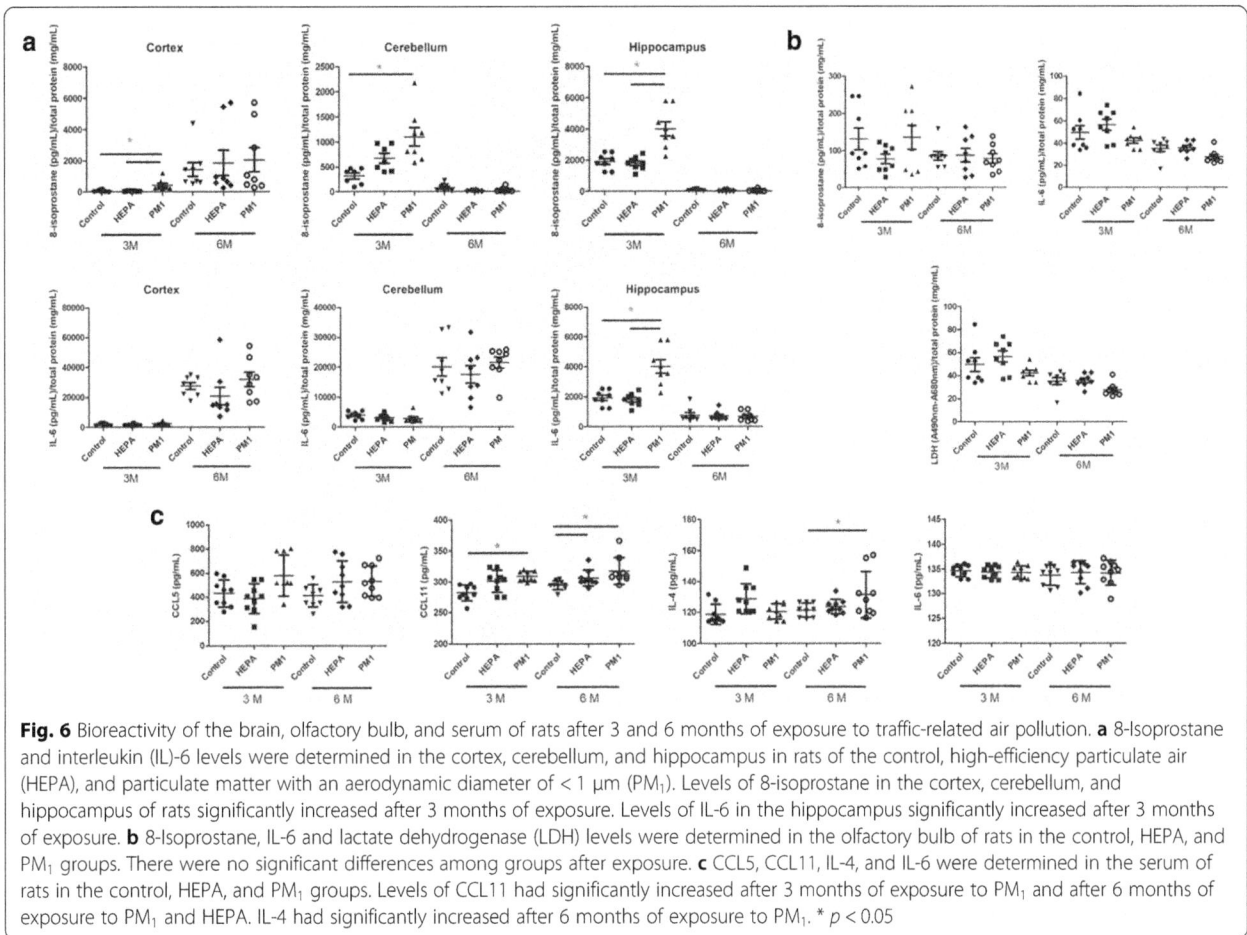

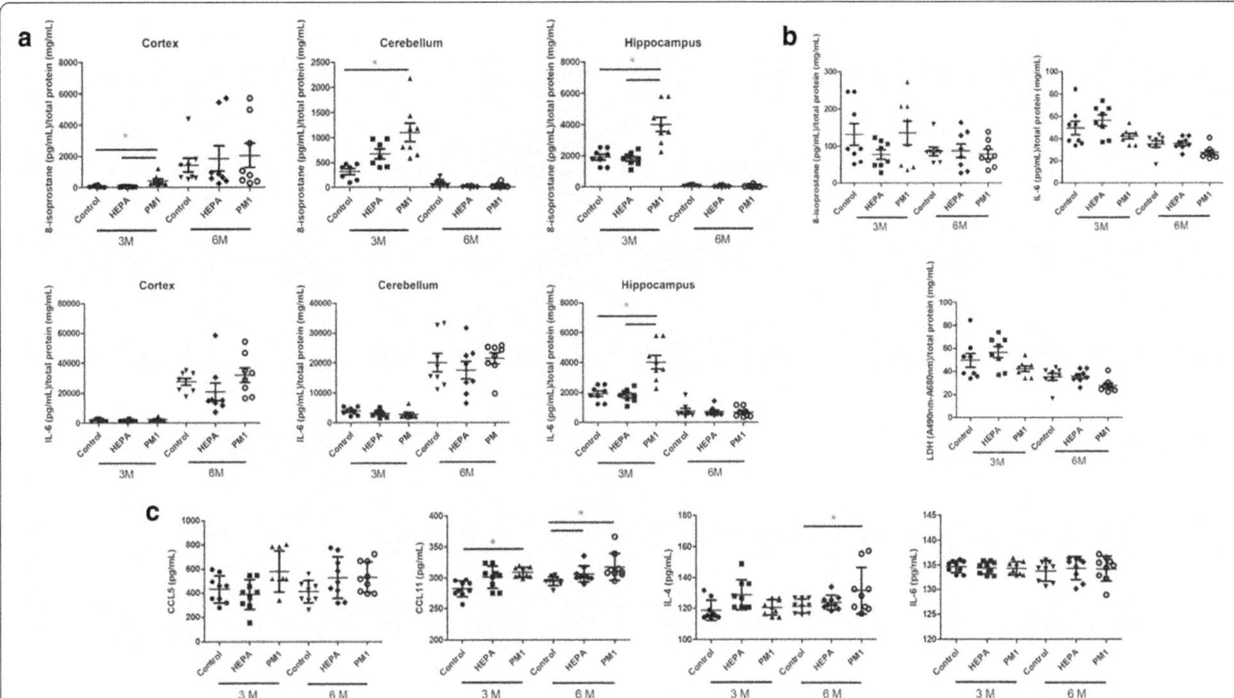

Fig. 6 Bioreactivity of the brain, olfactory bulb, and serum of rats after 3 and 6 months of exposure to traffic-related air pollution. **a** 8-Isoprostane and interleukin (IL)-6 levels were determined in the cortex, cerebellum, and hippocampus in rats of the control, high-efficiency particulate air (HEPA), and particulate matter with an aerodynamic diameter of < 1 μm (PM_1). Levels of 8-isoprostane in the cortex, cerebellum, and hippocampus of rats significantly increased after 3 months of exposure. Levels of IL-6 in the hippocampus significantly increased after 3 months of exposure. **b** 8-Isoprostane, IL-6 and lactate dehydrogenase (LDH) levels were determined in the olfactory bulb of rats in the control, HEPA, and PM_1 groups. There were no significant differences among groups after exposure. **c** CCL5, CCL11, IL-4, and IL-6 were determined in the serum of rats in the control, HEPA, and PM_1 groups. Levels of CCL11 had significantly increased after 3 months of exposure to PM_1 and after 6 months of exposure to PM_1 and HEPA. IL-4 had significantly increased after 6 months of exposure to PM_1. * $p < 0.05$

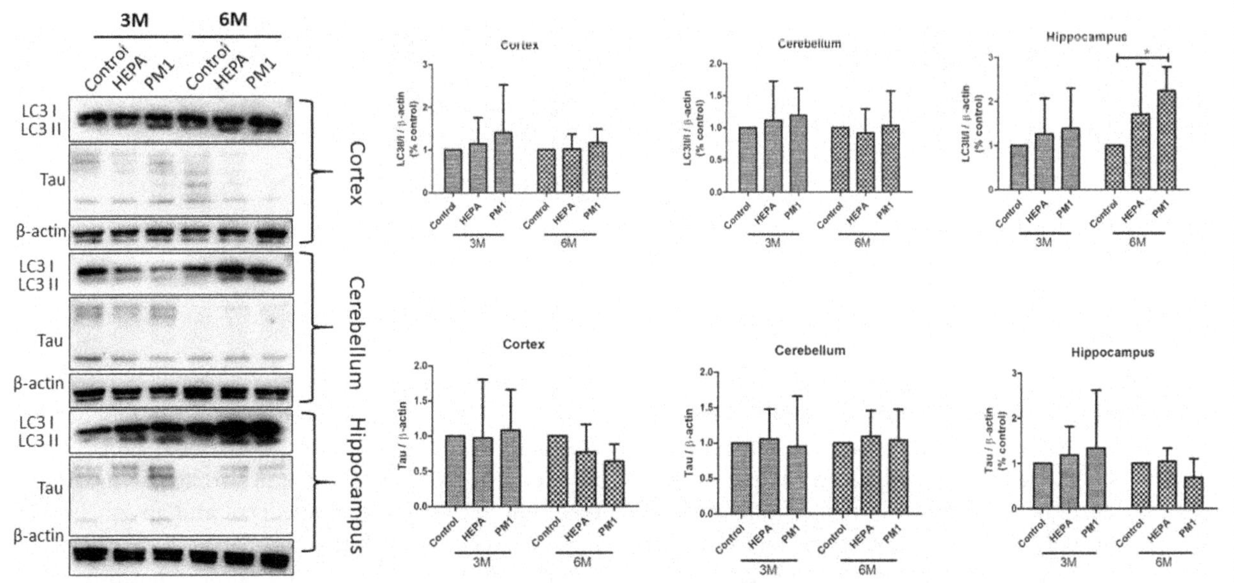

Fig. 7 Expressions of light chain 3II and I (LC3II/I) and total tau in the cortex, cerebellum, and hippocampus of rats after 3 and 6 months of exposure to traffic-related air pollution in the control, high-efficiency particulate air (HEPA), and particulate matter with an aerodynamic diameter of < 1 μm (PM_1) groups. LC3II/I expression in the hippocampus increased after 6 months of exposure to PM_1. * $p < 0.05$

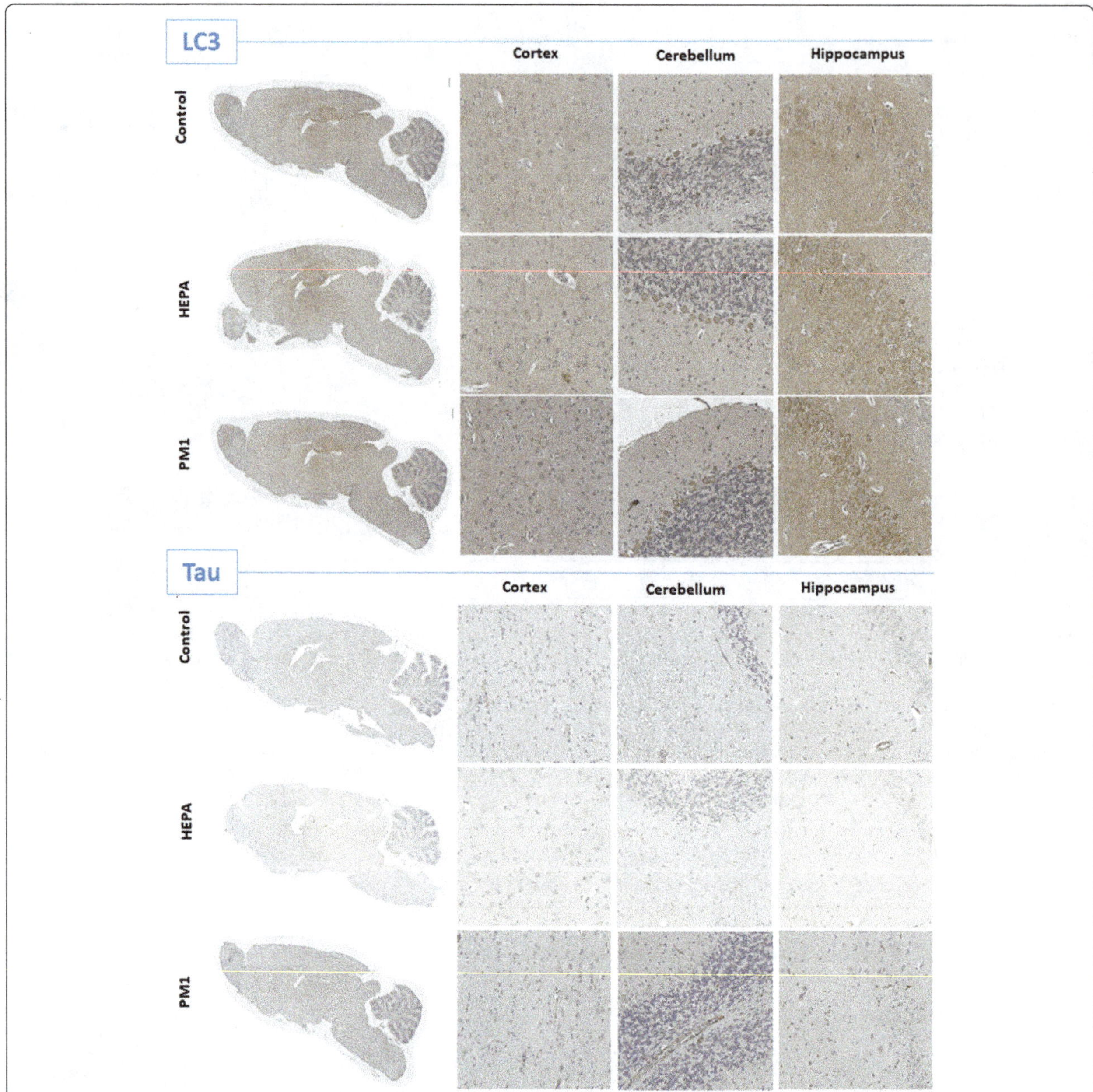

Fig. 8 IHC images of light chain 3 (LC3) and total tau in the cortex, cerebellum, and hippocampus of rats after 6 months of exposure to traffic-related air pollution in the control, high-efficiency particulate air (HEPA), and particulate matter with an aerodynamic diameter of < 1 μm (PM_1) groups. LC3 was more strongly positive in the hippocampus after 6 months of PM_1 exposure. Scar bar is 50 μm

by intracellular accumulation of fluid and Na^+ resulting in cell swelling. In contrast, cerebral atrophy is characterized by loss of neurons, shrinkage of neuronal cell bodies, or reductions in the number and extent of dendrites [30], leading to a decrease in the brain volume. Based on our MRI observations, 6 months of exposure to air pollution induced early-phase cerebral edema. Also, the occurrence of edema was followed by cerebral atrophy in the late stage as reported by epidemiological evidence. A neuroimaging study in individuals with mild cognitive impairment and early Alzheimer's disease (AD) showed BBB breakdown in the hippocampus [31] and several grey and white matter regions [32, 33], respectively. Alterations in the structural integrity of the brain, including cerebral edema and atrophy, may be hallmarks of pathophysiological changes for particulate air pollution-induced neurological disorders; however, further studies are required to examine the possible mechanisms.

Neuroimaging observations in our study showed that the brain and hippocampal volumes were enlarged by exposure

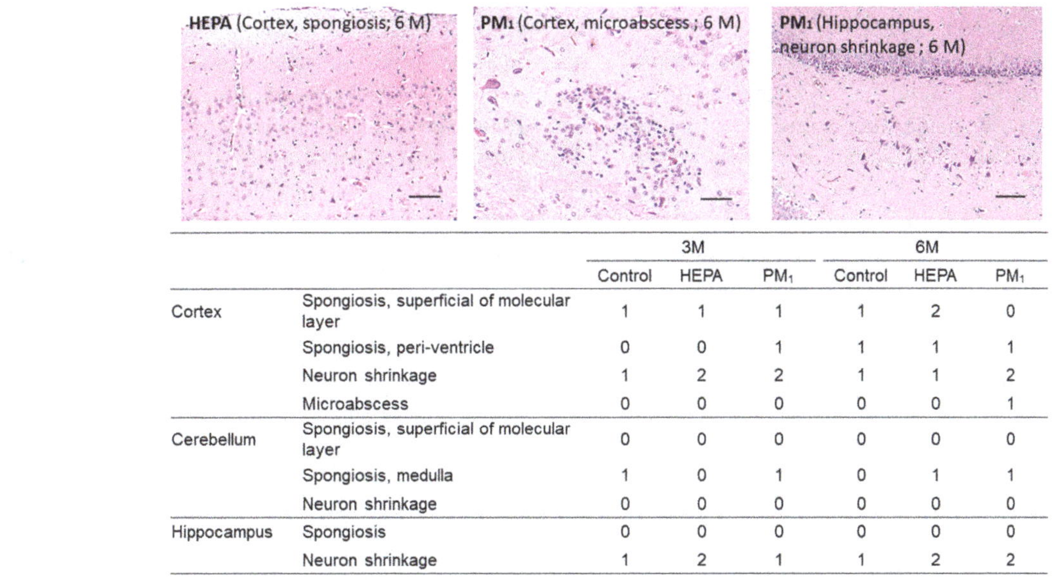

		3M			6M		
		Control	HEPA	PM_1	Control	HEPA	PM_1
Cortex	Spongiosis, superficial of molecular layer	1	1	1	1	2	0
	Spongiosis, peri-ventricle	0	0	1	1	1	1
	Neuron shrinkage	1	2	2	1	1	2
	Microabscess	0	0	0	0	0	1
Cerebellum	Spongiosis, superficial of molecular layer	0	0	0	0	0	0
	Spongiosis, medulla	1	0	1	0	1	1
	Neuron shrinkage	0	0	0	0	0	0
Hippocampus	Spongiosis	0	0	0	0	0	0
	Neuron shrinkage	1	2	1	1	2	2

Fig. 9 H&E staining and scoring of the cortex, cerebellum, and hippocampus after 3 and 6 months of exposure to traffic-related air pollution in the control, high-efficiency particulate air (HEPA), and particulate matter with an aerodynamic diameter of < 1 μm (PM_1) groups. Spongiosis and neuronal shrinkage were observed after 3 and 6 months of exposure to PM_1 (× 200). Microabscesses were identified in the cortex after 6 months of PM1 exposure (× 200). 0: No significant lesions. The extent of the lesions was graded from 1 to 5 depending on the severity: 1 = minimal (< 1%); 2 = slight, mild (1%~ 25%); 3 = moderate (26%~ 50%); 4 = moderate/severe (51%~ 75%); 5 = severe/high (76%~ 100%)

to traffic-related air pollution. Clinical complications of cerebral edema include behavioral and cognitive changes, memory loss, mental dysfunction, etc. [34]. Therefore, we next observed behavioral changes in rats by the NOR task (for short-term memory) and rotarod performance test (for motor function) (Fig. 4). We found that a short-term memory deficiency was caused by 3 months of exposure to PM_1 in rats. Consistently, associations between cognitive dysfunction and air pollution were previously reported. For example, exposure to PM was related to a decrease in cognition function [1] and faster cognitive declines [2]. Exposure to $PM_{2.5}$ and NO_2 was associated with decreased cognitive function [35]. Similarly, impairments in spatial learning and memory were also observed in mice after exposure to $PM_{2.5}$ [36]. A previous report showed that mild cognitive dysfunction is a prodromal syndrome of neurodegenerative dementia without significant dysfunction in activities of daily living [37]. Their observations support our finding of insignificant alteration in motor function after exposure to air pollution in rats. In the present study, the behavioral observations support the MRI results that PM caused neurotoxicity. However, the underlying mechanisms and pathophysiology of air pollution-induced cognitive dysfunction remain unclear.

Next, quantitative electroencephalography (qEEG) was carried out in rats after exposure (Fig. 5). qEEG measures are considered a reliable technique to examine neurodegenerative diseases, such as PD and AD, at the beginning of the dementing process, and can also be correlated with the extent of cognitive decline [38–40]. The presence of PD was correlated with an increase in theta power in the left temporal region and a decreasing median frequency [38]. Also, a human study was conduced to study alterations of the median power frequency and specific frequency bands of the qEEG after exposure to dilute diesel exhaust at 300 $\mu g/m^3$ [41]. The authors observed a significant increase in the median power frequency (fast wave activity of beta2) in the frontal cortex with 30 min of exposure. Therefore, we expected that the results of qEEG would confirm the behavioral observations in the present study. However, there was no significant difference in the relative or absolutely power of the frequency band in rats. EEG signals are produced by nonlinear coupling interactions between neuronal cells. Neuronal death and a deficiency of neurotransmitters such as acetylcholine and/or loss of connectivity of local neuronal networks are thought to be associated with a decrease in the dynamic complexity of the EEG in neurodegenerative disease [42]. But, we did not observe significant differences in the MSE among the control, HEPA, and PM_1 groups in the present study. The qEEG measurement reflects functional connections between different brain sections beneath the electrodes. The insignificant observation could have been due to a difference between the pathological location and the connected electrodes in the brain. Also, 6 months of exposure to air pollution will not cause fatal injuries to neuronal cells in the brain.

Neuroinflammation, a non-specific protective response, is recognized as an essential response to exposure to particulate air pollution [4, 5]. Chronic inflammation is observed in aged brains [43], and there are further increases in brain inflammation in neurodegenerative disorders. In the present study, we observed structural changes in the brain and behavioral alterations in rats after pulmonary exposure to traffic-related air pollution. It is important to further explore the bioreactivity of PM_1 on various brain sections, including the cortex, cerebellum, and hippocampus. We observed that PM_1 produced oxidative stress in the cortex, cerebellum, and hippocampus after 3 months of exposure in rats (Figure 6). Also, we found that hippocampal inflammation was caused by 3 months of exposure to PM_1. Oxidative stress is considered an important mechanism in regulating inflammatory responses [44, 45], which was observed in our study. Oxidative stress is commonly observed in neurodegenerative diseases, which is recognized to be neurodegenerative pathogenesis, and it is conceivable that the effects of PM exposure could induce a decrease in cognitive function [46]. Acute exposure to 250~ 300 $\mu g/m^3$ diesel exhaust particle for 6 h was found to induce oxidative stress, microglia activation, neuro-inflammation, and neurogenesis impairment in various brain regions, such as the hippocampal subgranular zone and subventricular zone [47]. Long-term exposure to $PM_{2.5}$ elevated hippocampal inflammatory cytokines in mice [36]. Campbell and colleagues (2005) observed that asthmatic mice exposed to concentrated ambient particles exhibited increased inflammatory cytokines, such as IL-1α and tumor necrosis factor (TNF)-α in brain tissues. Guerra and colleagues (2013) further showed that exposure to different-sized fractions of ambient particles caused distinct physiological changes, inflammation, oxidative stress, and unfolded protein responses in the CNS, particularly in the striatum. Although in vivo studies indicated that particulate air pollution causes neuroinflammation, possible lung-to-brain pathways of exposure to air pollution remain unclear. It was noted that ultrafine PM is capable of being translocated into the brain via the olfactory nerves [13]. Also, inhaled PM is able to damage the nasal epithelium [14]. To examine the effects of PM_1 on the olfactory bulb, oxidative stress, inflammation, and cytotoxicity were determined in rats after 3 and 6 months of PM_1 exposure. However, we did not observe significant alterations in 8-isoprostane, IL-6, or lactate dehydrogenase (LDH) levels with PM_1 exposure. A previous study showed that exposure to ambient PM induced olfactory bulb inflammatory gene expressions in C57BL/6 male mice [48]. The difference from the current study could have been due to different expression levels between proteins and genes. Notably, one study observed that exposure to traffic-related air pollution altered the brain's microvascular integrity in a high-fat diet animal model [26]. The authors suggested that particulate air pollution could cause BBB impairment, leading to local inflammation due to particles accumulating in the brain. If such BBB impairment is an important pathway of regulating air pollution-induced neurotoxicity, an increase in the permeability of the brain and systemic-to-local (brain) inflammation could explain the MRI observations of increased brain volumes. Additionally, we observed that CCL11 and IL-4 had increased after 3 and 6 months of exposure to PM_1 in rats. CCL11 was shown to pass the BBB and was identified as a crucial mediator of decreased neurogenesis and increased cognitive impairment in mice [49]. Mice lacking IL-4 demonstrated cognitive impairment in a spatial learning task [50]. Together, alterations in CCL11 and IL-4 could support the behavioral observations in the present study. However, additional mechanistic investigations should be conducted in the future.

Deposition of insoluble proteins in cells of the neuromuscular system is related to the development of neurological diseases. Clinically, intraneuronal accumulation of tau proteins is considered an important hallmark of the development of AD [51]. Tau overexpression in neuroblastoma cells can lead to tau aggregation and the appearance of smaller proteolytic fragments [52]. In the present study, we did not observe significant alterations in tau expression in the cortex, cerebellum, or hippocampus after 3 or 6 months of exposure to air pollution in rats (Figs. 7 and 8). Our results suggest that exposure of air pollution in rats did not produce significant development of neurodegenerative disease at the current stages. A previous study showed that phospho-tau (Ser199) increased after exposure to diesel exhaust at 992 and 311 $\mu g/m^3$ [53]. Notably, we observed autophagy activation in the hippocampus after 6 months of exposure to PM_1 in rats. Autophagy is one of the degradative mechanisms, which is able to remove tau aggregates [52]. Therefore, autophagy is considered an essential function for maintaining the brain's health. Autophagy dysfunction and loss of basal autophagy may lead to neurodegeneration, whereas activation of autophagy can remove aggregated oxidized/diseased proteins such as tau protein aggregates [54]. In the present study, we suspect that activation of autophagy may have played a critical role in maintaining the brain's health after exposure to air pollution.

Due to the rigidity of the skull, cerebral edema can lead to higher intracranial pressure, which subsequently decreases cerebral perfusion, ultimately leading to pathological changes in the brain [55]. In the present study, spongiosis and/or neuronal shrinkage were commonly observed in the cortex, cerebellum, and hippocampus of rats exposed to air pollution (Fig. 9). Fonken and colleagues [36] observed that exposure to $PM_{2.5}$ for

10 months caused changes in the hippocampal neuronal morphology, including apical dendritic spine density and dendritic branching, in mice. We further showed that microabscesses occurred in the cortex after 6 months of exposure to PM_1. Brain abscesses, defined as focal infections within the brain parenchyma, are caused by inflammation and the collection of infected material within brain tissues [56]. Therefore, the cortical microabscesses observed after 6 months of exposure to PM_1 may have resulted from particles crossing the BBB into the brain. However, more-direct evidence is required to examine the possible pathways of PM-related neurotoxicity.

Taken together, we hypothesized a theoretical model for the impacts of particulate air pollution on the brain as shown in Fig. 10. Inhaled particulate air pollution is able to induce oxidative stress and inflammation in the brain, leading to CNS impairment. The extracellular accumulation of fluid due to the increased permeability of the BBB results in the formation of cerebral edema. The air pollution-induced edematous brain is repaired by protective mechanisms, resulting in cerebral atrophy. Although our results support the hypothetical model of PM neurotoxicity, cerebral atrophy was not observed in the present study (due to the stage of pathological progression). Also, the pathways of PM from the lungs to the brain remain unclear. We found that gaseous pollution caused neurotoxicity after 6 months of exposure, including increase in whole and hippocampus volumes and systemic CCL5 levels in rats. The gaseous effect on brain is poorly unknown. Based on our findings, we hypothesize that some types of gaseous pollution is a source of free readcals that could cause systemic oxidative stress and inflammation, leading to brain impariement. However, the contributions of different gaseous pollutants were not investigated in the present study. Effects of metals and organics on neurotoxicity should be addressed in future work.

Conclusions

In conclusion, chronic exposure to air pollution caused brain impairment, leading to cerebral edema, behavioral changes, oxidative stress, inflammation, autophagy activation, and histological changes in the rat brain. Cerebral edema could be an early stage of progression for the development of neurological diseases caused by air pollution. Our findings provide further evidence that long-term exposure to particulate air pollution increases the risks of neurological disorders.

Materials

Animals

Animal experiments were performed in compliance with the animal and ethics review committee of the Laboratory Animal Center at Taipei Medical University (Taipei, Taiwan). Male 6-month-old SD rats obtained from the National Laboratory Animal Center (Taipei, Taiwan) were maintained at a constant temperature of 22 ± 2 °C and a relative humidity (RH) of 55% ± 10%. Rats were housed in plastic cages with a 12:12-h light: dark cycle throughout the study. Lab Diet 5001 (PMI Nutrition International, USA) and water were provided ad libitum during the study.

Whole-body exposure to traffic-related PM_1

As shown in Fig. 1a, rats were randomly divided into three groups: (1) a clean air control group (housed in the Specific Pathogen Free I (SPF I) level of Laboratory

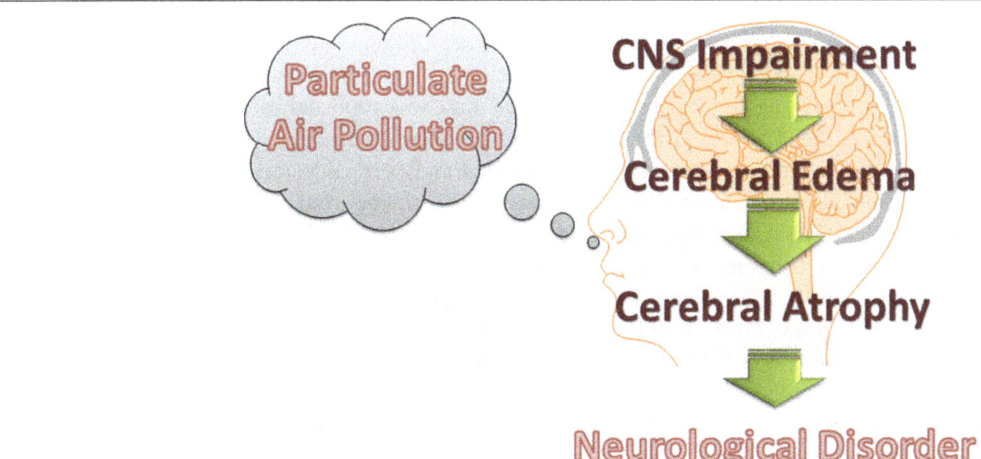

Fig. 10 Illustration of the hypothetical pathways of particulate air pollution involved in the development of neurological disorders. Inhaled particulate air pollution is able to induce oxidative stress and inflammation in the brain, leading to central nervous system (CNS) impairment. The extracellular accumulation of fluid due to increased permeability of the blood-brain barrier (BBB), results in formation of cerebral edema. The air pollution-induced edematous brain is repaired by protective mechanisms, leading to cerebral atrophy. Continuous exposure to particulate air pollution leads to the development of neurological disorders

Animal Center, Taipei City), (2) a high-efficiency particulate air (HEPA)-filtered air control group (exposed to gaseous pollution only), and (3) a PM_1 group (exposed to particulate and gaseous pollution). Because of ventilation of the animal centre was introduced from the outdoor ambient air with HEPA filtration, the clean air control group may be still exposed under the urban background levels of air pollution. The whole-body exposure system used to radent for PM_1 exposure was previously reported [22]. The whole-body exposure system was located in a traffic-dominated urban region (New Taipei City, Taiwan), which is near a highway and expressway. Briefly, ambient air was continuously sampled by an omnidirectional PM inlet located on the roof of a station and then introduced into whole-body exposure system as shown in Fig. 1b. A stream was sampled from an empty whole-body exposure cage (without rats) for characterization of PM's physical features. The whole-body exposure system had the higher penetration rate of PM (outdoor PM to system PM) with the particle size less than 1 μm (Additional file 2: Figure S2). The data suggested that PM_1 was the main size fraction for the whole-body exposure in this system. Mass concentrations were monitored using a tapered element oscillating microbalance (TEOM, Thermo Scientific 1400a). Additionally, a scanning mobility particle sizer (SMPS, TSI 3936), an aerodynamic particle sizer (APS; TSI 3321), and a nanoparticle surface area monitor (NSAM; TSI 3550) were respectively used to monitor the submicron particle size distribution (PSD), supermicron PSD, and LDSA concentrations. An aethalometer (Magee Scientific AE33, Berkeley, CA, USA) was simultaneously employed to measure the BC mass concentration. The details of these instrutemnts are provided in Additional file 2: Table S2. The onsite exposure experiment was conducted for 3 and 6 months.

Experimental design

The experimental design is shown in Fig. 1c. Rats in the HEPA ($n = 18$) and PM_1 groups ($n = 18$) were directly exposed to traffic-related air pollution for 3 and 6 months between November 2016 and May 2017. Simultaneously, rats in the clean air control group ($n = 18$) were housed in the Laboratory Animal Center for the same study period (3 and 6 months). After exposure for 3 and 6 months, nine rats in each group were randomly selected for an MRI analysis. Next, six rats in each group, after the MRI, were randomly selected for behavioral observations, including a novel object recognition (NOR) task and rotarod performance task. Electroencephalographic (EEG) implementation and monitoring were conducted in the remaining three rats from each group. Finally, an animal necropsy was performed, and serum and tissues were collected as described previously [57].

MRI

MRI experiments were performed on a custom-made 3 T MRI system. A gradient coil insert with an inner diameter of 115 mm and a maximum gradient strength of 670 mT/m (BFG 200–115, Resonance Research, Inc., USA) was installed and a home-made single-loop surface RF coil with a diameter of 4 cm was used for RF transmission. MRI sequences were executed by a 3 T spectrometer (MR Solutions, UK). For rat brain imaging, T2-weighted images (T2WIs) were acquired using a fast spin echo sequence with 10 coronal slices, a slice thickness of 2 mm without a gap, a repetition time (TR) of 4000 ms, an echo time (TE) of 63 ms, an echo train length (ETL) of 8, a field of view (FOV) of 40 × 40 mm, and a matrix size of 256 × 256, yielding an in-plane resolution of 156 × 156 μm, with 16 averages. All animals were fixed with a home-made magnetic resonance-compatible animal stereotaxic frame, made using a 3D printer (KINGSSEL3070+, MASTECH MACHINE CO., LTD., Taiwan), and they were anesthetized using an isoflurane vaporizer with the concentration adjusted to maintain 40~ 60 breaths/min of the breathing rate during the MRI scan. The total experiment time was around 1 h for each animal.

MRI data analysis

For the MRI volumetric analysis, the bilateral hippocampus and whole brain areas were manually selected using MRI analytical software, MRIcro (https://www.mccauslandcenter.sc.edu/crnl/). The region of interest (ROI) of the hippocampus was determined according to the rat brain atlas [58]. The voxel numbers of each ROI were automatically calculated using MRIcro. The volume calculation was based on the counted voxel numbers multiplied to the voxel size of the acquired image (0.156 × 0.156 × 2 mm).

NOR task

The NOR task was reported to be a useful approach for studying short-term memory, which is influenced by both hippocampal and cortical lesions. The procedure of NOR task was previously reported [59]. Briefly, the NOR sample and test sessions occurred in context A, an open field arena measuring 60 × 60 cm, with 40-cm-high black translucent walls and a white floor with black gridlines spaced 15 cm apart. Context A was 360° encompassed by a 180-cm-high black curtain in order to block distal sensory information; object locations inside the arena also remained constant between sessions. Over 3 days, each subject was transported in its home cage and allowed to explore context A for 5 min, after which it was returned to the vivarium. During the sample and test sessions, objects were taped to the floor to ensure that they could not be moved by the animal. The objects were a transparent green water bottle made of non-porous plastic (22 × 9 cm) and a semi-opaque, brown glass bottle (22 × 7 cm). The two objects were located 15 cm from the nearest arena wall and separated by 30 cm. For the sample session, each rat was placed near the center of the open field, facing away from the two identical objects (counter-balanced) and allowed to explore for 5 min. Rats were returned to the same context 20 or 240 min later. Using the same spatial locations within the arena, one familiar object (sample objective) and one novel object were presented, counter-balanced across the left-right position. The subject was again placed near the center of the open field, facing away from the objects and allowed to explore for 3 min. The recognition index, the proportion of time spent with the novel object/location compared to the total exploration time of both objects, was used to measure recognition memory. A recognition index significantly above 0.50 demonstrates a novelty preference and thus recognition memory [60].

Rotarod performance test

The rotarod performance test was carried out using the Rotarod system (Rotamex-5; Columbus Inst; Columbus, OH, USA) to evaluate motor function. Each rat was trained three times/day for 3 consecutive days before the real test. The training speed was from 4 to 20 revolutions/min (rpm) at a rate of 0.5 revolutions/s (rps). After completing the training, a rat was placed onto a rotating rod at a constant speed of 40 rpm over a period of 5 min essentially, acceleration Increments of 1.2 rpm per ten second. The duration time of staying on the rotating rod was recorded. Each rat was given three trials at 30-min intervals, and the average time of the three trials was recorded as the final result.

EEG implementation and monitoring

Stereotactic surgery was conducted under light anesthesia induced by 2% isoflurane vapor (2 ml/min) using a rodent anesthesia machine (Northern Vaporiser; Skipton, UK). EEG electrodes were secured to the skull using stainless steel screws, which were placed epidurally in the frontal cortex, parietal area (somatosensory cortex), and occipital cortex [61]. Electrodes were fixed to the skull with methyl methacrylate monomer together with two additional anchoring screws. Simultaneously, electromyography (EMG) was implemented and connected to a muscle. After surgery, rats were individually housed for 7 days in order to prevent damage to the electrode connectors. After recovery, EEG signals were continuously recorded for 24 h in freely moving rats, and the output was fed into a multi-channel amplifier (MP35, Biopac System, Goleta, CA, USA). The sampling frequency of raw EEG data was 200 Hz, and the digital resolution was 12 bits. A notch filter of 50/60 Hz was applied.

Power spectrum analysis of EEG

EEG data were mainly processed using MATLAB software (MATLAB, R2007a; MathWorks, Natick, MA, USA) to conduct further computations. First, raw EEG data were visually checked to exclude epochs with significant artifacts. Fast Fourier transformation of the EEG data was computed to obtain the power spectrum of the EEG signals. The absolute power and relative power of four frequency bands were calculated, including the delta (0.5~ 2 Hz), theta (2~ 8 Hz), alpha (8~ 12 Hz), and beta (12~ 30 Hz) bands.

Multiscale entropy (MSE) analysis

MSE was determined based on an analysis of sample entropy of EEG signals at different time scales. Signals at differential time scales were computed through a coarse-graining procedure of the original data. The coarse-graining procedure was conducted by dividing the original signal into non-overlapping segments of equal length corresponding to the scalar factor. The average of signals in each window was then calculated to yield a new time series. The sample entropy, calculated as the self-similarity of the signal based on the conditioned probability, was then calculated for each time series based on different scalar factors. We utilized the C -ode program developed by Goldberger et al. to calculate the MSE of the EEG signals [62].

Given a time series denoting the measured EEG:

$$x(n) = (\times 1, \times 2, \times 3, ..., xn); \quad (1)$$

the coarse-grain series was obtained by averaging variables by applying non-overlapping windows.

$$X(s) = (\text{mean}\,(\times 1, \times 2, \times 3, ..., xs), \\ \text{mean}\,(xs+1, xs+2, xs+3, ..., x2s), ...); \quad (2)$$

the MSE for each time scalar factor was computed according to the equation:

$$\text{MSE}\ (s) = \text{SpEn}\,(X(s), m, r); \quad (3)$$

where SpEn denotes the sample entropy, m denotes the vector of length, and r denotes the tolerance of similarity. In the present study, we selected m = 2 and $r = 0.15$ for MSE computations.

Brain and olfactory bulb tissue preparations

Rats from each group (control, HEPA, and PM_1) were transcardially perfused with 15 mL of phosphate-buffered saline (PBS) and immediately decapitated. The cortex, cerebellum, hippocampus, and olfactory bulb from each rat were collected, frozen in liquid nitrogen, and stored at − 80 °C. Tissues were homogenized in Cell lysis MT (Sigma, St. Louis, MO, USA) with a Complete™ protease inhibitor (Roche Diagnostics, Basel, Switzerland), according to the manufacturers' instructions. All preparation were conduced on ice, and centrifuged for 30 min at 12,000 *xg* and 4 °C. The supernatant was collected, and the total protein concentration was measured using a BCA Protein Assay Kit.

Enzyme-linked immunosorbent assay (ELISA)

8-Isoprostane (Cayman, USA), IL-6 (R&D System, Minneapolis, MN, USA) and Lactate dehydrogenase (LDH) Cytotoxicity Assay Kit (Thermo Scientific, Waltham, MA, USA) were determined using ELISA kits in accordance with the manufacturer's instructions. All data are presented after adjusting for the total protein.

Multiplex assay

Chemokine (C-C motif) ligand 5 (CCL5), CCL11, IL-4, and IL-6 in plasma were assayed with the AimPlex™ multiplex assay (St. Louis, MO, USA), according to the manufacturer's instructions. Complexes of beads and the studied proteins labeled with phycoerythrin antibodies were determined using a BD LSRFortessa™ cell analyzer (NJ, USA).

Western blot analysis

Details of the Western blot analyses were previously described [63]. Lysed tissue samples were electrophoresed through sodium dodecylsulfate polyacrylamide gel electrophoresis (SDS-PAGE) and transferred onto polyvinylidene difluoride (PVDF) membranes (Millipore, Darmstadt, Germany). Primary antibodies for light chain 3 (LC3; 1:1000), tau (1:1000), and β-catenin (1:1000) were obtained from Cell Signaling (Danvers, MA, US). Anti-rabbit (1:2000) and anti-mouse (1:2000) horseradish peroxidase (HRP)-conjugated secondary antibodies were obtained from Chemicon International (MA, USA) and Merck Millipore (MA, USA), respectively. PBST containing 5% skim milk was used to block blots, followed by probing with primary antibodies overnight at 4 °C. Samples were then incubated with an HRP-labeled secondary antibody at room temperature. Immunoreactivity was observed through enhanced chemiluminescence (ECL). Images were taken with the BioSpectrum Imaging System (UVP, Upland, CA, USA). Quantitative data were obtained using Image-Pro vers. 4 (Media Cybernetics, Inc., MD, USA) for Windorws. All data were adjusted to the control (multiples of change of the control).

Immunohistochemistry (IHC) of brain tissues

Tissues were fixed in 2% paraformaldehyde and were permeabilized with 0.1% Triton X-100 in 0.01 M PBS (pH 7.4; containing 0.2% bovine serum albumin). Incubation with polyclonal antibodies against LC3 (1:1000) and tau (1:1000), obtained from GeneTex (Irvine, CA, USA), in PBS and containing 3% normal goat serum, was performed, whereas incubation with PBS served as a negative control. An anti-rabbit immunoglobulin G (IgG) FITC-conjugated secondary antibody (Jackson ImmunoResearch, PA, USA; 1:500 dilution) was incubated with cells, followed by staining with 4′,6-diamidino-2-phenylindole (DAPI). Microphotographs were acquired using an AxioCam MRc digital video camera and the Zeiss AxioVision software (Carl Zeiss, NY, USA).

Histology

Brains were excised and washed with ice-cold PBS followed by fixation with 10% neutral buffered formalin, embedded in paraffin, sectioned, and stained with hematoxylin and eosin (H&E). Histological examinations were conducted under light microscopy by a histopathologist in a blinded manner.

Statistical analysis

Data are expressed as the mean ± standard deviation (SD). For comparisons among multiple values, a one-way analysis of variance (ANOVA) with Tukey's post-hoc test was used. Statistical analyses were performed using GraphPad vers. 5 for Windows. The level of significance was set to $p < 0.05$.

Additional files

Additional file 1: Figure S1. Alteration in body weight during the 6-months exposure of PM_1. (TIF 146 kb)

Additional file 2: Table S1. Meteorological and gaseous data measured by the traffic-related EPA Yonghe air quality monitoring stations during the study period. **Table S2.** Instruments used to characterize the exposure conditions for rats. **Figure S2.** Characterization of particle size and penetration distribution (between outdoor and whole-body exposure system) determined using a scanning mobility particle sizer (SMPS, TSI 3936; upper size limit: 710 nm). (a) The exposure cages (yellow marked: 1–1, 1–3, 1–5, 2–3, 3–1, 3–3 and 3–5) were measured for size-penetration distribution. (b) The individual cage for animal exposure showed a consistent size-penetration distribution. The geometric mean diameter (GMD) was 50 nm. (DOCX 152 kb)

Acknowledgements

The authors wish to thank Mr. Xiao-Yue Chen, Mr. Cheng-Ze Liao, Miss Shu-Hsien Wu and Miss Jei-Ping Li for technical assistance with this research.

Funding

This study was funded by the Ministry of Science and Technology of Taiwan (MOST105–2633-B-038-001 and 106–2633-B-038-001).

Authors' contributions

All authors contributed substantially to the concept and design of the study, drafting of the article, and critically revising the manuscript for important intellectual content. All authors have read and approved the final version of the manuscript for publication.

Competing interests
The authors declare that they have no competing interest.

Author details
[1]School of Respiratory Therapy, College of Medicine, Taipei Medical University, Taipei, Taiwan. [2]Institute of Biomedical Engineering & Nanomedicine, National Health Research Institutes, Miaoli, Taiwan. [3]Graduate Institute of Environmental Engineering, National Taiwan University, Taipei, Taiwan. [4]Department of Physical Medicine and Rehabilitation, Taipei Medical University Hospital, Taipei, Taiwan. [5]Department of Physical Medicine and Rehabilitation, School of Medicine, College of Medicine, Taipei Medical University, Taipei, Taiwan. [6]The Ph.D Program for Neural Regenerative Medicine, College of Medical Science and Technology, Taipei Medical University, Taipei, Taiwan. [7]School of Public Health, College of Public Health, Taipei Medical University, Taipei, Taiwan. [8]Department of Public Health, School of Medicine, College of Medicine, Taipei Medical University, Taipei, Taiwan. [9]Institute of Occupational Medicine and Industrial Hygiene, College of Public Health, National Taiwan University, Taipei, Taiwan. [10]Division of Pulmonary Medicine, Department of Internal Medicine, Shuang Ho Hospital, Taipei Medical University, New Taipei City, Taiwan.

References

1. Power MC, Weisskopf MG, Alexeeff SE, Coull BA, Spiro A 3rd, Schwartz J. Traffic-related air pollution and cognitive function in a cohort of older men. Environ Health Perspect. 2011;119(5):682–7.
2. Weuve J, Puett RC, Schwartz J, Yanosky JD, Laden F, Grodstein F. Exposure to particulate air pollution and cognitive decline in older women. Arch Intern Med. 2012;172(3):219–27.
3. Kioumourtzoglou MA, Schwartz JD, Weisskopf MG, Melly SJ, Wang Y, Dominici F, et al. Long-term PM Exposure and Neurological Hospital Admissions in the Northeastern United States. Environ Health Perspect. 2016;124(1):23–9.
4. Gerlofs-Nijland ME, van Berlo D, Cassee FR, Schins RP, Wang K, Campbell A. Effect of prolonged exposure to diesel engine exhaust on proinflammatory markers in different regions of the rat brain. Part Fibre Toxicol. 2010;7:12.
5. Campbell A, Oldham M, Becaria A, Bondy SC, Meacher D, Sioutas C, et al. Particulate matter in polluted air may increase biomarkers of inflammation in mouse brain. Neurotoxicology. 2005;26(1):133–40.
6. Tyler CR, Zychowski KE, Sanchez BN, Rivero V, Lucas S, Herbert G, et al. Surface area-dependence of gas-particle interactions influences pulmonary and neuroinflammatory outcomes. Part Fibre Toxicol. 2016;13(1):64.
7. Brook RD, Rajagopalan S, Pope CA 3rd, Brook JR, Bhatnagar A, Diez-Roux AV, et al. Particulate matter air pollution and cardiovascular disease: an update to the scientific statement from the American Heart Association. Circulation. 2010;121(21):2331–78.
8. Oberdorster G, Elder A, Rinderknecht A. Nanoparticles and the brain: cause for concern? J Nanosci Nanotechnol. 2009;9(8):4996–5007.
9. Block ML, Calderon-Garciduenas L. Air pollution: mechanisms of neuroinflammation and CNS disease. Trends Neurosci. 2009;32(9):506–16.
10. The Lancet Neurology. Air pollution and brain health: an emerging issue. Lancet Neurol. 2018;17(2):103.
11. Maher BA, Ahmed IA, Karloukovski V, MacLaren DA, Foulds PG, Allsop D, et al. Magnetite pollution nanoparticles in the human brain. Proc Natl Acad Sci U S A. 2016;113(39):10797–801.
12. Calderon-Garciduenas L, Reynoso-Robles R, Vargas-Martinez J, Gomez-Maqueo-Chew A, Perez-Guille B, Mukherjee PS, et al. Prefrontal white matter pathology in air pollution exposed Mexico City young urbanites and their potential impact on neurovascular unit dysfunction and the development of Alzheimer's disease. Environ Res. 2016;146:404–17.
13. Garcia GJ, Kimbell JS. Deposition of inhaled nanoparticles in the rat nasal passages: dose to the olfactory region. Inhal Toxicol. 2009;21(14): 1165–75.
14. Calderon-Garciduenas L, Torres-Jardon R, Kulesza RJ, Park SB, D'Angiulli A. Air pollution and detrimental effects on children's brain. The need for a multidisciplinary approach to the issue complexity and challenges. Front Hum Neurosci. 2014;8:613.
15. Lee K-Y, Cao J-J, Lee C-H, Hsiao T-C, Yeh C-T, Huynh T-T, et al. Inhibition of the WNT/β-catenin pathway by fine particulate matter in haze: roles of metals and polycyclic aromatic hydrocarbons. Atmos Environ. 2015;109:118–29.
16. Luttmann-Gibson H, Sarnat SE, Suh HH, Coull BA, Schwartz J, Zanobetti A, et al. Short-term effects of air pollution on oxygen saturation in a cohort of senior adults in Steubenville, Ohio. J Occup Environ Med. 2014;56(2):149–54.
17. Lee KY, Chiang LL, Ho SC, Liu WT, Chen TT, Feng PH, et al. Associations of autophagy with lung diffusion capacity and oxygen saturation in severe COPD: effects of particulate air pollution. Int J Chron Obstruct Pulmon Dis. 2016;11:1569–78.
18. Chen H, Kwong JC, Copes R, Hystad P, van Donkelaar A, Tu K, et al. Exposure to ambient air pollution and the incidence of dementia: a population-based cohort study. Environ Int. 2017;108:271–7.
19. Shen Y-L, Liu W-T, Lee K-Y, Chuang H-C, Chen H-W, Chuang K-J. Association of PM 2.5 with sleep-disordered breathing from a population-based study in Northern Taiwan urban areas. Environ Pollut. 2018;233:109–13.
20. WHO. WHO Air quality guidelines for particulate matter, ozone, nitrogen dioxide and sulfur dioxide: World Health Organization; 2006. Available from: http://apps.who.int/iris/handle/10665/69477.
21. Chuang HC, Lin YJ, Chou CCK, Hwang JS, Chen CC, Yan YH, et al. Alterations in cardiovascular function by particulate matter in rats using a crossover design. Environ Pollut. 2017;231(Pt 1):812–20.
22. Yan YH, CKC C, Wang JS, Tung CL, Li YR, Lo K, et al. Subchronic effects of inhaled ambient particulate matter on glucose homeostasis and target organ damage in a type 1 diabetic rat model. Toxicol Appl Pharmacol. 2014; 281(2):211–20.
23. Reche C, Viana M, Brines M, Perez N, Beddows D, Alastuey A, et al. Determinants of aerosol lung-deposited surface area variation in an urban environment. Sci Total Environ. 2015;517:38–47.
24. Casanova R, Wang X, Reyes J, Akita Y, Serre ML, Vizuete W, et al. A voxel-based morphometry study reveals local brain structural alterations associated with ambient fine particles in older women. Front Hum Neurosci. 2016;10:495.
25. Chen JC, Wang X, Wellenius GA, Serre ML, Driscoll I, Casanova R, et al. Ambient air pollution and neurotoxicity on brain structure: evidence from women's health initiative memory study. Ann Neurol. 2015;78(3):466–76.
26. Suwannasual U, Lucero J, McDonald JD, Lund AK. Exposure to traffic-generated air pollutants mediates alterations in brain microvascular integrity in wildtype mice on a high-fat diet. Environ Res. 2018;160:449–61.
27. Nag S, Manias JL, Stewart DJ. Pathology and new players in the pathogenesis of brain edema. Acta Neuropathol. 2009;118(2):197–217.
28. Michinaga S, Koyama Y. Pathogenesis of brain edema and investigation into anti-edema drugs. Int J Mol Sci. 2015;16(5):9949–75.
29. Liang D, Bhatta S, Gerzanich V, Simard JM. Cytotoxic edema: mechanisms of pathological cell swelling. Neurosurg Focus. 2007;22(5):E2.
30. Brooks PJ. Brain atrophy and neuronal loss in alcoholism: a role for DNA damage? Neurochem Int. 2000;37(5–6):403–12.
31. Montagne A, Barnes SR, Sweeney MD, Halliday MR, Sagare AP, Zhao Z, et al. Blood-brain barrier breakdown in the aging human hippocampus. Neuron. 2015;85(2):296–302.
32. van de Haar HJ, Burgmans S, Jansen JF, van Osch MJ, van Buchem MA, Muller M, et al. Blood-brain barrier leakage in patients with early Alzheimer disease. Radiology. 2016;281(2):527–35.
33. van de Haar HJ, Jansen JFA, van Osch MJP, van Buchem MA, Muller M, Wong SM, et al. Neurovascular unit impairment in early Alzheimer's disease measured with magnetic resonance imaging. Neurobiol Aging. 2016;45:190–6.
34. Chen Y, Garcia GE, Huang W, Constantini S. The involvement of secondary neuronal damage in the development of neuropsychiatric disorders following brain insults. Front Neurol. 2014;5:22.
35. Tallon LA, Manjourides J, Pun VC, Salhi C, Suh H. Cognitive impacts of ambient air pollution in the National Social Health and aging project (NSHAP) cohort. Environ Int. 2017;104:102–9.
36. Fonken LK, Xu X, Weil ZM, Chen G, Sun Q, Rajagopalan S, et al. Air pollution impairs cognition, provokes depressive-like behaviors and alters hippocampal cytokine expression and morphology. Mol Psychiatry. 2011; 16(10):987–95 73.
37. Albert MS, DeKosky ST, Dickson D, Dubois B, Feldman HH, Fox NC, et al. The diagnosis of mild cognitive impairment due to Alzheimer's disease: recommendations from the National Institute on Aging-Alzheimer's

Association workgroups on diagnostic guidelines for Alzheimer's disease. Alzheimers Dementia. 2011;7(3):270–9.
38. Benz N, Hatz F, Bousleiman H, Ehrensperger MM, Gschwandtner U, Hardmeier M, et al. Slowing of EEG background activity in Parkinson's and Alzheimer's disease with early cognitive dysfunction. Front Aging Neurosci. 2014;6:314.
39. Garn H, Waser M, Deistler M, Benke T, Dal-Bianco P, Ransmayr G, et al. Quantitative EEG markers relate to Alzheimer's disease severity in the prospective dementia registry Austria (PRODEM). Clin Neurophysiol. 2015; 126(3):505–13.
40. Czigler B, Csikos D, Hidasi Z, Anna Gaal Z, Csibri E, Kiss E, et al. Quantitative EEG in early Alzheimer's disease patients - power spectrum and complexity features. Int J Psychophysiol. 2008;68(1):75–80.
41. Cruts B, van Etten L, Tornqvist H, Blomberg A, Sandstrom T, Mills NL, et al. Exposure to diesel exhaust induces changes in EEG in human volunteers. Part Fibre Toxicol. 2008;5:4.
42. Lizio R, Vecchio F, Frisoni GB, Ferri R, Rodriguez G, Babiloni C. Electroencephalographic rhythms in Alzheimer's disease. Int J Alzheimers Dis. 2011;2011:927573.
43. Rosano C, Marsland AL, Gianaros PJ. Maintaining brain health by monitoring inflammatory processes: a mechanism to promote successful aging. Aging Dis. 2012;3(1):16–33.
44. BéruBé KA, Aufderheide M, Breheny D, Clothier R, Combes R, Duffin R, et al. In vitro models of inhalation toxicity and disease: the report of a FRAME workshop. ATLA. 2009;37(1):89.
45. Chen LC, Lippmann M. Effects of metals within ambient air particulate matter (PM) on human health. Inhal Toxicol. 2009;21(1):1–31.
46. Calderon-Garciduenas L, Reed W, Maronpot RR, Henriquez-Roldan C, Delgado-Chavez R, Calderon-Garciduenas A, et al. Brain inflammation and Alzheimer's-like pathology in individuals exposed to severe air pollution. Toxicol Pathol. 2004;32(6):650–8.
47. Coburn JL, Cole TB, Dao KT, Costa LG. Acute exposure to diesel exhaust impairs adult neurogenesis in mice: prominence in males and protective effect of pioglitazone. Arch Toxicol. 2018;92(5):1815–29.
48. Liu X, Qian X, Xing J, Wang J, Sun Y, Wang Q, et al. Particulate matter triggers depressive-like response associated with modulation of inflammatory cytokine homeostasis and brain-derived neurotrophic factor signaling pathway in mice. Toxicol Sci. 2018;164(1):278–288.
49. Hoefer J, Luger M, Dal-Pont C, Culig Z, Schennach H, Jochberger S. The "aging factor" Eotaxin-1 (CCL11) is detectable in transfusion blood products and increases with the Donor's age. Front Aging Neurosci. 2017;9:402.
50. Gadani SP, Cronk JC, Norris GT, Kipnis J. IL-4 in the brain: a cytokine to remember. J Immunol. 2012;189(9):4213–9.
51. Serrano-Pozo A, Frosch MP, Masliah E, Hyman BT. Neuropathological alterations in Alzheimer disease. Cold Spring Harb Perspect Med. 2011; 1(1):a006189.
52. Chesser AS, Pritchard SM, Johnson GV. Tau clearance mechanisms and their possible role in the pathogenesis of Alzheimer disease. Front Neurol. 2013;4:122.
53. Levesque S, Surace MJ, McDonald J, Block ML. Air pollution & the brain: subchronic diesel exhaust exposure causes neuroinflammation and elevates early markers of neurodegenerative disease. J Neuroinflammation. 2011;8:105.
54. Levine B, Kroemer G. Autophagy in the pathogenesis of disease. Cell. 2008; 132(1):27–42.
55. Mayer SA, Coplin WM, Raps EC. Cerebral edema, intracranial pressure, and herniation syndromes. J Stroke Cerebrovasc Dis. 1999;8(3):183–91.
56. Alvis Miranda H, Castellar-Leones SM, Elzain MA, Moscote-Salazar LR. Brain abscess: current management. J Neurosci Rural Pract. 2013;4(Suppl 1):S67–81.
57. Li N, Wang M, Bramble LA, Schmitz DA, Schauer JJ, Sioutas C, et al. The adjuvant effect of ambient particulate matter is closely reflected by the particulate oxidant potential. Environ Health Perspect. 2009;117(7):1116–23.
58. George Paxinos CW. The rat brain in stereotaxic coordinates: sixth edition-academic press; 2007.
59. Antunes M, Biala G. The novel object recognition memory: neurobiology, test procedure, and its modifications. Cogn Process. 2012; 13(2):93–110.
60. Fleming SA, Monaikul S, Patsavas AJ, Waworuntu RV, Berg BM, Dilger RN. Dietary polydextrose and galactooligosaccharide increase exploratory behavior, improve recognition memory, and alter neurochemistry in the young pig. Nutr Neurosci. 2017:18:1–14.
61. Sitnikova E, Hramov AE, Grubov V, Koronovsky AA. Rhythmic activity in EEG and sleep in rats with absence epilepsy. Brain Res Bull. 2015;120:106–16.
62. Goldberger AL, Amaral LA, Glass L, Hausdorff JM, Ivanov PC, Mark RG, et al. PhysioBank, PhysioToolkit, and PhysioNet: components of a new research resource for complex physiologic signals. Circulation. 2000;101(23):E215–20.
63. Chen BC, Chang YS, Kang JC, Hsu MJ, Sheu JR, Chen TL, et al. Peptidoglycan induces nuclear factor-kappaB activation and cyclooxygenase-2 expression via Ras, Raf-1, and ERK in RAW 264.7 macrophages. J Biol Chem. 2004; 279(20):20889–97.

13

Pulmonary exposure to carbonaceous nanomaterials and sperm quality

Astrid Skovmand[1,2], Anna Jacobsen Lauvås[2], Preben Christensen[3], Ulla Vogel[1,4], Karin Sørig Hougaard[1,5] and Sandra Goericke-Pesch[2*]

Abstract

Background: Semen quality parameters are potentially affected by nanomaterials in several ways: Inhaled nanosized particles are potent inducers of pulmonary inflammation, leading to the release of inflammatory mediators. Small amounts of particles may translocate from the lungs into the lung capillaries, enter the systemic circulation and ultimately reach the testes. Both the inflammatory response and the particles may induce oxidative stress which can directly affect spermatogenesis. Furthermore, spermatogenesis may be indirectly affected by changes in the hormonal milieu as systemic inflammation is a potential modulator of endocrine function. The aim of this study was to investigate the effects of pulmonary exposure to carbonaceous nanomaterials on sperm quality parameters in an experimental mouse model.

Methods: Effects on sperm quality after pulmonary inflammation induced by carbonaceous nanomaterials were investigated by intratracheally instilling sexually mature male NMRI mice with four different carbonaceous nanomaterials dispersed in nanopure water: graphene oxide (18 µg/mouse/i.t.), Flammruss 101, Printex 90 and SRM1650b (0.1 mg/mouse/i.t. each) weekly for seven consecutive weeks. Pulmonary inflammation was determined by differential cell count in bronchoalveolar lavage fluid. Epididymal sperm concentration and motility were measured by computer-assisted sperm analysis. Epididymal sperm viability and morphological abnormalities were assessed manually using Hoechst 33,342/PI flourescent and Spermac staining, respectively. Epididymal sperm were assessed with regard to sperm DNA integrity (damage). Daily sperm production was measured in the testis, and testosterone levels were measured in blood plasma by ELISA.

Results: Neutrophil numbers in the bronchoalveolar fluid showed sustained inflammatory response in the nanoparticle-exposed groups one week after the last instillation. No significant changes in epididymal sperm parameters, daily sperm production or plasma testosterone levels were found.

Conclusion: Despite the sustained pulmonary inflammatory response, an eight week exposure to graphene oxide, Flammruss 101, Printex 90 and the diesel particle SRM1650b in the present study did not appear to affect semen parameters, daily sperm production or testosterone concentration in male NMRI mice.

Keywords: Nanomaterials, Particles, Toxicity, Semen parameters, Pulmonary exposure, Computer-assisted sperm analysis, Inflammation

* Correspondence: Sandra.Goericke-Pesch@tiho-hannover.de
[2]Section for Veterinary Reproduction and Obstetrics, Department of Veterinary Clinical Sciences, University of Copenhagen, Dyrlægvej 68, DK-1870 Frederiksberg C, Denmark
Full list of author information is available at the end of the article

Background

The use and development of nanotechnology have been rapidly increasing. The ever expanding application of nanomaterials (NMs) includes areas such as cosmetics, electronics and food science, and as a result, men in the reproductive age are potentially exposed to nanomaterials both as workers in the various industries and as consumers. Likewise, the general public can also be exposed due to the release of nanoparticles (NPs) into the environment from natural and anthropogenic sources. The male germ line is highly sensitive to toxic insults and a number of environmental toxicants, such as ionizing radiation, organic solvents, and heavy metals, markedly decrease semen quality [1]. The apparent worldwide decline in semen quality, a controversial and often debated statement, has been reported by several researchers [2–4]. Linear regression analysis of 138 published reports from Europe, North and South America, and Asia between 1980 and 2015 showed a 57% decrease in mean sperm concentration in men [4]. Danish researchers, for example, have reported a decreasing trend and although recent monitoring programs now document a slight increase in semen quality in young Danish men, only one out of four has optimal semen quality [3]. Air pollution and its particulate constituents have been associated with several adverse health effects, mainly pulmonary and cardiovascular diseases [5]. Epidemiological studies of adult men have, however, also found that elevated levels of air pollution are associated with decreased sperm motility, increased percentages of morphologically abnormal sperm, and elevated levels of DNA damage in sperm [6, 7]. Consequently, the question of whether NMs can affect male fertility by decreasing semen quality parameters merits further investigation.

The mechanisms how inhaled NMs may affect semen quality are yet to be elucidated. It has been hypothesised that NMs may affect semen quality in several ways: when inhaled, particles are potent inducers of pulmonary inflammation, which may result in the release of inflammatory mediators into the blood stream. Small amounts of particles may also translocate from the lungs into the lung capillaries and enter the blood stream [8]. The systemic inflammation may weaken the integrity of the blood-testis-barrier and increase its permeability, ultimately allowing NMs that have deposited in the testis to enter the lumen of the seminiferous tubules [9]. An inflammatory response in the testis may be induced due to infection, trauma and/or environmental toxins. Accordingly, it may be possible that NMs in the testis may elicit a testicular inflammatory response and thus possibly activate resident macrophages or result in an influx of neutrophils and other leukocytes [10]. Particles and leukocytes may create a Reactive Oxygen Species (ROS)/antioxidant imbalance, as both the particles and the leukocytes are strong inducers of ROS [11]. High levels of oxidative stress have been hypothesised to be a major cause for male infertility, because spermatozoa are highly sensitive to oxidative damage [12].

Exposure to NMs may also indirectly affect spermatogenesis by affecting the hormonal milieu via effects on the hypathalamic-pituitay-gonadal axis, as this axis is sensitive to inflammation. In female mice, it has been recently shown that airway exposure to multi-walled carbon nanotubes can interfere with the estrous cycle by either direct action of the particles or indirectly by the influence of inflammatory and acute phase responses [13]. NP-rich diesel exhaust inhalation exposure (5 h/day, 5 days/week) of adult male Fisher 344 rats increased plasma testosterone levels, possibly due to the induction of testosterone biosynthesis through elevation of StAR and P450scc in the testis via growth hormone signaling. Interestingly, the NP-rich diesel exhaust did not show dose-dependent effects, high levels of testosterone were found at the low (2.27×10^5 /cm^3) and medium (5.11×10^5 /cm^3) exposure levels whereas testosterone concentrations remained unchanged at the high (1.36×10^6 /cm^3) exposure level [14]. In ICR mice, inhalation exposure (12 h/day for 6 months) to diesel exhaust at 0.3, 1 and 3 mg DEP/m^3, has been shown to cause degenerative and necrotic changes in the testis, desquamation of the seminiferous tubules and loss of spermatozoa, degenerative changes in Leydig cells such as the appearance of myelin, lipid droplets and secondary lysosomes, and a reduction in daily sperm production (DSP) [15]. In the same strain, 10 weekly exposures to 0.1 mg/mouse by intratracheal instillation (i.t.) of three different sizes of carbon black (CB) NPs (14, 56, and 95 nm) were shown to significantly decrease DSP, increase testosterone levels and cause vacuolation of the seminiferous tubules [16]. Following intratracheal instillation of 2 mg/kg (every 3 days for 45 days) of silica particles (57 nm), particles have been observed to cross the blood-testis-barrier in C57BL/6 mice using transmission electron microscopy. The silica NPs decreased sperm concentration and motility, and increased sperm abnormalities. Testicular malondialdehyde and 3-nitrotyrosine levels were increased, whereas SOD activity was impaired; suggesting that the damage may have arisen due to oxidative stress in the testis [17].

Based on these findings, we hypothesised that airway exposure to nanomaterials may interfere with normal spermatogenesis and decrease the quality of sperm, potentially altering male reproductive function. To further investigate and characterize these effects, sexually mature NMRI male mice were exposed to four carbonaceus NMs with different shape, size and surface chemistry and the effects on sperm quality parameters and testosterone concentrations were investigated.

Methods

Experimental design

One hundred and five male NMRI mice, purchased from Taconic Biosciences Inc. (Ejby, Denmark), were acclimatized for one week prior to the commencement of the experimental procedures, which began when the mice were eight weeks of age. The mice were randomly divided into 7 groups ($n = 15$): graphene oxide, Flammruss 101, Printex 90, SRM1650b, vehicle (nanopure water) controls, unhandled controls and high fat diet (HFD) controls. The graphene oxide, Flammruss 101, Printex 90 and SRM1650b exposed animals were intratracheally instilled with 50 μl of particle suspension followed by 200 μl of air under general anesthesia with 3–4% isoflurane mixed with sterile filtered air as described by Jackson et al. [18]. The mice were instilled once a week for seven consecutive weeks and the study was terminated six to eight days after the last exposure resulting in a total exposure time of 1.6 spermatogenic cycles, as one spermatogenic cycle corresponds to ~35 days in mice. All the mice in the CB and diesel exhaust particle groups received the same dose of 0.1 mg/mouse per instillation, corresponding to a cumulative dose of 0.7 mg during the study period. The current occupational exposure limit in Denmark is 3.5 mg/m^3 for CB. However, mean concentrations of 14.90 mg/m^3 of CB have been measured by personal air samplers in the workplace [19]. Based on the observed particle size distribution during aerosolisation of particles [20], at the current occupational exposure limit of 3.5 mg/m^3, the estimated deposited dose is 16.6 μg in mice, giving a weekly deposited dose of 83 μg. [20, 21]. The graphene oxide was administered at a lower dose of 18 μg/mouse per instillation, with a cumulative dose of 126 μg, to ensure that the animal's welfare was not affected, based on previous findings [22]. The vehicle control group was treated as the particle exposed group and received instillations of 50 μl of nanopure water without NMs. The unhandled and HFD control groups did not receive instillations or isoflurane at any time. All 105 animals were randomly euthanized by exsanguination under deep anaesthesia with a cocktail of ZRF (Zoletil 250 mg, Rompun 20 mg/ml and Fentanyl 50 mg/ml in sterile isotone saline) at a dose of 0.01 ml per g body weight. Due to logistical reasons half of the mice in each group were euthanized six or eight days after the last instillation. Testicles and epididymides were collected and weighed separately. The right testicle was snap frozen in liquid nitrogen and the left testicle was stored in Bouin's fixation solution. The head and tail of the epididymides were separated; the right and left head and the right tail were snap frozen individually. The left tail was used for sperm retrieval (see below).

The mice were housed individually in clear 1290D euro standard type 3 cages with aspen sawdust bedding (Tapvei, Estonia) and enrichment, nesting material (Enviro Dri, Lillico, Biotechnology, UK), mouse house (80-ACRE011, Techniplast, Italy) and small aspen blocks (Tapvei, Estonia). Housing conditions were kept constant, with a 12:12 h light and dark cycle at an average temperature of 22 °C and 55% humidity. Tap water and standard pellet diet Altromin no. 1324 (Brogaarden, Denmark) were provided ad libitum to all groups, except for the HFD control group which received a 60% kcal fat diet ad libitum upon arrival and throughout the study (RD Western Diet D12492, Open Source Diets, Brogaarden, Denmark). All experimental procedures followed the handling guidelines established by the Danish government and permits from the Experimental Animal Inspectorate (no. 201515-0201-00465 and 2015-15-0201-00569). Prior to the study, specific experimental protocols were approved by the local Animal Ethics Council.

Nanoparticles, preparation and characterization

The physico-chemical properties of the studied particles have been assessed and reported previously [23–25] and are summarized in Table 1. The graphene oxide in aqueous suspension was manufactured and supplied by Graphenea (San Sebastian, Spain) and has been previously characterized in detail in Bengtson et al. [23]. In suspension it appears as flat plates consisting of mainly two to three stacked graphene layers with a lateral size of 2–3 μm. The specific surface area has not been reported, but the corresponding reduced graphene oxide had a specific surface area of 338–411 m^2/g [23]. The Flammruss 101 and Printex 90 carbon black NPs in powder form were gifts from Boesens Fabrikker ApS (Denmark) and Degussa (Germany), respectively, and have been previously characterized in detail by Saber et al. [24]. Flammruss 101 consists of spherical particles with a primary particle diameter of 95 nm and a specific surface area of 23.8 m^2/g [24]. Printex 90 has a similar shape to that of the Flammruss 101, with a reported primary particle diameter of 14 nm and a specific surface area of 295–338 m^2/g [24]. The diesel exhaust particle (SRM1650b) is a standard reference material and the certificate of analysis is available from the National Institute of Standards & Technology (Gaithersburg, MD, USA, https://www.nist.gov/). It is an exhaust particle from a heavy duty diesel engine with a reported primary particle diameter of 18–30 nm and a specific surface area of 108 m^2/g [25]. Unlike the other three particles, the SRM1650b has a high content of adhered heavy metals and polycyclic aromatic hydrocarbons (PAHs) i.e.

Table 1 Summary of particle characteristics

Particle	Primary particle size	Shape	Surface area	Z-average (in nanopure water)	Reference
Graphene oxide	Lateral size: 2–3 μm Thickness: 2 nm	flat plates consisting of mainly two to three stacked graphene layers	338–411 m^2/g (reduced graphene oxide)	486.7 nm	[31]
Flammruss 101	95 nm	spherical	23.8 m^2/g	305.4 nm	[32]
Printex 90	14 nm	spherical	295–338 m^2/g	147.2 nm	[32]
SRM1650b	18–30 nm	spherical	108 m^2/g		[33]

a ~3000 fold higher content of PAHs compared to Printex 90 [25].

For instillation, the particles were dispersed in nanopure water at a concentration of 2 mg/ml and sonicated for 16 min on ice using a 400 W Branson Sonifier A-450D (Branson Ultrasonic Corp., Danbury, CT, USA) equipped with a disruptor horn (Model 101–147-037). The hydrodynamic particle size distribution in nanopure water was measured by dynamic light scattering using a Malvern Zetasizer Nano ZS equipped with a 633 nm He-Ne Laser (Malvern Inc., UK).

Bronchoalveolar lavage

Bronchoalveolar lavage fluid (BALF) differential cell counts were performed as previously described in Kyjovska et al. [26]. The BALF was collected for 12 of the 15 mice per particle exposed group as the lungs of 3 mice per group were collected for histology. The trachea of the mice ($n = 12$ per group) was exposed and cannulated with a 22 gauge BD Insyte catheter. The lungs were flushed twice with 0.8 ml of 0.9% saline in a 1 ml syringe. The BALF was centrifuged at 400 g at 4 °C for 10 min. The cell pellet was re-suspended in 100 μl of Ham's F-12 Nutrient Mix cell culture medium. Total cells were counted using a NucleoCounter (Chemometec, NucleoCounter NC-200). For the differential cell counts 50 μl of the BALF cell suspension were pipetted onto glass slides and spun at 1000 rpm for 4 min in a cytospin centrifuge. The slides were fixated and then stained with May-Grünwald Eosin-Methyleneblue and Giemsa Azur-Eosin-Methylene Blue solution. Differential cell counts were performed under a bright field microscope using oil immersion and a 1000× magnification.

Collection of epididymal sperm and computer-assisted sperm analysis of concentration, motility and viability

The left epididymal tail was placed in 500 μl warm (37 ° C) TCM199 medium (Sigma-Aldrich, Denmark) and minced with scissors. The sperm cells were allowed to swim out for 10 min and were then filtered through a stainless steel mesh. Samples were kept at 37 °C on a heating stage during the whole procedure including microscopy analysis. Computer-assisted sperm analysis (CASA) was performed using a negative phase contrast microscope (Olympus BX60, Tokyo, Japan) equipped with a heating stage and a high-speed GigE camera (avA21000-100gc) with a CCD sensor (aviator series, Basler, Germany) detecting 101 frames/s and the AndroVision software (Ref 12,500/0000, Software Version 1.0.0.9, Minitube, Tiefenbach, Germany). For analysis of concentration and motility, an aliquot of the diluted semen (2.0 μl) was pipetted into an evaluation chamber (Leja ® Standard Count 4 Chamber Slide, 10μm, Leja Products B. V., Nieuw Vennep, The Netherlands) and 10 randomly distributed fields were analysed at 200× magnification. The software calculated the sperm concentration per mL and analysed the sperm motility parameters. Motility results were presented as the total percentage of motile spermatozoa and the percentage of progressively motile spermatozoa. The following settings on the CASA system were used: sperm recognition area 10–100 μm^2, 10 fields per sample, TM = PM + LM, PM = CM+ slow motility + fast motility, LM: velocity curved line (VCL) < $80 \times 10^4 \mu/s$ and velocity straight line (VSL) < $20 \times 10^4 \mu/s$, Circular Motility: linearity <0.6000 and rotation >0.8000.

Additionally, another aliquot (50 μl) of the diluted semen was added to 1.5 μl of ready to use Hoechst 33,342/PI fluorescent stain (Minitube) and incubated at 37 °C for 15 min. The viability was analyzed manually by counting 200 sperm per sample using a fluorescent microscope fitted with a U-MU filter cube and a mercury burner. The results were presented as percentage of viable spermatozoa. Blue sperm were considered as viable, whereas red were considered as non-viable (www.minitube.com).

Sperm morphology

Native semen smears were prepared, air-dried, fixated and stained with Spermac® according to the manufacturer's instructions (Minitube). 200 spermatozoa were identified and categorized as normal or as having a morphological deviation. Deviations were differentiated into sperm acrosome, head, neck, mid-piece or tail defects, cytoplasmic droplets or loose heads. In case of several morphological deviations in one sperm, only the one considered as the most severe was recorded. The exposure status of the samples on morphology was blinded to the scorer. The results were presented as percentage of abnormal spermatozoa in the respective location as well as total percentage of normal spermatozoa as defined by 100% - each % of abnormalities in the respective locations.

Sperm DNA integrity

Neat epididymal semen samples were diluted 1:2 with TNE buffer (0.01 M Tris-Cl, 0.15 M NaCl, 1 mM EDTA, pH 7.4) and frozen directly at −196 °C in a dryshipper and transported to the laboratory. The fluorescent staining was performed according to the protocol for the sperm chromatin structure assay as described by Evenson and Jost 2000 [27]. Semen samples were thawed at 35 °C for 3 min and were then incubated on ice for 5 min [28]. An aliquot of the thawed sample was diluted to a concentration of 2×10^6 sperm/mL with TNE buffer to a total volume of 200 μL. DNA denaturation was induced by addition of 400 μL acid detergent solution (0.08 M HCl, 0.15 M NaCl, 0.1% *v*/v Triton X-100, pH 1.2). After 30 s, 1.20 mL of acridine orange staining solution (Citric acid 0.037 M, Na_2HPO_4 0.126 M, NaCl 0.15 M, Na_2EDTA 1 mM, pH 6.0) were added. The sample was immediately placed in the flow cytometer and run through the system to allow for equilibration prior to acquisition of data. The samples were blinded and analyzed using a FACSCalibur (BD Biosciences) flow cytometer with an air-cooled argon orthogonal laser operating at 488 nm with 15 mW of power. After transiting a 560 nm short-pass dichroic mirror, the green fluorescence (FL1) was collected through a 515 to 545 nm band-pass filter and the red fluorescence (FL3) through a 650 nm long-pass filter. The sheath/sample was set to "high" with an estimated flow rate of 60 μl/min. This flow rate resulted in analysis of approximately 200 events per second. Acquisition of 5000 events was started exactly 3 min after initiation of the acid detergent treatment at a point in time when the sample had been running through the flow system for approximately 2.5 min to achieve equilibration. To ensure good quality control, each analysis was run in duplicate and results were only accepted, if the standard deviation (SD) between duplicates was below 2.5%. If variation exceeded 2.5%, two new aliquots were analyzed. If the event rate was above the expected 200 events per second, a new dilution and staining cycle was performed to ensure an event rate below 200 and thus an optimal ratio between acridine orange molecules and DNA. The results of the analyses were reported as DFI% which describes the proportion of sperm with a detectable level of DNA damage after acid denaturation.

Daily sperm production

The adipose tissue from the frozen testes was trimmed and the tunica albuginea was peeled off with forceps after making a shallow longitudinal incision. The testes were weighed, placed into 4 ml of 0.05% TRITON-X100 and homogenized for 3 min using the IKAULTRA TURRAX T25 disperser S25 N-10G. Homogenates were kept on ice for 30 min. 200 μl of the homogenate were mixed with 200 μl of 0.04% Trypan blue and left for 5 min at room temperature. Sperm heads were counted using a Bürker counting chamber. DSP was calculated using the following formulas:

N = sperm number per μl x volume of lysis (buffer)

DSP = N / 4.84

where N is the total number of spermatids per sample. The DSP is then calculated by dividing the total number of spermatids per sample by 4.84, which is the number of days for a spermatid to develop through stages 14 to 16, i.e., the stages where spermatids are resistant to homogenization. The samples were blinded and counts were done in duplicates. If the two counts deviated by more than 20%, the procedure was repeated for the sample.

Testosterone measurement

Blood was collected from the heart, stabilized using K_2EDTA and then centrifuged at 2500 g for 10 min. The EDTA-plasma was pipetted into separate snapstrip PCR-vials and stored at −80 °C until analysis. The plasma samples were blinded and the testosterone concentrations were determined in duplicates and 1:2 dilutions with phosphate-buffered saline (PBS), using competitive ELISA (RTC001R, Biovendor, Brno, Czech Republic). Samples were analysed following the manufacturer's protocol, with a standard curve in the range of 0.1–25 ng/mL. All samples that fell outside the standard curve were diluted 1:4 in PBS and re-analyzed. (Interassay) coefficient of variance was 4.8–7.8%.

Statistical analysis

An ANOVA was used to test for the overall significance of the BALF counts and was followed by a Dunnett's test where particle exposed and unhandled control groups were compared to the vehicle control (SAS® software, version 9.4 of the SAS system for windows 7 (Cary, NC, USA)). All other data were analyzed by ANOVA, followed by post-hoc Fischer least statistical difference test when appropriate (Origin Pro, version 2016 (64-bit), OriginLab Corp (Northampton, MA, USA)). Results obtained from mice exposed to NMs were compared to those from vehicle-exposed mice, whereas results from HFD mice were compared to those of unhandled controls. The level of significance was set at 0.05. The *a priori* statistical power analysis had been calculated using the 33% ± SD difference in DSP between the Printex 90 and vehicle control exposed mice reported by Yoshida et al. 2008 (16) (G*Power software version 3.1.9.2, Düsseldorf, Germany).

Results

Nanoparticle characterization

The graphene oxide, Flammruss 101 and Printex 90 dispersed in nanopure water at a concentration of 2 mg/ml had a Z-average of 486.7 nm, 305.4 nm and 147.2 nm, respectively. Due to a lack of material the DLS was not performed on the SRM1650b, however, the SRM1650b dispersed in nanopure water at a concentration of 3.24 mg/ml was previously measured to have a Z-average of 167.8 nm (25). The particles characteristics are summarized in Table 1.

Body, testicular and epididymal weights

There was no difference in body weight and absolute and relative organ weight between the groups, except for the HFD controls which had a statistically significantly higher body weight compared to all other groups (Table 2). However, only five out of the 15 mice in the HFD group gained enough weight to be considered obese, which means mice weighing more than 51.27 g, based on the mean weight of the unhandled +2 SD.

Pulmonary inflammation

BALF neutrophil numbers were significantly elevated in the lungs from mice exposed to graphene oxide (51-fold increase), Flammruss 101 (61-fold increase), Printex 90 (329-fold increase) and SRM1650b (78-fold increase) compared to vehicle controls ($p < 0.001$) (Table 3). The unhandled and the HFD were not statistically different from the vehicle control group, confirming that the instillation procedure and the vehicle did not induce pulmonary inflammation. Interestingly, Printex 90 induced a stronger inflammatory response one week after the last instillation compared to the other three NMs. Neutrophil influx was plotted against deposited surface area since surface area may be a more biological relevant dose metric for spherical NMs than mass (see Additional file 1). Neutrophil cell numbers correlated with deposited surface area ($R^2 = 0.64$).

Epididymal sperm concentration, motility, viability, morphology and sperm DNA damage

There was no statistically significant difference between the groups for the epididymal sperm concentration, total and progressive motility, viability (Fig. 1) and sperm DNA damage (DFI, Fig. 2). Furthermore, there was no significant difference between the groups regarding sperm morphology (percentage of sperm acrosome, head, neck, mid-piece and tail defects, cytoplasmic droplets and loose heads) (Table 4).

Daily sperm production and testosterone

There was no statistically significant difference between groups for DSP (Fig. 3) and blood plasma testosterone concentrations (Fig. 4).

Discussion

Knowledge about the effect of NMs on sperm quality is limited, especially following pulmonary exposure. Although various NMs have been reported to induce testicular toxicity and decrease semen quality, mainly oral and intravenous exposures have been investigated [9, 29]. This is somehow striking as inhalation is the major exposure route for NMs in humans, and the systemic inflammation which is induced after a pulmonary exposure may be an important indirect mechanism for the induction of testicular toxicity. In the current study, male mice were exposed via the lungs to four different carbonaceous NMs and the effects of these NMs on sperm quality parameters, measured as epidydimal sperm concentration, viability, motility, morphology, sperm DNA damage, DSP, and plasma testosterone concentrations, were investigated.

At a final cumulative dose of 700 μg/mouse (126 μg for graphene oxide), the significant influxes of PMNs demonstrate pulmonary inflammation one week post exposure compared to the three control groups. Previous studies showed that instilled Printex 90 at a final cumulative dose of 268 μg/mouse induced lung inflammation in terms of increased neutrophil influx and expression of

Table 2 Body weight (g), and absolute (mg) and relative weights of left testis and epididymis at the time of euthanasia

	Body weight (g)	Testis weight (mg)	Testis relative weight	Epididymal weight (mg)	Epididymal relative weight
Vehicle control	39.39 ± 3.19	107.67 ± 6.61	2.75 ± 0.23	45.33 ± 6.21	1.15 ± 0.14
Graphene oxide	40.26 ± 3.82	103.10 ± 14.03	2.58 ± 0.37	43.29 ± 6.33	1.08 ± 0.14
Flammruss 101	39.91 ± 4.23	107.91 ± 15.43	2.71 ± 0.42	39.49 ± 9.32	0.98 ± 0.18
Printex 90	37.96 ± 2.15	107.91 ± 10.34	2.85 ± 0.25	43.71 ± 3.97	1.15 ± 0.11
SRM1650b	40.08 ± 3.50	103.14 ± 17.46	2.58 ± 0.42	41.09 ± 12.41	1.09 ± 0.13
Unhandled	42.97 ± 4.15	107.78 ± 11.14	2.53 ± 0.32	45.03 ± 2.48	1.06 ± 0.13
High fat diet	50.09 ± 6.34[a]	111.77 ± 7.45	2.26 ± 0.28	46.16 ± 3.09	0.93 ± 0.12

Mean ± SD ($n = 15$).
[a] < 0.001, compared with vehicle control

Table 3 Pulmonary inflammation presented as total cell, macrophage and neutrophil counts in the BALF 6 to 8 days after the last instillation

	Total cells ($\times 10^5$)	Macrophages ($\times 10^5$)	Neutrophils ($\times 10^5$)
Vehicle control	10.95 ± 0.73	10.58 ± 0.73	0.04 ± 0.02
Graphene oxide	16.21 ± 1.15[a]	13.39 ± 0.97	2.07 ± 0.39[b]
Flammruss 101	11.89 ± 2.09	8.85 ± 0.79	2.47 ± 1.46[b]
Printex 90	27.90 ± 2.96[b]	19.09 ± 2.06	13.19 ± 1.11[b]
SRM1650b	14.78 ± 1.24	10.90 ± 0.83	3.15 ± 0.56[b]
Unhandled	12.56 ± 1.25	12.07 ± 1.24	0.11 ± 0.02
High fat diet	10.92 ± 0.91	10.18 ± 0.92	0.07 ± 0.03

Mean ± SD (n = 13–15)
[a] < 0.05, [b] < 0.001, compared with vehicle control

inflammatory and acute phase response both at mRNA and protein levels in the lung, including increased expression of chemokine ligand 5 (Cxcl5), serum amyloid A 3 (Saa3), immunoglobulin joining chain (Igj) and lymphocyte antigen 6 complex, locus F (Ly6f) [30]. This reflects that at high levels of CB exposure there is a pro-inflammatory response and an adaptive immune response. Based on our previous results, the observed neutrophil influx would suggest systemic inflammation at the applied cumulative dose levels. Despite the pulmonary inflammatory response we did not identify statistically significant differences in the investigated sperm parameters and testosterone concentrations between the particle exposed and vehicle control group.

Our results are in direct contrast to those described by Yoshida et al. (2008) who, at similar dose levels as in the present study, reported reduced DSP, seminiferous tubules damage and increased testosterone concentrations in ICR mice following ten instillations of Printex 90, and reduced DSP and seminiferous tubules damage following ten instillations of Flammruss 101 NPs [16]. The reason for this discrepancy is not clear. There are, however, major differences between the two studies in reference to mouse strain (NMRI versus ICR), number of instillations (seven versus ten), sampling time (24 h versus 6–8 days after the last instillation), and the vehicle used for the dispersion of particles (nanopure water versus saline with 0.05% tween 80).

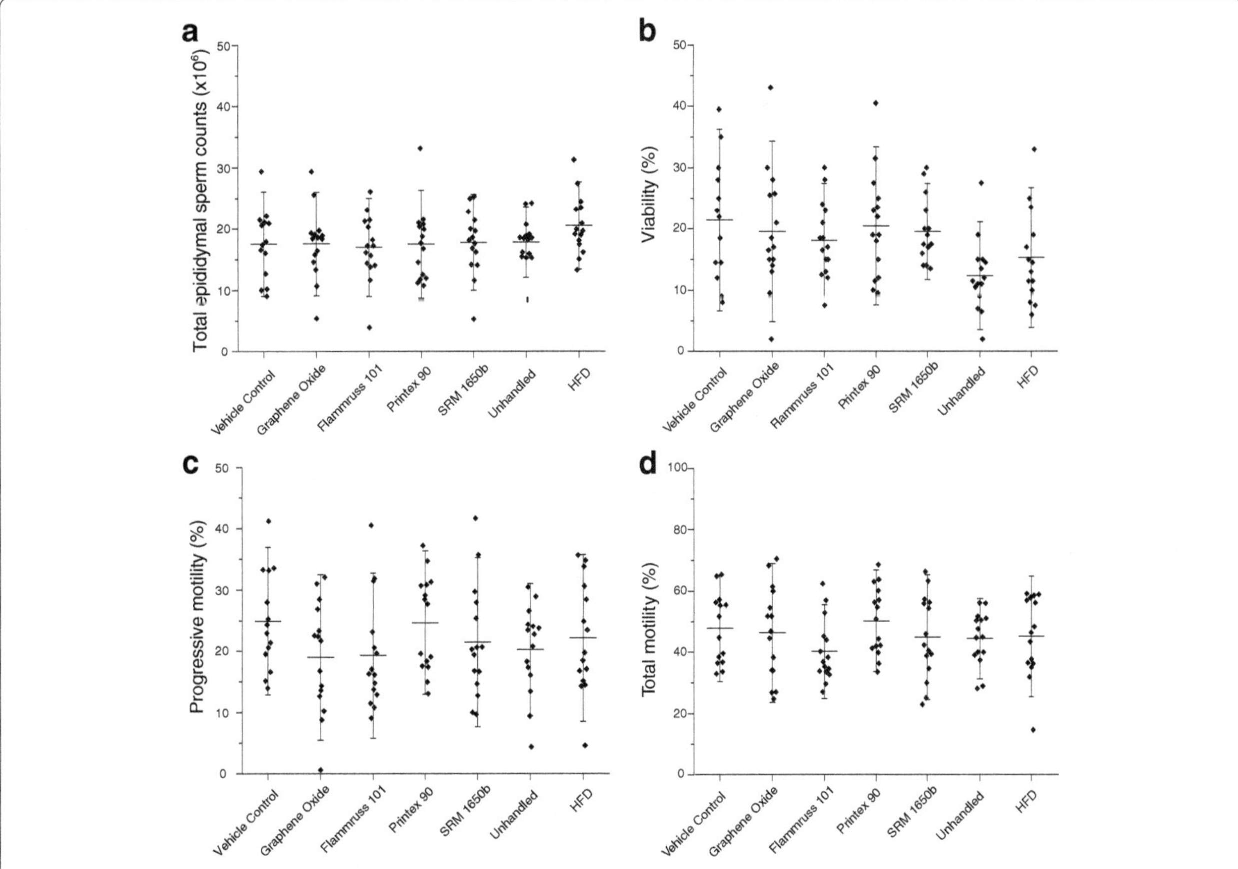

Fig. 1 Epididymal sperm parameters analysed from the left epididymal tail. **a** Total epididymal sperm counts ($\times 10^6$) **b** Viable sperm (%) **c** Progressive motility (%) **d** Total motility (%). Mean ± SD (n = 14–15)

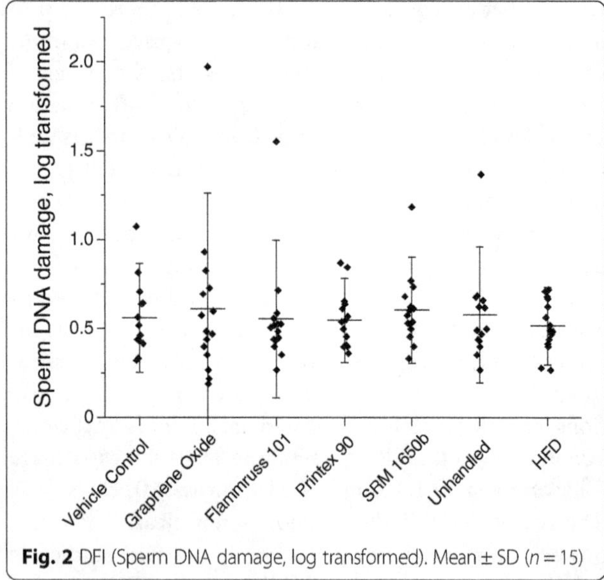

Fig. 2 DFI (Sperm DNA damage, log transformed). Mean ± SD ($n = 15$)

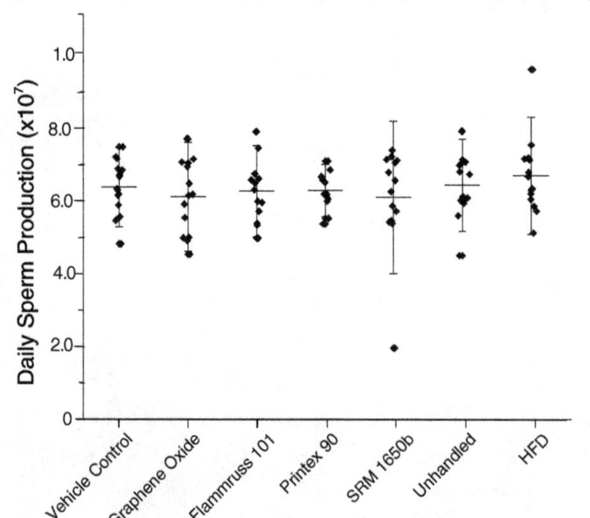

Fig. 3 Daily sperm production derived as spermatids in developmental stage 14 to 16 measured in the left testicle ($\times 10^7$ spermatids). Mean ± SD ($n = 13$–15)

The use of different vehicles and dispersants warrants important consideration in studies of male reproductive toxicity of NMs, because the vehicle can potentially change the chemical and physical properties of the particles and thereby influence their bioavailability and thus their potential for toxic insult. Surfactant molecules, like tween, have both lipophilic and hydrophilic properties and are therefore able to partition between lipid and protein structures; they are also known to enhance permeability because of their effects on tight junctions and cellular membranes [31]. Studies in male mice dosed intravenously with graphene oxide (1000 μg/ml) with or without 1% tween 80 showed that graphene oxide alone appeared to have a higher retention in the lungs compared to the graphene oxide with tween 80. In contrast, increased amounts of graphene oxide with tween 80 appeared to be retained in the liver. The authors concluded that tween 80 changes the zeta potential of particles and enables particles, like graphene oxide, to pass the capillary bed without massive deposition in the lungs [32]. Interestingly, no aggregates of graphene oxide or histopathological changes were found in the testis from mice in any of the graphene groups [32]. Nevertheless, Akhavan et al. [33] found accumulation of graphene oxide in the testis accompanied by significantly decreased epididymal sperm viability and motility, and increased sperm DNA damage and ROS generation in semen after an intravenous administration to BALB/c mice at a dose of 4 mg/kg of graphene oxide dispersed in PBS and DSPE-PEG-NH_2 polymers. On the other hand, Liang et al. [34] found that intravenous administration of graphene oxide dispersed in PBS alone at 6.25, 12.5 and 25 mg/kg to ICR mice had no effect on epididymal sperm motility, morphology, concentration, male endogenous sex hormone and histology in the testis. Similarly, 10 instillations of Printex 90 dispered in 0.05% tween 80 caused adverse effects on reproductive parameters [16], whereas 7 instillations of Printex 90 dispered in nanopure water alone did not (present study).

Table 4 Percentages of normal spermatozoa and of spermatozoa with morphological defects in the acrosome, head, neck, mid-piece or tail region, those having a cytoplasmic droplet and a loose head

	Normal (%)	Acrosome (%)	Head (%)	Neck (%)	Mid-piece (%)	Tail (%)	Cytoplasmic droplets (%)	Loose heads (%)
Vehicle control	30.64 ± 10.0	16.7 ± 10.3	3.00 ± 2.5	5.39 ± 2.4	3.07 ± 3.8	33.54 ± 8.2	3.29 ± 4.8	4.32 ± 3.5
Graphene oxide	24.50 ± 13.5	12.17 ± 12.2	2.77 ± 2.7	7.77 ± 7.7	4.83 ± 7.1	39.57 ± 15.2	2.37 ± 2.3	6.03 ± 5.6
Flammruss 101	29.86 ± 8.1	17.32 ± 12.1	4.32 ± 2.5	4.68 ± 2.4	0.82 ± 1.0	35.36 ± 12.0	2.28 ± 3.1	5.35 ± 2.5
Printex 90	28.23 ± 10.7	21.10 ± 9.6	2.56 ± 1.2	5.07 ± 3.3	2.00 ± 1.9	32.20 ± 12.4	2.17 ± 3.0	6.67 ± 3.9
SRM1650b	26.26 ± 9.5	23.50 ± 7.9	4.76 ± 4.1	6.17 ± 3.0	2.30 ± 1.7	29.23 ± 11.7	1.43 ± 1.7	6.33 ± 5.4
Unhandled	25.20 ± 12.8	18.87 ± 9.7	1.70 ± 1.2	4.37 ± 2.0	0.83 ± 1.0	36.83 ± 10.5	1.00 ± 1.5	10.80 ± 16.9
High fat diet	26.63 ± 10.1	21.56 ± 10.4	3.63 ± 1.6	4.46 ± 2.3	1.47 ± 1.5	36.16 ± 9.12	1.33 ± 1.4	4.73 ± 2.8

Mean ± SD ($n = 14$–15)

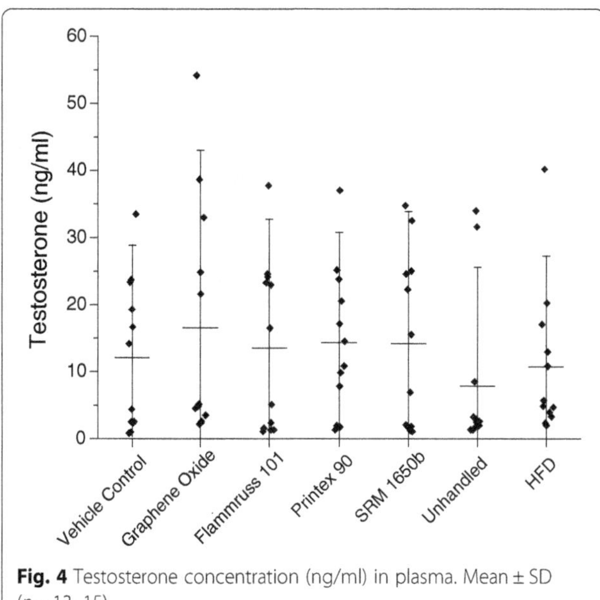

Fig. 4 Testosterone concentration (ng/ml) in plasma. Mean ± SD ($n = 13–15$)

Translocation of titanium dioxide nanoparticles from lung to secondary tissues including liver and heart has been shown after intratracheal instillation of nano-TiO_2 dispersed in 0.9% NaCl MilliQ water with 10% acellular BAL fluid [35] or water [36]. Therefore, we might expect some degree of translocation into the systemic circulation of nanosized particles that were deposited in the lungs. However, in the present study, microscopical examination of the testis revealed no gross morphological alterations between the groups and there was no apparent indication of particle deposition in the testis (data not shown). A more comprehensive comparison on the potentially increased bioavailability to reproductive organs and the potential disruption of the blood-testis-barrier as well as testicular toxicity of surfactant coated and non coated NMs remains to be investigated.

Apart from surface coating, other physicochemical properties of the nanomaterials, such as size and core chemistry, may influence their effects on the male reproductive system [37]. Size-dependent effects on plasma testosterone are apparent in the paper by Yoshida et al. (2008), as plasma testosterone was increased for Printex 90 (primary particle size of 14 nm) while it remained unchanged for Flammruss 101 (primary particles size of 95 nm). We failed to reproduce this dependency on particle size, despite the evident differences in primary particle size of the carbonaceous NMs as well as the particle-induced inflammation.

In the present study, the nanomaterials were deposited in the lungs by instillation, i.e., the materials were delivered as a bolus. This typically results in a higher dose rate than during inhalation, and instillation may therefore not compare directly to real-life exposure. Instillation is very convenient for conduction of proof of principle studies and comparison of toxicity between studies and particles, as it ensures that similar doses can be delivered for all assessed particles. For Printex 90, we have, however, previously shown that inhalation and instillation may both induce strong and long lasting lung inflammation at estimated comparable deposited dose levels [20]. Furthermore, studies of the pulmonary global transcriptional responses following inhalation and pulmonary exposure to two different nanomaterials suggest that the global transcriptional responses to inhaled and instilled or aspirated nanomaterials are very similar [38, 39].

Spermatogenesis is a steady state process and the ability to regenerate germ cell populations and recover functional spermatogonia after toxic insult are good. In fact, full recovery after an intratracheal instillation of 2 mg/kg of micelle coated silica NPs (57.66 nm) dispersed in saline has been observed [17]. Approximately thirty days after the last exposure, TEM images revealed that the silica particles could no longer be observed in the testis of C57 mice, and the reduced sperm motility and increased sperm abnormalities and apoptosis had been reversed [17]. Potentially, induced effects may have been reversed in our study one week after the last instillation, when the tissue samples were collected. However, at the time of necropsy, the observed pulmonary inflammation indicated pulmonary presence of the particles. Pulmonary translocation of NMs is an ongoing process and would still be occuring for days following the last instillation. Time dependent translocation has been shown in rats. Hence instilled radioisotopes of nanosized Cerium-141 were measured at significantly higher levels 28 days post-instillation in the blood, liver and spleen compared to day seven post-instillation [40]. With regards to time-dependent translocation to the testis, multiwalled carbon nanotubes dispersed in PBS and 0.1% tween 80 administered intravenously at a dose of 5 mg/kg to BALB/c mice showed an increased trend of translocation to the testis; 41, 61 and 151 ng were found in the testis 10 min, 60 min and 24 h post-exposure, respectively. The authors concluded that after repeated administration the multiwalled carbon nanotubes would continue to accumulate in the testis, and certain effects could be observed up to 15 days post-instillation. Furthermore, during week eight (day 56) when our experiment was terminated and organs were collected, the spermatids in the epididymides would correspond to those in the testis during the first and second instillations, as spermatogenesis in mice takes 35 days plus approximately 14 days for epididymal maturation. We therefore postulate that if there would have been significant testicular toxicity, either by direct effect of the particles or indirectly by the inflammation, it would have been detected one week after the last instillation in the present study.

The HFD was chosen as a positive control because it has been previously shown to have a negative impact on semen quality in mice, e.g. by decreasing sperm motility, increasing oxidative stress (measured by intracellular ROS) and increasing sperm DNA damage [41]. However, the selection of a HFD as a positive control is a critical limitation to the study. Only one third of the mice in the HFD control group gained sufficient weight to be regarded as obese and therefore the effects, for examples on motility, may have not been detected (see Additional file 2). Suceptibility to HFD based adipose tissue inflammation and lipid peroxidative damage in muscle and liver have been shown to be strain specific [41]. In addition, it has been previously reported that semen quality and suceptibility to toxic insult may vary greatly between mouse strains [42, 43]. For example, the inflammatory marker TNF-α was significantly upregulated in the epididymal adipose tissue of BALB/c and FVB/N mice fed a HFD, while TNF-α remained unchanged in BL/6, 129/X1 and DBA/2 mice fed with the same diet [41]. The use of different mouse strains and experimental models in studies of male reprotoductive toxicity may provide some explanation to the contradictive results often encountered in this field.

To our knowledge, the present study is the first to investigate male reproductive toxicity of carbonaceous NMs administered via the lung, without the use of surfactants like tween 80. The strength of the study is that all instilled mice, including the vehicle controls, underwent the same exposure procedure and received the same vehicle. We are therefore confident that there is no added effect from the procedure or the choice of vehicle, as confirmed by the similar low levels of neutrophils in the vehicle control compared to the unhandled and HFD groups reciving no instillation. Several of the assays presented here, such as the DSP [44], testosterone ELISA (unpublished data), and DNA damage [27, 28] assays were validated prior to this experiment. *An a priori* power analysis indicated that the chosen group size in this study ($n = 15$) provided a 95% chance of detecting approximately a one-fold difference at the 5% significance level.

Conclusion

In the present experiment, our results suggest that sperm quality parameters (epidydimal sperm concentration, sperm viability, sperm motility, sperm morphology, sperm DNA damage, DSP, and plasma testosterone concentration) were not altered in the exposed groups compared to the controls, neither by direct action of the NMs nor indirectly from the inflammatory response, after eight weeks of exposure to graphene oxide (18 mg/mouse/i.t.), Flammruss 101, Printex 90 and the SRM1650b (each 0.1 mg/mouse/i.t.) dispersed in nanopure water, in the NMRI mouse model. Standardization of experimental procedures, e.g. use of vehicle, in studies of male reproductive toxicity of NMs are needed in order to have a collective conclusion on the effects of NMs on male reproductive function. This may be imperative when determining legislative measures on workplace exposure levels for men in the reproductive age.

Abbreviations

BALF: Bronchoalveolar lavage fluid; CASA: Computer assisted sperm analysis; CB: Carbon black; DSP: Daily sperm production; HFD: High fat diet; i.t.: Intratracheal instillation; NMs: Nanomaterials; NPs: Nanoparticles; PAH: Polycyclic aromatic hydrocarbons; PBS: Phosphate-buffered saline; ROS: Reactive oxygen species; SD: Standard deviation; SRM: Standard reference material

Acknowledgements

The technical assistance from Michael Guldbrandsen, Eva Terrida, Natascha Synnøve Olsen and Inge Christensen was greatly appreciated.

Funding

The Danish Centre for Nanosafety II at the National Research Centre for the Working Environment and the Department of Large Animal Sciences/ Department of Veterinary Clinical Sciences, University of Copenhagen supported this PhD-study.

Authors' contributions

AS performed all exposures and most of the animal handling, participated in the semen analysis, performed the daily sperm production, analysed and interpreted the datasets and drafted the manuscript. AL performed the testosterone measurements. PC performed the analyses of sperm DNA integrity. SGP was overall responsible for the semen analysis. KSH conceived the idea and drafted the study protocol, with UV suggesting the particles to include. SGP, KSH and UV all contributed to the final study protocol and gave major guidance and input during the study and writing of the manuscript. All authors read and approved the final manuscript.

Competing interests

All authors declare that they have no competing interests.

Author details

[1]The National Research Center for the Working Environment, Lersø Parkallé, DK-2100 Copenhagen Ø, Denmark. [2]Section for Veterinary Reproduction and Obstetrics, Department of Veterinary Clinical Sciences, University of Copenhagen, Dyrlægvej 68, DK-1870 Frederiksberg C, Denmark. [3]SPZ Lab A/S, Fruebjergvej 3, DK-2100 København Ø, Denmark. [4]Department of Micro- and Nanotechnology, Technical University of Denmark, DK-2800 Kongens Lyngby, Denmark. [5]Department of Public Health, University of Copenhagen, Øster Farimagsgade 5, DK-1014 Copenhagen K, Denmark.

References

1. Bonde JP. Male reproductive organs are at risk from environmental hazards. Asian J Androl. 2009;12(2):152–6.
2. Sengupta P, Borges E, Dutta S, Krajewska-Kulak E. Decline in sperm count in European men during the past 50 years. Hum Exp Toxicol. 2017; https://doi.org/10.1177/0960327117703690.
3. Jørgensen N, Nordstrom Joensen U, Kold Jensen T, Blomberg Jensen M, Almstrup K, Ahlmann Olesen I, Juul A, Andersson AM, Carlsen E, Holm Petersen J, Toppari J, Skakkebæk NE. Human semen quality in the new millennium: a prospective cross-sectional population-based study of 4867 men. BMJ Open. 2012;62:1197–8.
4. Sengupta P, Dutta S, Krajewska-Kulak E. The disappearing sperms: analysis of reports published between 1980 and 2015. Am J Mens Health. 2016; https://doi.org/10.1177/1557988316643383.
5. World Health Organization. Air quality guidelines for particulate matter, ozone, nitrogen dioxide and sulfur dioxide: global update 2005: summary of risk assessment. Geneva World Heal Organ. 2006;1–22. http://apps.who.int/iris/bitstream/10665/69477/1/WHO_SDE_PHE_OEH_06.02_eng.pdf.
6. Selevan SG, Borkovec L, Slott VL, Zudová Z, Rubeš J, Evenson DP, Perreault SD. Semen quality and reproductive health of young Czech men exposed to seasonal air pollution. Environ Health Perspect. 2000;108(9):887–94.
7. Lafuente R, Garcia-Blaquez N, Jacquemin B, Checa MA. Outdoor air pollution and sperm quality. Fertil Steril. 2016;106:880–96.
8. Oberdörster G, Sharp Z, Atudorei V, Elder A, Gelein R, Lunts A, Kreyling W. Extrapulmonary translocation of ultrafine carbon particles following whole-body inhalation exposure of rats. J Toxicol Environ Health. 2002; 65:1531–43.
9. Lan Z, Yang WX. Nanoparticles and spermatogenesis: how do nanoparticles affect spermatogenesis and penetrate the blood–testis barrier. Nanomedicine. 2012;7:579–96.
10. Hedger MP. Testicular leukocytes: what are they doing? Rev Reprod. 1997;2:38–47.
11. Manke A, Wang L, Rojanasakul Y. Mechanisms of nanoparticle-induced oxidative stress and toxicity. Biomed Res Int. 2013; https://doi.org/10.1155/2013/942916.
12. Sharma R, Agarwal A. Role of reactive oxygen species in male infertility. Urology. 1996;48(6):835–50.
13. Johansson HKL, Hansen JS, Elfving B, Lund SP, Kyjovska ZO, Loft S, Barford KK, Jackson P, Vogel U, Hougaard KS. Airway exposure to multi-walled carbon nanotubes disrupts the female reproductive cycle without affecting pregnancy outcomes in mice. Part Fibre Toxicol. 2017; https://doi.org/10.1186/s12989-017-0197-1.
14. Ramdhan DH, Ito Y, Yanagiba Y, Yamagishi N, Hayashi Y, Li C, Taneda S, Suzuki A, Watanabe G, Taya K, Kamijima M, Nakajima T. Nanoparticle-rich diesel exhaust may disrupt testosterone biosynthesis and metabolism via growth hormone. Toxicol Lett. 2009;191:103–8.
15. Yoshida S, Sagai M, Oshio S, Umeda T, Ihara T, Sugamata M, Sugawara I, Takeda K. Exposure to diesel exhaust affects the male reproductive system of mice. Int J Androl. 1999;22:307–15.
16. Yoshida S, Hiyoshi K, Ichinose T, Takano H, Oshio S, Sugawara I, Takeda K, Shibamoto T. Effects of nanoparticles on the male reproductive system of mice. Int J Androl. 2008;32:337–42.
17. Ren L, Zhang J, Zou Y, Zhang L, Wei J, Shi Z, Li Y, Guo C, Sun Z, Zhou X. Silica nanoparticles induce reversible damage of spermatogenic cells via RIPK1 signal pathways in C57 mice. Int J Nanomedicine. 2016;11:2251–64.
18. Jackson P, Lund SP, Kristiansen G, Andersen O, Vogel U, Wallin H, Hougaard KS. An experimental protocol for maternal pulmonary exposure in developmental toxicology. Basic Clin Pharmacol Toxicol. 2011;108:202–7.
19. Zhang R, Dai Y, Zhang X, Niu Y, Meng T, Li Y, Duan H, Bin P, Ye M, Jia X, Shen M, Yu S, Yang X, Gao W, Zheng Y. Reduced pulmonary function and increased pro-inflammatory cytokines in nanoscale carbon black-exposed workers. Part Fibre Toxicol. 2014;11(1):73.
20. Jackson P, Hougaard KS, Boisen AMZ, Jacobsen NR, Jensen KA, Møller P, Brunborg G, Gutzkow KB, Andersen O, Loft S, Vogel U, Wallin H. Pulmonary exposure to carbon black by inhalation or instillation in pregnant mice: effects on liver DNA strand breaks in dams and offspring. Nanotoxicology. 2012;6(5):486–500.
21. The Danish Working Environment Authority. At-vejledning. Stoffer og Materiale. Danish Work Environ Auth. 2017AD;C.0.1.:1–84.
22. Bengtson S, Knudsen KB, Kyjovska ZO, Berthing T, Skaug V, Levin M, Koponen IK, Shivayogimath A, Booth TJ, Alonso B, Pesquera A, Zurutuza A, Thomsen BL, Troelsen JT, Jacobsen NR, Vogel U. Differences in inflammation and acute phase response but similar genotoxicity in mice following pulmonary exposure to graphene oxide and reduced graphene oxide. PLoS ONE. 2017; https://doi.org/10.1371/journal.pone.0178355.
23. Bengtson S, Kling K, Madsen AM, Noergaard AW, Jacobsen NR, Clausen PA, Alonso B, Pesquera A, Zurutuza A, Ramos R, Okuno H, Dijon J, Wallin H, Vogel U. No cytotoxicity or genotoxicity of graphene and graphene oxide in murine lung epithelial FE1 cells in vitro. Environ Mol Mutagen. 2016;57:469–82.
24. Saber AT, Jensen KA, Jacobsen NR, Birkedal R, Mikkelsen L, Møller P, Loft S, Wallin H, Vogel U. Inflammatory and genotoxic effects of nanoparticles designed for inclusion in paints and lacquers. Nanotoxicology. 2012;6:453–71.
25. Kyjovska ZO, Jacobsen NR, Saber AT, Bengtson S, Jackson P, Wallin H, Vogel U. DNA strand breaks, acute phase response and inflammation following pulmonary exposure by instillation to the diesel exhaust particle NIST1650b in mice. Mutagenesis. 2015;30:499–507.
26. Kyjovska ZO, Jacobsen NR, Saber AT, Bengtson S, Jackson P, Wallin H, Vogel UDNA. Damage following pulmonary exposure by instillation to low doses of carbon black (printex 90) nanoparticles in mice. Environ Mol Mutagen. 2010;51:229–35.
27. Evenson D, Jost L. Sperm chromatin structure assay for fertility assessment. Meth in Cell Sci. 2000;22:169–89.
28. Boe-Hansen GB, Ersbøll AK, Christiensen P. Variability and laboratory factors affecting the sperm chromatin structure assay in human semen. J Androl. 2005;26:360–8.
29. Ema M, Hougaard KS, Kishimoto A, Honda K. Reproductive and developmental toxicity of carbon-based nanomaterials: a literature review. Nanotoxicology. 2016;10:1–22.
30. Jackson P, Hougaard KS, Vogel U, Wu D, Casavant L, Williams A, Wade M, Yuak CL, Wallin H. Halappanavar. Exposure of pregnant mice to carbon black by intratracheal instillation: Toxicogenomic effects in dams and offspring. Mutat Res Genet Toxicol Environ Mutagen. 2012;745(1–2):73–83.
31. Kaur G, Mehta SK. Developments of Polysorbate (tween) based microemulsions: preclinical drug delivery, toxicity and antimicrobial applications. Int J Pharm. 2017;529:134–60.
32. Qu G, Wang X, Liu Q, Liu R, Yin N, Ma J, Chen L, He J, Liu S, Jiang G. The ex vivo and in vivo biological performances of graphene oxide and the impact of surfactant on graphene oxide's biocompatibility. J Environ Sci. 2013;25:873–81.
33. Akhavan O, Ghaderi E, Hashemi E, Akbari E. Dose-dependent effects of nanoscale graphene oxide on reproduction capability of mammals. Carbon 2015;95:309–17.
34. Liang S, Xu S, Zhang D, He J, Chu M. Reproductive toxicity of nanoscale graphene oxide in male mice. Nanotoxicology. 2015;9:1–14.
35. Husain M, Wu D, Saber AT, Decan N, Jacobsen NR, Williams A, Yuak CL, Wallin H, Vogel U, Halappanavar S. Intratracheally instilled titanium dioxide nanoparticles translocate to heart and liver and activate complement cascade in the heart of C57BL/6 mice. Nanotoxicology. 2015;9(8):1013–22.
36. Kreyling WG, Holzwarth U, Schleh C, Kozempel J, Wenk A, Haberl N, Hirn S, Schaffler M, Lipka J, Semmler-Behnke M, Gibson N. Quantitative biokinetics of titanium dioxide nanoparticles after oral application in rats: part 2. Nanotoxicology. 2017;11(4):443–53.
37. Campagnolo L, Massimiani M, Magrini A, Camaioni A, Pietroiusti A. Physico-chemical properties mediating reproductive and developmental toxicity of engineered nanomaterials. Curr Med Chem. 2012;19:4488–94.
38. Kinaret P, Ilves M, Fortino V, Rydman E, Karisola P, Lahde A, Koivisto J, Jokiniemi J, Wolff H, Savolainen K, Greco D, Alenius H. Inhalation and oropharyngeal aspiration exposure to rod-like carbon nanotubes Induse similar airway inflammation and biological responses in mouse lungs. ACS Nano. 2017;11:291–303.
39. Husain M, Saber A, Guo C, Jacobsen N, Jensen K, Yauk C, Willims A, Vogel U, Wallin H. Halappanavar. Pulmonary instillation of low doses of titation dioxide nanoparticles in mice leads to particle retention and gene expression changes in the absence of inflammation. Tox Appl Pharma. 2013; 269(3):250–02.
40. He X, He X, Zhang H, Ma Y, Bai W, Zhang Z, Lu K, Ding Y, Zhao Y, Chai Z. Lung deposition and extrapulmonary translocation of nano-ceria after

intratracheal instillation. Nanotechnology. 2010; https://doi.org/10.1088/0957-4484/21/28/285103.

41. Montgomery MK, Hallahan NL, Brown SH, Liu M, Mitchell TW, Cooney GJ, Turner N. Mouse strain-dependent variation in obesity and glucose homeostasis in response to high-fat feeding. Diabetologia. 2013;56:1129–39.
42. Krzanowska H. Sperm head abnormalities in relation to the age and strain of mice. J Reprod Fert. 1981;62:385–92.
43. Thurston LM, Watson PF, Holt WV. Semen cryopreservation: a genetic explanation for species and individual variation? CryoLetters. 2002;23: 255–62.
44. Kyjovska ZO, Boisen AMZ, Jackson P, Wallin H, Vogel U, Hougaard KS. Daily sperm production: application in studies of prenatal exposure to nanoparticles in mice. Reprod Toxicol. 2013;36:88–97.

14

Kinetics and dissolution of intratracheally administered nickel oxide nanomaterials in rats

Naohide Shinohara[1*], Guihua Zhang[1], Yutaka Oshima[2], Toshio Kobayashi[2], Nobuya Imatanaka[3], Makoto Nakai[3], Takeshi Sasaki[4], Kenji Kawaguchi[4] and Masashi Gamo[1]

Abstract

Background: The toxicokinetics of nanomaterials are an important factor in toxicity, which may be affected by slow clearance and/or distribution in the body.

Methods: Four types of nickel oxide (NiO) nanoparticles were single-administered intratracheally to male F344 rats at three doses of 0.67–6.0 mg/kg body weight. The rats were sacrificed under anesthesia and the lung, thoracic lymph nodes, bronchoalveolar lavage fluid, liver, and other organs were sampled for Ni burden measurement 3, 28, and 91 days post-administration; Ni excretion was measured 6 and 24 h after administration. Solubility of NiO nanoparticles was determined using artificial lysosomal fluid, artificial interstitial fluid, hydrogen peroxide solution, pure water, and saline. In addition, macrophage migration to trachea and phagosome-lysosome-fusion rate constants were estimated using pulmonary clearance and dissolution rate constants.

Results: The wire-like NiO nanoparticles were 100% dissolved by 24 h when mixed with artificial lysosomal fluid (dissolution rate coefficient: 0.18/h); spherical NiO nanoparticles were 12% and 35% dissolved after 216 h when mixed with artificial lysosomal fluid (1.4×10^{-3} and 4.9×10^{-3}/h). The largest irregular-shaped NiO nanoparticles hardly dissolved in any solution, including artificial lysosomal fluid (7.8×10^{-5}/h). Pulmonary clearance rate constants, estimated using a one-compartment model, were much higher for the NiO nanoparticles with a wire-shape (0.069–0.078/day) than for the spherical and irregular-shaped NiO nanoparticles (0–0.012/day). Pulmonary clearance rate constants of the largest irregular-shaped NiO nanoparticles showed an inverse correlation with dose. Translocation of NiO from the lungs to the thoracic lymph nodes increased in a time- and dose-dependent manner for three spherical and irregular-shaped NiO nanoparticles, but not for the wire-like NiO nanoparticles. Thirty-five percent of the wire-like NiO nanoparticles were excreted in the first 24 h after administration; excretion was 0.33 3.6% in that time frame for the spherical and irregular-shaped NiO nanoparticles.

Conclusion: These findings suggest that nanomaterial solubility differences can result in variations in their pulmonary clearance. Nanoparticles with moderate lysosomal solubility may induce persistent pulmonary inflammation.

Keywords: Toxicokinetics, Intratracheal administration, Clearance rate constant, Lymph node, Dissolubility, Artificial biological fluid (Gamble's solution)

* Correspondence: n-shinohara@aist.go.jp
[1]National Institute of Advanced Industrial Science and Technology (AIST), Tsukuba, Ibaraki 305-8569, Japan
Full list of author information is available at the end of the article

Background

There are growing concerns about the toxicity of nanomaterials owing to the lack of information on their potential risks in workers and the general population. Nanomaterials with the same chemical formula may exert different toxicities, depending on physicochemical characteristics such as size, shape, and crystalline structure. Studies have compared the toxicities of nanomaterials with different physicochemical properties [1]. Pulmonary clearance and translocation to extrapulmonary organs offer valuable insights into the inhalation toxicity of nanomaterials. Recently, we showed that six types of TiO_2 nanoparticles of different sizes and shapes had similar pulmonary clearance rate constants, while TiO_2 nanoparticles with an $Al(OH)_3$ coating had much lower pulmonary clearance rate constants [2] and displayed higher toxicity [3]. TiO_2 nanoparticle toxicity increases with decreasing particle size [3]. Extensive inflammation was observed in rats intratracheally instilled with nickel oxide (NiO) nanoparticles, but was minimal in rats intratracheally instilled with NiO submicron-sized particles [4, 5].

Although NiO is often considered a poorly soluble Ni compound, some NiO can be dissolved [6]. Inhaled soluble Ni compounds are rapidly cleared from the lung and exhibit higher toxicity, while inhaled insoluble NiO is slowly cleared from the lungs and exhibits lower toxicity [7–10]. Ni-containing compounds can induce pulmonary inflammation [11–13], which could be related to the dissolution rate [13]. Solubility and cytotoxicity are higher for black NiO than for green NiO, even though the particle size is identical [14, 15]. Therefore, the toxicity and pulmonary clearance of NiO nanoparticles could be associated with particle size and solubility. In addition, in vivo nanoparticle dissolution should be considered, as well as water solubility.

This study evaluated the relationship between the toxicokinetics and biological solubility of NiO using an artificial biological fluid, as biological solubility is difficult to determine in situ. Further, we measured pulmonary clearance kinetics, extrapulmonary translocation, and excretion of four NiO nanomaterials, which differed in particle size and biological solubility, after intratracheal administration in rats. Finally, the pulmonary clearance and lung-to-lymph translocation rate constants of these four nanomaterials were compared for a range of doses.

Methods

Preparation and characterization of NiO suspensions

Four NiO particles (A, B, C, and D) were used in the present study. The names and manufacturers of these NiO particles, as well as the suspension characteristics, including primary particle size, surface area, and size of the agglomerates in suspension, are shown in Table 1.

NiO particles (2 g) were sonicated in 50 mL pure water for 2 h, followed by centrifugation at 1000 *g* for 30 min at 20°C. The supernatant was collected as a stock suspension to remove the large aggregate of particles. Suspensions of 0.67, 2.0, and 6.0 mg/mL for animal tests and 2.0 mg/mL for biological solubility tests were prepared by diluting the stock suspension with pure water.

Table 1 Characteristics of the NiO particles used in the study

	Name (Manufacturer)	Crystalline	Shape	Primary particle size[a] [nm]	Specific surface area[b] [m^2/g]	Converted spherical primary particle size based on the specific surface area [nm]	Number-based agglomerate particle size[c] (DLS measurement) [nm]	SEM/TEM picture
A	US3352 (US Research Nanomaterials, Inc., TX, USA)	NaCl type	Spherical	20 ± 8	51	18	49	
B	NovaWireNiO1 (Novarials Co., MA, USA)	NaCl type	Wire	Length 240 Diameter 29	180	5.0	Impossible determination[e]	
C	I small particle (Kusaka Rare Metal Products Co., LTD., Tokyo, Japan)	NaCl type	Irregular	140 ± 67	6.6	140	1600	
D	Ni(II) Oxide Nanopowder (Sigma-Aldrich Co. LLC., MO, USA)	NaCl type	Spherical	Impossible observation[d]	93	9.6	39	

[a]Determined by SEM (scanning electron microscopy, S4800, Hitachi High-Technologies Co., Tokyo, Japan) or TEM (transmission electron microscopy, JEM-2010, JEOL, Tokyo, Japan) of 500 particles for each material

[b]Determined by Brunauer-Emmett-Teller (BET) surface area analysis (GEMINI VII, Shimadzu Co., Kyoto, Japan) after drying

[c]Determined by dynamic light scattering (DLS) (Zetasizer nano-ZS; Malvern Instruments Ltd., Worcestershire, UK)

[d] The small NiO D particle size, caused the particles to aggregate when the suspension was dried. Consequently, particle dimensions were difficult to ascertain even with suspension dilution and spraying

[e] Reproducibiliy of dynamic light scattering (DLS) measurement for NiO B was not feasible

The concentration of the stock suspension was determined by a standard weight analysis, where the weight-loss of the suspension was measured using a balance (AUW220D; Shimadzu Co., Kyoto, Japan) after drying at 200 °C in a thermostatic chamber (ON-300S; Asone Co., Osaka, Japan).

Biological solubility of NiO nanoparticles

For these experiments, six solutions were used as artificial biological fluids: Saline; hydrogen peroxide (266.7 and 13.3 μmol/L); artificial interstitium solution (Gamble's solution); artificial lysosomal solution; pure water. The final concentrations of the hydrogen peroxide solution (200 and 10 μmol/L) were selected based on previous studies [16–18]. The artificial interstitium and artificial lysosomal fluids were prepared using the method shown in Additional file 1.

The nanoparticle suspension (10 mL of 2.0 mg/mL) and artificial biological fluids (30 mL) were mixed and shaken at 200 rpm. At 0.5–216 h after the mixing period (12 time points), 2.5 mL fluid were sampled and filtered at 6000 *g* for 30 min with an ultrafilter (50,000 molecular weight cut off [MWCO]; VS2032, Sartorius Stedim Biotech, Aubagne, France) to separate the dissolved Ni ions; a molecular weight of 50,000 is equivalent to 6–7 nm. Ultrapure water (1 mL) was then added to the ultrafiltrate, and the samples were centrifuged at 6000 *g* for 15 min; these steps were performed twice. The Ni ion concentration (ng/mL) was then analyzed, fitted to the curve, and the solution equilibrium was expressed using the following equation:

$$\text{Solid} \underset{k'}{\overset{k_{\text{dis}}}{\rightleftarrows}} \text{ion} \tag{1}$$

The dissolution and solidification rate coefficients, k_{dis} (/h) and k' (/h), respectively, were estimated using the least-squares approach with the solver function in Excel 2007.

Experimental procedure for animal testing

Two hundred and forty male F344/DuCrlCrlj rats (12 weeks old; mean body weight 256 ± 11 g) obtained from Charles River Laboratories Japan, Inc. (Kanagawa, Japan) were anesthetized by isoflurane inhalation and intratracheally administered pure water (as the negative control) or NiO suspensions (0.67, 2.0, or 6.0 mg/kg body weight [BW]) at 1 mL/kg BW using a MicroSprayer® Aerosolizer (model IA-1B-R for Rat; Penn-Century, Inc., Wyndmoor, PA, USA). Five rats in each group were euthanized by exsanguination from the abdominal aorta under intraperitoneal pentobarbital anesthesia (50 mg/kg BW) on days 3, 28, and 91 post-NiO particle administration. Thereafter, the lungs were lavaged twice with 7 mL physiological saline, as previously described [2]. After the bronchoalveolar lavage fluid (BALF) sampling, the trachea, lungs, right and left posterior mediastinal lymph nodes, parathymic lymph nodes, liver, kidneys, spleen, and brain of each animal were dissected, rinsed with saline, and weighed. The observation period of 91 days was chosen because the fast clearance pathway could become less attributed to pulmonary clearance more than 91 days after administration. The effect of slow clearance can be evaluated in 91 days according to previous studies that reported the half time of fast clearance as 25–27 days [19] and 23–50 days [20], and half time of slow clearance as 224 days [19] and 75–845 days [20]. They found the differences in fast clearance rates, between doses and mammalian species, to be small.

Additional tests were conducted using metabolism cages to evaluate excretion in five rats from each group administered NiO particles (2.0 mg/kg BW). The feces and urine were collected between 0 and 6 h and 6–24 h post-NiO administration. The rats were euthanized and dissected 6 h and 24 h post-NiO administration. In addition to the organs listed above, the small intestine, large intestine, esophagus, and stomach were dissected after collection of BALF and gastrointestinal contents. Extracellular Ni ion fractions ([extracellular Ni ions]/[extracellular Ni particles + extracellular Ni ions + intracellular Ni particles + intracellular Ni ions]) in BALF were determined after ultrafiltration.

All animals were treated in accordance with the guidelines for animal experiments in our laboratory, which adhere to the guidelines of the Ministry of the Environment, Ministry of Health, Labour and Welfare, Ministry of Agriculture, Forestry and Fisheries, and Ministry of Education, Culture, Sports, Science and Technology. The experiments were approved by the Animal Care and Use Committee, Chemicals Evaluation and Research Institute, and the Institutional Animal Care and Use Committee of the National Institute of Advanced Industrial Science and Technology.

Pulmonary NiO clearance and translocation rate coefficients

We used the previously described [2] model shown in Fig. 1 to express the pulmonary clearance and translocation to thoracic lymph nodes. The rate constants (/day) for pulmonary clearance (k_{Lung}) and translocation from the lung to thoracic lymph node ($k_{\text{Lung} \to \text{Lym}}$) were estimated using eqs. (2) and (3), according to Shinohara et al. [2]:

$$\frac{dB_{\text{Lung}}}{dt} = -k_{\text{Lung}} B_{\text{Lung}} \qquad (t = 0 : B_{\text{Lung}} = rD) \tag{2}$$

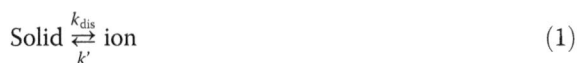

$$\frac{dB_{\text{Lym}}}{dt} = k_{\text{Lung}\to\text{Lym}} B_{\text{Lung}} \qquad (t = 0 : B_{\text{Lym}} = 0) \tag{3}$$

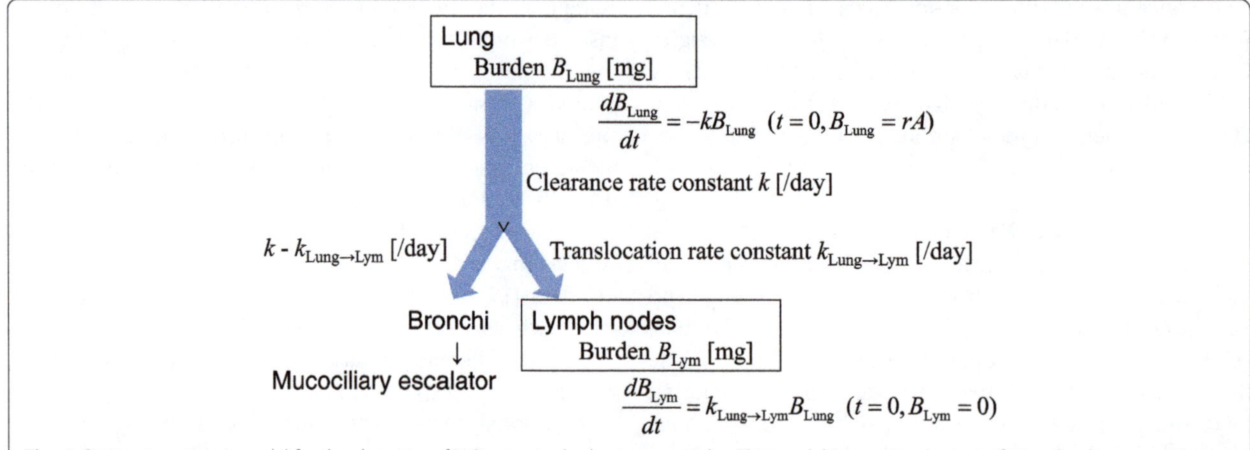

Fig. 1 One-compartment model for the clearance of NiO nano and submicron particles. This model is expressed using a first-order decay equation with rate constant k

where B_{Lung} and B_{Lym} were the lung and total thoracic lymph node burdens of NiO, respectively; D was the administered dose of NiO (μg); t was the time elapsed after administration (days), and r was the fraction that reached the alveolar region following NiO administration. The least-squares approach was used for curve-fitting.

Analysis

Samples were homogenized in ultrapure water and then acid-treated prior to determining the Ni content using inductively coupled plasma-mass spectrometry (ICP-MS), under the conditions shown in Table 2. We altered the acid-treatment methods for NiO C and D because the recovery efficiency for

Table 2 Instruments and conditions used for homogenization, acid treatment, and analysis

Homogenate		
Volume of pure water for homogenate	Liver	10 mL
	Other organs	2 mL
	Face	2 mL
	Food	2 mL
	Gastrointestinal contents	2 mL
Electric homogenizer	PT10–35 (Kinematica AG, NS-50, and NS-52; Microtec Co. Ltd., Chiba, Japan)	
Acid treatment for NiO A and B		
Volume of samples and acid	Homogenate sample	1.0 g
	HNO_3 (68%)	1.0 mL
Ashing	180 °C (2 h) ⇒ 350 °C (2 h) ⇒ 550 °C (3 h)	
Electric furnace	TFF45-C (Tokyo Technological Labo Co. Ltd., Kanagawa, Japan)	
Acid treatment for NiO C and D		
Volume of samples and acid	Homogenate sample	1.0 g
	HNO_3 (68%)	0.5 mL
	H_2O_2	0.2 mL
Heating	180 °C (20 min)	
Microwave sample preparation instrument	ETHOS 1 (Milestone Srl, Sorisole, Italy) or Speedwave 4 (Berghof, Eningen, Germany)	
Analysis		
ICP-MS	ELEMENT 2/ ELEMENT XR (Thermo Fisher Scientific, Waltham, MA, USA)	
RF output	1200 W	
Target mass (m/z)	^{60}Ni (mass: 59.9308)	

NiO C was not high when using the method for NiO A and B.

Good linearity of the calibration curves for Ni using ICP-MS was observed in a 0–20 ng/mL standard solution ($R^2 > 0.999$). Recovery efficiencies from Ni standard solution-spiked samples (5 ng/mL) were >90% for most of the samples (Additional file 2). Five nanograms per milliliter of Ni standard solution were added to organ samples every 10–20 samples, and the measured value were corrected by the recovery efficiency. Based on the operation blank for the organ tissue samples, the limit of quantification was 2 ng/g for most organ tissues, 1 ng/mL for BALF, 0.5 ng/mL for blood, and 0.5 ng for trachea and lymph nodes.

Statistical analysis

Two-way repeated analysis of variance (ANOVA) with Scheffe's test was used to compare the study group NiO concentrations following an F-test with SPSS 20.0 (IMD SPSS, Armonk, NY, USA). Since the administered doses differed depending on BW, the organ burdens are shown as normalized values where the organ burden was divided by the BW at the time of NiO administration. Percentages of administered doses are also shown for organ burdens.

Results

Biological solubility of NiO nanoparticles

The Ni ion concentrations increased over time for each NiO nanoparticle tested in each solution (Fig. 2). NiO B was 100% dissolved 24 h after mixing in lysosomal fluid, while only 3.5–6.5% of NiO B had dissolved after 216 h in the other five solutions. In contrast, approximately 11, 0.70, and 33% of NiO A, C, and D, respectively, had dissolved after 216 h in lysosomal fluid, while 2.3–3.7%, 0.14–0.51%, and 3.9–6.3% of NiO A, C, and D, respectively, had dissolved at 216 h in the other five fluids.

The dissolution rate coefficients in lysosomal fluid, k_{dis}, were 2–3 orders of magnitude higher for NiO B than for NiO A, C, and D (Table 3). With the exception of artificial interstitium fluid, the solidification rate coefficients, k', did not differ much between the NiO particles (approximately 1×10^{-2}/h).

Organ NiO burdens after intratracheal administration

NiO burdens in BALF and in the lung (after BALF sampling) were significantly higher ($P < 0.01$) in the NiO-treated rats than in the control group from days 3 to 91, except for rats treated with NiO B on day 91 (Fig. 3, Table 4, Additional files 3 and 4). These NiO burdens were dose-dependent. The lung burdens for NiO

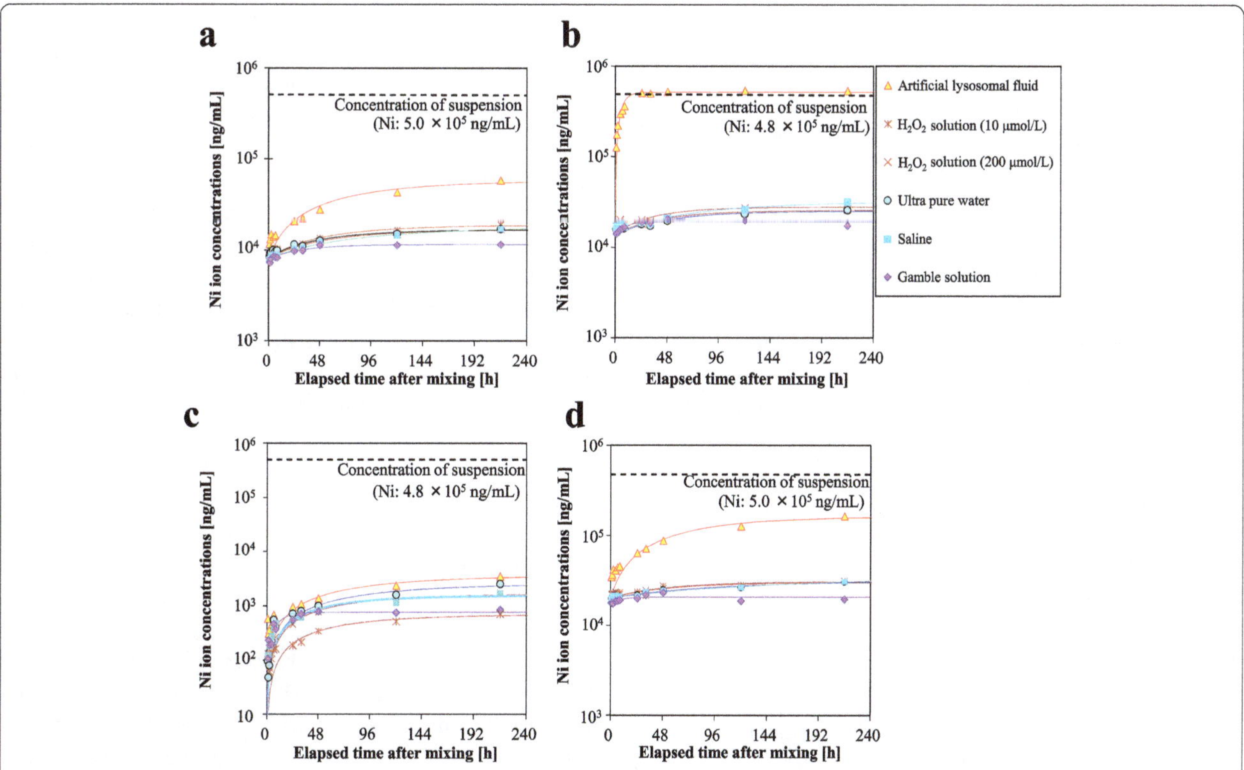

Fig. 2 Concentration of dissolved Ni ions in the artificial fluids for four types of NiO. Ultrapure water, saline, hydrogen peroxide (H_2O_2) solutions (10 and 200 μM), artificial lysosomal fluid, and Gamble's solution (artificial interstitium fluid) were used as the artificial fluids. The broken line indicates the Ni concentrations (both particle and ion) in the suspension. **a** NiO A. **b** NiO B. **c** NiO C. **d** NiO D

Table 3 Dissolution rate coefficient *k* and solidification rate coefficient *k'* of NiO nanoparticles in six solutions

NiO particles	Solutions	*k* (/h)	*k'* (/h)
NiO A	Saline	3.4×10^{-4}	8.8×10^{-3}
	Pure water	5.8×10^{-4}	1.7×10^{-2}
	H_2O_2 (200 μmol/L)	5.0×10^{-4}	1.4×10^{-2}
	H_2O_2 (10 μmol/L)	5.7×10^{-4}	1.5×10^{-2}
	Artificial lysosomal solution	1.4×10^{-3}	1.1×10^{-2}
	Artificial interstitium solution (Gamble's solution)	6.2×10^{-4}	2.6×10^{-2}
NiO B	Saline	6.5×10^{-4}	1.0×10^{-2}
	Pure water	8.0×10^{-4}	1.6×10^{-2}
	H_2O_2 (200 μmol/L)	1.2×10^{-3}	2.3×10^{-2}
	H_2O_2 (10 μmol/L)	9.3×10^{-3}	1.9×10^{-2}
	Artificial lysosomal solution	0.18	9.2×10^{-3}
	Artificial interstitium solution (Gamble's solution)	3.6×10^{-3}	9.8×10^{-2}
NiO C	Saline	5.4×10^{-5}	1.7×10^{-2}
	Pure water	5.5×10^{-5}	1.0×10^{-2}
	H_2O_2 (200 μmol/L)	2.0×10^{-5}	1.4×10^{-2}
	H_2O_2 (10 μmol/L)	4.7×10^{-5}	1.4×10^{-2}
	Artificial lysosomal solution	7.8×10^{-5}	1.0×10^{-2}
	Artificial interstitium solution (Gamble's solution)	1.5×10^{-4}	9.5×10^{-2}
NiO D	Saline	3.7×10^{-4}	4.4×10^{-3}
	Pure water	5.4×10^{-4}	7.3×10^{-3}
	H_2O_2 (200 μmol/L)	1.0×10^{-3}	1.5×10^{-2}
	H_2O_2 (10 μmol/L)	1.1×10^{-3}	1.5×10^{-2}
	Artificial lysosomal solution	4.9×10^{-3}	9.3×10^{-3}
	Artificial interstitium solution (Gamble's solution)	4.3×10^{-3}	9.4×10^{-2}

A, C, and D decreased slowly over time, whereas burdens for NiO B decreased rapidly to <1% of the administered dose by day 28 post-administration. Higher BALF-to-total lung burden ratios were observed at lower doses and with longer observation periods in rats treated with NiO B; this trend was not observed for NiO A, C, or D (Table 5).

The NiO burdens in most of the thoracic lymph nodes (total burden in the right and left posterior mediastinal lymph nodes and parathymic lymph nodes) were significantly higher in the groups dosed with NiO particles than in the control group (Fig. 3, Table 4, Additional files 3 and 4). Except for NiO B, the NiO burden in the thoracic lymph nodes increased in a dose- and time-dependent manner from day 3 to day 91, with percentage burdens (total burden in the thoracic lymph nodes relative to the administered dose) of 0.015–0.18% (day 3) to 0.12–12% (day 91). In most rats, a higher NiO burden was detected in the right and left mediastinal lymph nodes than in the parathymic lymph node (Additional file 5).

Although the liver NiO burdens in some rats were higher than those in the negative control group, no clear dose- or time-dependency was observed (Fig. 3). No significant differences were observed in the NiO levels of the kidney, spleen, and brain in the NiO-treated and control animals.

Pulmonary NiO clearance and translocation rate coefficients

The pulmonary NiO clearance rate coefficients, k_{Lung}, in animals treated with NiO B were much higher than those of animals treated with NiO A, C, or D (Fig. 4 and Table 6). k_{Lung} showed an inverse correlation with dose for NiO C, but this relationship was not observed for NiO A, B, or D. The translocation rate coefficients from lung to lymph nodes, $k_{Lung \rightarrow Lym}$, increased in a dose-dependent manner for NiO A, C, and D (Fig. 4 and Table 6). $k_{Lung \rightarrow Lym}$ was highest for NiO D, followed by NiO A, C, and B.

Evaluation of short-term excretion

The total organ, feces, urine, and gastrointestinal Ni content 6 h after administration of NiO A, B, C, and D was 96, 74, 44, and 92%, respectively. The distribution and excretion per initial (6-h) total NiO burden are shown in Fig. 5. Ni excretion in urine for up to 24 h was higher for NiO B (35%) than for NiO A (3.6%), while the Ni excretion of NiO D (2.1%) was much higher than that of NiO C (0.33%). Ni excretion levels in the feces for up to 24 h and in the gastrointestinal contents at 24 h were higher for animals treated with NiO B or C than for those exposed to NiO A or D. Although the Ni levels in the esophagus, stomach, small intestine, large intestine, liver, and blood were low (< 1%), the burdens in the kidneys and blood were significantly higher for NiO B than for the other NiO particles. In addition, the extracellular ion fractions in BALF were 8.3 and 9.7% for NiO B at 6 and 24 h after administration, respectively, whereas those for the other three NiO particles were below the detection limit.

Pulmonary inflammation

Representative images of H&E-stained lung tissue sections are shown in Fig. 6. Sustained pulmonary inflammation up to 13 weeks post-administration was observed in NiO A and D, and inflammatory cells (neutrophils and alveolar macrophages) tended to increase over time. For NiO B, inflammatory cells were observed 3 days post-administration, but decreased over time with almost no inflammation after 13 weeks. NiO C showed very mild lung effects at 3 days post-

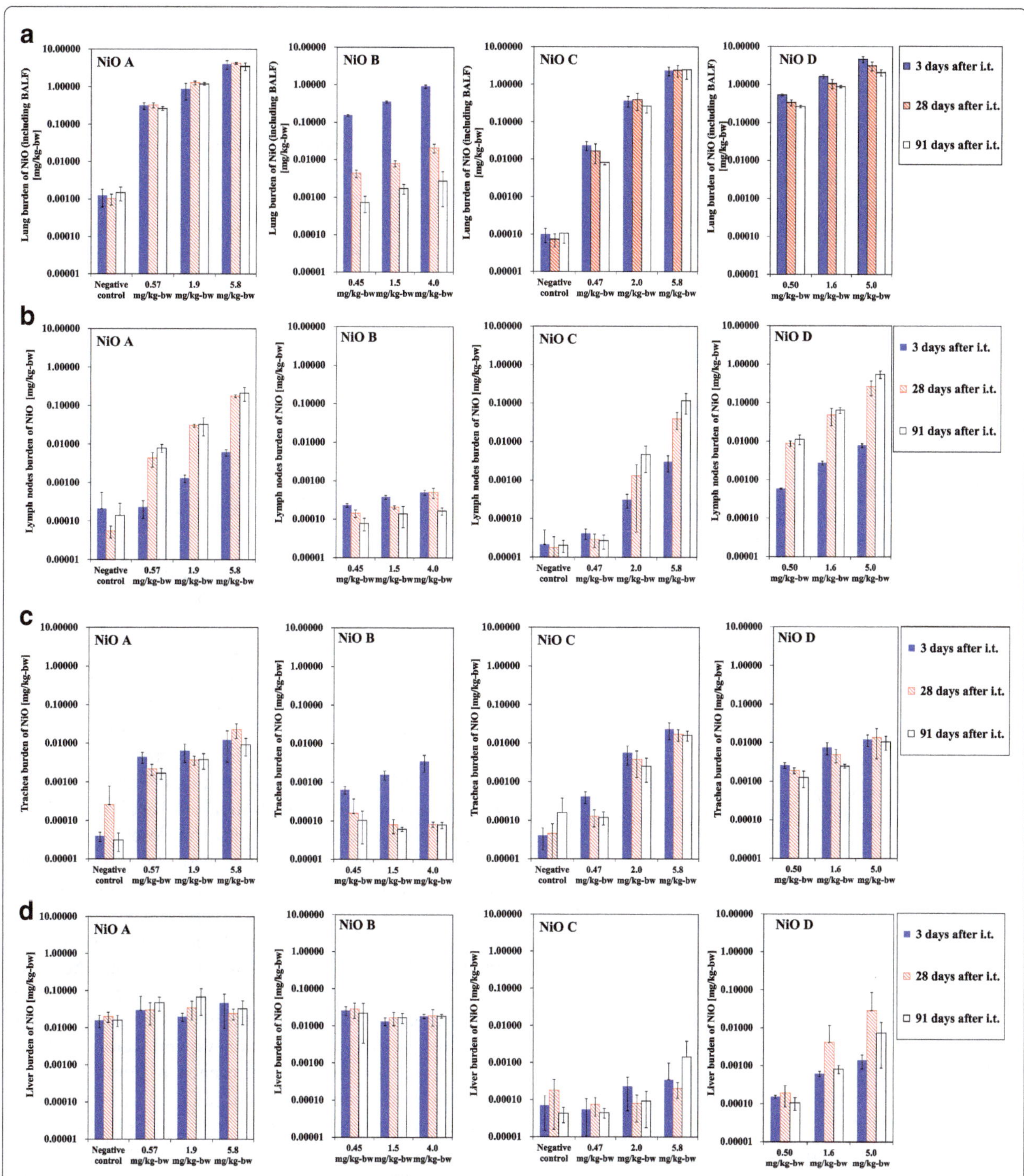

Fig. 3 NiO burden per initial body weight at the time of administration in the lung. Bronchoalveolar lavage fluid (BALF) (**a**), total thoracic lymph nodes (right mediastinal lymph node and left and right mediastinal lymph nodes) (**b**), trachea (**c**), and liver (**d**) following intratracheal NiO administration. Horizontal axis indicates the administered dose per initial body weight. The body weights of the rats were 256 ± 11 g. The column and error bars indicate the mean and standard deviation, respectively. Asterisks indicate statistically significant differences, compared with the control group (** $P < 0.01$, * $P < 0.05$). Samples with NiO levels below the quantification limit were assigned values corresponding to half the quantification limit

administration, and pulmonary inflammation disappeared 4 to 13 weeks post-administration. Neutrophil counts in BALF supported these trends in pulmonary inflammation for NiO A, B, C, and D (Table 7).

Discussion

In the dissolution test, only NiO B dissolved rapidly in artificial lysosomal fluid and more slowly in water, saline, and artificial interstitium fluid; this finding suggested that

Table 4 Percentage of NiO burden in each organ per administered dose. Values for the (A) lung, (B) bronchoalveolar lavage fluid (BALF), (C) trachea, and (D) lymph nodes are shown

(A) Lung

		Percentage of lung NiO burden per administered dose		
		3 days after i.t.	28 days after i.t.	91 days after i.t.
NiO A	0·57 mg/kg-bw	53% ± 11%	56% ± 8.7%	46% ± 5.3%
	1·9 mg/kg-bw	44% ± 21%	66% ± 8.0%	62% ± 4.8%
	5·8 mg/kg-bw	67% ± 17%	71% ± 3.0%	60% ± 14%
NiO B	0·45 mg/kg-bw	33% ± 1.6%	0.87% ± 0.051%	0.28% ± 0.032%
	1·5 mg/kg-bw	22% ± 1.5%	0.48% ± 0.10%	0.12% ± 0.020%
	4·0 mg/kg-bw	22% ± 2.1%	0.50% ± 0.12%	0.088% ± 0.049%
NiO C	0·47 mg/kg-bw	4.8% ± 1.3%	3.4% ± 1.9%	1.7% ± 0.22%
	2·0 mg/kg-bw	18% ± 5.5%	19% ± 9.3%	13% ± 4.5%
	5·8 mg/kg-bw	39% ± 10%	41% ± 14%	42% ± 19%
NiO D	0·50 mg/kg-bw	100% ± 6.3%	64% ± 12%	51% ± 3.8%
	1·6 mg/kg-bw	100% ± 11%	62% ± 16%	54% ± 4.0%
	5·0 mg/kg-bw	90% ± 16%	61% ± 16%	40% ± 7.9%

(B) Bronchoalveolar lavage fluid (BALF)

		Percentage of BALF NiO burden per administered dose		
		3 days after i.t.	28 days after i.t.	91 days after i.t.
NiO A	0·57 mg/kg-bw	1.2% ± 0.31%	0.51% ± 0.13%	0.59% ± 0.17%
	1·9 mg/kg-bw	0.28% ± 0.17%	0.61% ± 0.068%	0.39% ± 0.034%
	5·8 mg/kg-bw	0.51% ± 0.37%	1.9% ± 0.62%	0.57% ± 0.42%
NiO B	0·45 mg/kg-bw	1.1% ± 0.31%	0.35% ± 0.19%	0.15% ± 0.058%
	1·5 mg/kg-bw	0.94% ± 0.22%	0.11% ± 0.015%	0.058% ± 0.013%
	4·0 mg/kg-bw	0.65% ± 0.19%	0.050% ± 0.015%	0.016% ± 0.0049%
NiO C	0·47 mg/kg-bw	0.078% ± 0.021%	0.11% ± 0.053%	0.088% ± 0.031%
	2·0 mg/kg-bw	0.64% ± 0.81%	0.45% ± 0.20%	0.39% ± 0.092%
	5·8 mg/kg-bw	0.39% ± 0.098%	0.50% ± 0.42%	0.43% ± 0.34%
NiO D	0·50 mg/kg-bw	2.6% ± 0.39%	2.5% ± 1.1%	1.3% ± 0.13%
	1·6 mg/kg-bw	1.8% ± 0.49%	3.9% ± 1.6%	1.8% ± 0.46%
	5·0 mg/kg-bw	1.9% ± 0.63%	1.6% ± 0.74%	1.9% ± 0.54%

(C) Trachea

		Trachea NiO burden per initial body weight [mg/kg bw]		
		3 days after i.t.	28 days after i.t.	91 days after i.t.
NiO A	0·57 mg/kg-bw	0.77% ± 0.25%	0.38% ± 0.12%	0.30% ± 0.085%
	1·9 mg/kg-bw	0.33% ± 0.17%	0.19% ± 0.050%	0.20% ± 0.085%
	5·8 mg/kg-bw	0.21% ± 0.15%	0.39% ± 0.16%	0.16% ± 0.075%
NiO B	0·45 mg/kg-bw	0.14% ± 0.031%	0.035% ± 0.047%	0.023% ± 0.017%
	1·5 mg/kg-bw	0.10% ± 0.028%	0.0052% ± 0.0021%	0.0040% ± 0.00050%
	4·0 mg/kg-bw	0.086% ± 0.040%	0.0020% ± 0.00033%	0.0015% ± 0.0011%
NiO C	0·47 mg/kg-bw	0.087% ± 0.030%	0.027% ± 0.013%	0.026% ± 0.0097%
	2·0 mg/kg-bw	0.28% ± 0.14%	0.19% ± 0.13%	0.13% ± 0.078%
	5·8 mg/kg-bw	0.40% ± 0.19%	0.29% ± 0.097%	0.28% ± 0.079%
NiO D	0·50 mg/kg-bw	0.52% ± 0.084%	0.38% ± 0.065%	0.25% ± 0.12%
	1·6 mg/kg-bw	0.46% ± 0.16%	0.30% ± 0.12%	0.15% ± 0.017%
	5·0 mg/kg-bw	0.24% ± 0.078%	0.27% ± 0.19%	0.21% ± 0.084%

Table 4 Percentage of NiO burden in each organ per administered dose. Values for the (A) lung, (B) bronchoalveolar lavage fluid (BALF), (C) trachea, and (D) lymph nodes are shown *(Continued)*

(D) Lymph nodes

		Lymph nodes NiO burden per initial body weight [mg/kg bw]		
		3 days after i.t.	28 days after i.t.	91 days after i.t.
NiO A	0·57 mg/kg-bw	0.040% ± 0.019%	0.75% ± 0.30%	1.4% ± 0.32%
	1·9 mg/kg-bw	0.068% ± 0.015%	1.6% ± 0.14%	1.7% ± 0.84%
	5·8 mg/kg-bw	0.10% ± 0.050%	3.0% ± 0.26%	3.6% ± 1.4%
NiO B	0·45 mg/kg-bw	0.051% ± 0.0053%	0.031% ± 0.0069%	0.017% ± 0.0062%
	1·5 mg/kg-bw	0.025% ± 0.0029%	0.014% ± 0.0013%	0.0092% ± 0.0051%
	4·0 mg/kg-bw	0.012% ± 0.0018%	0.012% ± 0.0036%	0.0040% ± 0.00083%
NiO C	0·47 mg/kg-bw	0.0088% ± 0.0026%	0.0062% ± 0.0024%	0.0057% ± 0.0022%
	2·0 mg/kg-bw	0.015% ± 0.0061%	0.065% ± 0.063%	0.23% ± 0.15%
	5·8 mg/kg-bw	0.052% ± 0.023%	0.67% ± 0.31%	2.0% ± 1.1%
NiO D	0·50 mg/kg-bw	0.11% ± 0.0047%	1.7% ± 0.29%	2.2% ± 0.63%
	1·6 mg/kg-bw	0.17% ± 0.020%	3.0% ± 1.4%	4.0% ± 0.69%
	5·0 mg/kg-bw	0.15% ± 0.018%	5.2% ± 2.2%	11% ± 2.4%

dissolution may occur in macrophage lysosomes following phagocytosis, and would occur more rarely outside macrophages. Pulmonary clearance rates were much faster in rats treated with NiO B than in those treated with NiO A, C, or D. The clearance rates of NiO B were much faster than previously reported fast clearance rate constants for insoluble particles [19, 20]. This suggested that the clearance pathway of NiO B was different from the clearance pathways of other insoluble particles. For NiO B, the relative percentage of the Ni found in BALF to total lung burden correlated inversely with the dose and increased over time, whereas those values were stable for the other three NiO nanoparticles. NiO B was excreted in the urine within 24 h of administration to a greater extent than the other NiO particles tested. In addition, the Ni ion/total Ni in BALF fraction for NiO B was higher than the corresponding values for NiO A, C, and D. These data suggest that the Ni ions dissolved from NiO B translocated from the lungs to the blood and kidneys, and were excreted in the urine as excretion of intravenously administered Ni ions has been shown to be rapid [21].

The pulmonary half-life (= $\ln 2/k_{\text{Lung}}$) of NiO B was calculated as 4.4–4.5 days, and 310–410, 59–170, and 82–110 days for NiO A, C, and D, respectively. The half-life of NiO A, C, and D might be found to be longer if the observation period was set to be longer than that in the present study. This is because the effects of fast clearance decrease comparing to slow clearance over time. Previously, the pulmonary half-life of micron-sized, soluble $NiSO_4$ particles was determined to be 1.6 h, while that of micron-sized, insoluble NiO and Ni_3S_2 particles was 92 and 90 days, respectively [22]. Differences observed between $NiSO_4$ and NiO B might be attributable to the

Table 5 Percentage of Ni in bronchoalveolar lavage fluid (BALF) per Ni in total lung post-administration

		(Ni in BALF) / (Ni in lung and BALF)		
		3 days after i.t.	28 days after i.t.	91 days after i.t.
NiO A	0.57 mg/kg-bw	2.4% ± 1.2%	0.84% ± 0.11%	1.2% ± 0.24%
	1.9 mg/kg-bw	0.59% ± 0.043%	0.89% ± 0.043%	0.60% ± 0.041%
	5.8 mg/kg-bw	0.79% ± 0.52%	2.5% ± 0.70%	0.89% ± 0.48%
NiO B	0.45 mg/kg-bw	3.0% ± 0.88%	31% ± 13%	76% ± 17%
	1.5 mg/kg-bw	4.0% ± 1.0%	19% ± 5.0%	38% ± 2.9%
	4.0 mg/kg-bw	2.8% ± 0.82%	8.9% ± 1.8%	22% ± 5.8%
NiO C	0.47 mg/kg-bw	1.7% ± 0.72%	3.2% ± 1.4%	5.0% ± 1.5%
	2.0 mg/kg-bw	3.2% ± 1.4%	2.5% ± 0.86%	3.1% ± 1.1%
	5.8 mg/kg-bw	5.0% ± 1.5%	1.3% ± 1.4%	1.2% ± 0.93%
NiO D	0.50 mg/kg-bw	2.4% ± 0.29%	3.7% ± 1.7%	2.5% ± 0.33%
	1.6 mg/kg-bw	1.8% ± 0.61%	5.7% ± 1.1%	3.2% ± 0.68%
	5.0 mg/kg-bw	2.0% ± 0.42%	2.7% ± 1.3%	4.8% ± 1.5%

high solubility of $NiSO_4$ in water, whereas NiO B is highly soluble in lysosomal fluid but only slightly soluble in water, saline, and interstitium fluid. The pulmonary half-life of six types of insoluble TiO_2 particles has been reported as 34–44 days and 52–94 days for <2 mg/kg and 6 mg/kg, respectively, while that of $Al(OH)_3$-coated TiO_2 particles was 64, 141, and 907 days for 0.67, 2, and 6 mg/kg, respectively [2]. In addition, the slow clearance of NiO C and $Al(OH)_3$-coated TiO_2 particles may be explained by the toxicity of slightly dissolvable Ni or Al ions.

Particles in the alveolar region can be cleared by the following two routes: Route 1: Lung → phagocytosis by macrophage → macrophage transfer to the end of bronchi → tracheal ciliary motility after phagocytosis; route 2: Lung → phagocytosis by macrophage → phagosome-lysosome fusion in macrophage → dissolution in macrophage. NiO uptake via the alveoli into the pulmonary circulation was not assessed in the present study because intravenously administered insoluble TiO_2 nanoparticles have been reported to be trapped in the liver [20], and the NiO burden in blood and liver was not high in the present study. Routes 1 and 2 operate in parallel, and events within each route occur in tandem. Therefore, k_{Lung} (/h) can be expressed using the phagocytosis rate constant, k_{phar} (/h), the macrophage migration to the end of bronchi rate constant, k_{mig} (/h), the phagosome-lysosome fusion rate constant, k_{fusion} (/h), and the dissolution rate constant in lysosomes, k_{dis} (/h), using the following equation:

$$\frac{1}{k_{Lung}} = \frac{1}{k_{phar}} + \frac{1}{\frac{1}{1/k_{dis}+1/k_{fusion}} + k_{mig}} \tag{4}$$

In the present study, as NiO nanoparticles were not observed outside macrophages in the microscopic

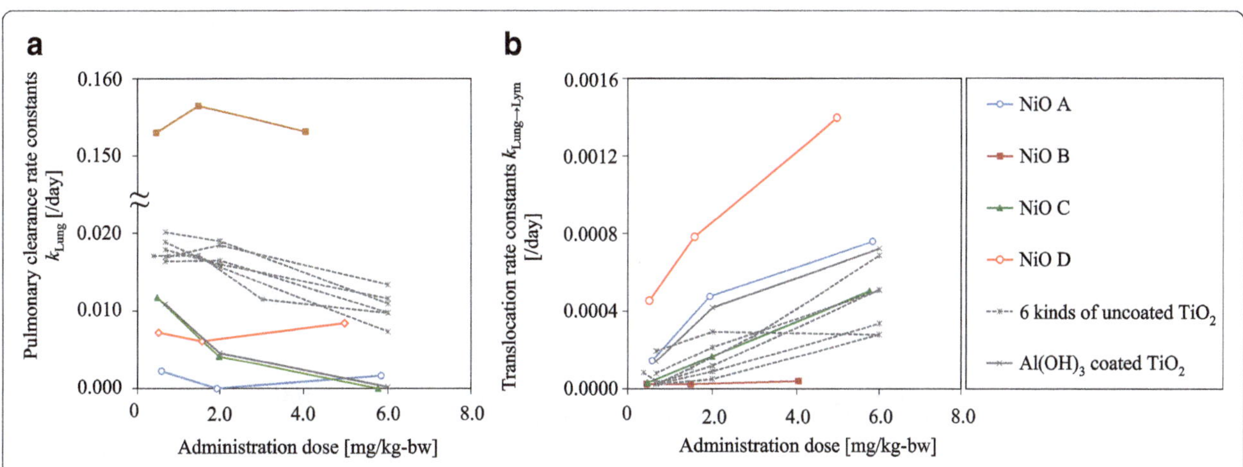

Fig. 4 Dose-dependent clearance rate constants (**a**) and lung-to-lymph nodes translocation rate constants (**b**). Broken line in (**a**) shows the 2-month half-life (0.0115/day). The rate constants of seven types of TiO_2 from a previous study [9] are also described in this figure

Table 6 Pulmonary clearance rate constants and initial fraction of administered NiO that reached the alveolar region

	Dose	Clearance rate constants k_{Lung} (1/day)	Half time $t_{1/2}$ (day)	Initial fraction reaching the alveolar region r	Translocation rate constants $k_{Lung \rightarrow Lym}$ (1/day)
NiO A	0.57 mg/kg-bw	0.0022	310 day	57%	0.00014
	1.9 mg/kg-bw	0.000	>690 day	58%	0.00048
	5.8 mg/kg-bw	0.0017	410 day	68%	0.00076
NiO B	0.45 mg/kg-bw	0.15	4.5 day	54%	0.000024
	1.5 mg/kg-bw	0.16	4.4 day	38%	0.000024
	4.0 mg/kg-bw	0.15	4.5 day	36%	0.000039
NiO C	0.47 mg/kg-bw	0.012	59 day	5.0%	0.000031
	2.0 mg/kg-bw	0.0041	170 day	20%	0.00017
	5.8 mg/kg-bw	0.000	>690 day	42%	0.00050
NiO D	0.50 mg/kg-bw	0.0073	96 day	97%	0.00045
	1.6 mg/kg-bw	0.0061	110 day	94%	0.00078
	5.0 mg/kg-bw	0.0084	82 day	88%	0.0014

Data estimated from the lung and bronchoalveolar lavage fluid (BALF) burden data, using a one-compartment model

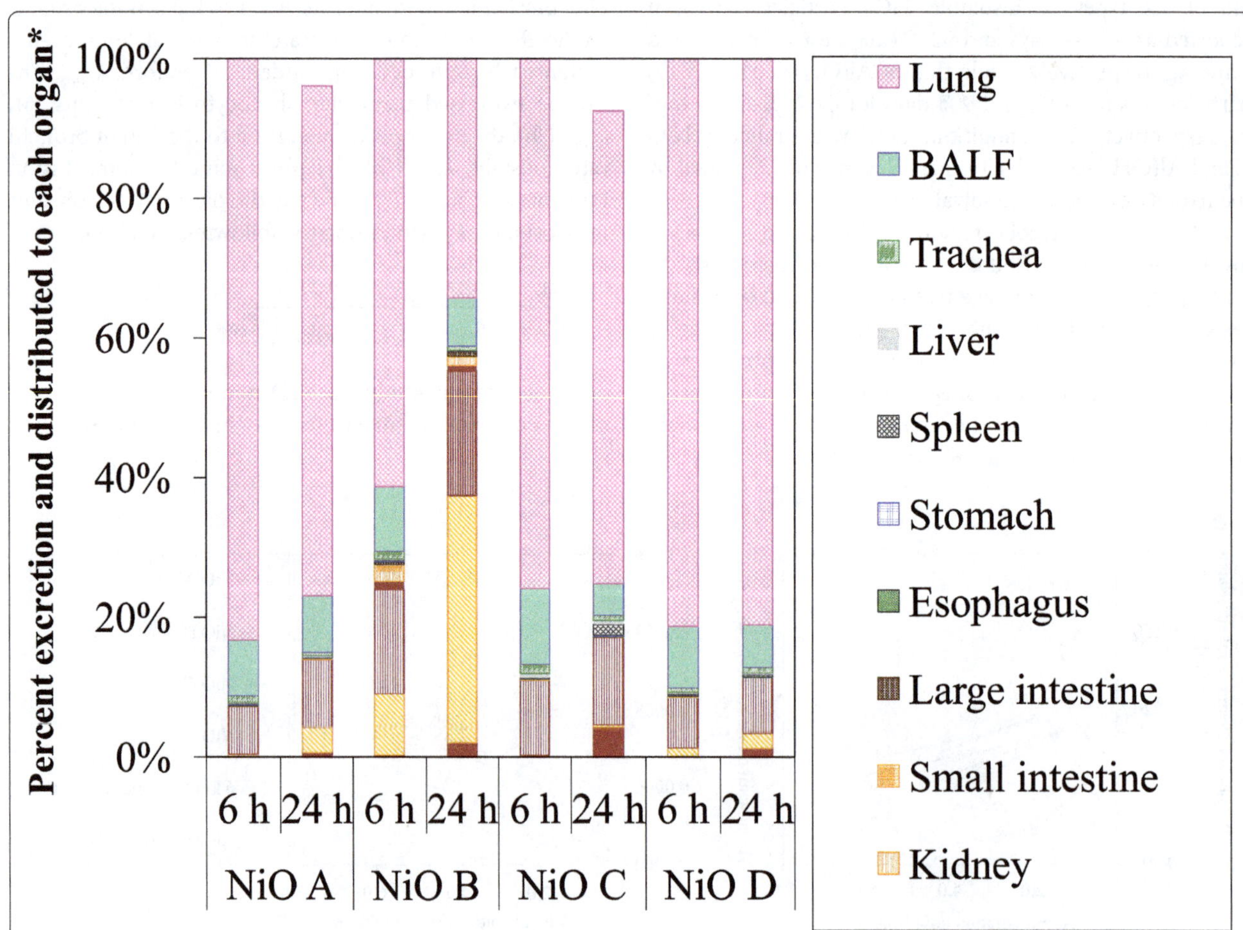

Fig. 5 Ni content in organs and excretion 6 h and 24 h post-administration. The total recovery 6 h post-administration was 94, 74, 41, and 90% for NiO A, B, C, and D, respectively

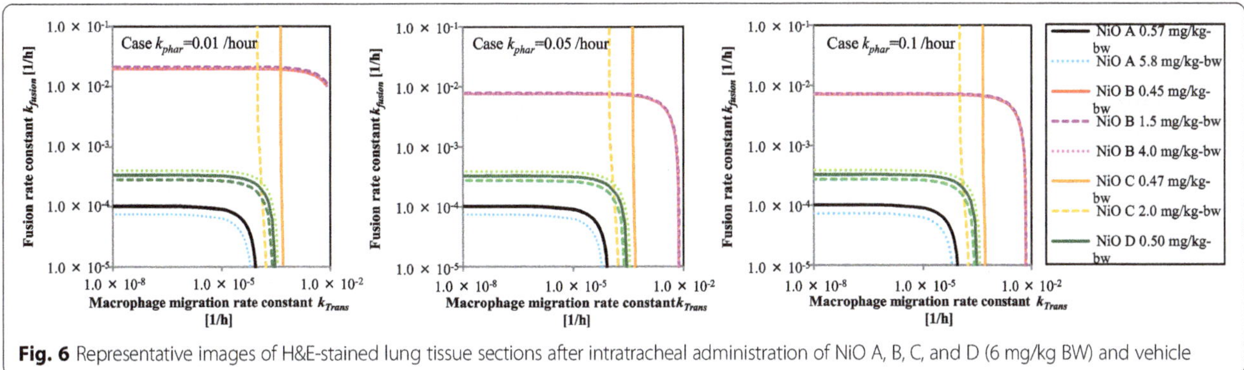

Fig. 6 Representative images of H&E-stained lung tissue sections after intratracheal administration of NiO A, B, C, and D (6 mg/kg BW) and vehicle

observation on day 3, k_{phar} was estimated to be approximately 0.05/h. Therefore, assuming that k_{phar} is 0.01, 0.05, or 0.1/h (52, 98, and >99% of particles are estimated to be ingested by macrophages 3 days after exposure), k_{fusion} and k_{mig} were estimated using the determined values of k_{Lung} and k_{dis}. Since k_{mig} was estimated to be constant with 1×10^{-1}–1×10^{-5}/h of k_{fusion} (Fig. 7) for NiO C only, the migration of macrophages after phagocytosis was suggested to be the rate-determining step (rate constant: 1×10^{-4}–5×10^{-4}/h). In other words, fusion and dissolution (Route 2) do not contribute to the pulmonary clearance of NiO C because of its low solubility in lysosomal fluid. This suggestion is in accordance with the dose-dependent overload observed for NiO C (only) in the animal experiment; this overload may reflect an inhibition of macrophage migration. For NiO A, B, and D, k_{fusion} or k_{mig} were estimated to increase in parallel with increasing solubility in lysosomal fluid (B > D > A) (Fig. 7). However, since overload was not observed in the animal experiment, particles located within macrophages did not affect k_{mig}. Therefore, increases in k_{mig} with solubility cannot be explained, whereas increases in k_{fusion} with solubility appear to be reasonable, indicating that phagosome-lysosome fusion represents the rate-determining step. The k_{fusion} values were estimated to be 1×10^{-4}, 1×10^{-2}, and 2×10^{-4} for any concentration of NiO A, B, and D, respectively. Inhibition and/or promotion of phagosome-lysosome fusion depends on the proteins around the particles [23–25].

Table 7 Neutrophil counts in bronchoalveolar lavage fluid after intratracheal administration to rats

	Neutrophil counts in BALF [cells/μL]		
	Day 3	Week 4	Week 13
NiO A (6 mg/kg BW)	374 ± 125	446 ± 113	767 ± 465
NiO B (6 mg/kg BW)	534 ± 186	94.2 ± 60.8	0.363 ± 0.725
NiO C (6 mg/kg BW)	10.1 ± 4.44	4.10 ± 2.89	4.17 ± 6.60
NiO D (6 mg/kg BW)	391 ± 171	693 ± 379	1240 ± 472
Control	0.55 ± 0.88	0.33 ± 0.35	0.61 ± 0.73

The adsorbed proteins on the particle can differ depending on the particle solubility.

For NiO B, the dissolution rate constant in lysosomal fluid (0.18/h) was much higher than that in interstitium solution (3.6×10^{-3}/h), suggesting that NiO B dissolved in macrophages immediately following fusion. This is consistent with the findings that extracellular ion fractions in BALF were much higher for NiO B than for NiO A, C, or D. The elevated Ni concentrations in blood, kidney, and urine of animals treated with NiO B, compared with those receiving NiO A, C, or D, suggested that dissolved Ni was cleared via blood to the kidney and excreted in urine. The fairly low blood Ni level (< 1% 6 h after administration) indicated that this process occurred rapidly.

NiO translocation to thoracic lymph nodes increased in a time- and dose-dependent manner for NiO A, C, and D; this observation has also been reported for other insoluble particles (TiO_2) [2, 26–28], but not for NiO B. These data suggest that dissolved Ni ions are distributed in the blood, but are not transferred to the lymph or immediately cleared from the lymph nodes.

The translocation of particles to lymph nodes indicates an overload due to damaged epithelial cells, as previously described [29]; particles that are cleared more slowly are transferred to the lymph nodes. In the present study, however, translocation to the lymph nodes was faster for NiO D than for NiO A, although pulmonary clearance rates were faster for NiO D than for NiO A. These phenomena are likely attributable to the greater solubility of NiO D in lysosomal fluid. Since Ni ions were not transferred to the lymph or immediately cleared from the lymph nodes, a possible mechanism for translocation to lymph nodes includes damage to epithelial cells, attributable to the Ni ion from NiO A and D, as well as from overloaded particles dissolving in the lysosome.

Particles that are soluble outside macrophages (e.g. $NiSO_4$) have been shown to induce greater acute pulmonary inflammation than Ni compounds with lower solubility (e.g. Ni_3S_2, NiO, and $Ni(OH)_2$) [13]. Ag ions are rapidly and directly toxic to organs, while nanoparticles induce toxicity more slowly, after dissolution in the

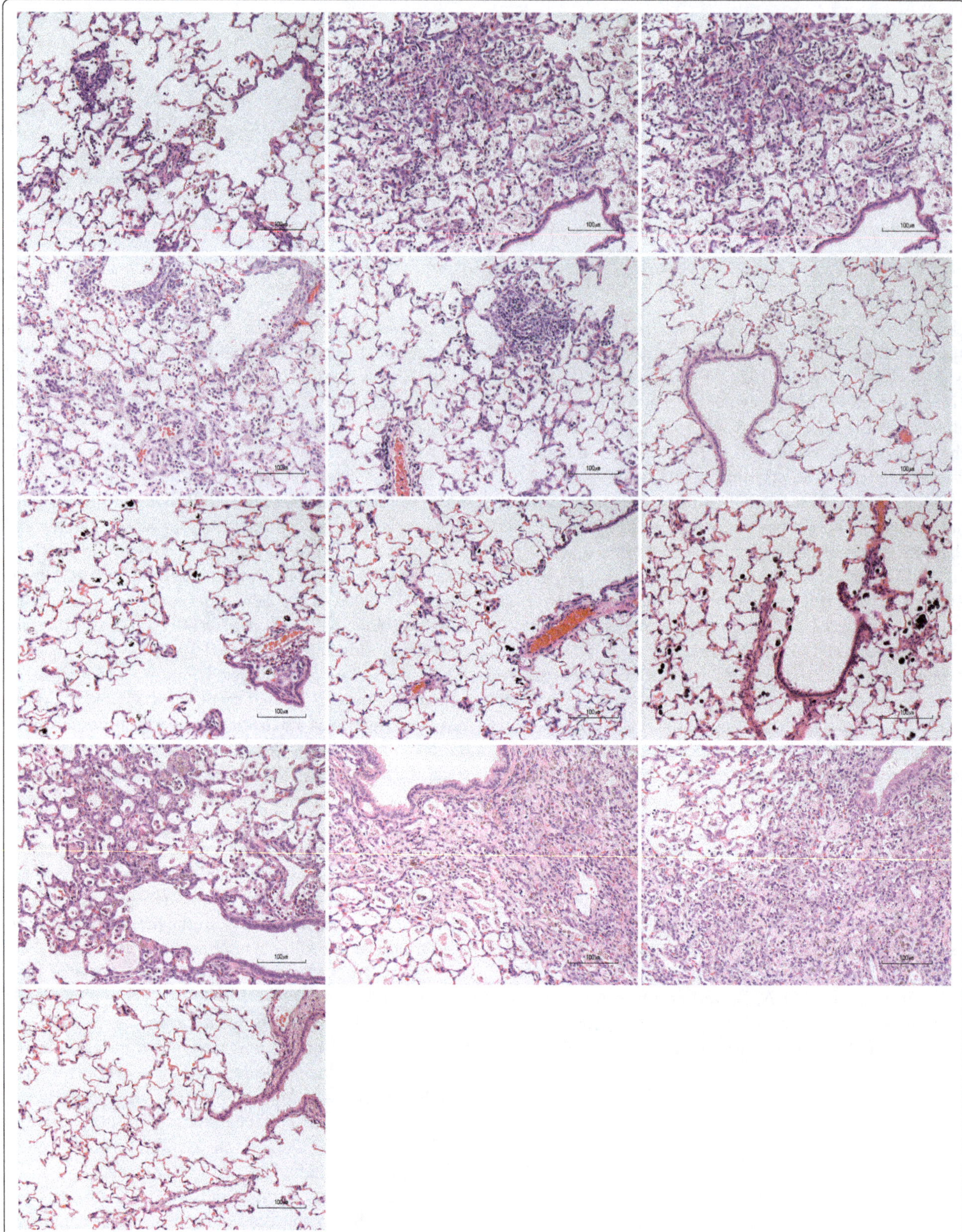

Fig. 7 Estimated macrophage migration to end of the bronchi rate constant and phagosome-lysosome fusion rate constant. The estimate was calculated for 0.01, 0.05, and 0.1 /h dissolution rate constants in the lysosome

lysosome [30]. Nanoparticles that are located within the macrophage and are rapidly soluble, such as NiO B, may induce acute pulmonary inflammation if the ion is toxic. Soluble nanoparticles located outside the macrophage can induce more severe inflammation than those within macrophages because the ion concentrations are much higher for the nanoparticles located outside the macrophage. However, this acute inflammation would decrease rapidly over time, because the dissolved Ni ions are rapidly cleared from the lungs [7, 8, 31]. In contrast, moderately soluble nanoparticles located within the macrophage, such as NiO A and D, may induce persistent pulmonary inflammation because of their longer retention and continual release of Ni ions in the lysosome. NiO particles that showed low solubility accumulated and induced chronic pulmonary effects in rats and mice, while water-soluble $NiSO_4$ did not produce these effects [8]. In addition, nanoparticles such as NiO D, which dissolve slowly within macrophages induced only mild acute and persistent pulmonary inflammation. These results suggest that dissolution tests in biological fluids and ion toxicity data can provide valuable information on the acute and chronic toxicity of nanoparticles. However, nanoparticles with moderate solubility and highly toxic ions (such as NiO A and D) require animal testing using a relevant exposure route such as intratracheal administration to obtain toxicity and toxicokinetic data.

In the present study, we conducted intratracheal administration of nanomaterials on rats for the evaluation of inhalation exposure. There are some differences between rats and humans and between inhalation exposure and intratracheal administration. The fast clearance rate was not different between humans and rats, while the slow clearance rate was 2 or 3 times higher for rats than for humans [19] and the fast clearance rate was 1-order higher than the slow clearance rate [19]. Therefore, at least the magnitude relationship of the clearance rate did not switch under overload-level doses. In a previous study, there were no significant differences in multi-wall carbon nanotube retention between intratracheal administration and inhalation [32] and the treatment groups had the same ranking whether measured after intratracheal inhalation or after instillation of tracer particles [33]. Therefore, we can compare the clearance rate constants between different nanoparticles using intratracheal instillation test on rats.

Conclusion

The present study measured the dissolution of nanoparticles in six different solutions, including artificial lysosomal fluid and artificial interstitium fluid. The tissue distribution and clearance of four types of NiO nanoparticles with different characteristics were determined 3, 28, and 91 days after intratracheal administration in rats. In particular, NiO nanoparticles that dissolve rapidly in artificial lysosomal fluid can be easily cleared from the lungs. With the exception of submicron NiO particles, pulmonary clearance overload was not observed, suggesting that the clearance mechanisms are not associated with macrophage migration to the end of bronchi, but involve dissolution in macrophage lysosomes.

Additional files

Additional file 1: Contents of artificial lung interstitium fluid and artificial lysosomal fluid. The reagents were dissolved in pure water one by one beginning at the top (DOCX 20 kb)

Additional file 2: Recovery efficiencies from Ni-spiked samples (DOCX 18 kb)

Additional file 3: NiO burdens per initial body weight at the time of administration. Values for (A) lung, (B) bronchoalveolar lavage fluid (BALF), (C) trachea, and (D) lymph nodes are shown (DOCX 33 kb)

Additional file 4: NiO burdens per organ tissue weight. Values for (A) lung, (B) bronchoalveolar lavage fluid (BALF), (C) trachea, and (D) lymph nodes are shown (DOCX 33 kb)

Additional file 5: Percentage of Ni in each lymph node out of the total Ni in all lymph nodes (DOCX 19 kb)

Abbreviations

ANOVA: Analysis of variance; BALF: Bronchoalveolar lavage fluid; BW: Body weight; ICP-MS: Inductively coupled plasma-mass spectrometry; NiO: Nickel oxide

Acknowledgements

This work is part of the research program "Development of innovative methodology for safety assessment of industrial nanomaterials", supported by the Ministry of Economy, Trade and Industry (METI) of Japan.

Funding

Ministry of Economy, Trade and Industry (METI) of Japan.

Authors' contributions

NS and MG conceived the hypothesis and designed the study. SM, YO, TK, NI, and MN performed the animal experiments. TS and KK prepared and characterized the NiO suspension. NS and GZ analyzed the samples using ICP-MS. NS analyzed the data. NS and MG wrote the manuscript. All authors have read and approved the final manuscript.

Competing interests

The authors declare that they have no competing interests.

Author details

[1]National Institute of Advanced Industrial Science and Technology (AIST), Tsukuba, Ibaraki 305-8569, Japan. [2]Chemicals Evaluation and Research Institute (CERI), Hita, Oita 877-0061, Japan. [3]Chemicals Evaluation and Research Institute (CERI), Bunkyo, Tokyo 112-0004, Japan. [4]National Institute of Advanced Industrial Science and Technology (AIST), Tsukuba, Ibaraki 305-8565, Japan.

References

1. Borm PJ, Robbins D, Haubold S, Kuhlbusch T, Fissan H, Donaldson K, et al. The potential risks of nanomaterials: a review carried out for ECETOC. Particle fibre. Toxicology. 2006;3:11.
2. Shinohara N, Oshima Y, Kobayashi T, Imatanaka N, Nakai M, Ichinose T, et al. Pulmonary clearance kinetics and extrapulmonary translocation of seven titanium dioxide nano and submicron materials following intratracheal administration in rats. Nanotoxicology. 2015;9:1050–8.
3. Hashizume N, Oshima Y, Nakai M, Kobayashi T, Sasaki T, Kawaguchi K, et al. Categorization of nano-structured titanium dioxide according to physicochemical characteristics and pulmonary toxicity. Toxicol Reports. 2016;3:490–500.
4. Ogami A, Morimoto Y, Myojo T, Oyabu T, Murakami M, Todoroki M, et al. Pathological features of different sizes of nickel oxide following intratracheal instillation in rats. Inhal Toxicol. 2009;21:812–8.
5. Horie M, Nishio K, Fujita K, Kato H, Nakamura A, Kinugasa S, et al. Ultrafine NiO particles induce cytotoxicity in vitro by cellular uptake and subsequent Ni(II) release. Chem Res Toxicol. 2009;22:1415–26.
6. Yamada M, Takahashi S, Sato H, Kubota Y, Kikuchi T, Furuya K. Solubility of nickel oxide particles in various solutions and rat alveolar macrophages. Biol Trace Element Res. 1993;36:89–98.
7. Benson JM, Barr EB, Bechtold WE, Cheng Y-S, Dunnick JK, Eastin WE. Fate of inhaled nickel-oxide and nickel subsulfide in F344/N rats. Inhal Toxicol. 1994; 6:167–83.
8. Benson JM, Chang IY, Cheng YS, Hahn FF, Kennedy CH, Barr EB, et al. Particle clearance and histopathology in lungs of F344/N rats and B6C3F1 mice inhaling nickel oxide or nickel sulfate. Fundam Appl Toxicol. 1995;28: 232–44.
9. Hsieh TH, CP Y, Oberdorster G. Deposition and clearance models of Ni compounds in the mouse lung and comparisons with the rat models. Aerosol Sci Technol. 1999;31:358–72.
10. Dunnick JK, Elwell MR, Benson JM, Hobbs CH, Hahn FF, Haly PJ, et al. Lung toxicity after 13-week inhalation exposure to nickel oxide, nickel subsulfide, or nickel sulfate hexahydrate in F344/N rats and B6C3F1 mice. Fundam Appl Toxicol. 1989;12:584–94.
11. IARC. IARC Monographs on the evaluation of carcinogenic risk of chemicals to humans, nickel and nickel compounds. 1990;100C:169–208.
12. NTP NTP. Toxicology and carcinogenesis studies of nickel oxide (CAS no. 1313-99-1) in F344 rats and B6C3F1 mice (inhalation studies). Natl Toxicol Program Tech Rep Ser. 1996;451:1–381.
13. Kang GS, Gillespie PA, Gunnison A, Rengifo H, Koberstein J, Chen LC. Comparative pulmonary toxicity of inhaled nickel nanoparticles; role of deposited dose and solubility. Inhal Toxicol. 2011;23:95–103.
14. Takahashi S, Oishi M, Takeda E, Kubota Y, Kikuchi T, Furuya K. Physicochemical characteristics and toxicity of nickel oxide particles calcined at different temperatures. Biol Trace Element Res. 1999;69:161–74.
15. Takahashi S, Yamada M, Kondo T, Sato H, Furuya K, Tanaka I. Cytotoxicity of nickel oxide particles in rat alveolar macro phages cultured in vitro. J Toxicol Sci. 1992;17:243–51.
16. Test ST, Weiss SJ. Quantitative and temporal characterization of the extracellular H_2O_2 pool generated by human neutrophils. J Biol Chem. 1984; 259:399–405.
17. Millonig G, Ganzleben I, Peccerella T, Casanovas G, Brodziak-Jarosz L, Breitkopf-Heinlein K, et al. Sustained submicromolar H_2O_2 levels induce hepcidin via signal transducer and activator of transcription 3 (STAT3). J Biol Chem. 2012;287:37472–82.
18. Ji G, O'Brien CD, Feldman M, Manevich Y, Lim P, Sun J, et al. PECAM-1 (CD31) regulates a hydrogen peroxide-activated nonselective cation channel in endothelial cells. J Cell Biol. 2002;157:173–84.
19. Hsieh TH, Yu CP. Two-phase pulmonary clearance of insoluble particles in mammalian species. Inhal Toxicol. 1998;10:121–30.
20. Shinohara N, Danno D, Ichinose T, Sasaki T, Fukui H, Honda K, Gamo M. Tissue distribution and clearance of intravenously administered titanium dioxide (TiO_2) nanoparticles. Nanotoxicology. 2014;8:132–41.
21. Onkelinx C, Becker J, Sunderman FW Jr. Compartmental analysis of metabolism of Ni-63(II) in rats and rabbits. Res Commun Chem Pathol Pharmacol. 1973;6:663–76.
22. Hsieh TH, CP Y, Oberdorster G. A dosimetry model of nickel compounds in the rat lung. Inhal Toxicol. 1999;11:229–48.
23. Liebl D, Griffiths G. Transient assembly of F-actin by phagosomes delays phagosome fusion with lysosomes in cargo overloaded macrophages. J Cell Sci. 2009;122:2935–45.
24. Kim GHE, Dayam RM, Prashar A, Terebiznik M, Botelho RJ. PIKfyve inhibition interferes with phagosome and endosome maturation in macrophages. Traffic. 2014;15:1143–63.
25. Tjelle TE, Lùvdal T, Berg T. Phagosome dynamics and function. BioEssays. 2000;22:255–63.
26. Bermudez E, Mangum JB, Wong BA, Asgharian B, Hext PM, Warheit DB, et al. Pulmonary responses of mice, rats, and hamsters to subchronic inhalation of ultrafine titanium dioxide particles. Toxicol Sci. 2004;77:347–57.
27. van Ravenzwaay B, Landsiedel R, Fabian E, Burkhardt S, Strauss V, Ma-Hock L. Comparing fate and effects of three particles of different surface properties: Nano-TiO_2, pigmentary TiO_2 and quartz. Toxicol Lett. 2009;186:152–9.
28. Shinohara N, Oshima Y, Kobayashi T, Imatanaka N, Nakai M, Ichinose T, et al. Dose-dependent clearance kinetics of intratracheally administered titanium dioxide nanoparticles in rat lung. Toxicology. 2014;325:1–11.
29. Cullen RT, Tran CL, Buchanan D, Davis JM, Searl A, Jones AD, et al. Inhalation of poorly soluble particles. I. Differences in inflammatory response and clearance during exposure. Inhal Toxicol. 2000;12:1089–111.
30. Arai Y, Miyayama T, Hirano S. Difference in the toxicity mechanism between ion and nanoparticle forms of silver in the mouse lung and in macrophages. Toxicology. 2015;328:84–92.
31. Ghezzi I, Baldasseroni A, Sesana G, Boni C, Cortona G, Alessio L. Behaviour of urinary nickel in low-level occupational exposure. Med Lav. 1989;80:244–50.
32. Silva RM, Doudrick K, Franzi LM, Teesy C, Anderson DS, Wu ZQ, et al. Instillation versus inhalation of multiwalled carbon Nanotubes: exposure-related health effects, clearance, and the role of particle characteristics. ACS Nano. 2014;8:8911–31.
33. Oberdorster G, Cox C, Gelein R. Intratracheal instillation versus intratracheal inhalation of tracer particles for measuring lung clearance function. Exp Lung Res. 1997;23:17–34.

15

Association of pulmonary, cardiovascular, and hematologic metrics with carbon nanotube and nanofiber exposure among U.S. workers

Mary K. Schubauer-Berigan[1*], Matthew M. Dahm[1], Aaron Erdely[2], John D. Beard[1,3,5], M. Eileen Birch[4], Douglas E. Evans[4], Joseph E. Fernback[4], Robert R. Mercer[2], Stephen J. Bertke[1], Tracy Eye[2] and Marie A. de Perio[1]

Abstract

Background: Commercial use of carbon nanotubes and nanofibers (CNT/F) in composites and electronics is increasing; however, little is known about health effects among workers. We conducted a cross-sectional study among 108 workers at 12 U.S. CNT/F facilities. We evaluated chest symptoms or respiratory allergies since starting work with CNT/F, lung function, resting blood pressure (BP), resting heart rate (RHR), and complete blood count (CBC) components.

Methods: We conducted multi-day, full-shift sampling to measure background-corrected elemental carbon (EC) and CNT/F structure count concentrations, and collected induced sputum to measure CNT/F in the respiratory tract. We measured (nonspecific) fine and ultrafine particulate matter mass and count concentrations. Concurrently, we conducted physical examinations, BP measurement, and spirometry, and collected whole blood. We evaluated associations between exposures and health measures, adjusting for confounders related to lifestyle and other occupational exposures.

Results: CNT/F air concentrations were generally low, while 18% of participants had evidence of CNT/F in sputum. Respiratory allergy development was positively associated with inhalable EC (p=0.040) and number of years worked with CNT/F (p=0.008). No exposures were associated with spirometry-based metrics or pulmonary symptoms, nor were CNT/F-specific metrics related to BP or most CBC components. Systolic BP was positively associated with fine particulate matter (p-values: 0.015-0.054). RHR was positively associated with EC, at both the respirable (p=0.0074) and inhalable (p=0.0026) size fractions. Hematocrit was positively associated with the log of CNT/F structure counts (p=0.043).

Conclusions: Most health measures were not associated with CNT/F. The positive associations between CNT/F exposure and respiratory allergies, RHR, and hematocrit counts may not be causal and require examination in other studies.

Keywords: Epidemiology, Pulmonary function, Blood pressure, Heart rate, Occupational, Nanomaterials, Advanced manufacturing, Nanotoxicology

* Correspondence: zcg3@cdc.gov
[1]National Institute for Occupational Safety and Health (NIOSH), Division of Surveillance, Hazard Evaluations, and Field Studies, 1090 Tusculum Ave MS-R15, Cincinnati, OH 45226, USA
Full list of author information is available at the end of the article

Background

Carbon nanotubes and nanofibers (CNT/F) are small, high-aspect-ratio (>5 μm long, <100 nm diameter) engineered nanomaterials of increasing commercial importance; e.g., they are used in conductive film and ink development in the electronics industry, and as strong, lightweight components of composites used in aircraft. Toxicological evidence suggests possible health effects from exposure to CNT/F, which were among the first engineered nanomaterials to reach commercialization [1]. Pulmonary inflammation and fibrotic changes or malignant transformation have been observed in animal models [2–4], as well as immunological, neurological, and cardiovascular effects, due to particle translocation or response to an inflammatory cascade [5–9].

Pulmonary function has been studied among workers exposed to engineered nanomaterials [10–12], and lung fibrosis was identified as the primary target outcome in a toxicology-based risk assessment for CNT/F [13]. However, the cardiovascular system may be more sensitive to adverse effects of engineered nanomaterials [14, 15], given findings from ambient ultrafine and fine particulate (U/FP) studies. Resting heart rate (RHR), a marker of changes in the autonomic nervous system, has been related to particulate air pollution [16] and found to be predictive of overall mortality risk [17]. Hypertension has been associated with ambient U/FP exposure in humans [18, 19]. Systemic inflammation can also be assessed by hematologic measures: increased neutrophil counts following exposure have been observed in welders [20]. Increased total leukocyte and neutrophil counts were found to be associated with ambient U/FP exposure in humans [18, 21] and with multiwalled CNT (MWCNT) in an animal model [9, 22].

The aim of this analysis was to evaluate whether there are associations between health-relevant metrics and exposure to CNT/F in a cross-sectional population of 108 U.S. workers. We did not employ an explicit "exposed" and "control" group design, but considered exposure-outcome associations across the full range of exposure in the study group. This approach both provides more statistical power and is more useful for risk assessment. We examined (1) self-reported respiratory illness or symptoms (after initiation of work with CNT/F); (2) spirometric lung function metrics; (3) cardiovascular health metrics; and (4) hematologic metrics. Lung function metrics were forced vital capacity (FVC) as one measure of potential restrictive lung disease, the ratio of forced expiratory volume in the first second (FEV1) to FVC and peak expiratory flow (PEF) as two metrics of potential obstructive lung disease, and forced expiratory flow at 25-75% of the pulmonary volume (FEF25-75%) as a potential indicator of small airways disease. Cardiovascular metrics were resting systolic and diastolic blood pressure (BP) and RHR. Hematologic measures were leukocyte counts and absolute concentrations of three leukocyte subcomponents (neutrophils, lymphocytes, and monocytes), platelets, hemoglobin, and hematocrit. Analyses of other markers of early effect (e.g., inflammatory cytokines, oxidative stress biomarkers, and endothelial activation products) in blood and sputum collected from this population are described elsewhere [23].

Methods

Selection of companies and participants

U.S. facilities handling CNT/F were eligible for inclusion in this study. Typical properties of CNT/Fs are described elsewhere [24]. We identified companies based on their participation in a survey to enumerate the engineered carbonaceous nanomaterial industry [1], supplemented with additional companies. Among 59 companies, 19 were considered for recruitment for the cross-sectional study, based on willingness to be interviewed about details related to their operations or participation in previous NIOSH exposure investigations [24, 25]. Four of the 19 companies were ineligible because they had stopped working with CNT/F (n=2) or were operating at purely research scale (n=2). Three eligible companies refused to participate. Thus, 80% of invited companies agreed to participate. For 11 of the 12 participating facilities, all employees working in a CNT/F unit were invited to participate. For one facility, due to its large size and study feasibility limitations, a subset of employees representing the widest variety of tasks was invited. Overall, 75% of eligible workers participated in the study (see Additional file 1: Table S1).

Exposure assessment for CNT/F and U/FP

We visited participating companies from 12/2012-9/2014 and conducted at least two days of full-shift, personal breathing zone exposure monitoring for each study participant (except one participant who was unavailable during the period of exposure monitoring and was assigned the exposure level of a co-worker performing similar tasks), as described elsewhere [24, 26]. In summary, each participant wore three air sampling pumps connected to filters located in the participant's breathing zone to measure the mass concentration of elemental carbon (EC) [13], for both the respirable and inhalable size fractions. A third set of air samples was collected for examination using transmission electron microscopy (TEM), which allowed the enumeration and size-binning of each particle with associated CNT/F, referred to as a CNT/F "structure" [27]. Air concentrations were calculated for total CNT/F structures (total structures/cm^3), and for size-specific structures [single fibers/cm^3, structures <1 μm (in diameter)/cm^3, structures <2 μm/cm^3, structures <5 μm/cm^3, and structures <10 μm/cm^3]. We evaluated multiple size bins for the structure counts because the most relevant size class of CNT/F for each health outcome is uncertain.

We used three direct-reading instruments to collect total ambient U/FP and ultrafine particulate (UP) count and U/FP mass, using general area samples contemporaneously collected with the CNT/F-specific measurements [26, 28, 29]. These metrics are: total U/FP counts (per cm^3), defined as 10-1000 nm in diameter [collected with a condensation particle counter (CPC 3007; TSI, Inc., Shoreview, MN)], total UP particulate counts (per cm^3), defined as 23-96 nm (collected with an electrical low-pressure impactor Dekati, Ltd, Tampere, Finland), and particulate mass ($\mu g/m^3$) less than 2.5 µm (collected with a DustTrak® photometer; DRX Model 8533; TSI, Inc., Shoreview, MN). Estimates of each participant's exposure were made, for each day of sampling, using professional judgment of the locations of the participant throughout their sampling day [26].

Questionnaire administration

Mid-shift during a mid-week workday (concurrently with exposure assessment), each participant was administered a standardized questionnaire by a trained interviewer. Questions were included on demographics, medical history, current and past exposure to CNT/F and other physical and chemical agents, and smoking and alcohol consumption (see Additional file 2). Questions pertaining to respiratory symptoms and illnesses were obtained from the American Thoracic Society (ATS) 1978 Adult Questionnaire [30]. Questions related to fitness for undergoing spirometry were drawn from the National Health and Nutrition Examination Survey (NHANES) Respiratory Health Spirometry Procedures Manual [31].

Medical examination, blood pressure and heart rate measurement, and spirometry

Immediately after questionnaire administration, participants were examined in a mobile examination unit by a study physician, who reviewed medical histories to determine eligibility for spirometry, sputum induction, and phlebotomy. Height without shoes (using a stadiometer) and waist circumference (using a tape measure) were measured to the nearest 0.5 cm, and weight was measured using a digital scale to the nearest 0.1 kg. Systolic and diastolic BP and RHR were ascertained after resting for five minutes, using the method described in NHANES [32, 33]. Readings were obtained with an OMRON™ HEM-907XL digital sphygmomanometer, which was calibration-checked weekly against an analog instrument. Three readings were collected for each metric, and the second and third readings were averaged for analysis. Two participants who completed the exposure assessment and questionnaire declined to participate in the medical examination and subsequent procedures.

We used a volume-based spirometer and standard methodology recommended by the ATS [34, 35] to collect spirometry metrics for all participants (n=103) not refusing or excluded based on medical exclusion criteria. Spirometry tests were conducted by a certified technician, who followed quality guidelines noted by ATS, and were interpreted clinically using ATS recommendations [35]. We used the percent predicted (PP) values for FVC, FEV1/FVC% (using the largest valid FEV1 and FVC), FEF25-75%, and PEF. Further details on the collection and interpretation of the spirometry data are provided in Additional file 3.

Collection of whole blood and complete blood count measurement

Whole blood was obtained through venipuncture for the CBC analysis, as well as for serum and plasma biomarker analyses described elsewhere [23]. A 3-mL ethylene-diaminetetraacetic acid tube of whole blood was collected, inverted 10 times, and stored at room temperature until the end of the day, when each batch was sent to a clinical laboratory (Quest Diagnostics or LabCorp) for CBC analyses using an automated cell counter. A shipping error resulted in the loss of samples for four participants. CBC analyses were available for 98 participants.

Sputum induction and processing

Sputum induction methodology is detailed in Additional file 3. In summary, seven participants were excluded based on contraindications. Ninety other participants agreed to provide sputum, which was induced by breathing aerosolized isotonic saline generated with a compressed-air nebulizer. Isotonic saline was used to reduce the likelihood of bronchial spasm induction and because previous research suggested that sputum of acceptable quality could be obtained [36]. However, we found the percentage of squamous epithelial cells, determined by manual counting, to be very high (>80% for all but one participant), likely due to the use of isotonic saline and the processing of the entire sputum specimen (rather than selecting sputum plugs from each specimen). Sputum cellular fractions were preserved at 4°C.

After arrival in the NIOSH laboratory, we prepared a cytospin of the cell pellet on ultrasonically cleaned, laser cut slides (Schott North America, Inc, Elmsford, NY). To enhance the contrast of nanomaterials, cytospin slides were stained with Sirius Red. Sections were briefly counterstained in freshly filtered Mayer's hematoxylin for 2 minutes, dehydrated, and coverslipped. Approximately 3,000 cells per slide (<1% of each specimen) were examined for evidence of CNT/F structures using dark-field microscopy [37].

Statistical methods

From the questionnaire, we estimated the length of time each participant worked with CNT/F (not always concordant with length of employment in the industry) as an integrative metric of past CNT/F exposure. We also estimated self-reported exposure to a variety of physical and chemical agents in the workplace (Additional file 1: Table S2). For most outcomes, the following were considered as potential confounders: age, sex, race/ethnicity, cigarette pack-years, self-reported current or past occupational exposures to solvents, polymers, strong acids, "other" (non-CNT/F) forms of nanomaterials, and a general category of particulates, termed "other dusts". Other potential confounders for some outcomes included childhood pneumonia, current self-reported respiratory diseases, alcohol consumption, use of certain medications, and a modified cardiovascular health metric (CHM) score (after [38], except using six metrics: body mass index, waist circumference, hypertension diagnosis, diabetes diagnosis, cigarette smoking, and use of antihypercholesterolemic medication; see Additional file 1: Tables S3 and S4).

Five CNT/F exposure variables were evaluated in exposure-response analyses: respirable and inhalable EC mass concentrations in air, TEM structure concentrations in air, presence/absence of CNT structures in induced sputum, and duration of exposure to any form of CNT/F. All EC samples were background-corrected to account for other (naturally occurring and anthropogenic) sources of EC [24]. Arithmetic means of all sampled days were used for these metrics.

We used a prevalent case-control analysis for binary outcomes (i.e., self-reported chest symptoms and respiratory allergies) that permitted evaluation of whether the illness started before or after the start of work with CNT/F (e.g., [39]). We used logistic regression to model the odds of exposure among those who exhibited the outcome (cases) after the start of exposure to CNT/F compared to those who did not (controls), among those who were outcome-free before exposure began. Due to the small number of cases, we did not adjust for confounding for these outcomes, but we evaluated associations of potential confounders with the outcomes. For continuous metrics (i.e., systolic and diastolic BP, RHR, lung function metrics, CBC measures), we used multiple linear regression [40] to model the association between the exposure metrics and outcomes, adjusted for important confounders. Log-transforms (for FEF25-75%, leukocyte and its differential counts, and platelet counts) or square transforms (for hemoglobin and hematocrit concentrations) were used to improve normality of the model residuals. We evaluated log-transformation of the highly skewed CNT/F exposure metrics. Potential covariates were treated as continuous or categorical variables. Because some covariates were highly correlated, their inclusion could lead to poor parameter estimation [40], and the small sample size limited the number of covariates that could be included. Therefore, covariates were screened for each outcome metric in a model with no CNT/F metrics: the best-fitting model from among all possible combinations of up to 10 covariates was identified using Schwarz's Bayesian Criterion (SBC), where a smaller SBC value indicates better model fit [41]. Use of SBC to select model predictors for outcomes in small studies has been shown to be superior to other methods at identifying the "true" underlying model, given correlated covariates [41]. Covariates so selected were retained if they changed the parameter estimate for the best-fitting CNT/F exposure metric by >10%. Model fit for alternative exposure metrics (e.g., log-transformed metrics; different TEM size bin cut points) was determined using SBC values. Parameter estimates and two-sided p-values were reported. CNT/F effect modification for each outcome was evaluated for sex, race/ethnicity (white non-Hispanic compared to all whites), age (<40 compared to ≥40), education level (college degree or higher compared to no college degree), smoking status (ever compared to never), reported respiratory disease or allergy, and CHM score (5-6 compared to 0-4). Fit was evaluated in the multiple regression models by evaluating residual patterns for heteroscedasticity or other fit problems [40]. All analyses were conducted using SAS ver. 9.4 (Cary, NC).

Results

Descriptive information

Table 1 shows the demographic characteristics of the study participants. The majority were male and of white race and non-Hispanic ethnicity. Age followed a bimodal distribution, with modes in the mid-30s and mid-50s. Most (65.8%) participants had at least a college degree, with 38% having a post-graduate education. Participants mostly reported never smoking cigarettes (63%) and currently drinking alcohol (65.7%).

Sputum was obtained from 90 participants. CNT/F was detected, via dark-field microscopy, in the sputum of 16 (17.7%) of these participants (typical images are provided in Fig. 1). Multi-day mean CNT/F exposure concentrations are shown in Table 2. Median concentrations for inhalable and respirable EC were low, at 0.24 and 0.096 μg/m^3, respectively, while mean concentrations were substantially higher (6.22 and 1.00 μg/m^3) due to a few outlying observations. Only 7 participants had background-corrected respirable EC levels above the NIOSH recommended exposure limit (REL) of 1 μg/m^3.

Table 1 Demographic and lifestyle characteristics of 108 cross-sectional study participants

Characteristic	Group	N (%)
Sex	Male	85 (78.7%)
	Female	23 (21.3%)
Ethnicity and Race	Non-Hispanic White alone	87 (80.6%)
	Non-Hispanic Asian alone	10 (9.3%)
	African-American, American Indian/Alaska Native, Multiple races, and Hispanic combined	11 (10.2%)
Age (years)	<25	6 (5.6%)
	25-<35	33 (30.6%)
	35-<45	16 (14.8%)
	45-<55	28 (25.9%)
	55-<65	20 (18.5%)
	65-<75	5 (4.6%)
Highest education level	High school, Trade or vocational	13 (12.1%)
	Some college	24 (22.2%)
	College graduate	30 (27.8%)
	Postgraduate	41 (38.0%)
Cigarette smoking status	Never	68 (63.0%)
	Former	24 (22.2%)
	Current	16 (14.8%)
Alcohol consumption status	Never	7 (6.5%)
	Former	30 (27.8%)
	Current	71 (65.7%)

The mean and median TEM structure count concentrations (all sizes) were 0.128 and 0.0073 structures/cm^3, respectively. Most structures (60%) were in the 2-10 μm size range, and just 20% of participants had any single fibers detected. Nearly all workers who directly worked with CNT/F handled them in unpurified form; for >80% of workers in our study, CNT/F had been manufactured with a Fe-based catalyst. The mean and median duration of time working with CNT/F were 4.07 and 3.66 years, respectively (Table 2). Sixteen participants (15%) indicated they had never worked with CNT/F.

Pulmonary outcomes and metrics

A minority of study participants reported respiratory illnesses (allergy: 41%, asthma: 8%, COPD: 6%) or symptoms (42%) before their start of CNT/F work (Additional file 1: Table S5). No participants reported asthma or COPD after the start of CNT/F work, while 21% reported the initiation of one or more chest symptoms and 14% reported the development of respiratory allergies after beginning work with CNT/F (Table 3). 89% of those reporting respiratory allergies after the start of CNT/F work stated that their allergies had been confirmed by a physician. No CNT/F exposure metrics were significantly associated with development of chest symptoms after starting CNT/F work. No demographic, lifestyle, or occupational covariates were significantly associated with development of respiratory allergy (Additional file 1: Table S6), but both the inhalable EC concentration (OR=1.1 at mean exposure of 4 μg/m^3; p=0.04) and duration of work with CNT/F (OR=1.2 at 1 year duration; p=0.008) were significantly positively associated with self-reported development of respiratory allergies (Table 3).

Spirometry metrics indicated an overall healthy respiratory profile among participants (Table 4): 92 participants (89%) exhibited normal expiratory flows and a normal FVC. Five participants (4.9%) had restrictive patterns, and four participants (3.9%) showed obstructive patterns. No participants exhibited mixed obstructive and restrictive patterns. Results were not clinically interpretable for two participants (1.9%). Few covariates (namely, race/ethnicity, cigarette smoking, and current or past exposure to solvents, dust, or strong acids) were significantly related to any of the PP values for FVC, FEV1/FVC, FEF25-75%, or PEF (Additional file 1: Table S7). After adjusting for covariates, no lung function metric was significantly negatively associated with any of the CNT metrics (Table 5). However, duration of employment with CNT/F was positively associated with FEV1/FVC, FEF25-75%, and PEF. Use of a log-transform for the EC and TEM exposure metrics showed similar results. No significant effect modification was observed by sex, race, age, education, prior lung disease, or CHM score (Table 5).

Cardiovascular metrics

A majority (58%) of subjects had BP in a range associated with pre-hypertension or hypertension (i.e., systolic BP ≥120 or diastolic BP ≥80), while 13% had BP in a range associated with hypertension (i.e., systolic BP ≥140 or diastolic BP ≥90) (Table 4). Several covariates were significantly positively associated with systolic BP, diastolic BP, or RHR (Additional file 1: Table S8). U/FP counts were significantly positively associated only with systolic BP. Both before and after adjusting for confounding, none of the CNT/F metrics was significantly associated with systolic or diastolic BP, and point estimates tended to be negative for most exposure metrics (Additional file 1: Table S6 and S8). After adjusting for confounding, RHR was significantly positively associated with inhalable and respirable EC and significantly negatively associated with duration of time worked with CNT/F. (Table 6). Use of a log-transform for the EC and TEM exposure metrics showed similar results except for respirable EC, which was no longer significantly associated with RHR. While no significant effect modification was observed for BP by age, sex, race, education, prior

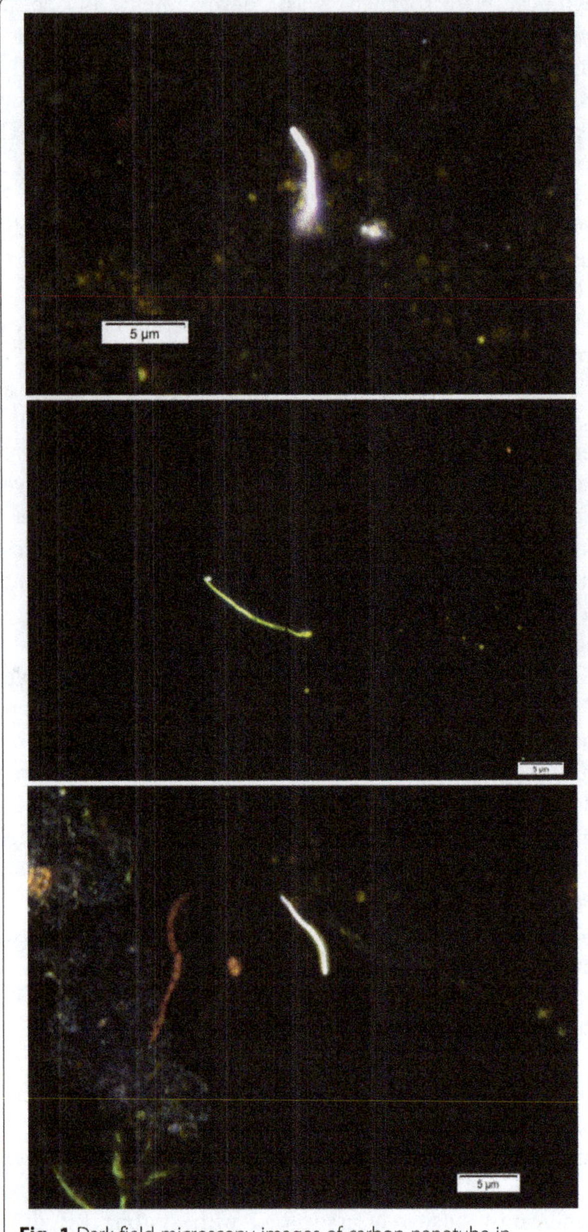

Fig. 1 Dark-field microscopy images of carbon nanotube in biospecimen of sputum/saliva

lung disease, or CHM score, we found a significant interaction between inhalable EC and sex (p=0.063) for RHR: its positive association with EC was restricted to men (Table 6).

Hematologic metrics

Most participants had blood component counts within the normal range (Table 4); however, absolute lymphocyte count was elevated for 8.2% of participants. U/FP count concentration was significantly positively associated with total leukocyte, neutrophil and lymphocyte counts (Additional file 1: Table S9). Several covariates (including sex, race/ethnicity, alcohol consumption, current respiratory infection, CHM score, and past exposure to solvents or "other" nanomaterials) were significantly associated with one or more blood components (Additional file 1: Tables S9 and S10). After adjusting for confounding, none of the CNT/F metrics was significantly associated with leukocyte counts or platelets. Log-transformed TEM structure concentration was positively associated with hematocrit (p=0.04) (Table 7). Significant interactions were seen with TEM structure concentrations and race/ethnicity (Hispanic and non-white participants had a stronger negative association between TEM structure concentrations and both leukocytes and neutrophils than other participants) and with the log of TEM structure counts and education (participants with college degrees had a stronger positive relationship between the log of TEM structure counts and both hemoglobin and hematocrit than other participants; Table 7). There were also significant interactions between the log of TEM structure counts and sex (females had stronger negative associations between the log of TEM structure counts and platelets than males), age (participants less than age 40 years had stronger negative associations between the log of TEM structure counts and platelets than participants age 40 years or older), and CHM score (participants with lower CHM scores had stronger negative associations between the log of TEM structure counts and platelets than participants with higher CHM scores; Table 7).

Regression model diagnostics

Model residuals for all outcomes were reasonably normally distributed, and no apparent patterns were observed between residuals and predictors. For RHR, a highly influential observation was detected. Removal of this observation decreased the association between (untransformed) inhalable EC and heart rate, but the log-transformed inhalable EC remained significantly associated with heart rate, and the pattern of effect modification with sex remained.

Discussion

Since the commercialization of carbon nanotubes and nanofibers over the past 10-15 years, concern has been raised about their possible human health effects, due to their pulmonary and cardiovascular toxicity in animal models and through analogy with fibrous structures such as asbestos [3, 42]. In this study, we observed little evidence of associations between different metrics of CNT/F exposure and clinically relevant outcomes, including pulmonary function, BP, and most hematologic elements, among 108 U.S. workers exposed routinely to CNT/F. Few workers showed evident pulmonary function decrement (below the lower limit of normal) for the age, sex, race and height-adjusted population, and no

Table 2 Descriptive statistics for carbon nanotube or nanofiber (CNT/F) exposure variables among 108 study participants

Exposure Variable[a]	Mean	Median	Standard deviation	25th, 75th %-ile
Multi-day mean EC (background-corrected) concentration (μg/m³)				
Respirable size fraction	1.00	0.096	4.94	0.018, 0.33
Inhalable size fraction	6.22	0.24	41.2	0.027, 1.32
Multi-day mean TEM structure count concentration (structures/cm³)				
All CNT/F-containing structures	0.128	7.29E-3	0.469	9.02E-4, 8.30E-2
Structures < 10 μm diameter	0.121	6.03E-3	0.440	3.80E-4, 8.34E-2
Structures <5 μm diameter	0.0865	3.04E-3	0.316	9.60E-5, 6.52E-2
Structures <2 μm diameter	0.0443	3.08E-4	0.201	0, 3.33E-3
Structures <1 μm diameter	0.0398	0	0.194	0, 7.12E-4
Single fiber structures	0.0324	0	0.193	0, 0
Duration worked with CNT/F (years)	4.07	3.66	4.01	1.05, 5.61

[a]Abbreviations: *CNT/F* carbon nanotubes or nanofibers, *EC* elemental carbon, *TEM* transmission electron microscopy

negative associations were found between these metrics and sub-clinical pulmonary function levels. We found that a relatively high percentage of the CNT/F workers were pre- or hypertensive: when including those who self-reported a physician diagnosis of hypertension, the percentage rose from 58% to 62%. However, the percentage by age group was similar to that in the general U.S. population (Fig. 2), as reported in NHANES [33], and BP was not associated with CNT/F exposure.

We identified a few health measures significantly associated with some metrics of CNT/F exposure: 14% of workers developed respiratory allergy after starting work with CNT/F, and the odds of reporting respiratory allergies increased with length of time spent working with CNT/F. Both respiratory allergy development and RHR were significantly positively associated with inhalable EC concentration. Respirable EC concentration was positively associated with RHR, whereas length of time spent working with CNT/F was negatively associated with RHR. While the overall reporting of any chest symptom (49%) and respiratory allergy (54%) was relatively high in our study, such participants did not exhibit greater sensitivity to CNT/F for the pulmonary, cardiovascular, or hematologic metrics we evaluated. The negative association between total leukocyte and total TEM structure concentrations was stronger for Hispanic and non-white workers than for white workers. Hemoglobin concentration and hematocrit percentage were positively associated with CNT/F structure count concentrations (log-transformed), particularly among workers with higher education levels, and negative associations between the same metric and platelet concentrations were significantly stronger among

Table 3 Associations of occupational exposure metrics with chest symptom and respiratory allergy development among 108 workers

	Chest symptom	Respiratory allergy
N outcome-free at start of work	63	64
N (%) reporting outcome after start of CNT/F work	13 (21%)	9 (14%)
Unadjusted OR (p-value[a]) from logistic regression		
Duration of CNT/F work (OR at 1 year)	1.07 (0.36)	1.20 (0.0081)
Presence of CNT in sputum (OR yes:no)	NA[b]	0.91 (0.94)
EC – inhalable (OR at 1 μg/m³)	1.02 (0.34)	1.02 (0.040)
EC – respirable (OR at 1 μg/m³)	1.11 (0.19)	1.08 (0.096)
TEM structure count (OR at 0.1 structure/cm³)	1.03 (0.47)	1.07 (0.33)
Fine particulate counts (OR at 2000 per cm³)[c]	1.07 (0.31)	0.85 (0.095)
Nanoscale particulate counts (OR at 2000 per cm³)[d]	1.05 (0.63)	0.98 (0.85)
Fine particulate matter mass (OR at 10 μg/m³)[e]	0.84 (0.67)	0.61 (0.31)

Abbreviations: *CNT/F* carbon nanotubes or nanofibers, *EC* elemental carbon, *NA* not available, *OR* odds ratio, *TEM* transmission electron microscopy
[a]maximum-likelihood based
[b]no sputum CNT was detected among those reporting chest symptoms since start of CNT/F work
[c]measured with condensation particle counter (10-1000 nm diameter)
[d]measured with electrical low-pressure impactor (23-96 nm diameter)
[e]measured with photometer (<2.5 μm diameter)

Table 4 Descriptive statistics for outcome variables among 108 study participants

Outcome Variable	N available	Mean	Median	Standard deviation	25th-75th %-ile	Min.-Max.	N (%) outside normal range[a]
Spirometry measures							
FVC PP	103	98.6%	99.6%	11.5%	90.7-105%	66.8-133%	5 (5.0%)
FEV1/FVC ratio PP	103	99.6%	100%	7.56%	93.9-105%	78.6-116%	8 (7.8%)[b]
FEF25-75 PP	103	100%	96.7%	31.5%	75.0-125%	35.6-185%	8 (7.8%)
PEF PP	103	107%	107%	14.6%	96.9-117%	69.8-142%	1 (1.0%)
Cardiovascular measures							
Systolic BP (mmHg)	106	122	122	14.2	112-130	92-164	13 (12.3%)
Diastolic BP (mmHg)	106	75.1	74.5	10.1	69-82	42.5-106	6 (5.7%)
Heart rate (BPM)	106	69.9	69.8	11.2	61.5-77	45.5-108	1 (0.9%)
Blood component measures							
Leukocyte count (x10^3/μL)	98	7.01	6.80	1.70	5.9-8.0	3.5-12.2	2 (2.0%)
Abs. neutrophils	98	3.99	3.80	1.24	3.2-4.7	1.6-7.3	1 (1.0%)
Abs. lymphocytes	98	2.33	2.30	0.69	1.8-2.6	1.1-4.8	8 (8.2%)[c]
Abs. monocytes	98	0.50	0.50	0.15	0.4-0.6	0.20-0.83	2 (2.0%)
Platelet (x10^3/μL)	98	249.8	238.5	53.2	212-279	157-460	1 (1.0%)
Hemoglobin (g/dL)	98	15.1	15.3	1.18	14.3-16	12.1-17.5	2 (2.0%)
Hematocrit	98	44.8%	45.1%	2.98%	42.5-47.3%	37.3-49.9%	0

Abbreviations: *BP* blood pressure, *BPM* beats per minute, *FEV1* forced expiratory volume in one second, *FVC* forced vital capacity, *PP* percent predicted, *FEF25-75* forced expiratory flow at 25-75-% of the pulmonary volume, *PEF* peak expiratory flow

[a]Below the lower limit of normal for pulmonary function measures (two subjects' tests were not interpretable with respect to this criterion); above 139 and 89 mm Hg for systolic and diastolic (respectively) BP; above 100 beats per minute for heart rate; above or below the reference range for blood component measures

[b]Includes three participants determined clinically to have normal spirometry pattern and one participant with clinically uninterpretable spirometry

[c]All were above the reference range

female workers, younger workers, and workers with worse cardiovascular health.

There have been few studies of clinically relevant health metrics among workers exposed to CNT/F. A small study in Korea of nine workers manufacturing MWCNT [11] found none had depressed (<80% predicted) FVC or FEV1. Two workers exhibited abnormal monocyte counts, and several others showed abnormal levels of certain hepatic enzymes. The Korean workers had inhalable EC exposure levels in a range about ten times higher than the median level observed in our study. Liou et al. [10] measured pulmonary function among a group of 227 workers handling a variety of engineered nanomaterials (23% were exposed only to CNT), compared to a group of unexposed workers. No association was found between exposure and lung function metrics. That study team did observe evidence of respiratory and dermal symptoms (sneezing and dermatitis) in the more highly exposed workers in this population [39]. No association was observed between CNT/F exposure and pulmonary function in a small European study [12].

No human studies, to our knowledge, have evaluated the association of CNT/F exposure with RHR or resting BP. RHR, measured cross-sectionally, was associated strongly with mortality in a healthy male population: risk of death in a 16-year period rose 16% (95% confidence interval: 10-22%) per 10 beat-per-minute heart rate level, after adjusting for physical fitness and other covariates [17]. Therefore, it is important to identify environmental or occupational contributors to high RHR. We consider our finding of an association between RHR and inhalable EC to be preliminary until it is replicated in other groups, particularly because a study of MWCNT exposure in spontaneously hypertensive rats found a depression in RHR [9]. The positive association we observed between CNT/F exposure and hematocrit could reflect less hydration among CNT/F-exposed workers, as the tasks associated with this work can involve heat exposure.

It is important to note that very few workers (n=7) had background-corrected, respirable EC exposure concentrations above the NIOSH REL of 1 μg/m^3 [13]. However, a much larger percentage had inhalable concentrations above this level (although there is no REL established for the inhalable EC air concentration). Therefore, it is of considerable interest whether the inhalable or respirable fraction of EC is a more health-relevant metric. We found that inhalable EC or total structure count concentration tended to relate more strongly to the few pulmonary, cardiovascular, or hematologic endpoints that were associated with a

Table 5 Results of multiple linear regression modeling of pulmonary function metrics

	CNT/F metric β estimate (*p*-value)			
	FVC PP[a]	FEV1/FVC PP[b]	ln(FEF25-75 PP)[c]	PEF PP[d]
Exposure variable - untransformed				
EC–inhalable (μg/m³)	-1.78E-4 (0.478)	2.53E-4 (0.155)[e]	2.65E-4 (0.754)	8.17E-5 (0.810)
EC-respirable (μg/m³)	-6.12E-4 (0.772)	1.87E-3 (0.208)	2.12E-3 (0.771)	1.76E-4 (0.950)
TEM-total (structures/cm³)	1.02E-2 (0.651)	-4.80E-4 (0.976)	3.97E-2 (0.555)	-2.54E-2 (0.398)
CNT/F found in sputum	-1.61E-2 (0.558)	-5.15E-3 (0.804)	-3.14E-2 (0.707)	1.57E-2 (0.700)
CNT/F duration employed (years)	-2.30E-4 (0.930)	2.83E-3 (0.125)	1.98E-2 (0.0148)	5.32E-3 (0.130)
Exposure variable – log-transformed				
ln(EC-inhalable)	1.63E-6 (0.999)	1.27E-3 (0.598)	1.08E-2 (0.288)	-4.41E-3 (0.334)
ln(EC-respirable)	6.79E-3 (0.172)[e]	6.28E-4 (0.857)	1.77E-2 (0.224)	-9.24E-3 (0.159)[e]
ln(TEM-total)	5.34E-3 (0.203)	2.55E-3 (0.376)	2.14E-2 (0.0746)[e]	3.23E-3 (0.554)
Effect modification[f]				
Male	6.86E-3	2.51E-4	2.27E-2	-9.40E-3
Female	6.55E-3	6.12E-4	1.73E-2	-8.72E-3
p for interaction	0.968	0.869	0.689	0.948
White race, non-Hispanic	8.02E-3	2.50E-4	2.04E-2	-7.76E-3
All other races and Hispanic	-8.48E-4	-1.53E-3	2.83E-2	-1.54E-2
p for interaction	0.533	0.907	0.592	0.496
Age <40	3.81E-3	-1.32E-4	1.35E-2	-1.16E-2
Age ≥40	8.66E-3	2.74E-4	2.56E-2	-7.41E-3
p for interaction	0.468	0.587	0.304	0.635
Education < college degree	1.11E-2	-1.65E-3	3.09E-2	-1.83E-3
Education ≥ college degree	5.57E-3	2.80E-4	1.58E-2	-1.11E-2
p for interaction	0.457	0.149	0.212	0.349
No lung disease[g]	6.38E-3	1.69E-4	1.84E-2	-1.82E-2
Has lung disease	6.99E-3	2.56E-4	2.23E-2	-3.90E-3
p for interaction	0.927	0.928	0.726	0.0985
CHM score <5	7.91E-4	2.54E-4	3.00E-2	-9.74E-3
CHM score ≥5	1.41E-2	3.03E-6	1.80E-2	-8.87E-3
p for interaction	0.186	0.908	0.287	0.922

Abbreviations— *CHM* cardiovascular health metric, *CNT/F* carbon nanotubes or nanofibers, *EC* elemental carbon, *FEV1* forced expiratory volume in one second, *FVC* forced vital capacity, *FEF25-75* forced expiratory fraction between 25 and 75% of maximal, *PEF* peak expiratory flow, *PP* percent predicted, *TEM* transmission electron microscopy

[a]FVC percent predicted adjusted for race/ethnicity, high CHM score, and self-reported current exposure to strong acids

[b]FEV1/FVC percent predicted unadjusted

[c]FEF25-75% adjusted for cigarette pack-years, self-reported current solvent exposure, and duration of exposure to CNT/F

[d]PEF adjusted for self-reported past exposure to dust

[e]CNT/F exposure metric associated with the lowest Schwarz's Bayesian Criterion value (best fit)

[f]Parameter estimates and p-values are shown for the CNT/F exposure metric identified as having the best fit

[g]Self-reported respiratory allergy, asthma, or chronic obstructive pulmonary disease

CNT/F metric. This finding is similar to that observed for blood and sputum biomarkers of early effect in the same study group [23], and an *in vivo* study of MWCNT that primarily deposited in the conducting airways [43]. These findings suggest that protective standards should also consider aerosol size fractions larger than respirable, such as the inhalable or thoracic fractions.

No outcomes were significantly associated with the presence of CNT/F in sputum, and this metric showed little association with biomarker levels in blood or sputum [23]. The sensitivity of this metric is probably low, given the poor quality of the sputum (which indicates that much of it may have originated in the oral cavity) and the small percentage (<1%) of the specimen that was inspected using the dark-field microscopy method. It is notable that, in contrast to the air sampling results [24, 26] all CNT/F structures observed in sputum were single fibers (e.g., Fig. 1), suggesting that some

Table 6 Results of multiple linear regression modeling of cardiovascular metrics

	CNT/F metric β estimate (*p*-value)		
	Systolic BP[a]	Diastolic BP[b]	Heart rate[c]
Exposure variable – untransformed			
EC–inhalable (μg/m^3)	-2.65E-2 (0.386)	-2.85E-2 (0.213)[d]	8.63E-2 (0.0026)[d]
EC-respirable (μg/m^3)	-0.255 (0.317)[d]	-0.221 (0.251)	0.667 (0.0074)
TEM-total (structures/cm^3)	-0.321 (0.905)	-0.992 (0.624)	0.929 (0.688)
CNT/F found in sputum	1.03 (0.779)	1.02 (0.712)	1.20 (0.695)
CNT/F duration employed (years)	0.181 (0.575)	-9.46E-3 (0.968)	-0.777 (0.0029)
Exposure variable – log-transformed			
ln(EC-inhalable)	0.187 (0.653)	-5.72E-2 (0.856)	0.958 (0.0055)
ln(EC-respirable)	-0.588 (0.331)	-0.367 (0.416)	0.190 (0.705)
ln(TEM-total)	0.349 (0.469)	-2.59E-4 (0.999)	0.216 (0.597)
Effect modification[e]			
Male	-0.238	-0.0270	0.0870
Female	-3.52	-0.241	-0.454
p for interaction	0.350	0.459	0.063
White race, non-Hispanic	-0.259	-0.0284	0.0860
All other races and Hispanic	-11.6	0.417	-1.81
p for interaction	0.398	0.819	0.352
Age <40	-0.195	-5.88E-2	1.55E-2
Age ≥40	-0.279	-2.69E-2	8.79E-2
p for interaction	0.881	0.740	0.483
Education < college degree	-0.206	-6.38E-2	9.86E-2
Education ≥ college degree	-0.257	-2.81E-2	8.60E-2
p for interaction	0.966	0.837	0.945
No lung disease[f]	-0.254	-7.14E-4	9.03E-2
Has lung disease	-0.255	-2.94E-2	8.63E-2
p for interaction	1.00	0.814	0.976
CHM score <5	-0.254	-0.0263	0.0867
CHM score ≥5	-5.49	-0.315	-0.383
p for interaction	0.133	0.309	0.112

Abbreviations—*BP* blood pressure, *CHM* cardiovascular health metric, *CNT/F* carbon nanotubes or nanofibers, *EC* elemental carbon, *TEM* transmission electron microscopy

[a]Systolic BP adjusted for age, sex, and total 10-1000 nm particulate counts per cm^3 (measured with condensation particle counter)

[b]Diastolic BP adjusted for sex, cigarette pack-years, and CHM score

[c]Heart rate adjusted for employment duration and CHM score

[d]CNT/F exposure metric associated with the lowest Schwarz's Bayesian Criterion value (best fit)

[e]Parameter estimates and *p*-values are shown for the CNT/F exposure metric identified as having the best fit

[f]Self-reported respiratory allergy, asthma, or COPD

dissociation of agglomerates may occur after oral cavity or respiratory tract intake.

We observed several other occupational exposures to be associated with some respiratory, cardiovascular, and hematologic metrics: polymers, solvents and strong acids were the most commonly self-reported. Measured U/FP concentrations in the workplace were more important predictors of blood pressure and leukocyte components than CNT/F exposure. The ambient air quality metric most consistently associated with health measures was the U/FP count concentration, measured with a CPC. While U/FP concentration was only weakly correlated with CNT/F exposure, it was significantly positively associated with systolic BP and leukocyte, neutrophil, and lymphocyte counts. (Additional file 1: Tables S8 and S9). This finding, if indicative of a causal association, could have utility for the health of the workers, as it confirms the importance of minimizing exposure to U/FP in the workplace, aside from specific concern about CNT/F. U/FP are common in workplaces and can be caused by a

Table 7 Results of multiple linear regression modeling of complete blood count components

	CNT/F metric β estimate (*p*-value)						
	ln(Leukocytes)[a]	ln(Neutrophils)[b]	ln(Lymphocytes)[c]	ln(Monocytes)[d]	ln(Platelets)[e]	Hemoglobin[2f]	Hematocrit[2g]
Exposure variable – untransformed							
EC–inhalable (μg/m^3)	-2.17E-4 (0.692)	-9.34E-5 (0.899)	-3.74E-4 (0.577)	-5.94E-3 (0.364)	2.09E-5 (0.965)	-1.80E-2 (0.775)	-0.237 (0.618)
EC-respirable (μg/m^3)	-3.92E-3 (0.468)	-3.78E-3 (0.533)	-3.32E-3 (0.556)	-4.39E-3 (0.428)	1.59E-3 (0.692)	-0.294 (0.578)	-2.33 (0.563)
TEM-total (structures/ cm^3)	-8.30E-2 (0.080)[h]	-9.06E-2 (0.154)[h]	-7.51E-2 (0.201)[h]	-3.03E-2 (0.612)	-3.76E-3 (0.929)	-4.08 (0.463)	-26.9 (0.533)
CNT/F found in sputum	5.75E-2 (0.380)	8.21E-2 (0.355)	1.90E-2 (0.980)	4.79E-2 (0.542)	-8.40E-2 (0.109)	2.17 (0.332)	32.4 (0.566)
CNT/F emp. duration (years)	-5.78E-3 (0.316)	-7.34E-2 (0.340)	1.70E-3 (0.814)	3.78E-3 (0.594)	-1.27E-3 (0.804)	0.400 (0.548)	5.28 (0.308)
Exposure variable – log-transformed							
ln(EC-inhalable)	4.05E-3 (0.592)	8.15E-3 (0.419)	-4.31E-3 (0.646)	1.34E-2 (0.149)[h]	-3.74E-3 (0.575)	1.44 (0.103)	10.3 (0.127)
ln(EC-respirable)	-1.06E-2 (0.373)	-1.43E-2 (0.371)	-2.40E-3 (0.869)	-9.98E-3 (0.494)	1.30E-2 (0.206)	-0.460 (0.738)	6.02E-3 (0.999)
ln(TEM-total)	-1.28E-3 (0.885)	6.89E-3 (0.560)	-1.14E-2 (0.303)	-3.20E-3 (0.771)	-1.28E-2 (0.101)[h]	1.82 (0.0788)[h]	15.9 (0.0433)[h]
Effect modification[i]							
Male	-8.24E-2	-9.31E-2	-7.85E-2	1.45E-2	-6.60E-3	1.85	18.5
Female	-9.14E-2	-5.31E-2	-2.50E-2	-5.96E-3	-3.59E-2	1.74	7.51
p for interaction	0.9596	0.867	0.805	0.531	0.001	0.965	0.553
White race, non-Hispanic	-8.29E-2	-9.27E-2	-7.52E-2	6.66E-4	-1.23E-2	1.86	14.8
All other races and Hispanic	-6.23	-6.54	-4.44	1.46E-2	-2.02E-2	1.33	34.0
p for interaction	0.009	0.041	0.124	0.646	0.803	0.898	0.542
Age <40	-9.04E-2	-0.111	-6.72E-2	5.27E-3	-2.19E-2	1.50	16.0
Age ≥40	1.39E-2	0.178	-2.17E-1	1.76E-2	-8.10E-3	1.95	15.9
p for interaction	0.529	0.191	0.478	0.461	0.067	0.649	0.995
Education < college degree	-8.91E-2	-1.06E-1	-1.18E-1	1.64E-2	-1.64E-2	0.530	4.27
Education ≥ college degree	-7.65E-2	-7.45E-2	-2.81E-2	1.23E-2	-1.11E-2	2.55	22.7
p for interaction	0.890	0.796	0.427	0.836	0.513	0.056	0.020
No lung disease[j]	-8.87E-2	-1.18E-1	-1.19E-2	1.41E-2	-5.11E-3	1.72	14.0
Has lung disease	-7.96E-2	-6.86E-2	-1.11E-1	1.27E-2	-1.58E-2	1.85	16.5
p for interaction	0.924	0.733	0.388	0.934	0.170	0.900	0.747
CHM score <5	-8.85E-2	-9.98E-2	-8.42E-2	1.45E-2	-2.20E-2	2.25	17.4
CHM score ≥5	2.86E-2	9.34E-2	6.90E-2	1.28E-2	-8.79E-3	1.42	14.5
p for interaction	0.547	0.458	0.533	0.920	0.085	0.688	0.856

Abbreviations—*CNT/F* carbon nanotubes or nanofibers, *CHM* cardiovascular health metric, *EC* elemental carbon, *TEM* transmission electron microscopy
[a]Leukocytes adjusted for total U/FP counts per cm^3 and self-reported current dust exposure
[b]Neutrophils adjusted for total U/FP counts per cm^3 and self-reported current dust exposure
[c]Lymphocytes adjusted for NSAID use, CHM score, and self-reported past exposure to nanomaterials other than CNT/F
[d]Monocytes adjusted for race/ethnicity, current respiratory infection, total U/FP counts per cm^3 and self-reported past polymer exposure
[e]Platelets adjusted for race/ethnicity
[f]Hemoglobin adjusted for sex, race/ethnicity, and CHM score
[g]Hematocrit adjusted for sex, race/ethnicity, CHM score, and current respiratory infection
[h]CNT/F exposure metric associated with the lowest Schwarz's Bayesian Criterion value (best fit)
[i]Parameter estimates and p-values are shown for the CNT/F exposure metric identified as having the best fit
[j]Self-reported respiratory allergy, asthma, or chronic obstructive pulmonary disease

variety of combustion sources such as vehicle exhaust and reactor byproducts, as well as industrial dryers, compressors, and vacuum cleaners. The CPC is a relatively inexpensive, easy-to-use instrument for measuring real-time concentrations of 10-1000 nm-diameter particulates in the workplace.

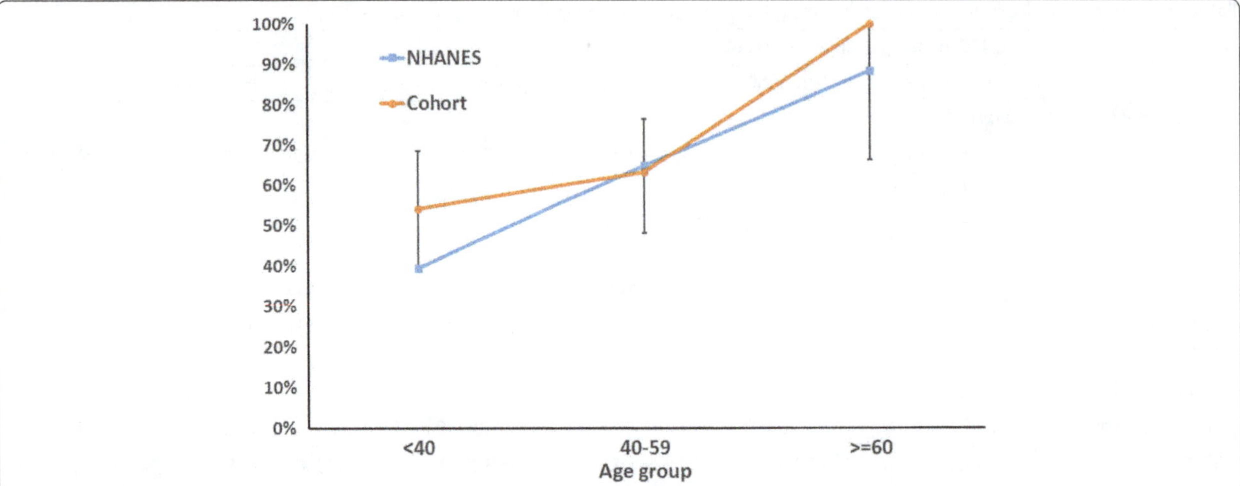

Fig. 2 Percent of population hypertensive or pre-hypertensive. Abbreviations: CNT/F – carbon nanotubes and nanofiber; NHANES – National Health and Nutrition Examination Survey. NHANES data from NHANES 2013. 95% confidence intervals were estimated for the CNT/F workers, assuming an exact binomial distribution

Strengths of this study include the consistent exposure and outcome assessment methodologies, the use of a wide range of CNT/F exposure metrics, and the large number of facilities included, with a nationally representative range of CNT/F types. This study is subject to a number of important limitations. We were unable to verify the accuracy of self-reported chest symptoms and respiratory diseases. The cross-sectional design hampers interpretability of temporality of any observed associations and is subject to selection bias, in that more susceptible workers may have dropped out of the CNT/F workforce. The positive association between CNT/F duration and lung function suggests such selection could exist in this workforce. The design also limits the ability to estimate respiratory symptom or allergy development, given the potential correlation of these events with follow-up time (although we found that age was not related to risk of development of symptoms or allergies). The small study size and generally low exposure levels limit the statistical power to detect subclinical effects on the outcomes. This limitation might be reduced through pooling of these data with similarly conducted studies worldwide (e.g., [12]). Variability in the types of CNT/F included in this study presented a challenge, as the toxic potential of carbon nanotubes varies substantially by material characteristics [44]. Most facilities in our study were using CNTs of a "tangled" morphology, not the rigid form deemed to be "possibly carcinogenic" [45]. Given the very recent commercialization of CNT/F, there is short latency for developing restrictive or obstructive lung disease: the average duration of time these participants worked with CNT/F was 4 years. The exposure metrics did not account for use of protective equipment, such as respirators, as we could not assess the efficacy of use on an individual basis. It is uncertain to what degree our cross-sectionally measured air concentrations of EC or CNT/F structures accurately reflect past exposure for workers in our study. The mean and median exposures measured here were lower than in previous studies of the same workforce (e.g., in [24]). However, this likely was influenced by differences in participant selection for these studies: 37% of participants in this study reported not directly handling CNT/F, whereas our previous studies [24] focused on workers directly handling these materials. Lastly, the representativeness of the facilities included in this study is uncertain, as only 1/3 responded to our initial request for information about their use of CNT/F. However, our study targeted companies with the highest volume of CNT/F handling in the U.S., and the overall non-selective and high employee participation rate suggests that within-facility representativeness was high.

Conclusions

We found that most pulmonary, cardiovascular and hematologic measures were unrelated to metrics of CNT/F exposure in U.S. workplaces. Respiratory allergy development and resting heart rate were positively associated with inhalable concentrations of EC. Hemoglobin and hematocrit concentrations were positively related to CNT/F structure count concentrations. These findings require confirmation in other exposed populations, preferably with longitudinal designs. The low exposure levels and lack of substantive clinical impairment suggest that the CNT/F industry is responsibly handling these materials, and efforts should continue to use a comprehensive approach to minimize exposure to CNT/F, fine particulates and other potentially hazardous agents in these workplaces.

Additional files

Additional file 1: Table S1. Participation rates by facility. **Table S2.** Current and past self-reported exposure frequency among cross-sectional study participants. **Table S3.** Scoring method for risk factors used in cardiovascular health metrics score. **Table S4.** Distribution of cardiovascular health metric (CHM) score values, where a higher score implies better cardiovascular health. **Table S5.** Frequency of chest symptoms or respiratory illnesses among 108 study participants. **Table S6.** Results of univariable logistic regression modeling of personal characteristics and occupational exposures for development of chest symptoms or respiratory allergy after the start of CNT/F work. **Table S7.** Results of univariable linear regression modeling of pulmonary function metrics (highlight indicates selected in "best model" by Schwarz Bayesian Criterion and considered as potential confounder in multiple linear regression model with main exposure variables). **Table S8.** Results of univariable linear regression modeling of cardiovascular metrics (highlight indicates selected in "best model" by Schwarz Bayesian Criterion and considered as potential confounder in multiple linear regression model with main exposure variables). **Table S9.** Results of univariable linear regression modeling of natural log (ln)-transformed WBC and differential metrics (highlight indicates selected in "best model" by Schwarz Bayesian Criterion and considered as potential confounder in multiple linear regression model with main exposure variables). **Table S10.** Results of univariable linear regression modeling of other transformed CBC metrics (highlight indicates selected in "best model" by Schwarz Bayesian Criterion and considered as potential confounder in multiple linear regression model with main exposure variables). (DOCX 41 kb)

Additional file 2: Questionnaire. (DOCX 37 kb)

Additional file 3: Supplementary information. (DOCX 24 kb)

Acknowledgements

The authors thank D. Booher, K. Sparks, D. Trout, K.L. Dunn, C. Toennis, D. Sammons, J. Clark, C. Striley, and V. Burkel for assistance with field work, L. Luo for help with data management, and K. Cummings for advice on clinical interpretation of spirometry. We are grateful for the assistance of the participating companies and individuals in the study. Mention of trade names does not imply endorsement by the U.S. Government. The findings and conclusions of this report are those of the authors and do not necessarily reflect those of NIOSH.

Funding

The research reported in this manuscript was funded by the Nanotechnology Research Center of the National Institute for Occupational Safety and Health (NIOSH), as well as the National Institute of Environmental Health Sciences (Interagency Agreement AES 12029-001).

Authors' contributions

MS-B, MMD, AE, MEB, DEE, and MAdP designed the study; these authors and JEF, RRM, and TE conducted the field work or laboratory analyses; MS-B, MMD, JDB and SJB conducted the analysis of data. All authors contributed to the interpretation of data. MS-B was the primary drafter of the manuscript. All authors reviewed and revised the manuscript critically for content. Each author gave approval of the version submitted.

Competing interests

The authors declare that they have no competing interests.

Author details

[1]National Institute for Occupational Safety and Health (NIOSH), Division of Surveillance, Hazard Evaluations, and Field Studies, 1090 Tusculum Ave MS-R15, Cincinnati, OH 45226, USA. [2]NIOSH, Health Effects Laboratory Division, Morgantown, WV, USA. [3]Centers for Disease Control and Prevention, Epidemic Intelligence Service, Atlanta, GA, USA. [4]NIOSH, Division of Applied Research and Technology, Cincinnati, OH, USA. [5]Present address: Department of Public Health, College of Life Sciences, Brigham Young University, Provo, UT, USA.

References

1. Schubauer-Berigan MK, Dahm MM, Yencken MS. Engineered carbonaceous nanomaterials manufacturers in the United States: workforce size, characteristics and feasibility of epidemiologic studies. J Occup Environ Med. 2011;53(Suppl 6):S62–7.
2. Sargent LM, Shvedova AA, Hubbs AF, Solisbury JJ, Benkovic SA, Kashon ML, et al. Induction of aneuploidy by single-walled carbon nanotubes. Environ Mol Mutagen. 2009;50:708–17.
3. Oberdorster G, Castranova V, Asgharian B, Sayre P. Inhalation exposure to carbon nanotubes (Cnt) and carbon nanofibers (Cnf): methodology and dosimetry. J Toxicol Environ Health B Crit Rev. 2015;18:121–212.
4. Kasai T, Umeda Y, Ohnishi M, Mine T, Kondo H, Takeuchi T, et al. Lung carcinogenicity of inhaled multi-walled carbon nanotube in rats. Part Fibre Toxicol. 2016;13:53.
5. Seaton A, Donaldson K. Nanoscience, nanotechnology, and the need to think small. Lancet. 2005;365:923–4.
6. Mitchell LA, Lauer FT, Burchiel SW, McDonald JD. Mechanisms for how inhaled multiwalled carbon nanotubes suppress systemic immune function in mice. Nat Nanotechnol. 2009;4:451–6.
7. Simeonova PP, Erdely A. Engineered nanoparticles respiratory exposure and potential risks for cardiovascular toxicity: predictive tests and biomarkers. Inhal Toxicol. 2009;21(Suppl 1):68–73.
8. Aragon MJ, Topper L, Tyler CR, Sanchez B, Zychowski K, Young T, et al. Serum-borne bioactivity caused by pulmonary multiwalled carbon nanotubes induces neuroinflammation via blood-brain barrier impairment. Proc Natl Acad Sci USA. 2017;114:E1968–76.
9. Chen R, Zhang L, Ge C, Tseng MT, Bai R, Qu Y, et al. Subchronic toxicity and cardiovascular responses in spontaneously hypertensive rats after exposure to multiwalled carbon nanotubes by intratracheal instillation. Chem Res Toxicol. 2015;28:440–50.
10. Liou S-H, Tsou T-C, Wang S-L, Li L-A, Chiang H-C, Li W-F, et al. Epidemiological study of health hazards among workers handling engineered nanomaterials. J Nanopart Res. 2012;4:878.
11. Lee JS, Choi YC, Sin JH, Lee JH, Lee Y, Park SY, et al. Health surveillance study of workers who manufacture multi-walled carbon nanotubes. Nanotoxicol. 2015;9:802–11.
12. Vlaanderen J, Pronk A, Rothman N, Hildesheim A, Silverman D, Hosgood HD, et al. A cross-sectional study of changes in markers of immunological effects and lung health due to exposure to multi-walled carbon nanotubes. Nanotoxicol. 2017;11:395–404.
13. National Institute for Occupational Safety and Health (NIOSH). Current Intelligence Bulletin 65: Occupational Exposure to Carbon Nanotubes and Nanofibers. Department of Health and Human Services (NIOSH) Publication Number 2013-145. 2013. https://www.cdc.gov/niosh/docs/2013-145/default.html . Accessed 9 May 2018.
14. Nurkiewicz TR, Porter DW, Barger M, Millecchia L, Rao KM, Marvar PJ, et al. Systemic microvascular dysfunction and inflammation after pulmonary particulate matter exposure. Environ Health Perspect. 2006;114:412–9.
15. Nurkiewicz TR, Porter DW, Hubbs AF, Cumpston JL, Chen BT, Frazer DG, et al. Nanoparticle inhalation augments particle-dependent systemic microvascular dysfunction. Part Fibre Toxicol. 2008;12:5–1.
16. Peters A, Perz S, Doring A, Stieber J, Koenig W, Wichmann H-E. Increases in heart rate during an air pollution episode. Am J Epidemiol. 1999;150:1094–8.
17. Jensen MT, Suadicani P, Hein HO, Gyntelberg F. Elevated resting heart rate, physical fitness and all-cause mortality: a 16-year follow-up in the Copenhagen Male Study. Heart. 2013;99:882–7.

18. Brook RD, Urch B, Dvonch JT, Bard RL, Speck M, Keeler G, et al. Insights into the mechanisms and mediators of the effects of air pollution exposure on blood pressure and vascular function in healthy humans. Hypertension. 2009;54:659–67.
19. Fuks KB, Weinmayr G, Basagaña X, Gruzieva O, Hampel R, Oftedal B, et al. Long-term exposure to ambient air pollution and traffic noise and incident hypertension in seven cohorts of the European study of cohorts for air pollution effects (ESCAPE). Eur Heart J. 2017;38:983–90.
20. Kim JY, Chen JC, Boyce PD, Christiani DC. Exposure to welding fumes is associated with acute systemic inflammatory responses. Occup Environ Med. 2005;62:157–63.
21. Olsen Y, Karottki DG, Jensen DM, Bekö G, Kjeldsen BU, Clausen G, et al. Vascular and lung function related to ultrafine and fine particles exposure assessed by personal and indoor monitoring: a cross-sectional study. Environ Health. 2014;13:112.
22. Erdely A, Hulderman T, Salmen R, Liston A, Zeidler-Erdely PC, Schwegler-Berry D, et al. Cross-talk between lung and systemic circulation during carbon nanotube respiratory exposure. Potential biomarkers. Nano Lett. 2009;9:36–43.
23. Beard JD, Erdely A, Dahm MM, de Perio MA, Birch ME, Evans DE, Fernback JE, Eye T, Kodali V, Mercer RR, Bertke SJ, Schubauer-Berigan MK. Carbon nanotube and nanofiber exposure and sputum and blood biomarkers of early effect among U.S. workers. Environ Int. 2018;116:214–28. https://doi.org/10.1016/j.envint.2018.04.004.
24. Dahm MM, Schubauer-Berigan MK, Evans DE, Birch ME, Fernback JE, Deddens JA. Carbon nanotube and nanofiber exposure assessments: an analysis of 14 site visits. Ann Occup Hyg. 2015;59:705–23.
25. Birch ME, Ku BK, Evans DE, Ruda-Eberenz T. Exposure and emissions monitoring during carbon nanofiber production–part I: elemental carbon exposure marker. Ann Occup Hyg. 2011;55:1016–36.
26. Dahm MM, Schubauer-Berigan MK, Evans DE, Birch ME, Bertke SJ, Beard JD, et al. Exposure assessments for a cross-sectional epidemiologic study of US carbon nanotube and nanofiber workers. Int J Hyg Environ Health. 2018;221: 429–40.
27. Birch ME, Wang C, Fernback JE, Feng HA, Birch QT, Dozier AK. Analysis of carbon nanotubes and nanofibers on mixed cellulose ester filters by transmission electron microscopy. In: Ashley K, O'Connor PF, eds. NIOSH Manual of Analytical Methods. 5th ed. Cincinnati,. Department of Health and Human Services, Centers for Disease Control and Prevention, National Institute for Occupational Safety and Health, DHHS (NIOSH) Publication No. 2014-151. 2017; Chapter CN. www.cdc.gov/niosh/nmam. Accessed 9 May 2018.
28. Dahm MM, Evans DE, Schubauer-Berigan MK, Birch ME, Deddens JA. Occupational exposure assessment in carbon nanotube and nanofiber primary and secondary manufacturers: mobile direct-reading sampling. Ann Occup Hyg. 2013;57:328–44.
29. Evans DE, Ku BK, Birch ME, Dunn KH. Aerosol monitoring during carbon nanofiber production: mobile direct-reading sampling. Ann Occup Hyg. 2010;54:514–31.
30. Ferris BG. Epidemiology standardization project. II. Recommended respiratory disease questionnaires for use with adults and children in epidemiologic research. Am Rev Respir Dis. 1978;118(Suppl 6):7–53.
31. National Health and Nutrition Examination Survey (NHANES). Respiratory Health Spirometry Procedures Manual. 2008. http://www.cdc.gov/nchs/data/nhanes/nhanes_07_08/spirometry.pdf . Accessed 9 May 2018.
32. Egan BM, Zhao Y, Axon RN. US trends in prevalence, awareness, treatment, and control of hypertension, 1988-2008. JAMA. 2010;303:2043–50.
33. National Health and Nutrition Examination Survey. 2011-2012 Data Documentation, Codebook, and Frequencies: Blood Pressure. 2013. https://wwwn.cdc.gov/nchs/nhanes/2011-2012/BPX_G.htm. Accessed 9 May 2018.
34. Miller MR, Crapo R, Hankinson J, Brusasco V, Burgos F, Casaburi R, et al. General considerations for lung function testing. Eur Respir J. 2005;26:153–61.
35. Pellegrino R, Viegi G, Brusasco V, Crapo RO, Burgos F, Casaburi R, et al. Interpretive strategies for lung function tests. Eur Respir J. 2005;26:948–68.
36. Loh LC, Eg KP, Puspanathan P, Tang SP, Yip KS, Vijayasingham P, et al. A comparison of sputum induction methods: ultrasonic vs. compressed-air nebulizer and hypertonic vs. isotonic saline inhalation. Asian Pac J Allergy Immunol. 2004;22:11–7.
37. Mercer RR, Hubbs AF, Scabilloni JF, Wang L, Battelli LA, Friend S, et al. Pulmonary fibrotic response to aspiration of multi-walled carbon nanotubes. Part Fibre Toxicol. 2011;8:21.
38. Shockey TM, Sussell AL, Odom EC. Cardiovascular health status by occupational group - 21 states, 2013. MMWR Morb Mortal Wkly Rep. 2016; 65:793–8.
39. Liao H-Y, Chung Y-T, Lai C-H, Lin M-H, Liou S-H. Sneezing and allergic dermatitis were increased in engineered nanomaterial handling workers. Ind Health. 2014;52:199–215.
40. Neter J, Kutner MH, Nachtsheim CJ, Wasserman W. Applied Linear Statistical Models. 4th ed. Chicago: Irwin; 1996.
41. Beal DJ. 2007. Information criteria methods in SAS for multiple linear regression models. SESUG Proceedings 2007, SA05, pp. 1-10. http://analytics.ncsu.edu/sesug/2007/SA05.pdf. Accessed 9 May 2018.
42. Laney AS, McCauley LA, Schubauer-Berigan MK. Workshop summary: epidemiologic design strategies for studies of nanomaterial workers. J Occup Environ Med. 2011;53(Suppl 6):S87–90.
43. Bishop L, Cena L, Orandle M, Yanamala N, Dahm MM, Birch ME, et al. In vivo toxicity assessment of occupational components of the carbon nanotube life cycle to provide context to potential health effects. ACS Nano. 2017;11: 8849–63.
44. Sharma M, Nikota J, Halappanavar S, Castranova V, Rothen-Rutishauser B, Clippinger AJ. Predicting pulmonary fibrosis in humans after exposure to multi-walled carbon nanotubes (MWCNTs). Arch Toxicol. 2016;90:1605–22.
45. International Agency for Research on Cancer (IARC). Some Nanomaterials and Some Fibres. IARC Monogr Eval Carcinog Risk Hum. 2017;111:35–192.

Permissions

All chapters in this book were first published in P&FT, by BioMed Central; hereby published with permission under the Creative Commons Attribution License or equivalent. Every chapter published in this book has been scrutinized by our experts. Their significance has been extensively debated. The topics covered herein carry significant findings which will fuel the growth of the discipline. They may even be implemented as practical applications or may be referred to as a beginning point for another development.

The contributors of this book come from diverse backgrounds, making this book a truly international effort. This book will bring forth new frontiers with its revolutionizing research information and detailed analysis of the nascent developments around the world.

We would like to thank all the contributing authors for lending their expertise to make the book truly unique. They have played a crucial role in the development of this book. Without their invaluable contributions this book wouldn't have been possible. They have made vital efforts to compile up to date information on the varied aspects of this subject to make this book a valuable addition to the collection of many professionals and students.

This book was conceptualized with the vision of imparting up-to-date information and advanced data in this field. To ensure the same, a matchless editorial board was set up. Every individual on the board went through rigorous rounds of assessment to prove their worth. After which they invested a large part of their time researching and compiling the most relevant data for our readers.

The editorial board has been involved in producing this book since its inception. They have spent rigorous hours researching and exploring the diverse topics which have resulted in the successful publishing of this book. They have passed on their knowledge of decades through this book. To expedite this challenging task, the publisher supported the team at every step. A small team of assistant editors was also appointed to further simplify the editing procedure and attain best results for the readers.

Apart from the editorial board, the designing team has also invested a significant amount of their time in understanding the subject and creating the most relevant covers. They scrutinized every image to scout for the most suitable representation of the subject and create an appropriate cover for the book.

The publishing team has been an ardent support to the editorial, designing and production team. Their endless efforts to recruit the best for this project, has resulted in the accomplishment of this book. They are a veteran in the field of academics and their pool of knowledge is as vast as their experience in printing. Their expertise and guidance has proved useful at every step. Their uncompromising quality standards have made this book an exceptional effort. Their encouragement from time to time has been an inspiration for everyone.

The publisher and the editorial board hope that this book will prove to be a valuable piece of knowledge for researchers, students, practitioners and scholars across the globe.

List of Contributors

Maja Hullmann, Catrin Albrecht, Tina Wahle and Roel P. F. Schins
IUF - Leibniz Research Institute for Environmental Medicine, Auf'm Hennekamp 50, 40225 Düsseldorf, Germany

Agnes W. Boots
IUF - Leibniz Research Institute for Environmental Medicine, Auf'm Hennekamp 50, 40225 Düsseldorf, Germany
Department of Pharmacology and Toxicology, NUTRIM School of Nutrition and Translational Research in Metabolism, Maastricht University, Maastricht, The Netherlands

Jean Krutmann
IUF - Leibniz Research Institute for Environmental Medicine, Auf'm Hennekamp 50, 40225 Düsseldorf, Germany
Medical Faculty, Heinrich-Heine-University, Düsseldorf, Germany

Damiën van Berlo
IUF - Leibniz Research Institute for Environmental Medicine, Auf'm Hennekamp 50, 40225 Düsseldorf, Germany
Triskelion BV Utrechtseweg 48, 3704 HE Zeist, The Netherlands

Miriam E. Gerlofs-Nijland
National Institute for Public Health and the Environment, Bilthoven, The Netherlands

Flemming R. Cassee
National Institute for Public Health and the Environment, Bilthoven, The Netherlands
Institute of Risk Assessment Sciences, Utrecht University, Utrecht, The Netherlands

Thomas A. Bayer
Department of Psychiatry and Psychotherapy, Division of Molecular Psychiatry, Georg-August-University Göttingen, University Medicine Göttingen, Göttingen, Germany

Paul J. A. Borm
Borm Nanoconsult Holding BV, Proost Willemstraat 1, 6231 CV Meerssen, The Netherlands

Paul Fowler
FSToxconsulting Ltd.,Raunds, UK

David Kirkland
Kirkland Consulting,Tadcaster, UK

Sarah Robertson
Centre for Radiation, Chemical and Environmental Hazards, Public Health England, Harwell Science and Innovation Campus, Didcot, Oxfordshire OX11 0RQ, UK

Mark R. Miller
University/BHF Centre of Cardiovascular Science, University of Edinburgh, Edinburgh, UK

Deniz Öner, Manosij Ghosh, Katrien Luyts and Peter HM Hoet
Laboratory of Toxicology, Unit of Environment and Health, Department of Public Health and Primary Care, KU Leuven, 3000 Leuven, Belgium

Jeroen AJ Vanoirbeek
Laboratory of Toxicology, Unit of Environment and Health, Department of Public Health and Primary Care, KU Leuven, 3000 Leuven, Belgium
Laboratory for Occupational and Environmental Hygiene, Unit of Environment and Health, Department of Public Health and Primary Care, KU Leuven, 3000 Leuven, Belgium

Eveline Putzeys
Laboratory of Toxicology, Unit of Environment and Health, Department of Public Health and Primary Care, KU Leuven, 3000 Leuven, Belgium
Department of Oral Health Sciences, Unit of Biomaterials (BIOMAT), KU Leuven, 3000 Leuven, Belgium

Hannelore Bové
Centre for Surface Chemistry and Catalysis, KU Leuven, Celestijnenlaan 200F, 3001 Leuven, Belgium
Biomedical Research Institute, Agoralaan Building C, Hasselt University, 3590 Diepenbeek, Belgium

Marcel Ameloot
Biomedical Research Institute, Agoralaan Building C, Hasselt University, 3590 Diepenbeek, Belgium

Matthieu Moisse, Bram Boeckx and Diether Lambrechts
Laboratory for Translational Genetics, Department of Human Genetics, KU Leuven, 3000 Leuven, Belgium
Laboratory for Translational Genetics, VIB Centre for Cancer Biology, VIB, 3000 Leuven, Belgium

Radu C. Duca and Katrien Poels
Laboratory for Occupational and Environmental Hygiene, Unit of Environment and Health, Department of Public Health and Primary Care, KU Leuven, 3000 Leuven, Belgium

Lode Godderis
Laboratory for Occupational and Environmental Hygiene, Unit of Environment and Health, Department of Public Health and Primary Care, KU Leuven, 3000 Leuven, Belgium
External Service for Prevention and Protection at Work, IDEWE, B-3001, Leuven, Belgium

Kirsten Van Landuydt
Department of Oral Health Sciences, Unit of Biomaterials (BIOMAT), KU Leuven, 3000 Leuven, Belgium

Jie Ji, Swapna Upadhyay, Xiaomiao Xiong and Lena Palmberg
Institute of Environmental Medicine, Karolinska Institute, SE-171 77 Stockholm, Sweden

Maria Malmlöf and Per Gerde
Institute of Environmental Medicine, Karolinska Institute, SE-171 77 Stockholm, Sweden
Inhalation Sciences Sweden AB, Stockholm, Sweden

Thomas Sandström
Department of Public Health and Clinical Medicine, University Hospital, Umeå, Sweden

Dalibor Breznan, Patrick Goegan, Julie S. O'Brien and Subramanian Karthikeyan
Inhalation Toxicology Laboratory, Environmental Health Science and Research Bureau, Health Canada, Ottawa, ON K1A 0K9, Canada

Ngoc Q. Vuong and Renaud Vincent
Inhalation Toxicology Laboratory, Environmental Health Science and Research Bureau, Health Canada, Ottawa, ON K1A 0K9, Canada
Department of Biochemistry, Faculty of Science, University of Ottawa, Ottawa, ON K1H 8M5, Canada

Premkumari Kumarathasan
Analytical Biochemistry and Proteomics, Environmental Health Science and Research Bureau, Health Canada, Ottawa, ON K1A 0K9, Canada

Andrew Williams
Biostatistics Section, Population Studies Division, Environmental Health Science and Research Bureau, Health Canada, Ottawa, ON K1A 0K9, Canada

Françoise Rogerieux, Bénédicte Trouiller, Anne Braun and Ghislaine Lacroix
Institut National de l'Environnement Industriel et des Risques (INERIS), (DRC/ VIVA/TOXI), Parc Technologique ALATA - BP 2, F-60550 Verneuil-en-Halatte, France

Thomas Loret
Institut National de l'Environnement Industriel et des Risques (INERIS), (DRC/ VIVA/TOXI), Parc Technologique ALATA - BP 2, F-60550 Verneuil-en-Halatte, France
Université de Technologie de Compiègne (UTC), Laboratoire BioMécanique et BioIngénierie (BMBI), UMR CNRS 7338, 60205 Compiègne, France

Christophe Egles
Université de Technologie de Compiègne (UTC), Laboratoire BioMécanique et BioIngénierie (BMBI), UMR CNRS 7338, 60205 Compiègne, France
Department of Biomedical Engineering, Tufts University, Medford, MA, USA

Christian Monsé, Olaf Hagemeyer, Monika Raulf, Birger Jettkant, Vera van Kampen, Benjamin Kendzia, Vitali Gering, Tobias Weiss, Nadin Ulrich, Eike-Maximilian Marek, Jürgen Bünger, Thomas Brüning and Rolf Merget
Institute for Prevention and Occupational Medicine of the German Social ccident Insurance, Institute of the Ruhr-Universität Bochum (IPA), Bürkle-de-la-Camp-Platz 1, 44789 Bochum, Germany

Günther Kappert
Gerinnungszentrum Rhein-Ruhr, Königstraße 13, 47051 Duisburg, Germany

Siqi Zhang, Susanne Breitner, Annette Peters and Alexandra Schneider
Institute of Epidemiology, Helmholtz Zentrum München, Ingolstädter Landstr.1, 29, D-85764 Neuherberg, Germany

Wayne E Cascio, Robert B Devlin, Lucas M Neas and David Diaz-Sanchez
National Health and Environmental Effects Research Laboratory, US Environmental Protection Agency, Research Triangle Park, Durham, NC, USA

William E Kraus and Elizabeth R Hauser
Duke Molecular Physiology Institute, School of Medicine, Duke University, Durham, NC, USA

Joel Schwartz
Department of Environmental Health, Harvard T.H. Chan School of Public Health, Boston, MA, USA

P. A. Stapleton
Department of Pharmacology and Toxicology, Ernest Mario School of Pharmacy, Rutgers University, Piscataway, NJ, USA
Environmental and Occupational Health Sciences Institute, Piscataway, NJ, USA

M. V. Pinti and D. L. Shepherd
Division of Exercise Physiology, West Virginia University School of Medicine, Morgantown, WV, USA
Mitochondria, Metabolism & Bioenergetics Working Group, West Virginia University School of Medicine, Morgantown, WV, USA

Q. A. Hathaway and J. M. Hollander
Division of Exercise Physiology, West Virginia University School of Medicine, Morgantown, WV, USA
Mitochondria, Metabolism & Bioenergetics Working Group, West Virginia University School of Medicine, Morgantown, WV, USA
Toxicology Working Group, West Virginia University School of Medicine, Morgantown, WV, USA

T. R. Nurkiewicz
Mitochondria, Metabolism & Bioenergetics Working Group, West Virginia University School of Medicine, Morgantown, WV, USA
Toxicology Working Group, West Virginia University School of Medicine, Morgantown, WV, USA
Department of Physiology, Pharmacology, and Neuroscience, Robert C. Byrd Health Sciences Center, West Virginia University School of Medicine, 1 Medical Center Drive, Morgantown, WV 26506-9229, USA

C. E. Nichols
Immunity, Inflammation, and Disease Laboratory, National Institute of Environmental Health Sciences, Research Triangle Park, NC, USA

A. B. Abukabda and V. C. Castranova
Toxicology Working Group, West Virginia University School of Medicine, Morgantown, WV, USA
Department of Pharmaceutical Sciences, West Virginia University School of Pharmacy, Morgantown, USA

C. R. McBride and J. Yi
Toxicology Working Group, West Virginia University School of Medicine, Morgantown, WV, USA
Department of Physiology, Pharmacology, and Neuroscience, Robert C. Byrd Health Sciences Center, West Virginia University School of Medicine, 1 Medical Center Drive, Morgantown, WV 26506-9229, USA

Rupa Biswas, Kevin L. Trout, Forrest Jessop and Andrij Holian
Center for Environmental Health Sciences, Department of Biomedical and Pharmaceutical Sciences, University of Montana, Missoula, MT 59812, USA

Jack R.Harkema
Department of Pathobiology and Diagnostic Investigation, Michigan State University, East Lansing, MI 48824, USA

Chi-Hsiang Shih, Zhe-Wei Lin and Yi-Syuan Lin
School of Respiratory Therapy, College of Medicine, Taipei Medical University, Taipei, Taiwan

Hsiao-Chi Chuang
School of Respiratory Therapy, College of Medicine, Taipei Medical University, Taipei, Taiwan
School of Public Health, College of Public Health, Taipei Medical University, Taipei, Taiwan
Division of Pulmonary Medicine, Department of Internal Medicine, Shuang Ho Hospital, Taipei Medical University, New Taipei City, Taiwan

Jen-Kun Chen, Li-Wei Kuo and Kuan-Hung Cho
Institute of Biomedical Engineering & Nanomedicine, National Health Research Institutes, Miaoli, Taiwan

Ta-Chih Hsiao
Graduate Institute of Environmental Engineering, National Taiwan University, Taipei, Taiwan

Jiunn-Horng Kang
Department of Physical Medicine and Rehabilitation, Taipei Medical University Hospital, Taipei, Taiwan
Department of Physical Medicine and Rehabilitation, School of Medicine, College of Medicine, Taipei Medical University, Taipei, Taiwan

Yu-Chun Lo
The Ph.D Program for Neural Regenerative Medicine, College of Medical Science and Technology, Taipei Medical University, Taipei, Taiwan

Kai-Jen Chuang
School of Public Health, College of Public Health, Taipei Medical University, Taipei, Taiwan
Department of Public Health, School of Medicine, College of Medicine, Taipei Medical University, Taipei, Taiwan

Tsun-Jen Cheng
Institute of Occupational Medicine and Industrial Hygiene, College of Public Health, National Taiwan University, Taipei, Taiwan

Astrid Skovmand
The National Research Center for the Working Environment, Lersø Parkallé, DK-2100 Copenhagen Ø, Denmark
Section for Veterinary Reproduction and Obstetrics, Department of Veterinary Clinical Sciences, University of Copenhagen, Dyrlægvej 68, DK-1870 Frederiksberg C, Denmark

Ulla Vogel
The National Research Center for the Working Environment, Lersø Parkallé, DK-2100 Copenhagen Ø, Denmark
Department of Microand Nanotechnology, Technical University of Denmark, DK-2800 Kongens Lyngby, Denmark

Karin Sørig Hougaard
The National Research Center for the Working Environment, Lersø Parkallé, DK-2100 Copenhagen Ø, Denmark
Department of Public Health, University of Copenhagen, Øster Farimagsgade 5, DK-1014 Copenhagen K, Denmark

Anna Jacobsen Lauvås and Sandra Goericke-Pesch
Section for Veterinary Reproduction and Obstetrics, Department of Veterinary Clinical Sciences, University of Copenhagen, Dyrlægvej 68, DK-1870 Frederiksberg C, Denmark

Preben Christensen
SPZ Lab A/ S, Fruebjergvej 3, DK-2100 København Ø, Denmark

Naohide Shinohara, Guihua Zhang and Masashi Gamo
National Institute of Advanced Industrial Science and Technology (AIST), Tsukuba, Ibaraki 305-8569, Japan

Yutaka Oshima and Toshio Kobayashi
Chemicals Evaluation and Research Institute (CERI), Hita, Oita 877-0061, Japan

Nobuya Imatanaka and Makoto Nakai
Chemicals Evaluation and Research Institute (CERI), Bunkyo, Tokyo 112-0004, Japan.

Takeshi Sasaki and Kenji Kawaguchi
National Institute of Advanced Industrial Science and Technology (AIST), Tsukuba, Ibaraki 305-8565, Japan

Mary K. Schubauer-Berigan, Matthew M. Dahm, M. Stephen J. Bertke and Marie A. de Perio
National Institute for Occupational Safety and Health (NIOSH), Division of Surveillance, Hazard Evaluations, and Field Studies, 1090 Tusculum Ave MS-R15, Cincinnati, OH 45226, USA

Index

www.ingramcontent.com/pod-product-compliance
Lightning Source LLC
Chambersburg PA
CBHW061251190326
41458CB00011B/3638
9781632418609